Core Readings in Psychiatry

*An Annotated Guide
to the Literature*

Second Edition

Core Readings in Psychiatry

*An Annotated Guide
to the Literature*

Second Edition

Edited by

Michael H. Sacks, M.D.
William H. Sledge, M.D.
Catherine Warren, M.L.S.

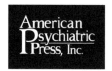

American
Psychiatric
Press, Inc.

Washington, DC
London, England

Copyright © 1995 American Psychiatric Press, Inc.
ALL RIGHTS RESERVED
Manufactured in the United States of America on acid-free paper
98 97 96 95   4 3 2 1
Second Edition

American Psychiatric Press, Inc.
1400 K Street, N.W., Washington, DC   20005

Library of Congress Cataloging-in-Publication Data
Core readings in psychiatry : an annotated guide to the literature /
   edited by Michael H. Sacks, William H. Sledge, and Catherine Warren.
   — 2nd ed.
      p.   cm.
   Includes bibliographical references and index.
   ISBN 0-88048-559-0
   1. Psychiatry—Abstracts.   2. Psychology, Pathological—Abstracts.
3. Psychotherapy—Abstracts.   4. Developmental psychology—
Abstracts.   I. Sacks, Michael H.   II. Sledge, William H., 1945–   .
III. Warren, Catherine, 1952–   .
   [DNLM: 1. Mental Disorders—abstracts.   2. Psychiatry—abstracts.
ZWM 100 C797 1995]
RC454.C655   1995
616.89—dc20
DNLM/DLC
for Library of Congress   95-10613
                                                                        CIP

British Library Cataloguing in Publication Data
A CIP record is available from the British Library.

To Phyllis Rubinton (1927–1985)

In appreciation of her dedication to the importance of the world of bibliography, which inspired the first edition of *Core Readings in Psychiatry*, and whose memory inspired the second edition.

Contents

PART I

BASIC SCIENCES:
BIOLOGICAL, PSYCHOLOGICAL, AND SOCIAL

PART II

PSYCHOPATHOLOGY

PART III

ASSESSMENT

PART IV

TREATMENT

PART V

NORMALITY AND DEVELOPMENT

PART VI

SPECIAL TOPICS

Contributors

Gerard Addonizio, M.D., Associate Professor of Clinical Psychiatry, Cornell University Medical College, New York, New York

George Alexopoulos, M.D., Professor of Psychiatry, Cornell University Medical College, New York, New York

Carol M. Anderson, Ph.D., Professor of Psychiatry, University of Pittsburgh School of Medicine, Pittsburgh, Pennsylvania

Nancy C. Andreasen, M.D., Ph.D., Andrew H. Woods Professor of Psychiatry, University of Iowa Hospitals and Clinics, Iowa City, Iowa

Boris M. Astrachan, M.D., Professor and Head, Department of Psychiatry, University of Illinois College of Medicine, Chicago, Illinois

Harriet Baldwin, M.A., Literature Committee Chair, National Alliance for the Mentally Ill, Arlington, Virginia

Gordon G. Ball, Ph.D., Associate Professor in Psychiatry, Columbia University College of Physicians and Surgeons, New York, New York

Aaron T. Beck, M.D., Professor of Psychiatry, University of Pennsylvania, School of Medicine, Philadelphia, Pennsylvania

Vajramala Bhatia, M.D., M.A., M.Ed., Senior Resident in Psychiatry, Middletown Psychiatric Center, Middletown, New York

Howard C. Blue, M.D., Assistant Professor, Yale University School of Medicine, New Haven, Connecticut

Daniel J. Buysse, M.D., Assistant Professor of Psychiatry, University of Pittsburgh, School of Medicine, Pittsburgh, Pennsylvania

Eric D. Caine, M.D., Professor of Psychiatry and Neurology, University of Rochester, School of Medicine, Rochester, New York

Deborah Clark, B.A., Research Coordinator, University of Pennsylvania, Philadelphia, Pennsylvania

John F. Clarkin, Ph.D., Professor of Clinical Psychology in Psychiatry, Cornell University Medical College, New York, New York

Francine Cournos, M.D., Associate Clinical Professor of Psychiatry, Columbia University College of Physicians and Surgeons, New York, New York

David L. Cutler, M.D., Professor of Psychiatry, Oregon Health Sciences University, Portland, Oregon

Leah J. Dickstein, M.D., Professor of Psychiatry and Behavioral Sciences, University of Louisville, School of Medicine, Louisville, Kentucky

Willie Earley, M.D., Assistant Professor of Clinical Psychiatry, University of Illinois at Chicago, Chicago, Illinois

Marshall Edelson, M.D., Ph.D., Professor of Psychiatry, Yale University School of Medicine, New Haven, Connecticut

Joseph T. English, M.D., Chairman, Department of Psychiatry, St. Vincent's Hospital, New York, New York

Aaron H. Esman, M.D., Professor of Clinical Psychiatry, Cornell University Medical College, New York, New York

Michael Flaum, M.D., Assistant Professor of Psychiatry, University of Iowa Hospitals and Clinics, Iowa City, Iowa

Mark Fleisher, M.D., Attending Psychiatrist, Dual Diagnosis Clinic, Creighton-Nebraska Department of Psychiatry, University of Nebraska Medical Center, Omaha, Nebraska

Allen Frances, M.D., Chairman, Department of Psychiatry, Duke University Medical Center, Durham, North Carolina

Richard J. Frances, M.D., Chairman of Psychiatry, Hackensack Medical Center, Hackensack, New Jersey

Deborah Fried, M.D., Assistant Professor of Psychiatry, Yale University School of Medicine, New Haven, Connecticut

William A. Frosch, M.D., Professor of Psychiatry, Cornell University Medical College, New York, New York

Albert C. Gaw, M.D., Associate Professor of Psychiatry, Boston University School of Medicine, Boston, Massachusetts

Joel E. Gelernter, M.D., Associate Professor of Psychiatry, Yale University School of Medicine, West Haven DVA Medical Center, West Haven, Connecticut

Ira D. Glick, M.D., Professor of Psychiatry, Stanford University School of Medicine, Stanford, California

Carlos Gonzalez, M.D., Assistant Professor of Psychiatry, Yale University School of Medicine, New Haven, Connecticut

Ezra E. H. Griffith, M.D., Professor of Psychiatry and of African and Afro-American Studies, Yale University School of Medicine, New Haven, Connecticut

Leonard C. Groopman, M.D., Ph.D., Clinical Instructor in Psychiatry, Cornell University Medical College, New York, New York

Hillel Grossman, M.D., Assistant Professor in Psychiatry, Tufts University School of Medicine, Boston, Massachusetts

John G. Gunderson, M.D., Associate Professor of Psychiatry, Harvard Medical School, Boston, Massachusetts

Richard C. Haaser, M.D., Rochester Park Medical Group, Rochester, New York

Seymour L. Halleck, M.D., Professor of Psychiatry and Adjunct Professor of Law, University of North Carolina, School of Medicine, Chapel Hill, North Carolina

Eric Hollander, M.D., Associate Professor of Psychiatry, Columbia University College of Physicians and Surgeons, New York, New York

Ewald Horwath, M.D., Associate Clinical Professor of Psychiatry, Columbia University College of Physicians and Surgeons, New York, New York

Selby Jacobs, M.D., Professor of Psychiatry, Yale University School of Medicine, New Haven, Connecticut

Robin Johnson, M.D., Clinical Instructor in Psychiatry, Yale University School of Medicine, New Haven, Connecticut

David R. Jones, M.D., Clinical Professor of Psychiatry, University of Texas Health Sciences Center in San Antonio, San Antonio, Texas

Helen Singer Kaplan, M.D., Ph.D., Director, Human Sexuality Program, Cornell University Medical College, New York, New York

Charles A. Kaufmann, M.D., Associate Professor of Clinical Psychiatry, Columbia University College of Physicians and Surgeons, New York, New York

Howard D. Kibel, M.D., Associate Professor of Clinical Psychiatry, Cornell University Medical College, New York, New York

Kathleen Kim, M.D., Assistant Professor of Psychiatry, Yale University School of Medicine, New Haven, Connecticut

James H. Kocsis, M.D., Professor of Psychiatry, Cornell University Medical College, New York, New York

Nathan M. Kravis, M.D., Clinical Assistant Professor of Psychiatry, Cornell University Medical College, New York, New York

Penelope Krener, M.D., Associate Professor of Psychiatry and Pediatrics, University of California at Davis, Sacramento, California

David J. Kupfer, M.D., Professor and Chairman in the Department of Psychiatry, University of Pittsburgh School of Medicine, Pittsburgh, Pennsylvania

Howard B. Levine, M.D., Faculty, Boston Psychoanalytic Institute and Massachusetts Institute of Psychoanalysis, Boston, Massachusetts

Ruth E. Levine, M.D., Assistant Professor, Department of Psychiatry and Behavioral Sciences, University of Texas Medical Branch, Galveston, Texas

Victor Lidz, Ph.D., Assistant Professor, Department of Mental Health Sciences, School of Medicine, Hahnemann University, Philadelphia, Pennsylvania

James W. Lomax, M.D., Professor of Clinical Psychiatry, Baylor College of Medicine, Houston, Texas

M. Philip Luber, M.D., Assistant Professor of Psychiatry in Medicine, Cornell University Medical College, New York, New York

Avram H. Mack, A.B., Medical Student, Cornell University Medical College, New York, New York

Kevin M. Malone, M.D., Visiting Assistant Professor of Psychiatry, Western Psychiatric Institute and Clinic, University of Pittsburgh, Pittsburgh, Pennsylvania

John T. Maltsberger, M.D., Lecturer in Psychiatry, Harvard Medical School, Boston, Massachusetts

John C. Markowitz, M.D., Assistant Professor of Psychiatry, Cornell University Medical College, New York, New York

Steven Mattis, Ph.D., Director of Psychological Services, Hillside–Long Island Jewish Medical Center, Glen Oaks, New York

Linda C. Mayes, M.D., Arnold Gessel Associate Professor of Child Development, Pediatrics and Psychology, Yale Child Study Center, New Haven, Connecticut

Richard G. McCarrick, M.D., M.H.A., Assistant Clinical Professor, Yale University School of Medicine, New Haven, Connecticut

David A. Mrazek, M.D., F.R.C.Psych., Professor of Psychiatry and Pediatrics, The George Washington University, Washington, DC

Stephen D. Mullins, M.D., M.P.H., Assistant Professor of Psychiatry, Western Psychiatric Institute and Clinic, University of Pittsburgh School of Medicine, Pittsburgh, Pennsylvania

Richard L. Munich, M.D., Professor of Clinical Psychiatry, Cornell University Medical College, New York, New York

J. Craig Nelson, M.D., Professor of Psychiatry, Yale University School of Medicine, New Haven, Connecticut

Eric J. Nestler, M.D., Ph.D., Elizabeth Mears and House Jameson Associate Professor of Psychiatry and Pharmacology, Connecticut Mental Health Center, Yale University, New Haven, Connecticut

Bradley M. Pechter, M.D., Assistant Professor of Clinical Psychiatry, University of Illinois at Chicago, Chicago, Illinois

Samuel W. Perry, M.D., Professor of Psychiatry, Cornell University Medical College, New York, New York

Katharine A. Phillips, M.D., Instructor in Psychiatry, Harvard Medical School, Boston, Massachusetts

Robert S. Pynoos, M.D., M.P.H., Associate Professor in Psychiatry, UCLA/Neuropsychiatric Institute, Los Angeles, California

Donald M. Quinlan, Ph.D., Professor of Psychiatry and Psychology, Moorse College, New Haven, Connecticut

Charles F. Reynolds III, M.D., Professor of Psychiatry and Neurology, University of Pittsburgh School of Medicine, Pittsburgh, Pennsylvania

Jay B. Rohrlich, M.D., Assistant Clinical Professor of Psychiatry, Cornell University Medical College, New York, New York

Michael H. Sacks, M.D., Professor of Psychiatry, Cornell University Medical College, New York, New York

Carl Salzman, M.D., Professor of Psychiatry, Harvard Medical School, Boston, Massachusetts

Shawn Christopher Shea, M.D., Director of the Continuous Treatment Team, Monadnock Family Services, Keene, New Hampshire

Roger C. Sider, M.D., Professor of Psychiatry, College of Human Medicine, Michigan State University, Grand Rapids, Michigan

David A. Silbersweig, M.D., Assistant Professor of Psychiatry and Neurology, Cornell University Medical College, New York, New York

Daphne Simeon, M.D., Research Fellow in Psychiatry, Columbia University College of Physicians and Surgeons, New York, New York

Jerome L. Singer, Ph.D., Professor of Psychology, Yale University, New Haven, Connecticut

William H. Sledge, M.D., Professor of Psychiatry, Yale University School of Medicine, New Haven, Connecticut

Alan M. Steinberg, Ph.D., Visiting Lecturer in Biomedical Ethics, Department of Developmental and Cell Biology, University of California at Irvine, Irvine, California

Fred D. Strider, Ph.D., Clinical Professor of Psychiatry, Creighton University School of Medicine, Omaha, Nebraska

John A. Sweeney, Ph.D., Assistant Professor of Psychiatry and Neurology, University of Pittsburgh School of Medicine, Pittsburgh, Pennsylvania

Rajiv Tandon, M.D., Associate Professor of Psychiatry, University of Michigan Medical Center, Ann Arbor, Michigan

Kenneth Tardiff, M.D., M.P.H., Professor of Psychiatry and Public Health, Cornell University Medical School, New York, New York

Kenneth S. Thompson, M.D., Assistant Professor of Psychiatry, Western Psychiatric Institute and Clinic, University of Pittsburgh, School of Medicine, Pittsburgh, Pennsylvania

George E. Vaillant, M.D., Professor of Psychiatry, Harvard Medical School, Boston, Massachusetts

Milton Viederman, M.D., Professor of Clinical Psychiatry, Cornell University Medical College, New York, New York

William J. Waked, Ph.D., Instructor of Physical Medicine and Rehabilitation, New Jersey Medical School, University of Medicine and Dentistry of New Jersey, Newark, New Jersey

Joel J. Wallack, M.D., Clinical Associate Professor, New York University School of Medicine, New York, New York

Catherine Warren, M.L.S., Librarian, Medical Library, Children's Hospital National Medical Center, Washington, DC

Myrna M. Weissman, Ph.D., Professor of Epidemiology in Psychiatry, Columbia University College of Physicians and Surgeons, New York, New York

Renee Welner, M.D., Clinical Assistant Professor of Psychiatry, Cornell University Medical College, New York, New York

Joel Yager, M.D., Professor of Psychiatry, University of California at Los Angeles, Los Angeles, California

Foreword

Perhaps the most difficult, and certainly the most guilt-provoking, aspect of being a mental health professional is the never-ending struggle to keep up with the literature. The research in psychiatry is expanding exponentially (believe it or not, there are studies showing this), and in many areas it has become too specialized and too technical for generalists to follow with any degree of confidence. The paradox is that research findings are increasingly crucial for carrying on an intelligent clinical practice, but the research is increasingly overwhelming and inaccessible to the nonspecialist.

Thus lies the value and delight of this unusual gem of a book. Leading figures from across the four corners of psychiatric practice, education, research, and administration walk us through the most important works in their respective fields. With the great leverage provided by their expertise and guidance, the reader can in a convenient way catch up on the wealth of new methods and findings that are emerging so rapidly and in so many directions. Not only does one learn a great deal in this process, but one also learns what one does not know and needs to find out. The great virtue of this book is that it provides a broad survey, but it also promotes and directs one's own further and deeper inquiry. The book also provides an archival "time capsule" portrait of our field at this time. It is fascinating to compare this edition with its earlier counterpart, and this edition will, in its turn, serve as a source for comparison as the field advances with later editions.

I would also like to acknowledge my own very personal debt to Phyllis Rubinton, to whom this book is dedicated. Phyllis and I began work at the Payne Whitney Clinic at about the same time—she as keeper of the library and me as a junior faculty member who had been told to write papers. Phyllis helped a great deal in all sorts of practical ways, but most important was her love of the knowledge contained in the psychiatric literature and of the process of sharing it with others. It is in her spirit, and with her radiance, that this book has been compiled.

Allen Frances, M.D.

Introduction

Editing the second edition of *Core Readings in Psychiatry* has been both interesting and exhilarating. To be sure there were the usual frustrations of persuading, annoying, and even threatening a large number of busy and hard-working people to meet our deadlines, but it was not without its compensations. All the authors finally came in with their chapters, and what an adventure it has been to follow them into the nooks and corners of their special expertise.

The experience in editing the first edition was a delight in meeting old companions and an excitement in learning about areas that, although unfamiliar, we were aware of as acquaintances. It was like listening to a familiar piece of music; it brought pleasure in revisiting familiar themes and excitement in discovering new passages that we had not noticed or paid attention to previously. Editing the second edition has been like listening to an entirely new piece of music. In the intervening years since the prior edition, the profession's knowledge base has changed immensely. We had expected change; it was this expectation that motivated the undertaking of a new edition. But as the chapters came in, again and again we were impressed both in terms of the recent citations and the numbers of new topics that were not in the earlier edition. We felt educated in reading these chapters in a way that we did not in the first edition. We also felt a sense of awe at how far the field of psychiatry has expanded and matured in such a brief period of time.

Several dimensions of what has changed can be noted. Not only are there new areas of study—which are represented by chapters such as those on acquired immunodeficiency syndrome, neuropsychiatry, models of psychoanalytic thought, child development, and medical economics—but there are new topics in the traditionally central topics of psychiatry such as psychopathology and treatment. Change is also evident in the paradigms used in the selection of articles in each chapter. A recurrent editorial problem in the earlier edition was to address the bias of the author and to ask the author either to balance the reading list or to describe the bias in the introduction. In this current edition, the contributors seemed comfortable with approaches that involved social-family, personal-intrapsychic, and biological-genetic aspects. In fact, there seemed a remarkable disinterest in establishing the importance or centrality of a single perspective. This earlier doctrinaire type of approach has been replaced by an interest and curiosity in what can be learned from each of the different models and their cross-fertilization. There is a clear sense from our contributors that the arguments over which approach is the correct one has been replaced by what can we learn from each approach.

The most important function of the editors has been in the choice of the chapter authors. We selected those from the first edition who remained active within the area they had developed in the first edition. We had chosen those who were experienced educators and academicians and whose work we knew well. For this edition, we broadened our range, but the number of authors from Cornell and Yale indicates that we did not have to go very far from familiar communities to find experts.

As in the prior edition, the instructions to the authors were to select the sources that they believed were "most central" to their field. These source were to include citations that identified and effectively dealt with the major issues within their topic. They were also to identify the classical citations and those that make up the core readings within the areas; citations the authors considered essential are indicated by an asterisk (*). We recognized the subjective and personal element in such a selection and encouraged the authors to express their particular vision of what was central. However, we insisted that they try to state explicitly in the chapter introduction what their selection process was, or what we have called their "selection paradigm."

Once the experts were identified and their cooperation secured, our role became more one of adviser and time keeper. We attempted to keep "self citations" to a respectable minimum; we made a few suggestions that we thought might add to the balance or range of the authors' selections; and we tried to ensure a format and stylistic continuity that renders the book more accessible without inhibiting the authors' creativity and vision. We permitted multiple citations by different authors of the same reference because the citations were often used differently in different chapters and our authors have different perspectives on the same well-known reference. For those who like to puzzle over frequency distributions, the five most cited authors were Sigmund Freud, Gerald L. Klerman, Myrna M. Weissman, Aaron T. Beck, and Donald F. Klein.

Once the final text and citations were agreed on, we instituted a rigorous independent bibliographic checking process to ensure accuracy and consistency. Any errors that occur in the book are our responsibility.

A subject index is included that addresses the issue of topic overlap and cross-referencing of citations. An author index including all authors cited is also included. Citations are referred to in the indexes by the chapter number plus a decimal and then the reference number within that chapter (e.g., "15.59" refers to Chapter 15, reference 59). Citations that consist of a chapter number plus "I" (e.g., "24I") refer to the introduction to that chapter.

What we have as a final product is a selected, annotated view of the essential English-language publications that define the field of psychiatry, particularly as it is viewed in the United States. We hope that this book will open bibliographic doors for academicians as well as for providers, shapers, managers, and consumers of psychiatric services and knowledge. It is designed to be an introduction and guide to the entire psychiatric literature. Our hope is that our readers will be well served by this book.

Michael H. Sacks, M.D.
William H. Sledge, M.D.
Catherine Warren, M.L.S.

I

Basic Sciences
Biological, Psychological, and Social

1

Neuroscience

Eric J. Nestler, M.D., Ph.D.

A s the reality that severe mental disorders are caused by diseases of the brain becomes increasingly acknowledged and accepted among psychiatrists, the importance of the neurosciences in psychiatric teaching and research has increased.

The neurosciences have witnessed unparalleled advances in recent years. Whereas the brain was once viewed as a collection of minute batteries with a relatively fixed (albeit complex) wiring diagram, we now know that the brain is a remarkably plastic organ. It adapts to a wide variety of circumstances, forms memories of experiences, and learns procedures; it can become dependent on drugs or produce disabling psychopathology; and it can recover. The plasticity of our brains, and therefore our ability to learn and adapt, is at the heart of our evolutionary success in nature and of our cultural evolution as well.

The brain is so extraordinarily complex that the mechanisms by which it functions have frequently been declared unknowable. The brain, however, is an organ, and, like any organ, it is composed of cells. All of the brain's functions are carried out by nerve cells called neurons (and supportive glial cells), which communicate with each other in networks of remarkably complex, but precise, connections. The heart of modern neuroscience is to understand the mechanisms that control these connections and their plasticity in response to external and physiological cues, at the multicellular, single cellular, and intracellular levels.

It is impossible to represent the full spectrum of neuroscience research in 60 publications. The emphasis in this chapter is given to specific areas of molecular and cellular neuroscience because advances in these fields have laid the foundation for a fundamentally new neuroscience of psychiatry. In addition, representative publications that attempt to understand cellular and molecular phenomena within a behavioral and clinical context are listed.

This chapter is divided into several sections. First, basic texts are given for those individuals interested in elementary, broad-based information of the nervous system. Second, selections in molecular neurobiology are listed. Molecular neurobiology has provided one of the primary driving forces behind recent advances in the neurosciences and will no doubt continue to do so. Third are selections covering mechanisms of synaptic transmission, the processes by which individual neurons communicate with one another. The references are divided into subsections on neurotransmitters, receptors, postreceptor mechanisms, growth factors, and neurophysiology. This section includes the largest number of citations based on the view that mechanisms of synaptic transmission are likely central to the etiology, pathophysiology, and treatment of severe mental disorders. Fourth, articles concerned with the long-term effects of drugs on the nervous system are presented. A relatively large number of citations are offered due to the belief that studies of drugs provide a unique strategy by which to probe and understand brain function. Fifth, a small number of references that introduce the reader to research in neural systems and networks are given. Ultimately, molecular and cellular analyses of the nervous system must be synthesized with neural systems research to obtain a more complete and functional view of the brain. Finally, representative publications in the large field of clinical psychiatric neuroscience are presented.

Basic Texts

1. **Cooper JR, Bloom FE, Roth RH:** *The Biochemical Basis of Neuropharmacology*, 6th Edition. New York, Oxford, 1991

   This book provides an excellent overview of neuropharmacology—namely, the types of chemicals that serve as neurotransmitters in the brain and their specific receptors. Emphasis is placed on acetylcholine and the monoamines, dopamine, norepinephrine, epinephrine, and serotonin. The book is accessible to those without extensive prior knowledge of the field; however, background knowledge of biochemistry is helpful.

2. *Hyman SE, Nestler EJ:** *The Molecular Foundations of Psychiatry*. Washington, DC, American Psychiatric Press, 1993

This book introduces psychiatrists to the basic neurosciences. It includes reviews of molecular biology and genetics, synaptic transmission and signal transduction pathways, neuropharmacology, and neural plasticity. Implications of these fields for psychiatric practice and research are discussed. Material is presented in two levels of difficulty. This makes the book readable for clinical psychiatrists with little prior knowledge of neuroscience and sufficiently detailed for individuals seeking more advanced information.

3. **Kandel ER, Schwartz JH, Jessel T** (eds): *Principals of Neural Science*, 3rd Edition. New York, Elsevier, 1991

An excellent general textbook for the neurosciences, this book is comprehensive and authoritative. It can be used as a reference to gain detailed knowledge of most important aspects of neuroscience. Sections on electrophysiology and neural networks are particularly strong.

4. **Siegel GJ, Agranoff B, Alber RW, Molinoff P** (eds): *Basic Neurochemistry*, 5th Edition. New York, Raven, 1994

This textbook of neurochemistry provides a detailed and comprehensive overview of the chemical makeup of the nervous system. The book offers more detailed information, compared with Kandel et al. (1991) above, on specific proteins in the nervous system and their roles in brain function.

Molecular Neurobiology

The references described in this section offer detailed and up-to-date information concerning the mechanisms underlying gene expression in the nervous system. This includes the mechanisms by which genes contained within DNA are transcribed into messenger RNAs, which in turn are translated into the proteins that underlie virtually all aspects of brain function.

5. **Hyman SE, Nestler EJ:** Basic molecular neurobiology, in *Comprehensive Textbook of Psychiatry/VI*, 6th Edition. Edited by Kaplan HI, Sadock BJ. Baltimore, MD, Williams & Wilkins (in press)

This chapter provides an overview of the process of gene transcription and messenger RNA translation. It is written at an elementary level and is suitable for individuals with little prior knowledge of the field.

6. **Mitchell PJ, Tjian R:** Transcriptional regulation in mammalian cells by sequence-specific DNA binding proteins. *Science* 245:371–378, 1989

The authors of this reference review the classes of proteins that serve as transcription factors. Transcription factors are proteins that bind to specific sequences of DNA within certain genes and thereby increase or decrease the rate at which those genes are transcribed. This article is written at a highly technical level and is meant as a review for those individuals with considerable background knowledge.

7. *__Morgan JI, Curran T:__ Stimulus-transcription coupling in the nervous system. *Annu Rev Neurosci* 14:421–451, 1991

Focusing on one particular family of transcription factors, products of the immediate early genes, and the role they play in signal transduction in the nervous system, this article provides readable advanced information for those with some background in the neurosciences.

8. **Treacy MN, Rosenfeld MG:** Expression of a family of POU-domain protein regulatory genes during development of the central nervous system. *Annu Rev Neurosci* 15:139–165, 1992

This article reviews a class of transcription factors, POU proteins, that appear to play a central role in neuronal differentiation. Given the fact that the brain contains thousands, probably tens of thousands, of distinct neuronal cell types, each with distinct synaptic connections, an understanding of the processes by which the specialized features of neurons form during development and are maintained through adulthood is of profound importance to neuroscience and psychiatry.

9. **Watson JD, Hopkins NH, Roberts JW, Steitz JA, Weiner AM:** *Molecular Biology of the Gene,* 4th Edition. Menlo Park, CA, Benjamin/Cummings, 1987

This standard textbook in molecular biology includes elementary and advanced information suitable for individuals with college- and graduate-level knowledge of the biomedical sciences.

Synaptic Transmission

The primary feature of brain function is the process by which information, perceived from the environment by sensory neurons, is passed intercellularly to other neurons in the brain and spinal cord and passed intracellularly to modify the functioning of individual neurons to environmental and physiological cues. This section is divided into several parts: consideration of neurotransmitters and their life cycle, receptors for neurotransmitters, postreceptor mechanisms that mediate the effects of neurotransmitter-receptor interactions, and trophic factors in the nervous system.

Neurotransmitters: Synthesis, Storage, Release, and Reuptake

10. **De Camilli P, Jahn R:** Pathways to regulated exocytosis in neurons. *Annu Rev Physiol* 52:625–645, 1990

    This article reviews the process of neurotransmitter release with particular emphasis on proteins associated with synaptic vesicles. Synaptic vesicles are subcellular organelles in which the neurotransmitter is stored; in response to specific physiological stimuli, these vesicles move toward and fuse with the nerve terminal plasma membrane and release their contents into the synaptic cleft.

11. **Uhl GR:** Neurotransmitter transporters (plus): a promising new gene family. *Trends Neurosci* 15:265–268, 1991

    It has been known for years that the monoamines released into synaptic clefts are inactivated functionally via their reuptake back into nerve terminals, where they are repackaged into synaptic vesicles and readied for subsequent release. However, the specific proteins that subserve this reuptake function have only recently been characterized at the biochemical and molecular level. This information is summarized in concise form in this review. Particular attention has been given to these proteins in psychiatric neuroscience research because important psychotropic drugs (tricyclic antidepressants, cocaine) are potent inhibitors of the proteins.

12. *Valtorta F, Benfenati F, Greengard P:** Structure and function of the synapsins. *J Biol Chem* 267:7195–7198, 1992

    This article focuses on the synapsins, a major family of synaptic vesicle-associated proteins that mediate the actions of many physiological stimuli in regulating neurotransmitter release. In conjunction with De Camilli and Jahn (1990) above, this article provides an advanced and timely review of the field.

13. **Zigmond RE, Schwarzschild MA, Rittenhouse AR:** Acute regulation of tyrosine hydroxylase by nerve activity and by neurotransmitter via phosphorylation. *Annu Rev Neurosci* 12:415–461, 1989

    Tyrosine hydroxylase is the rate-limiting enzyme in the biosynthesis of the catecholamine neurotransmitters dopamine, norepinephrine, and epinephrine. The high degree of regulation of this enzyme, which is the focus of this well-written review article, plays an important role in maintaining catecholaminergic function commensurate with physiological needs.

Neurotransmitter Receptors

Neurotransmitter receptors can be divided into two major classes: ligand-gated ion channels and G protein–coupled receptors. Ligand-gated ion channels are receptors that contain ion channels within their multisubunit structure; the binding of neurotransmitter to the receptor opens or closes this intrinsic channel. As a result, these receptors can mediate very rapid effects in the nervous system, because intervening steps are not required at least for their initial actions. G protein–coupled receptors, in contrast, produce their effects by binding to G proteins, which then influence a variety of neural processes.

14. **Burt DR, Kamatchi GL:** GABA$_A$ receptor subtypes: from pharmacology to molecular biology. *FASEB J* 5:2916–2923, 1991

   This review summarizes current knowledge of the major type of receptor for the neurotransmitter GABA (gamma-aminobutyric acid). These ligand-gated receptors, termed GABAA receptors, mediate a majority of the inhibitory synaptic transmission in the brain. These receptors also mediate the actions of the benzodiazepines and all sedative-hypnotic agents.

15. *Gasic GP, Heinemann S:** Receptors coupled to ionic channels: the glutamate receptor family. *Current Opinion in Neurobiology* 1:20–26, 1991

   Glutamate is the major excitatory neurotransmitter in the brain. Most of its receptors, covered in this informative review article, are ligand-gated ion channels. Particular attention has been given to the *N*-methyl-D-aspartate (NMDA) subtype of glutamate receptors for its apparent role in mediating neural plasticity.

16. **Huganir RL, Greengard P:** Regulation of neurotransmitter receptor desensitization by protein phosphorylation. *Neuron* 5:555–567, 1990

   This article reviews an important mechanism by which receptor function is regulated in the nervous system: protein phosphorylation (see section "Postreceptor Mechanisms" in this chapter). Phosphorylation of receptors appears to be the predominant mechanism by which desensitization and sensitization of receptor function are achieved.

17. **Julius D:** Molecular biology of serotonin receptors. *Annu Rev Neurosci* 14:335–360, 1991

   This article provides an overview of serotonin receptors. To date, seven types of serotonin receptors have been identified on the basis of pharmacological and molecular cloning studies. Most are G protein–coupled. The diversity of serotonin receptors holds potential importance for psychiatry:

agonists and antagonists of these various receptors are being developed as therapeutic agents for a variety of neuropsychiatric disorders.

18. *Kobilka B:* Adrenergic receptors as models for G protein–coupled receptors. *Annu Rev Neurosci* 15:87–114, 1992

Adrenergic receptors, which mediate the actions of norepinephrine and epinephrine, are among the best characterized G protein–coupled receptors. The structure of adrenergic receptors and the mechanisms by which receptor function is regulated are reviewed in this article.

19. **Meador-Woodruff JH, Mansour A, Bunzow JR, Van Tol HH, Watson Jr SJ, Civelli O:** Distribution of D2 dopamine receptor mRNA in rat brain. *Proc Natl Acad Sci U S A* 86:7625–7628, 1989

Dopamine receptors are the topic of this research publication. Whereas classic pharmacological studies have revealed the existence of two types of dopamine receptor (D1 and D2), molecular cloning studies have to date demonstrated the existence of at least six, all of which are G protein coupled. This large number of dopamine receptors has important implications for psychiatry: drugs with specific actions at a particular dopamine receptor might be an effective antipsychotic drug without the troubling side effects of traditional neuroleptics.

Postreceptor Mechanisms

The mechanisms by which neurotransmitters bind to receptors located extracellularly on the plasma membrane and produce changes in neuronal function by altering intracellular processes have been among the most intensely investigated areas in the neurosciences. We now know that neurotransmitters (which can be called first messengers) produce intraneuronal changes by influencing levels of second messengers in target neurons. In the case of G protein–coupled receptors, neurotransmitter-receptor interactions lead to changes in second messenger levels through G proteins, which couple the receptors to enzymes that control the synthesis or degradation of specific second messengers. (G proteins also couple receptors directly to ion channels; see the section "Neurophysiology" in this chapter.) In the case of ligand-gated ion channels, neurotransmitter-receptor interactions also lead to changes in second messengers, but indirectly via their effects on ion channels.

20. **Berridge MJ, Irvine RF:** Inositol phosphates and cell signaling. *Nature* 341:197–205, 1989

The phosphatidylinositol (PI) system plays an important second messenger role in the brain. The major metabolites of PI, inositol triphosphate (IP₃) and diacylglycerol, influence many neural processes. The metabolism of PI and its physiological roles are reviewed in this article.

21. *Bredt DS, Snyder SH:** Nitric oxide, a novel neuronal messenger. *Neuron* 8:3–11, 1992

This article focuses on nitric oxide, which has been recognized recently as an important second messenger in the nervous system.

22. *Nestler EJ, Greengard P:** *Protein Phosphorylation in the Nervous System.* New York, Wiley, 1984

This book provides a comprehensive discussion of protein phosphorylation. Included are chapters on protein kinases (the enzymes that phosphorylate proteins), protein phosphatases (the enzymes that dephosphorylate proteins), and neuronal phosphoproteins (examples of proteins whose phosphorylation underlies important aspects of regulation in the nervous system). It provides information from elementary to advanced levels.

23. **Nestler EJ, Hyman SE:** Intraneuronal signaling pathways, in *Comprehensive Textbook of Psychiatry/VI,* 6th Edition. Edited by Kaplan HI, Sadock BJ. Baltimore, MD, Williams & Wilkins (in press)

This chapter provides an overview of postreceptor mechanisms in the brain. It is intended for readers with little prior knowledge of the field.

24. **Piomelli D, Greengard P:** Lipoxygenase metabolites of arachidonic acid in neuronal transmembrane signalling. *Trends Pharmacol Sci* 11:367–373, 1990

The metabolites of arachidonic acid, which include the prostaglandins, prostacyclins, thromboxanes, and leukotrienes, subserve numerous second messenger functions in the nervous system. The metabolic pathways for these messengers and their physiological actions are reviewed in this article.

25. **Simon MI, Strathman MP, Gautam N:** Diversity of G proteins in signal transduction. *Science* 252:802–808, 1991

Close to 20 distinct G proteins have been cloned to date from mammalian tissues. The molecular structure of these proteins, their classification into distinct families, and their hypothesized physiological roles are the subject of this well-written review article.

Trophic Factors

Trophic factors contribute to the growth and differentiation of neurons during development and to the maintenance of differentiated characteristics of adult neurons. In recent years, great strides have been made in identifying peptides (small proteins) that serve as trophic factors in the nervous system and in characterizing their receptors.

26. **Barde YA:** Trophic factors and neuronal survival. *Neuron* 2:1525–1534, 1989

    This article reviews our current knowledge of trophic factors in the nervous system. Particular attention is given to nerve growth factor, a prototypical neurotrophic factor.

27. **Russell D:** Neurotrophins: mechanisms of action. The Neuroscientist 1:3–6, 1994

    This mini-review provides the most current and detailed review of neurotrophic factors and neurotrophic factor receptors. It is concise and contains a minimum of detail but provides numerous recent publications where in-depth information can be obtained.

Neurophysiology

One primary mechanism of synaptic transmission is the ability of neuro-transmitter-receptor interactions to influence the electrical properties of their target neurons. This is achieved through three main mechanisms: 1) through ligand-gated ion channels, 2) through the regulation of channel function via the binding of specific G proteins to the channels, or 3) through the regulation of channel function via the phosphorylation of the channels by specific second messenger and protein phosphorylation pathways.

28. *Aghajanian GK, Alreja M:** Basic electrophysiology, in *Comprehensive Textbook of Psychiatry/VI*, 6th Edition. Edited by Kaplan HI, Sadock BJ. Baltimore, MD, Williams & Wilkins (in press)

    This chapter is a good start for readers interested in an introduction to electrophysiology. It presents the basic principles of electrophysiology and of commonly used electrophysiological techniques. Also reviewed are electrophysiological properties of particular neuronal cell types implicated in psychiatry, namely, monoaminergic and cholinergic neurons.

29. **Birnbaumer L:** G proteins in signal transduction. *Annu Rev Pharmacol Toxicol* 30:675–705, 1990

    In addition to providing a general review of G proteins, this article focuses on the role played by G proteins in mediating the effects of certain neurotransmitters and receptors on the function of specific ion channels.

30. **Catterall WA:** Structure and function of voltage-sensitive ion channels. *Science* 242:50–61, 1988

    The author reviews the structural and functional classification of ion channels and the role played by protein phosphorylation in the regulation of channel function.

31. *Neher E, Sakmann B:** Single-channel currents recorded from membrane of denervated frog muscle fibres. *Nature* 260:799–802, 1976

    The development of patch clamp recording techniques represented a major advance in the field of electrophysiology. The authors of this review article are credited with developing this important methodology. Patch clamp techniques, which enable the introduction of large molecules directly into neurons while maintaining electrical recordings from the cells, have provided a more complete understanding, at the molecular level, of the regulation of a neuron's electrical properties.

Mechanisms of Psychotropic Drug Action

The field of neuropharmacology continues to play an important role in psychiatric neuroscience. This is because drugs provide a link between basic science studies in animals (for which it is difficult if at all possible to assess emotion and thought) and clinical psychiatric phenomena (for which it is difficult to study the basic underlying mechanisms). It is generally thought that a better understanding of how drugs influence brain function in animals will shed light on how they influence brain function in people. Because most psychotropic drugs produce their clinical effects only after prolonged exposure, the articles listed focus on mechanisms of *chronic* drug actions. In the sense that chronic exposure to a drug is prototypical of chronic exposure to other external stimuli (e.g., stress, trauma), a better understanding of drug action on the brain should provide important information as to how the brain responds to many types of long-term perturbations. Some representative research publications of a large literature that is growing geometrically are provided here.

32. *Avissar S, Schreiber G, Danon A, Belmaker RH: Lithium inhibits adrenergic and cholinergic increases in GTP binding in rat cortex. *Nature* 331:440–442, 1988

This was the first article to demonstrate a direct effect of lithium on G proteins. Acute and chronic lithium regulation of specific types of G protein is proposed to contribute to lithium's antidepressant and antimanic actions.

33. Baraban JM, Worley PF, Snyder SH: Second messenger systems and psychoactive drug action: focus on the phosphoinositide system and lithium. *Am J Psychiatry* 146:1251–1260, 1989

In addition to a general discussion of intracellular second messenger pathways, this citation concerns itself with the mechanisms of action of lithium. Electrophysiological evidence for the effects of lithium on the phosphatidylinositol system is presented.

34. Bunney BS, Sesack SR, Silva NL: Midbrain dopaminergic systems: neurophysiology and electrophysiological pharmacology, in *Psychopharmacology: Third Generation of Progress.* Edited by Meltzer HY. New York, Raven, 1987, pp 81–94

Classic antipsychotic drugs are dopamine receptor antagonists, but the drugs exert complex effects on the brain after prolonged administration. This article reviews the long-term actions of antipsychotic drugs on the brain's dopamine neurons.

35. Chappell PB, Smith MA, Kilts CD, Bissette G, Ritchie J, Anderson C, Nemeroff CB: Alterations in corticotropin-releasing factor-like immunoreactivity in discrete rat brain regions after acute and chronic stress. *J Neurosci* 6:2908–2914, 1986

The hypothalamic-pituitary-adrenal axis has been given considerable attention as a mediator of many stress-related responses. This axis consists of corticotropin-releasing factor, which controls the release of corticotropin (adrenocorticotropic hormone) from the pituitary, which in turn stimulates the release of glucocorticoid steroid hormones from the adrenal gland. This study examines the regulation of corticotropin-releasing factor in response to acute and chronic stress.

36. Colin SF, Chang HC, Mollner S, Pfeuffer T, Reed RR, Duman RS, Nestler EJ: Chronic lithium regulates the expression of adenylate cyclase and Gi-protein a subunit in rat cerebral cortex. *Proc Natl Acad Sci U S A* 88:10634–10637, 1991

This article is the first to report the influence of chronic lithium administration on the expression of G proteins and adenylyl cyclase (the enzyme that catalyzes the synthesis of the second messenger cyclic adenosine monophosphate).

37. **DeMontigny C:** Electroconvulsive shock treatments enhance responsiveness of forebrain neurons to serotonin. *J Pharmacol Exp Ther* 228:230–234, 1984

The brain's serotonin systems have been implicated in contributing to the mood-elevating effects of electroconvulsive seizures and of many types of antidepressant medications. This article was one of the first reports of the influence of chronic antidepressant treatments on serotonin function.

38. **Gellman RL, Aghajanian GK:** Serotonin$_2$ receptor–mediated excitation of interneurons in piriform cortex: antagonism by atypical antipsychotic drugs. *Neuroscience* 58:515–525, 1994

The serotonin 5-HT$_2$ and 5-HT$_{1c}$ receptors have received increasing attention for a possible role in the treatment of psychosis. Many antipsychotic drugs, including the atypical drug clozapine, are antagonists at these receptors (in addition to antagonizing various dopamine receptors), and all known hallucinogens are partial agonists at these receptors. This research article is focused on physiological and pharmacological mechanisms underlying 5-HT$_2$ and 5-HT$_{1c}$ receptor function.

39. **Hosoda K, Duman RS:** Regulation of β_1-adrenergic receptor mRNA and ligand binding by antidepressant treatments and norepinephrine depletion in rat frontal cortex. *J Neurochem* 60:1335–1342, 1993

To date, most studies of the effects of psychotropic drugs on neurotransmitter receptors have used ligand binding as a measure of receptor number. The recent cloning of numerous receptors and the development of specific antibodies directed against them has made it possible for the first time to study drug regulation of the receptors with more direct methodologies. The importance of this is highlighted by this article, which shows that the effects of some antidepressant drugs on messenger RNA of the β-adrenergic receptor would not have been predicted on the basis of earlier binding studies.

40. *Koob GF, Bloom FE:** Cellular and molecular mechanisms of drug dependence. *Science* 242:715–723, 1988

This article reviews our current knowledge concerning the neural pathways involved in drug addiction. It includes discussion of the opiates, psychostimulants, and alcohol. It is an excellent and comprehensible entrance to a large and complicated literature.

41. *Nestler EJ:* Molecular mechanism of drug addiction. *J Neurosci* 12:2439–2450, 1992

This review article presents the results of recent studies that have begun to establish molecular mechanisms of opiate and psychostimulant addiction. Emphasis is placed on long-term adaptations in intracellular messenger pathways in specific neuronal cell types.

42. **Nguyen TV, Kosofsky BE, Birnbaum R, Cohen BM, Hyman SE:** Differential expression of c-Fos and Zif268 in rat striatum after haloperidol, clozapine and amphetamine. *Proc Natl Acad Sci U S A* 89:4270–4274, 1992

Although typical and atypical antipsychotic drugs antagonize dopamine and other neurotransmitter receptors acutely, their antipsychotic effects are seen only after chronic administration. This research article presents the types of long-term mechanisms involving the regulation of gene expression that might be expected to be involved in such chronic drug action.

43. **Sulser F:** New perspectives on the molecular pharmacology of affective disorders. *Eur Arch Psychiatry Neurol Sci* 238:231–239, 1989

The acute effects of some antidepressant drugs are well established; for example, the tricyclic antidepressants are monoamine reuptake blockers and the monoamine oxidase inhibitors inhibit monoamine oxidase. However, the therapeutic effects of these and all other known antidepressants require their long-term administration, indicating that monoamine reuptake blockade or monoamine oxidase inhibition per se does not mediate the drugs' clinical effects. This article discusses hypothetical mechanisms that could contribute to the long-term effects of these antidepressants.

44. *Wise RA:* The role of reward pathways in the development of drug dependence. *Pharmacol Ther* 35:227–263, 1987

The brain's mesolimbic dopamine system appears to be an important neural substrate of drug reward. In fact, as discussed in this review article, the rewarding actions of many types of drugs of abuse, including opiates, stimulants, and alcohol, may be achieved at least in part via this neural pathway.

Neural Networks

A complete understanding of brain function can be achieved only when the complex mechanisms of intracellular regulation of individual neurons can be integrated within the complex web of enumerable intercellular connections (or neural networks) that form between the brain's 10^{10}–10^{12} neurons. Neural networks are the subject of a vast literature. Only selected examples, with possible direct relevance to psychiatry, are given here.

45. **Davis M:** The role of the amygdala in fear and anxiety. *Annu Rev Neurosci* 15:353–375, 1992

    This article reviews the neural pathways, at the center of which is the amygdala, that underlie animal models of fear and anxiety.

46. *Gerfen CR:** The neostriatal mosaic: multiple levels of compartmental organization in the basal ganglia. *Annu Rev Neurosci* 15:285–320, 1992

    The cellular composition of the neostriatum is the subject of this review. This brain region has been extensively investigated and implicated in several neuropsychiatric disorders.

47. **Harris-Warrick RM, Marder E:** Modulation of neural networks for behavior. *Annu Rev Neurosci* 14:39–57, 1991

    This article provides an overview of the relationship between neural networks and the modulation of behavior in laboratory animals.

48. *Madison DV, Malenka RC, Nicoll RA:** Mechanisms underlying long-term potentiation of synaptic transmission. *Annu Rev Neurosci* 14:379–397, 1991

    Long-term potentiation is viewed by many as a cellular model of memory. The presynaptic and postsynaptic mechanisms thought to underlie long-term potentiation are reviewed in this article.

49. **Papez JW:** A proposed mechanism of emotion. *Archives of Neurology and Psychiatry* 38:725–743, 1937

    This classic article offers one of the first descriptions of a hypothesized role of the limbic system in mediating mood and emotional states.

50. **Penfield W:** Functional localization in temporal and deep Sylvian areas. *Res Publ Assoc Res Nerv Ment Dis* 36:210–226, 1958

    This is a description of classic neurosurgical research that localized higher cortical functions to specific brain regions.

51. **Sperry RW:** Mental unity following surgical disconnection of the cerebral hemispheres. *Harvey Lect* 62:293–323, 1968

    This is a review of pioneering research on the integration of the right and left cerebral hemispheres.

52. **Swanson LW, Sawchenko PE:** Hypothalamic integration: organization of the paraventricular and supraoptic nuclei. *Annu Rev Neurosci* 6:269–324, 1983

    This reference offers a good review of the key role played by the hypothalamus in the body's homeostatic control of peripheral and central functions.

Clinical Psychiatric Neuroscience

One of the greatest challenges in psychiatry today is to study effectively neurobiological mechanisms of mental illness and its treatment in living people. This is made difficult by the inaccessibility of living brain tissue (brain biopsies remain rare) and our current inability to understand higher-order brain processes (e.g., emotion and thought) in neurobiological terms. Nevertheless, a detailed knowledge of inter- and intracellular communication in the nervous system will lead to a gradually more complete understanding of brain function, including behavior. Clinical psychiatric neuroscience is covered by a vast literature. Representative research publications and some recent review articles are given here.

53. *Choi DW, Rothman SM:** The role of glutamate neurotoxicity in hypoxic-ischemic neuronal death. *Annu Rev Neurosci* 13:171–182, 1990

    Glutamate-induced neurotoxicity, the subject of this review, has been given a great deal of attention recently as a possible mechanism for neuronal death seen under a variety of clinical circumstances. This includes neurodegenerative disorders in addition to cerebrovascular events.

54. *Delgado PL, Charney DS, Price LH, Aghajanian GK, Landis H, Heninger GR:** Serotonin function and the mechanism of action of antidepressant action: reversal of antidepressant induced remission by rapid depletion of plasma tryptophan. *Arch Gen Psychiatry* 47:411–418, 1990

    The tryptophan depletion procedure presented in this research publication has provided some of the most direct evidence for a role of the brain's serotonin systems in the treatment of depression.

55. **Edelman RR:** Magnetic resonance imaging of the nervous system. *Discussions in Neurosciences* 7:11–63, 1990

    Magnetic resonance imaging techniques provide detailed information concerning the anatomical structure of the brain with resolution of a few millimeters. It is being used to identify abnormalities in the brain associated with schizophrenia and other neuropsychiatric disorders.

56. **Gold PW, Goodwin FK, Chrousols GP:** Clinical and biochemical manifestations of depression. *N Engl J Med* 319:348–353, 1988

Measurement of monoamine metabolites and neuroendocrine parameters in body fluids has been one strategy by which to reveal neurobiological mechanisms of depression. Preliminary classifications of subtypes of depression based on these types of measurements are presented.

57. **Heninger GR, Charney DS:** Mechanism of action of antidepressant treatments: implications for the etiology and treatment of depressive disorders, in *Psychopharmacology: The Third Generation of Progress.* Edited by Meltzer HY. New York, Raven, 1987, pp. 535–544

The pharmacological challenge paradigm is one strategy used to assess the function of specific neurotransmitter and receptor systems in the brains of normal individuals and those with specific mental disturbances. A progress report of these studies is provided in this review.

58. *Malison RT, Innis RB:** Principles of neuroimaging, in *Comprehensive Textbook of Psychiatry/VI,* 6th Edition. Edited by Kaplan HI, Sadock BJ. Baltimore, MD, Williams & Wilkins (in press)

This chapter reviews brain-imaging techniques and their possible applications one day to psychiatric practice and research. It offers cogent discussions of positron-emission tomography, single photon emission computed tomography, and magnetic resonance imaging.

59. **Meltzer HY** (ed): *Psychopharmacology: The Third Generation of Progress.* New York, Raven, 1987

This large volume includes chapters by many leading researchers in the field of basic and clinical biological psychiatry. Reviews of numerous topics can be found in this volume. It also serves as a useful reference of the state of psychiatric neuroscience research circa 1987.

60. *Wexler NS, Rose EA, Housman DE:** Molecular approaches to hereditary diseases of the nervous system: Huntington's disease as a paradigm. *Annu Rev Neurosci* 14:503–529, 1991

Molecular genetics offers a strategy of great potential importance to psychiatric neuroscience. The identification of genes that contribute to specific psychiatric disorders will represent a revolutionary advance in the diagnosis, treatment, and prevention of mental illness. Although this approach has not, to date, been successful for the major psychiatric disorders, it has revolutionized medical research and practice in general. The identification of the gene that causes Huntington's disease provides a useful model of this approach.

Genetics

Joel E. Gelernter, M.D.

enetics includes clinical studies (e.g., twin studies and family studies, in which patterns of transmission of illness are studied primarily through obtaining diagnostic information about patients and their relatives) and molecular genetics (e.g., linkage and association studies, generally laboratory studies of genetic markers or DNA from patients and their relatives about whom diagnostic information is available). Studies in genetics have been growing in importance in all fields of medicine, psychiatry included. This is happening because of the enormous explosion of methods and techniques appearing roughly in the last two decades, culminating in the present situation in which cloning and DNA sequencing are relatively common procedures. Gene cloning—the isolation of a DNA sequence and its duplication in vitro—was considered grounds for science fiction two decades ago. Now you can buy a commercial cloning kit and do it in a couple of hours.

One new technique, the polymerase chain reaction (PCR), allows amplification of millions of pieces of DNA from very few pieces of template. This method has come into wide use in molecular biology worldwide essentially in the past 8 years, although it was described earlier. The growth in molecular methods (such as the PCR) has provided the motivation for

This work was supported in part by NIMH SDA-C Grant MH00931 and by U.S. Department of Veterans Affairs (the VA Medical Research Program).

development of new statistical methods. Application to real problems also would not be possible without similar attention to such clinical issues as ascertainment and diagnosis.

The papers listed in this chapter are biased toward recent publication date. Several of these studies simply could not have been done 5 years ago because the methods had not been invented yet. I have consequently included some of the more important "methods" papers that do not relate directly to problems in psychiatry. This selection is intended to be only a sample of the literature and therefore omits many important and interesting papers.

Some of these papers are especially important for the student interested in psychiatric genetics. As a basic set, I would recommend the following: Bouchard et al. (1990), Brunner et al. (1993), Gershon et al. (1982), Goate et al. (1991), Gottesman and Bertelsen (1989), Kety et al. (1967), Pauls and Leckman (1986), and Risch (1990).

DNA Structure and General Methods

1. **Botstein D, White RL, Skolnick M, Davis RW:** Construction of a genetic linkage map in man using restriction fragment length polymorphisms. *Am J Hum Genet* 32:314–331, 1980

   Botstein et al. presented a compelling rationale for the wide use of restriction fragment length polymorphisms (RFLPs) in genetic research, primarily for linkage. Many of the predictions made in the article have already been borne out. RFLPs were the dominant method of generating genetic data for most of the 1980s and are only now being replaced by other methods of marker analysis (primarily short tandem repeats).

2. **Kidd KK, Matthysee S:** Research designs for the study of gene-environment interactions in psychiatric disorders. *Arch Gen Psychiatry* 35:925–932, 1978

   Here is an early blueprint for the sort of study design that grew to dominate psychiatric genetics in the 1980s and is still important.

3. **Ott J:** *Analysis of Human Genetic Linkage,* Revised Edition. Baltimore, MD, Johns Hopkins University Press, 1991

   Ott is one of the leading investigators of our time in methods of genetic analysis. This book is the standard handbook for methods of linkage analysis. It is clearly written and relatively easy to understand, although not without some effort on the student's part.

4. *Risch N: Genetic linkage and complex diseases, with special reference to psychiatric disorders. *Genet Epidemiol* 7:3–16, 1990

   Risch's article can help you understand why replications of linkage results in psychiatry have been so hard to come by. One might find this article very depressing because of the systematic way difficulties encountered by investigators in the field are enumerated. On the other hand, it is easier to negotiate a minefield if you have a map.

5. Saiki RK, Gelfand DH, Stoffel S, Scharf SJ, Higuchi R, Horn GT, Mullis KB, Erlich HA: Primer-directed amplification of DNA with a thermostable DNA polymerase. *Science* 239:487–491, 1988

   The method described in this article, the polymerase chain reaction performed with a thermostable DNA polymerase, has revolutionized molecular biology research. This method permits enzymatic amplification of many copies of a DNA sequence when oligonucleotides flanking the sequence can be synthesized.

6. Watson JD, Crick FHC: Molecular structure of nucleic acids: a structure for deoxyribose nucleic acid. *Nature* 171:737–738, 1953

   This research effectively launched the modern era of DNA research. The article is widely considered a model of elegant scientific writing. It is hard to believe that there was a time when the DNA double helix was unknown; it is now familiar to most anyone with a high school education; Watson and Crick introduced something of surpassing importance. Moreover, because the article is only a couple of columns long, there is no excuse for anyone to not read it.

Schizophrenia

7. Gershon ES, DeLisi LE, Hamovit J, Nurnberger JI Jr, Maxwell ME, Schreiber J, Dauphinais D, Dingman CW 2nd, Guroff JJ: A controlled family study of chronic psychoses: schizophrenia and schizoaffective disorder. *Arch Gen Psychiatry* 45:328–336, 1988

   This family study from Gershon's group at the National Institute of Mental Health provides evidence for the range of illness that bears a genetic relationship to schizophrenia. It follows a rigorous family study design: direct interview, using a standardized instrument, of subjects and relatives by an interviewer blind to whether the person being interviewed is an ill proband, a control subject, or a relative of an ill proband or control subject; and blind diagnoses based on those interviews plus other data that can be collected about each individual (through information from relatives and hospital records). Rates of illness are then compared for relatives of probands and relatives of control subjects. Risk of the illness studied to different classes of relatives (e.g., first degree, second degree) can be assessed. Other diagnoses seen more in relatives of probands than in relatives of control subjects may well be genetically related to the illness being studied.

8. *Gottesman II, Bertelsen A:** Confirming unexpressed genotypes for schizophrenia: risks in the offspring of Fischer's Danish identical and fraternal discordant twins. *Arch Gen Psychiatry* 46:867–872, 1989

Suppose you had two copies of the same genetic individual, one of whom had schizophrenia and one who did not (i.e., discordant monozygotic twins). If they really had the same genetic liability for developing schizophrenia, then the children of the nonschizophrenic person should be at the same risk for schizophrenia as the schizophrenic person's children. If this were found to be true, it would provide powerful evidence for genetic vulnerability underlying the ill twin's schizophrenia, rather than purely environmental factors: it would demonstrate the genetic basis for schizophrenia hidden in the well twins of the monozygotic twin pairs. This Gottesman et al. study (building on the work of Margit Fischer) compares rates of schizophrenia in offspring of discordant monozygotic twin pairs (where the well twin is an obligate carrier) and discordant dizygotic twin pairs (where the well twin may be a carrier but also may not be).

9. *Kety SS, Rosenthal D, Wender PH, Schulsinger F:** The types and prevalence of mental illness in the biological and adoptive families of adopted schizophrenics, in *The Transmission of Schizophrenia*. Edited by Rosenthal D, Kety SS. London, Pergamon, 1967, pp. 345–362

The Kety et al. adoption study is a classic: the study that showed definitively that genetic factors are important for schizophrenia. It is rather long. If done today, it would certainly have somewhat different methodology, but it is still widely quoted and was enormously influential.

10. **Suddath RL, Christison GW, Torrey EF, Casanova MF, Weinberger DR:** Anatomical abnormalities in the brains of monozygotic twins discordant for schizophrenia. *N Engl J Med* 322:789–794, 1990

It is widely appreciated that schizophrenia is not an entirely genetic disorder. One way this is provable is through the observation that only about 50% of monozygotic (identical) twins are concordant for schizophrenia. What about those twin pairs in which one twin is schizophrenic and the other is normal? The twins are genetically identical, so environmental factors (e.g., birth trauma, exposure to toxins or infectious agents, injury, family influences—we really do not know what exactly) must be responsible for the difference. In the discordant pairs we have in effect the same genetic individual developing in two different ways: the nonschizophrenic twin is the control for the ill one and lets us know what the schizophrenic twin would have been like if he or she had not become schizophrenic. This article compares magnetic resonance imaging brain images of discordant twin pairs and demonstrates that in most cases the schizophrenic twins have wider ventricles.

Bipolar Affective Disorder

11. **Egeland JA, Gerhard DS, Pauls DL, Susses JN, Kidd KK, Allen CR, Hostetter AM, Housman DE:** Bipolar affective disorder linked to DNA markers on chromosome 11. *Nature* 325:783–787, 1987

Unfortunately, the finding of this article could never be replicated and is now considered to be probably incorrect. In its time it made people very optimistic about using linkage methods to tackle mental illness; Blum et al. (1990) has had a similar effect at encouraging association studies. Despite the fact that the result is not now accepted, the methodology is sound.

12. *Gershon ES, Hamovit J, Guroff JJ, Dibble E, Leckman JF, Sceery W, Targum SD, Nurnberger JI, Goldin LR, Bunney WE Jr:** A family study of schizoaffective, bipolar I, bipolar II, unipolar, and normal control probands. *Arch Gen Psychiatry* 39:1157–1167, 1982

The design of this study is analogous to the family study by this group for schizophrenia (Gershon et al. 1988). One use for this type of data is in helping prospective parents to understand the risk of transmitting illness to their offspring; for example, a parent with an affective disorder has a 27% chance of transmitting illness, according to this article.

Personality and Intelligence

13. *Bouchard TJ Jr, Lykken DT, McGue M, Segal NL, Tellegen A:** Sources of human psychological differences: the Minnesota Study of Twins Reared Apart. *Science* 250:223–228, 1990

Bouchard et al. provide evidence for a genetic contribution to the development of many personality traits and intelligence. The design is elegant and easy to understand: monozygotic twins separated at an early age were evaluated independently on intelligence and personality measures, and concordance on those measures was examined (and compared with similar measures for monozygotic twins reared together). The authors summarize their findings and the literature: "For almost every behavioral trait so far investigated, from reaction time to religiosity, an important fraction of the variation among people turns out to be associated with genetic variation" (p. 227).

Tourette's Syndrome

14. **Gelernter J, Pakstis AJ, Pauls DL, Kurlan R, Gancher S, Civelli O, Grandy D, Kidd KK:** Gilles de la Tourette syndrome is not linked to D_2 dopamine receptor. *Arch Gen Psychiatry* 47:1073–1077, 1990

    We cannot tell you where the gene is so we might as well try to make telling you where it is not as interesting as possible. This article is a "candidate gene" study: the point was to find out if a gene for which there was a high prior level of suspicion for involvement in pathophysiology of the disorder was actually involved. In this case, linkage could be excluded with a high level of confidence. The problem with this approach for psychiatry is that virtually any central nervous system gene, and many noncentral nervous system genes, could be imagined to be involved in illness. The challenge is to make guesses that are as good as possible or that, even if incorrect, can still shed some light on research strategies worth pursuing for the disorder. People have been suspicious about primary D_2 dopamine receptor abnormalities in Tourette's syndrome for years.

15. **Pakstis AJ, Heutink P, Pauls DL, Kurlan R, van de Wetering M, Leckman JL, Sandkuyl LA, Kidd JR, Breedveld GJ, Castiglione CM, Weber J, Sparkes RS, Cohen DJ, Kidd KK, Oostra BA:** Progress in the search for genetic linkage with Tourette syndrome: an exclusion map covering more than 50% of the autosomal genome. *Am J Hum Genet* 48:281–294, 1991

    This article is a good example of the "genome scanning" method (testing many genetic markers throughout the genome) of using linkage analysis to attempt to locate disease susceptibility loci (or "disease genes"). No gene for Tourette's syndrome has been identified yet, but, under the genetic parameters used as assumptions for these analysis, a large fraction of the genome has been excluded from harboring that gene.

16. *Pauls DL, Leckman JF:** The inheritance of Gilles de la Tourette's syndrome and associated behaviors. *N Engl J Med* 315:993–997, 1986

    Pauls and Leckman's article helped establish a view of the genetic range of the "TS gene," which is thought to be capable of causing the full

Tourette's syndrome, chronic multiple tics, or obsessive-compulsive disorder. (Whether or not the same gene may also cause a host of other disorders as well, including, for example, attention-deficit/hyperactivity disorder, is presently controversial.)

Alcoholism

17. **Blum K, Noble EP, Sheridan PJ, Montgomery A, Ritchie T, Jagadeeswaran P, Nogami H, Briggs AH, Cohn JB:** Allelic association of human dopamine D_2 receptor gene in alcoholism. *JAMA* 263:2055–2060, 1990

    This article, although considered problematic, has been very influential in directing the field (of psychiatric genetics, not just alcohol research) toward genetic association studies, as opposed to genetic linkage studies. Nevertheless, the reader is encouraged to evaluate the data presented here critically (for help, see Gelernter et al. 1993 below). At the time of this writing, association studies attempted without strong prior physiological knowledge have not yet added substantially to our knowledge of the pathophysiology of psychiatric illness.

18. **Gelernter J, Goldman D, Risch N:** The A1 allele at the D_2 dopamine receptor gene and alcoholism: a reappraisal. *JAMA* 269:1673–1677, 1993

    We attempted a comprehensive critique of the association strategy, especially as it has been applied in the case of DRD2 alleles and alcoholism, and concluded that no pathophysiologically important genetic association has been proven.

19. **Goodwin DW, Schulsinger F, Hermansen L, Guze SB, Winokur G:** Alcohol problems in adoptees raised apart from alcoholic biological parents. *Arch Gen Psychiatry* 28:238–243, 1973

    This Danish adoption study provided good evidence for a genetic contribution to inheritance of alcoholism: biological children of alcoholic persons who were adopted away had a higher rate of alcohol-related problems than biological children of control subjects who were adopted away.

20. **Kendler KS, Heath AC, Neale MC, Kessler RC, Eaves LJ:** A population-based twin study of alcoholism in women. *JAMA* 268:1877–1882, 1992

    This article describes a superb recent twin study. The authors were able to determine that, depending on the disease definition of alcoholism used, the genetic contribution to liability to develop alcoholism in women is between 50% and 60%. Surprisingly, the rest of the variance is accounted for by individual environmental differences, as opposed to family differences.

21. **Thomasson HR, Edenberg HJ, Crabb DW, Mai XL, Jerome RE, Li TK, Wang SP, Lin YT, Lu RB, Yin SJ:** Alcohol and aldehyde dehydrogenase genotypes and alcoholism in Chinese men. *Am J Hum Genet* 48:677–681, 1991

   Although this was not the first study demonstrating a genetic association between alleles at alcohol-metabolizing enzymes and alcohol dependence in Asian populations, it is the most comprehensive.

Alzheimer's Disease

22. *Goate A, Chartier-Harlin MC, Mullan M, Brown J, Crawford F, Fidani L, Giuffra L, Haynes A, Irving N, James L, Mant R, Newton P, Rooke K, Roques P, Talbot C, Pericak-Vance M, Roses A, Williamson R, Rosser M, Owen M, Hardy J:** Segregation of a missense mutation in the amyloid precursor protein gene with familial Alzheimer's disease. *Nature* 349:704–706, 1991

   There are, fortunately, some clear success stories for genetics of psychiatric illness, in the case of familial Alzheimer's disease, for example. In this research, Goate et al. demonstrated that a rare mutation in the gene coding for amyloid precursor protein (APP), located on chromosome 21, is sometimes associated with familial Alzheimer's disease. The finding has now been replicated by several other groups. At this point it seems like the mutation could account for only a small percentage of cases (a chromosome 14 gene accounts for most early-onset familial Alzheimer's disease [see Schellenberg et al. 1992 below]) but the significant factor is that it accounts for some and begins to provide a way to examine the molecular mechanism of this kind of dementia.

23. **Schellenberg GD, Bird TD, Wijsman EM, Orr HT, Anderson L, Nemens E, White JA, Bonnycastle L, Weber JL, Alonso ME, Potter H, Heston LL, Martin GM:** Genetic linkage evidence for a familial Alzheimer's disease locus on chromosome 14. *Science* 258:668–671, 1992

   The data presented here established that familial Alzheimer's disease may be caused by a (not yet characterized) gene on chromosome 14 and, considered with a series of papers published soon after this one, that this autosomal dominant gene may account for *most* early-onset Alzheimer's disease. Familial Alzheimer's disease has thus now been demonstrated to be genetically heterogeneous, with known susceptibility loci mapped to chromosomes 21 and 14 (and some families with linkage to neither locus). The article also illustrates use of polymerase chain reaction–based (short tandem repeat) genetic markers and the limitations of current multipoint linkage mapping methods (which could not be employed for this work because of the complexity of the analyses and the amount of computer time they were projected to require).

Fragile X

24. **Kremer EJ, Pritchard M, Lynch M, Yu S, Holman K, Baker E, Warren ST, Schlessinger D, Sutherland GR, Richards RI:** Mapping of DNA instability at the fragile X to a trinucleotide repeat sequence p(CCG)n. *Science* 252:1711–1714, 1991

Here is an explanation for psychiatric abnormality in terms of base pairs of DNA. Fragile X was one of the earlier examples of a disorder with symptomatology in the psychiatric sphere (heritable mental retardation and possibly autism) with a clear genetic basis. It was mapped comparatively easily because symptoms were accompanied by a cytogenetic abnormality: a little constriction on the X chromosome that could be induced under certain circumstances. This was a clear structural variation in the morphology of the chromosome. (There are other fragile sites known on other chromosomes also.) The actual genetic defect giving rise to the fragile site on the X chromosome is now known and described in this article.

Violence and Impulsivity

25. **Brunner HG, Nelen M, Breakefield XO, Ropers HH, van Oost BA:** Abnormal behavior associated with a point mutation in the structural gene for monoamine oxidase A. *Science* 262:578–580, 1993

Here is a very clear example of a mutation in a gene with a role in monoamine metabolism associated with a specific behavioral outcome, consistent with what was already known about monoamine systems and behavior. In the family described in this article, a syndrome of abnormal behavior characterized by violence, impulsivity, and mild mental retardation segregates as an X-linked trait. Linkage analysis led the authors to the monoamine oxidase A and B genes, located together on the X chromosome. Affected individuals were shown to have complete deficiency of monoamine oxidase A activity; sequencing of the gene in family members demonstrated that every affected individual (they are all males) carries a mutation that introduces a termination codon into the monoamine oxidase A gene and therefore results in inactive gene product. This article provides one of the strongest links yet between a particular mutation and a particular behavior. It is so far unclear if this mutation is a common cause of these behaviors in the population; it could also be a "private" mutation, specific to the one family studied.

┌─────┐
│ 3 │
└─────┘

Psychoanalysis

Marshall Edelson, M.D., Ph.D.

The major problems facing psychoanalysis as a behavioral science are systematizing psychoanalytic theory, clarifying the relation of the theory to other bodies of knowledge and other theories in behavioral science, and deciding what kind of empirical evidence will test it and how. Therefore, the following list of references gives priority to works that 1) explicate or attempt to systematize psychoanalytic theory; 2) relate psychoanalytic theory to conceptual developments in such behavioral sciences as linguistics, sociology, and learning theory; 3) consider features of the psychoanalytic situation that have bearing on the kind of evidence obtained in it; or 4) raise questions about, point out where the need exists for, or suggest how to obtain evidence that is relevant to an evaluation of the scientific credibility of psychoanalytic hypotheses. In a first introduction to psychoanalysis, one cannot do better than to let Freud speak for himself. He remains his own most able expositor.

Works are organized into the following sections: 1) introduction to psychoanalysis, 2) the essential Freud, 3) psychoanalytic theory, 4) psychoanalysis and other disciplines, 5) psychoanalytic situation and method, and 6) scientific status of psychoanalysis.

Introduction to Psychoanalysis

1. **Brenner C:** An Elementary Textbook of Psychoanalysis, Revised and Expanded Edition. New York, International Universities Press, 1973

   This book is for students who want a relatively authoritative, up-to-date exposition of the fundamentals of psychoanalytic theory as it now stands, to serve as an introduction to, and a guide in reading, the primary sources.

2. **Clark R:** *Freud: The Man and the Cause.* New York, Random House, 1980

3. **Jones E:** *The Life and Work of Sigmund Freud,* Vols. 1–3. New York, Basic Books, 1953–1957

4. **Sulloway FJ:** *Freud, Biologist of the Mind: Beyond the Psychoanalytic Legend.* New York, Basic Books, 1979

5. **Wollheim R:** *Sigmund Freud.* New York, Cambridge University Press, 1971

   Clark's focus is on Freud as the charismatic political leader of a movement. The book by Jones is the definitive biography for those interested in a detailed account of the relation between the personal life and the work of Freud, for it scants neither. Sulloway, asserting against Jones that Freud remained in his work and aims a biologist, contributes some interesting material about the intellectual influences on Freud of psychophysics, sexual biology and sexology, and the Darwinian revolution. Wollheim's intellectual biography is one of the best introductions to Freud's thought and is appropriate for a general audience. Wollheim is a philosopher of mind, whose sympathetic appreciation and insight into the nature and developmental vicissitudes of Freud's work are unusual for a philosopher.

6. ****Freud S:** Introductory lectures on psycho-analysis (1915–1916), in *The Standard Edition of the Complete Psychological Works of Sigmund Freud,* Vol. 15. Translated and edited by Strachey J. London, Hogarth Press, 1961; **Freud S:** Introductory lectures on psycho-analysis (1916–1917), in *The Standard Edition of the Complete Psychological Works of Sigmund Freud,* Vol. 16. Translated and edited by Strachey J. London, Hogarth Press, 1963

7. ****Freud S:** New introductory lectures on psychoanalysis (1933), in *The Standard Edition of the Complete Psychological Works of Sigmund Freud,* Vol. 22. Translated and edited by Strachey J. London, Hogarth Press, 1964, pp. 5–182

The "Introductory Lectures" are the best relatively brief introduction to Freud's work. His anticipation of the reader's questions and objections is a powerful rhetoric. Lecture II ("Parapraxes"), among others, exemplifies his mode of argument about necessary and sufficient causes. Lecture XVII ("The Sense of Symptoms"), among others, exemplifies his use of questions to focus on distinctive problems. (What is the sense of an apparently senseless phenomenon? How can it be discovered?) Lecture XXIII ("The Paths to the Formation of Symptoms") presents a sophisticated causal model for explaining neurotic symptoms; his use of a complemental series (constitutional dispositions and experiences) at different stages of symptom formation is often neglected in reductions of psychoanalytic theory. If, in an introduction to Freud's thinking, it is desirable to avoid mixing in early and subsequently rejected formulations, then Lectures XXXI ("The Dissection of the Psychical Personality") and XXXII ("Anxiety and Instinctual Life") from the "New Introductory Lectures" can be substituted for the earlier XXIV ("The Common Neurotic State") and XXV ("Anxiety") in a reading of the "Introductory Lectures." It can also be useful to substitute Freud's "Three Essays on the Theory of Sexuality" as a more completed formulation of a difficult subject for Lectures XX and XXI on sexuality and libido.

8.   ***Freud S:** The question of lay analysis: conversations with an impartial person (1926), in *The Standard Edition of the Complete Psychological Works of Sigmund Freud,* Vol. 20. Translated and edited by Strachey J. London, Hogarth Press, 1959, pp. 183–258

The polemic about the relation between medicine and psychoanalysis aside (it certainly has its own interest), this nontechnical presentation of psychoanalysis is one of Freud's most delightful and rhetorically effective expositions; it was written after significant theoretical developments had taken place in his work.

9.   **Groddeck G:** *The Book of the It* (1923). New York, Vintage, 1961 (available from New York, International Universities Press, 1976)

Partly incredible but still enjoyable, this book includes lively, witty, didactic letters from "Patrick Troll" to "dearest friend" about the marvelous contents and manifestations of unconscious mental life. Each of us is lived by his or her It. The It, if rejected, expresses itself, believe it or not, in every kind of bodily illness. One must give up trying to subdue or master the It. Instead, one must make peace with the It. Besides being fun to read and giving a good feel for the kind of phenomena of central interest for psychoanalysis, this work is an antidote to current overestimation of the activity and strength of "the ego" in relation to "the id," and also to the popular (if not indeed at times, professional) misconception that conflict is the inevitable relation between a good achievement-oriented and reality-oriented "ego" and a bad chaotic and demonic "id" and that therapy is a process of getting rid of the latter in favor of the former.

10. **Nemiah JC:** *Foundations of Psychopathology.* New York, Oxford University Press, 1961 (available from New York, Jason Aronson, 1973)

This presentation of psychopathology emphasizes the role of conflict and defense, the unconscious and repression, and the childhood roots of emotional disorder in symptom formation; it also considers the relevance of these concepts—which are illustrated by many vivid, detailed clinical examples—to the practice of medicine. This is especially appropriate for use as part of an introduction of psychoanalysis to medical students.

The Essential Freud

11. *****Freud S:** The interpretation of dreams (1900), in *The Standard Edition of the Complete Psychological Works of Sigmund Freud,* Vol. 4. Translated and edited by Strachey J. London, Hogarth Press, 1953; **Freud S:** The interpretation of dreams (1900–1901), in *The Standard Edition of the Complete Psychological Works of Sigmund Freud,* Vol. 5. Translated and edited by Strachey J. London, Hogarth Press, 1953

This is a classic in behavioral science, which—like Durkheim's *Suicide* (see Lidz, Chapter 8, this volume)—unites formulation of a theory of broad scope and an unexpected body of data. This work exemplifies (throughout) the kind of argument Freud used as a scientist. It presents his method of free association (Chapter II), his way of relating hypotheses and evidence (Chapters III–VI), and his model of the mind (Chapter VII). Chapter II should be related to the account of the "theorems" presupposed in using the method of free association given in Chapter VII (part A). Chapter I, a masterful but neglected review of the literature, locates problems and paradoxical findings; in Chapter VII (part D), Freud summarizes the way in which his work resolves them. If one were to read only one work by Freud, this should be the one.

12. *****Freud S:** The psychopathology of everyday life (1901), in *The Standard Edition of the Complete Psychological Works of Sigmund Freud,* Vol. 6. Translated and edited by Strachey J. London, Hogarth Press, 1960

13. *****Freud S:** Jokes and their relation to the unconscious (1905), in *The Standard Edition of the Complete Psychological Works of Sigmund Freud,* Vol. 8. Translated and edited by Strachey J. London, Hogarth Press, 1960

These two works should be read together with "The Interpretation of Dreams," which are Freud's three most seminal, innovative, and ground-breaking works, and the core of his extension of his theory to empirical realms other than the neuroses.

14. ***Freud S:** Three essays on the theory of sexuality (1905), in *The Standard Edition of the Complete Psychological Works of Sigmund Freud,* Vol. 7. Translated and edited by Strachey J. London, Hogarth Press, 1953, pp. 130–243

This work is essential for understanding Freud's thinking about infantile sexuality. His use of information about the perversions in explicating infantile sexuality is often overlooked. In general, as readers of this work (including the footnotes) discover, what Freud actually wrote about sexuality differs considerably from the views sometimes attributed to him.

15. ***Freud S:** Formulations on the two principles of mental functioning (1911), in *The Standard Edition of the Complete Psychological Works of Sigmund Freud,* Vol. 12. Translated and edited by Strachey J. London, Hogarth Press, 1958, pp. 218–226

This work provides an important clarification of the difference between primary and secondary mental processes, one of Freud's major discoveries, in terms of the difference between the principles (pleasure principle and reality principle) regulating these processes, or the aims (maximizing immediate gratification and maximizing accommodation to external reality) governing them. This can profitably be read with "The Interpretation of Dreams" (Chapter VII).

16. ***Freud S:** Instincts and their vicissitudes (1915), in *The Standard Edition of the Complete Psychological Works of Sigmund Freud,* Vol. 14. Translated and edited by Strachey J. London, Hogarth Press, 1957, pp. 117–140

17. ***Freud S:** The unconscious (1915), in *The Standard Edition of the Complete Psychological Works of Sigmund Freud,* Vol. 14. Translated and edited by Strachey J. London, Hogarth Press, 1957, pp. 166–215

These two papers are examples of Freud's efforts to clarify central theoretical concepts. Both reveal Freud as a scientist thinking about the relation between phenomena and concepts. The first can profitably be read with "Three Essays on Sexuality," and the second with "The Interpretation of Dreams" (Chapter VII).

18. ***Freud S:** The ego and the id (1923), in *The Standard Edition of the Complete Psychological Works of Sigmund Freud,* Vol. 19. Translated and edited by Strachey J. London, Hogarth Press, 1961, pp. 12–66

19. *Freud S: Inhibitions, symptoms and anxiety (1926), in *The Standard Edition of the Complete Psychological Works of Sigmund Freud*, Vol. 20. Translated and edited by Strachey J. London, Hogarth Press, 1959, pp. 87–172

These are major revisions of psychoanalytic theory. The psychological system is described in terms of subsystems (ego, id, superego) with different characteristics and aims. Anxiety, rather than a transformation of dammed-up libido, serves the ego as a signal of, first, external and, ultimately, inner or instinctual danger. Both works suggest that, however determined Freud was not to give up the fundamental discoveries of psychoanalysis about mental life, when it came to the theoretical superstructure, he was responsive to data, especially data obtained in the psychoanalytic situation, and that his attempts to incorporate observations and to mitigate conceptual inconsistencies in dealing with observations motivated whatever major revisions of psychoanalytic theory he proposed.

Psychoanalytic Theory

20. **Abraham K:** A short study of the development of the libido viewed in light of mental disorders (1924), in *Selected Papers*. Edited by Abraham K. London, Hogarth Press, 1949, pp. 418–501

Abraham's hypothesis is that what kind of psychopathology occurs depends on the stage of libidinal development to which regression has occurred.

21. **Arlow J, Brenner C:** *Psychoanalytic Concepts and the Structural Theory.* New York, International Universities Press, 1964

22. **Gill M:** Topography and systems in psychoanalytic theory (Monogr. No. 10). *Psychol Issues* 3:1–179, 1963

23. **Lewin BD:** Phobic symptoms and dream interpretation. *Psychoanal Q* 21:295–322, 1952

What is the relationship between the terminology and model of the mind of Freud's "The Interpretation of Dreams" and the terminology and model of the mind of his major works of revision "The Ego and the Id" and "Inhibitions, Symptoms and Anxiety"? Gill, in an exemplary scholarly monograph of conceptual clarification, makes important distinctions and documents that the relationship between the two terminologies and models is subtle and complex and that significant problems have been left unsolved by the revision. For Arlow and Brenner, everything is settled. The relationship between the two is simple and straightforward. They are incompatible, and the former should be rejected in favor of the latter. Lewin argues that the two, each having its own purposes and advantages, may with profit be used interchangeably; he gives an account of phobic symptoms in the language of dream interpretation.

24. **Erikson EH:** *Childhood and Society,* 2nd Edition, Revised and Enlarged. New York, WW Norton, 1963

This restatement of the theory of infantile sexuality (Chapter 2) describes stages of development in terms of dominant bodily zones, characteristic modes of action or approach to objects, and typical nuclear conflicts.

25. **Fairbairn W:** *Psychoanalytic Studies of the Personality.* London, Tavistock, 1952

In "Schizoid Factors in the Personality" (1940), schizoid characterology and symptomatology are determined by a libidinal oral attitude; the themes, preoccupations, attitudes, and object relations found in work with schizoid characters are vividly captured. In "A Revised Psychopathology of the Psychoses and Psychoneuroses" (1941), however, Fairbairn rejects Abraham's hypothesis that regression to different stages of libidinal development determines the form of psychopathology. In fact, he rejects in its entirety the conception of libidinal phases presented by Abraham, and by Freud in "Three Essays on Sexuality." In an object relations formulation, Fairbairn proposes that it is the disposition (externalization or internalization) of good and bad objects that determines the variety of symptomatology that may be associated with either a fundamental schizoid or depressive position.

26. **Federn P:** *Ego Psychology and the Psychoses.* New York, Basic Books, 1952

Federn focuses on the patient's introspective-subjective experience of ego and nonego and concludes that schizophrenia arises from a disturbance in the distribution of ego feeling, in what is felt (which may conflict with what is thought) to be part of the ego and what is felt to be outside the ego, in what the ego feels and does not feel is real and significant. Federn draws conclusions about treatment. The chapters on ego feeling (1, 3), psychoanalysis and psychotherapy of psychoses (6, 7), and the ego aspects of schizophrenia (10, 11, 12) are more accessible than the others.

27. **Fenichel O:** *The Psychoanalytic Theory of Neurosis.* New York, WW Norton, 1945

Although clearly written, this encyclopedic summary of and attempt to systematize the psychoanalytic theory of neurosis is so comprehensive that it is difficult to read through. It is, however, an invaluable reference.

28. **Freud A:** *The Ego and the Mechanisms of Defense,* Revised Edition. New York, International Universities Press, 1966

    In this classic work, psychoanalysis shifts in its study of the vicissitudes of intrapsychic conflict from a focus on detecting derivatives of instinctual impulses to a detailed examination of defensive operations.

29. **Hartmann H:** *Ego Psychology and the Problem of Adaptation.* New York, International Universities Press, 1958

    This is a seminal effort to increase the scope of psychoanalytic theory so that, as a general psychology, it encompasses those structures and processes of personality serving adaptation and achievement, which are neither derived from nor necessarily involved in conflict.

30. **Hartmann H, Kris E, Loewenstein R:** The function of theory in psychoanalysis (Monogr. No. 14). *Psychol Issues* 4:117–143, 1964

    Addressing psychoanalysts who distrust theory, Hartmann et al. identify the difficulties and misunderstandings leading to that distrust and sources of dissatisfaction with psychoanalytic theory. They comment at length on the interdependence of theory and clinical work and observations in psychoanalysis.

31. **Isaacs S, Riviere J:** The nature and function of phantasy, in *Developments in Psycho-Analysis.* Edited by Riviere J. London, Hogarth Press, 1952, pp. 67–121

32. **Schafer R:** The mechanisms of defence. *Int J Psychoanal* 49:49–62, 1968

33. **Segal H:** *Introduction to the Work of Melanie Klein.* New York, Basic Books, 1964 (New and Revised Edition, New York, Basic Books, 1973)

    Freud discovered that psychic reality has causal efficacy: that is, mere phantasies (as distinct from physical lesions or features of an experienced situation) produce psychopathology. This discovery underlies his theory of instinctual drives, for such phantasies appear to be relatively independent of accidents of experience. Phantasy is central to psychoanalytic thought and practice, and these three works focus on its nature and function. All three question in different ways the sharp conceptual distinction between instinctual impulses and "mechanisms" of defense in conflict, and not only because a defense may serve instinctual gratification. A defense is far from being a contentless mechanism, but itself is in its essence the expression or manifestation of a phantasy.

34. **Jones E:** *Papers on Psycho-Analysis*, 5th Edition. Baltimore, MD, Williams & Wilkins, 1948

The paper on anal-erotic character traits (Chapter 24), in addition to elaborating one of Freud's startling findings (the unexpected correlation of certain traits), illuminates and makes vivid the theoretical paper on the important subject of symbolism (Chapter 8).

35. **Loewald HW:** Internalization, separation, mourning, and the superego. *Psychoanal Q* 31:483–504, 1962

36. **Loewald HW:** The superego and the ego-ideal, II: superego and time. *Int J Psychoanal* 43:264–268, 1962

These evocative essays on psychic structure emphasize its essential temporal nature and, especially, a view of the superego in terms of internal representations of, or orientation to, the future.

37. **Rapaport D:** *The Collected Papers of David Rapaport.* Edited by Gill MM. New York, Basic Books, 1967

This work includes papers on the conceptual model of psychoanalysis (1951) and on the psychoanalytic theory of thinking (1950), affects (1953), and motivation (1960); these make a major contribution to the effort to systematize psychoanalytic theory and to integrate and contrast it with other streams of psychological science. The 1960 paper on motivation can profitably be read in conjunction with a reading of Freud's "Three Essays on Sexuality." Important contributions to ego psychology include two papers on autonomy of the ego (1951, 1957) and one on activity and passivity (1953).

38. **Waelder R:** The principle of multiple function, observations on overdetermination. *Psychoanal Q* 5:45–62, 1936

Every psychic act is an attempt, at one and the same time, with varying degrees of success, to achieve multiple purposes, arising, for example, from the necessity to meet simultaneously claims of the instinctual drives, of the outer world, and of internalized commands and prohibitions, and to meet them in certain ways (e.g., by means resulting in active mastery of, rather than mere submission to, these claims). Any psychic act responds to different demands, serves or is exploited to achieve different ends, and therefore has multiple meanings or significances. Waelder here points to an ineluctable characteristic of the subject matter of psychoanalysis. Theory in psychoanalysis must take into account the multiple causation of, and the multiple meanings possessed by, phenomena of interest to it.

Psychoanalysis and Other Disciplines

39. **Edelson M:** *Language and Interpretation in Psychoanalysis.* New Haven, CT, Yale University Press, 1975 (University of Chicago Press paperback edition, 1984)

    Edelson explores some analogies between aspects of Chomsky's linguistic theory and some transformational-generative properties of Freud's theory of dreams, compares interpretations in the psychoanalytic situation with detailed interpretations of a Bach prelude and Wallace Stevens's poem "The Snow Man," and in general demystifies the psychoanalytic clinical instrument by arguing that "empathy" and "clinical intuition" might in part be the result of the psychoanalyst's unwitting response to complex syntactic, semantic, and phonetic patterns in the analysand's speech.

40. *****Freud S:** Totem and taboo (1913), in *The Standard Edition of the Complete Psychological Works of Sigmund Freud,* Vol. 13. Translated and edited by Strachey J. London, Hogarth Press, 1953, pp. xiii–162

41. *****Freud S:** Group psychology and the analysis of the ego (1921), in *The Standard Edition of the Complete Psychological Works of Sigmund Freud,* Vol. 18. Translated and edited by Strachey J. London, Hogarth Press, 1955, pp. 67–143

    Both of these works have influenced attempts to explain social and group phenomena, especially the relations between a group and its leader.

42. **Klein GS:** Consciousness in psychoanalytic theory: some implications for current research in perception. *J Am Psychoanal Assoc* 7:5–34, 1959

    This is an illustration of the impact of psychoanalytic theory on research in another discipline.

43. **Mahl G:** *Psychological Conflict and Defense.* Edited by Janis IL. New York, Harcourt Brace Jovanovich, 1971

    Mahl brings the perspective of learning theory to an introduction of the mechanisms of defense. This book can be usefully read with A. Freud's book on the same subject (1966 above).

44. **Parsons T:** Social structure and the development of personality: Freud's contribution to the integration of psychology and sociology. *Psychiatry* 21:321–340, 1958

Read together with Freud's "Three Essays on Sexuality," this sociological perspective on the same subject will provoke thought and discussion.

45. **Redl F:** Group emotion and leadership. *Psychiatry* 5:573–596, 1942

A development of Freud's ideas on group psychology, this article describes 10 types of group formation distinguished by differences in the relation to a central person, who is an object of identification, an object of drives, or an ego support. The assuagement of guilt and fear by the initiatory act of a seducer and the infection, with respect to expressing a particular drive, of a conflicted personality by a nonconflicted personality are two mechanisms postulated to operate in processes of group formation around a leader. Examples are provided from and applied to teacher-students relations.

46. **Reiser MF:** *Mind, Brain, Body: Toward a Convergence of Psychoanalysis and Neurobiology.* New York, Basic Books, 1984

47. **Reiser MF:** *Memory in Mind and Brain: What Dream Imagery Reveals.* New York, Basic Books, 1990

Reiser argues for the value of attending to the way in which psychoanalytic and neuroscientific empirical findings converge. In the first book, an especially vivid account of observable processes in the psychoanalytic situation is connected to what has become known about the brain. In the second book, an intriguing discussion of memory and dreams draws on knowledge from both domains.

Psychoanalytic Situation and Method

48. **Fenichel O:** *Problems of Psychoanalytic Technique.* New York, Psychoanalytic Quarterly, 1941

To evaluate the data obtained in the psychoanalytic situation, one must be clear about the nature of the psychoanalyst's interventions. Fenichel's theory of psychoanalytic therapy is distinguished by its use of metapsychological concepts to consider the dynamic, economic, and structural aspects of interpretation. He is lucid and pithy. The psychoanalytic task is "reversing displacements, abolishing isolations, or guiding traces of affect to their proper relationships" (pp. 42–43). The patient's childhood "is still actively present . . . in the behavior of the patient today; otherwise it would not interest us at all. If only we put the present in order correctly and understand it, we shall thereby make new impulses possible for the patient, until the childhood material comes of itself" (p. 49). A classic.

49. *Freud S: Papers on technique (1911–1915), in *The Standard Edition of the Complete Psychological Works of Sigmund Freud,* Vol. 12. Translated and edited by Strachey J. London, Hogarth Press, 1958, pp. 89–171

50. **Stone L:** *The Psychoanalytic Situation: An Examination of Its Development and Essential Nature.* New York, International Universities Press, 1961

The establishment and maintenance of the psychoanalytic situation are essential not only for treatment but for obtaining unique data hard to come by otherwise. Stone responds to Freud's technical recommendations as they are frequently interpreted by characterizing the multiple dilemmas the psychoanalyst traverses in creating and maintaining the psychoanalytic situation.

51. **Kris E:** On some vicissitudes of insight in psychoanalysis. *Int J Psychoanal* 37:445–455, 1956

The acquisition of insight is generally held to be not only a necessary condition for therapeutic success in psychoanalysis, but when insight leads to therapeutic success, it is also regarded as evidence justifying provisional acceptance of psychoanalytic hypotheses. Kris makes clear that the conditions leading to insight are very complex indeed. He emphasizes the role of preceding analytic work, preparatory preconscious mental activity, and the integrative capacity and functioning of the ego; questions that the occurrence of negative transference is always an obstacle; distinguishes between compliance with the analyst and compliance with the treatment process; and contrasts the characteristics of insight, partial or pseudo-insight, and the insight used in the service of defense and resistance. Influential individual differences have to do with capacities to control regression, to view the self objectively, and to control the discharge of affects.

52. **Kris A:** *Free Association: Method and Process.* New Haven, CT, Yale University Press, 1982

53. **Searl MN:** Some queries on principles of technique. *Int J Psychoanal* 17:471–493, 1936

Both authors approach the psychoanalytic process—with what they consider to be a minimal theoretical apparatus—from the point of view of free association, the unique method of investigation of psychoanalysis. The focus of the psychoanalyst's attention is on the vicissitudes of the analysand's reluctances and resistances, which appear in the course of attempting to report whatever comes to mind. These works are invaluable, from the point of view of interest in psychoanalysis as science, for understanding in what ways a psychoanalyst with a disciplined technique evaluates and does influence the data obtained in the psychoanalytic situation, and in what ways such a psychoanalyst does not influence these data.

54. Strachey J: The nature of the therapeutic action of psycho-analysis. *Int J Psychoanal* 15:127–159, 1934

That the past lives again in the transference is essential to the claim that data obtained in the psychoanalytic situation can serve to support psychoanalytic hypotheses. Strachey characterizes a mutative interpretation as one leading to awareness that a particular impulse is directed to the psychoanalyst, that anxiety and defense are responses to the occurrence of the impulse, that directing the impulse to the psychoanalyst is in some way inexplicable in terms of what is otherwise known about the psychoanalyst, and that the determinants of both impulse and conflict lie in unconscious phantasy and memory from infancy and childhood.

Scientific Status of Psychoanalysis

55. *Breuer J, Freud S: Studies on hysteria (1893–1895), in *The Standard Edition of the Complete Psychological Works of Sigmund Freud,* Vol. 2. Translated and edited by Strachey J. London, Hogarth Press, 1955

56. *Freud S: Constructions in analysis (1937), in *The Standard Edition of the Complete Psychological Works of Sigmund Freud,* Vol. 23. Translated and edited by Strachey J. London, Hogarth Press, 1964, pp. 257–269

57. Kris E: The recovery of childhood memories in psychoanalysis. *Psychoanal Study Child* 11:54–88, 1956

These works represent the move from the position that the patient suffers from unconscious memories of recent traumatic experiences and that successful therapeutic outcome depends on the recovery of these memories, to the position that what is etiologic are unconscious memories of infancy and childhood, which often cannot be recovered and must be reconstructed, and that the recovery of childhood memories is not essential to successful therapeutic outcome. The implication of this change for the scientific status of psychoanalysis has been discussed by Edelson (1988) below and Grunbaum (1984) below, who come to different conclusions about it.

58. **Edelson M:** *Psychoanalysis: A Theory in Crisis.* Chicago, IL, University of Chicago Press, 1988 (1990 paperback edition)

59. **Edelson M:** Can psychotherapy research answer this psychotherapist's questions? *Contemporary Psychoanalysis* 28:118–151, 1992

60. **Edelson M:** Telling and enacting stories in psychoanalysis, in *Interface of Psychoanalysis and Psychology.* Edited by Barron J, Eagle M, Wolitzky D. Washington, DC, American Psychological Association Press, 1992, pp. 99–124

In these works, Edelson attempts to define what he regards as an essential distinctive core in psychoanalytic theory, those concepts and propositions least likely to be found in other theories about the workings of the mind. He argues that, given this core and the nature of the theory, case studies are an appropriate method of research, and, in contrast to the belief of Grunbaum and others, are not simply a heuristic aid for generating psychoanalytic ideas. Instead, case studies are capable of testing psychoanalytic ideas. In part II of the 1988 book, he presents many arguments that might be used to justify rejecting or believing psychoanalytic assertions on the basis of data from the clinical situation. In the two 1992 papers, he turns more and more to a narrative paradigm to illuminate features of psychoanalytic process and to provide an observational unit (the "story" told or enacted) the description of which need not be contaminated by any of the competing theories in psychoanalysis.

61. **Freud S:** Notes upon a case of obsessional neurosis (1909), in *The Standard Edition of the Complete Psychological Works of Sigmund Freud,* Vol. 10. Translated and edited by Strachey J. London, Hogarth Press, 1955, pp. 155–318

62. **Glymour C:** Freud, Kepler, and the clinical evidence, in *Freud A: Collection of Critical Essays.* Edited by Wollheim R. New York, Anchor, 1974, pp. 285–304

Freud uses a case study (the Rat Man) to test and revise his theory. Glymour argues that Freud's methods here are essentially those of other scientists. Glymour's discussion of the Rat Man case suggests a way of thinking about testing theoretical hypotheses in a clinical case study.

63. **Freud S:** Analysis terminable and interminable (1937), in *The Standard Edition of the Complete Psychological Works of Sigmund Freud,* Vol. 23.

Translated and edited by Strachey J. London, Hogarth Press, 1964, pp. 216–253

This is a dark paper. Because it focuses on factors that unavoidably limit the efficacy of psychoanalysis as therapy, it constrains excessive therapeutic zeal, ambition, and optimism—and implies that the ultimate value of psychoanalysis lies in making, through its method of investigation, contributions to human knowledge.

64. **Glover E:** The therapeutic effect of inexact interpretation: a contribution to the theory of suggestion. *Int J Psychoanal* 12:397–411, 1931

This is an important contribution to consideration of the problem of suggestion, as it influences what data are obtained in the psychoanalytic situation—a topic also discussed by Edelson (1988) above and Grunbaum (1984) below, who come to different conclusions about the extent to which these data are unavoidably contaminated by suggestion, and therefore about their value for testing psychoanalytic hypotheses.

65. **Grunbaum A:** *The Foundations of Psychoanalysis: A Philosophical Critique.* Berkeley, CA, University of California Press, 1984

This is an incisive critique of the empirical foundations for psychoanalysis. The clarity and strength of Grunbaum's arguments for his claims—that the evidence is insufficient to provide support for the scientific credibility of psychoanalytic theory, and that such evidence is unlikely to be forthcoming from the psychoanalytic situation itself—make this book valuable. The necessity to respond should provoke more cogent rigorous thinking than has been characteristic of discussions by either philosophers or psychoanalysts about these problems. For one response, see Edelson (1988) above.

66. **Luborsky L:** Momentary forgetting during psychotherapy and psychoanalysis (Monogr. No. 18/19). *Psychol Issues* 5:177–217, 1967

67. **Luborsky L:** Forgetting and remembering (momentary forgetting) during psychotherapy: a new sample (Monogr. No. 30). *Psychol Issues* 8:29–55, 1973

68. **Luborsky L, Mintz J:** What sets off momentary forgetting during a psychoanalysis? investigations of symptom-onset conditions. *Psychoanalysis and Contemporary Science* 3:233–268, 1975

These papers describe stages in the invention of the symptom-context method, which uses data obtained from the psychoanalytic situation and is capable of testing, according to canons of scientific reasoning and method, many psychoanalytic hypotheses other than those mentioned in these studies. Luborsky's work decisively demonstrated that data from the psychoanalytic situation can be used as evidence to test psychoanalytic hypotheses.

69. **Waelder R:** *Basic Theory of Psychoanalysis.* New York, International Universities Press, 1960

This introduction to psychoanalytic theory is written by an author who knows science. He begins with a section on the validation of psychoanalytic interpretations and theories. Throughout his presentation of the historical development of psychoanalytic thought and his discussion of basic concepts, the author raises questions he believes require further study and research.

Models of Psychoanalysis

Renee Welner, M.D.

The focus of Sigmund Freud's psychology was the individual and intrapsychic life. He saw interpersonal relations as largely determined by the disposition of drive and defense. In this chapter I present the key work of those theorists who have come after him.

Ego psychologists, like Anna Freud, Hartmann, Arlow, and Brenner, have stayed mostly within Freud's framework, expanding our understanding of the ego's functioning in defense, conflict, adaptation, and compromise formation. Other psychoanalysts have shifted their emphasis from the primacy of the individual's drives and conflicts to the significance of the individual's relationships to important others. Beginning with Melanie Klein and then Fairbairn and Guntrip, they proposed a new model of personality conceived in terms of internalized object relations. Interpersonal theorists like Sullivan, Fromm, and Horney additionally focused on social and cultural influences on personality.

Freud's emphasis on the centrality of the Oedipus complex led to a relative neglect of pre-Oedipal experiences and conflicts as sources of character and psychopathology. With the work of Melanie Klein, Mahler, Spitz, Bowlby, and Jacobson, attention shifted to development during the pre-Oedipal period, to appreciation of the mother's role in the first years of life, and to direct infant observation to supplement the data obtained from the psychoanalytic situation.

Pre-Oedipal phenomena also came under greater scrutiny as analysts began to treat more patients with borderline and narcissistic pathology and sought to understand the nature of these disturbances. In his work, Kernberg has attempted to integrate classic metapsychology with an object relations approach derived from the work of Jacobson and Melanie Klein. On the other hand, Kohut's treatment of these patients led him to formulate a new model of the mind that employs the concept of a self and disorders of the self and that emphasizes needs and frustrations instead of the conflict model.

Recent years have also seen challenge to the scientific qualities of psychoanalysis. Some theorists, such as Spence, have taken the position that analysis is a hermeneutic endeavor, a search for narrative consistency rather than scientific or historical truth. The language of psychoanalytic discourse itself is of great interest to those like George Klein, Gill, and Schafer, who find metapsychological terms inadequate and suggest we replace them with clinically based ones. The readings conclude with the work of Lacan, who also focused on the psychoanalytic dialogue, reinterpreting Freudian metapsychology within a linguistic context.

Ego Psychology

The current version of Freud's "classical" theory reflects the contributions of those ego psychologists who have supplemented his work, as well as Jacobson, Mahler, and Spitz.

1. *Arlow JA, Brenner C: *Psychoanalytic Concepts and the Structural Theory.* New York, International Universities Press, 1964

   This work is an attempt to bring all the central concepts of psychoanalysis, including Freud's earlier "topographic" model of the mind, under the framework of the structural theory and thereby to provide the greatest possible coherence to "modern" psychoanalytic theory.

2. **Brenner C:** *The Mind in Conflict.* New York, International Universities Press, 1982

   Brenner emphasizes the ubiquitous nature of intrapsychic conflict and presents correlations of theory with clinical data.

3. *Freud S: The ego and the id (1923), in *The Standard Edition of the Complete Psychological Works of Sigmund Freud,* Vol. 19. Translated and edited by Strachey J. London, Hogarth Press, 1961, pp. 12–66

   The structural theory of the mind—the ego, the id, and the superego—was first clearly delineated here.

4. **Freud A:** (1936) *The Ego and the Mechanisms of Defense,* Revised Edition. New York, International Universities Press, 1966

This is the classic description of the various defense mechanisms and their role in personality.

5. **Hartmann H:** *Ego Psychology and the Problem of Adaptation.* New York, International Universities Press, 1958

Hartmann has been called the "father" of modern ego psychology. In his focus on ego functioning other than that involved in defense, he described the concept of adaptation, the dynamic interaction between the individual and the environment mediated by the individual's ego. He also introduced the idea that certain aspects of ego functioning, including consciousness, perception, motility, and memory, develop relatively autonomously from the instinctual drives and are therefore not involved in intrapsychic conflict. These functions have "primary autonomy" from the drives and are distinguished from those that become secondarily so.

Melanie Klein

The central focus of Klein's thought was on the joined vicissitudes of the instinctual drives (particularly the aggressive drive) and internalized object relations. From birth on, instinctual impulses are expressed in unconscious fantasies representing the self, the object, and primitive emotions, which are the forerunners of love and hate. Early objects are "part objects"—the breast, the penis—and are characteristic of the "paranoid-schizoid position." Only later do they become the whole objects, which characterize the "depressive position."

6. *Klein M:** The Oedipus complex in the light of early anxieties (1945), in *Love, Guilt, and Reparation.* London, Hogarth Press, 1975, pp. 370–419

This is Klein's delineation of the Oedipus complex, whose onset she places in the second half of the first year of life and links with the onset of the depressive position.

7. *Klein M:** Notes on some schizoid mechanisms (1946), in *Envy and Gratitude.* New York, Delacorte, 1975, pp. 1–24

In her presentation of the paranoid-schizoid position, Klein discusses splitting and introduces the term *projective identification*.

8. **Klein M:** Envy and gratitude (1957), in *Envy and Gratitude.* New York, Delacorte, 1975, pp. 176—235

Envy is described as an especially destructive form of inborn aggression because it is directed toward good objects rather than bad ones. This is distinguished from hatred, in which it is bad objects that are destroyed, and from greed, in which the primary motive is to possess all the goodness, and destruction is secondary. Envy is also distinguished from jealousy, a developmentally later phenomenon.

9. **Segal H:** *Introduction to the Work of Melanie Klein.* New York, Basic Books, 1973

   This is a useful and concise primer to Klein's work.

The British Object Relations Theorists

W. R. D. Fairbairn

Fairbairn replaced Freud's dual instinct theory with an idea of attachment to other people as the central motivational force in development. Libido, in this conceptualization, is object-seeking, rather than primarily pleasure-seeking, and aggression arises from frustration, rather than being innate. He described the development of intrapsychic structure from an original unitary ego with its own libidinal energy, as a consequence of a defensive internalization of three aspects of the original relationship with the mother, resulting in the establishment of internal objects: the ideal object from gratifying aspects of the mother, the exciting object from potentially gratifying aspects of the mother, and the frustrating object. The ego is then split, as different "parts" of the ego become bound to different internal objects, leading to the development of the "central ego," the "libidinal ego," and the "anti-libidinal ego."

10. *Fairbairn WRD: A synopsis of the development of the author's views regarding the structure of the personality (1951), in *Object-Relations Theory of the Personality.* New York, Basic Books, 1954, pp. 162–179

    This is Fairbairn's own review of his significant papers, with particular attention to the evolution of his thinking.

11. *Fairbairn WRD: Synopsis of an object-relations theory of the personality. *Int J Psychoanal* 44:224–225, 1963

    This is the condensed version of Fairbairn (1951/1954) above.

12. **Kernberg OF:** Fairbairn's theory and challenge, in *Internal World and External Reality.* New York, Jason Aronson, 1980, pp. 57–84

This is Kernberg's thoughtful summary and critique of one of the sources of his own theory.

D. W. Winnicott

Winnicott was concerned with the fundamental question of how one becomes a person: an integrated, stable self available for interactions with others. He described how the earliest structuring of the psyche is accomplished through the experience of the relationship between mother and infant. Mother provides a "holding environment" within which the infant is contained and the developing self is allowed to emerge. Failures in that early relationship lead to a "split," with profound consequences for development, between a "true" self and a "false" self. He also emphasized the importance of creativity and play as crucial for health and dependent on the quality of the mother's love from the start.

13. *Winnicott DW: Transitional objects and transitional phenomena. *Int J Psychoanal* 34:89–97, 1953

    Winnicott presents the idea that the "transitional object" represents a developmental step between a state of illusory omnipotence, in which infants feel they control their world, to a state in which infants objectively perceive the limits of their control of others. The transitional object is neither under the infant's illusory control nor is it out of the infant's control, as the mother is.

14. Winnicott DW: The capacity to be alone (1958), in *The Maturational Processes and the Facilitating Environment.* New York, International Universities Press, 1980, pp. 29–36

    Winnicott describes the capacity to be alone as representative of emotional maturity. This occurs through the gradual introjection of the ego-supportive mother, so that ultimately and unconsciously one has the experience of being alone in the presence of someone else.

15. Winnicott DW: Ego distortion in terms of true and false self (1960), in *The Maturational Processes and the Facilitating Environment.* New York, International Universities Press, 1980, pp. 140–152

    The "good-enough mother" responds to the infant's need for omnipotence and allows the infant to experience the illusion of omnipotent creating and controlling, which can later be gradually relinquished. This allows the infant to develop a "true self." Conversely, the "false self" arises because the "not good-enough mother" fails to do this, instead requiring the infant's compliance with her needs.

Harry Guntrip

Guntrip theorized that the core of psychopathology lay in the concept of the "regressed ego." He thought that profound maternal deprivation led to a devouring need so intense and so frightening that a part of the ego withdrew from all relationships, all objects—external and internal—and sought to return to the womb. Intrapsychic processes and interpersonal relationships, however pathological, thus essentially serve as defenses against regression and depersonalization.

16. **Guntrip H:** *Personality Structure and Human Interaction.* New York, International Universities Press, 1961

    Chapter 18 provides Guntrip's critical survey of psychoanalytic thought from its neurophysiologic origins with Freud to his own object relations approach, emphasizing the contributions of Klein and Fairbairn.

17. *****Guntrip H:** *Schizoid Phenomena, Object Relations and the Self.* New York, International Universities Press, 1969

    This book is useful clinically as a description of schizoid phenomena.

John Bowlby

Bowlby's approach was extra-analytic in its use of ethological principles and its shift from the individual to the species. His focus was the concept of "attachment," the repertoire of behaviors by which the infant is tied to the mother. For Bowlby, attachment was a central and primary phenomenon that serves species survival rather than a consequence of the gratification of the drives. Psychopathology was then seen as derivative of disturbances in attachment.

18. **Bowlby J:** The nature of the child's tie to his mother. *Int J Psychoanal* 39:350–373, 1958

    In this seminal article, Bowlby offers his theory of a primary attachment that challenges classic psychoanalytic thinking about early object relations, particularly the idea that the infant's connection to the mother develops only secondarily to the satisfaction of his or her physiological needs.

19. **Bowlby J:** Pathological mourning and childhood mourning. *J Am Psychoanal Assoc* 11:500–541, 1963

    Bowlby argues that it is childhood loss or separation from the mother that is a primary source of psychopathology in the adult.

Hans Loewald

For Loewald, interactional processes, both intrapsychic and interpsychic—as epitomized in the psychoanalytic situation—were the core of psychoanalytic theory and the subject of investigation. He retained Freudian terminology but reinterpreted much of it within an object relational approach. Loewald did not discard the drives, for example, but saw them as originating in and organized by interactions between the infant and the infant's environment, primarily the mother. Similarly, psychic structure results from the internalization of interactions in which the child identifies with certain parental functions. In analysis, as well, the analysand internalizes the (ego) "integrative experiences" provided by the analyst's interpretations.

20. *Loewald H: On the therapeutic action of psychoanalysis (1960), in *Papers on Psychoanalysis*. New Haven, CT, Yale University Press, 1980, pp. 221–256

    This is a landmark paper in which Loewald states his central idea that therapeutic change comes about through the interaction between patient and analyst.

21. **Loewald H:** Instinct theory, object relations, and psychic structure formation (1978), in *Papers on Psychoanalysis*. New Haven, CT, Yale University Press, 1980, pp. 207–218

    Loewald discusses how instincts, ego, and superego all come into being as a consequence of internalization of interaction between the child and the child's human environment.

22. *Loewald H: The waning of the Oedipus complex (1979), in *Papers on Psychoanalysis*. New Haven, CT, Yale University Press, 1980, pp. 383–404

    The Oedipal complex is viewed both in its conflictual triangular constellation and in its position as inheritor of pre-Oedipal development. The superego thus represents the resolution of triangular and, significantly, more archaic dyadic separation-individuation processes.

Rene Spitz

23. **Spitz RA:** *The First Year of Life*. New York, International Universities Press, 1965

24. **Spitz RA, Wolf KM:** Anaclitic depression: an inquiry into the genesis of psychiatric conditions in early childhood. *Psychoanal Study Child* 2:313–342, 1946

Spitz's work centered on the role of the mother in the mother-child dyad in the psychic development of the infant. He introduced the concept of the anaclitic depression, which was the result of an absence or inadequacy of mothering.

Margaret Mahler

25. *Mahler MS, Pine F, Bergman A: *The Psychological Birth of the Human Infant.* New York, Basic Books, 1975

Mahler, although working within an ego-psychological framework, was concerned with separation and individuation, issues that had not received emphasis in earlier discussions of ego development. Rather than seeing maturity simply in terms of successful resolution of the Oedipus complex and the establishment of genital primacy, her conceptualization viewed successful development as a process of separation and individuation from the mother-baby symbiotic unit to the achievement of object constancy, a stable sense of autonomous identity within an environment of discrete and realistically perceived objects.

Edith Jacobson

26. *Jacobson E: *The Self and the Object World (1964).* New York, International Universities Press, 1980

Jacobson formulated a model of psychological development and structure formation using classic metapsychological theory as well as object relations concepts. She described the beginnings of internal object relations, based on the baby's repeated experiences of pleasure or unpleasure (satisfaction or frustration of the drives), which lead to the formation of representations of the gratifying (good) or frustrating (bad) mother and of the self. Psychic structures evolve under the influence of interactions between self and object representations, and, reciprocally, the level of ego and superego development influence the nature of representational interaction.

Otto Kernberg

Kernberg has attempted to integrate object relations and ego psychological theory in an effort to describe and treat adequately the borderline and narcissistic patients with whom he worked. In essence, he has retained concepts like the tripartite model of the mind, defense mechanisms like repression and isolation, and phases of psychosexual development to discuss Oedipal development and pathology. He uses object relations theory to describe phenomena of the pre-Oedipal period or of pathology he sees as consequent to disturbances during that period.

27. **Kernberg O:** *Borderline Conditions and Pathological Narcissism.* New York, Jason Aronson, 1975

28. **Kernberg O:** *Object Relations Theory and Clinical Psychoanalysis.* New York, Jason Aronson, 1976

29. *Kernberg O, Selzer M, Koenigsberg H, Carr AR, Applebaum AH:* *Psychodynamic Psychotherapy of Borderline Patients.* New York, Basic Books, 1989

These works provide an excellent integration of theory and clinical application.

Self Psychology: Heinz Kohut

Heinz Kohut's work with patients with narcissistic pathology led him to a conceptualization of the self whose functions replace those of Freud's structures of id, ego, and superego. He formulated the idea that there is a separate line of development for narcissism independent of that for object relations, with the consequence that conceptualization of "healthy narcissism" is then possible. This is characterized by a cohesive self with appropriate self-esteem regulation and the possession of values, ideals, and ambition. Psychopathology reflects deficits in the self structure and arises primarily from "self object failures" in childhood: failures of parental empathy with the child, and the lack of provision of mirroring and opportunities for forming an idealized parent image, so that archaic grandiosity is maintained and self-cohesiveness is not established. Analysis seeks to have the patient acquire selfobject functions through "transmuting internalization" of the analyst's selfobject functions. This comes about through the appropriate management of the optimal failures of the basic selfobject transference to the analyst.

30. **Cooper A:** The place of self psychology in the history of depth psychology, in *The Future of Psychoanalysis.* Edited by Goldberg A. New York, International Universities Press, 1983, pp. 3–17

This is a discussion of the divergent theoretical positions of Freudian depth psychology and self psychology regarding questions about human nature and intrapsychic experience.

31. **Kohut H:** Introspection, empathy, and psychoanalysis. *J Am Psychoanal Assoc* 7:459–483, 1959

Kohut considers how the data of psychoanalytic observation are obtained via introspection in ourselves and vicarious introspection, or empathy, with others.

32. **Kohut H:** Forms and transformations of narcissism. *J Am Psychoanal Assoc* 14:243–272, 1966

    Here Kohut begins his study of the self, although it is still conceived of as a structure within the ego, similar to the classic model.

33. *__Kohut H:__ The two analyses of Mr. Z. *Int J Psychoanal* 60:3–27, 1979

    This is the case that demonstrates the shift in Kohut's thinking: his "two-installment" analysis of a patient with narcissistic pathology, the first employing a classic approach, which he felt led to a "transference cure," and the second, which began when he was writing "Forms and Transformations of Narcissism" (Kohut 1966), using a self psychological approach.

34. *__Kohut H, Wolfe E:__ The disorders of the self and their treatment: an outline. *Int J Psychoanal* 59:413–425, 1978

    This is a classic description of the etiology and treatment of disorders of the self, distinguished from a conceptualization of neurotic disorders that arise from intrapsychic conflict.

Metapsychology Versus Clinical Observation: George Klein, Merton Gill, and Roy Schafer

35. **Gill M:** Metapsychology is not psychology, in *Psychology Versus Metapsychology: Psychoanalytic Essays in Memory of George S. Klein.* Edited by Gill M, Holzman P. New York, International Universities Press, 1976, pp. 71–105

    Gill argues that Freud's metapsychology refers to a natural science model that is incompatible with psychoanalytically derived data and that psychoanalytic theory must be reformulated in psychological terms.

36. **Klein G:** Freud's two theories of sexuality (1969), in *Psychoanalytic Theory: An Exploration of Essentials.* New York, International Universities Press, 1976, pp. 72–120

    Klein's discussion of Freud's clinical and drive-discharge "theories" is representative of his attempt to formulate a psychoanalytic theory that discards metapsychological concepts like drives and instead focuses on motivation. His solution is "sensuality," a primary, physical experience of pleasure that, once experienced, continues to serve as a framework to structure current and future sensual experiences.

37. **Schafer R:** *A New Language for Psychoanalysis.* New Haven, CT, Yale University Press, 1976

    Schafer calls for the replacement of the "physico-chemical and biological language of Freudian metapsychology" with "action" language, an attempt to express all behavior and psychological functioning through verbs and adverbs and essentially to eliminate the use of all nouns and adjectives for this purpose.

Science Versus Hermeneutics: Donald Spence

38. **Spence DP:** *Narrative Truth and Historical Truth.* New York, WW Norton, 1982

    Spence challenges the veracity of psychoanalytically obtained historical truths or reconstructions and instead argues that the psychoanalytic process results in the creation or construction by the analyst and patient of a coherent and compelling narrative truth. The analyst is thus something of an artist, rather than an archaeologist.

Interpersonal Psychoanalysis

The chief interpersonal theorists—Harry Stack Sullivan, Erich Fromm, Karen Horney, Clara Thompson, and Frieda Fromm-Reichmann—share the belief that drive theory does not adequately describe motivation, which they see as derived from changing configurations of objects. They also believe that drive theory does not sufficiently address social and cultural influences on personality development and structure. This cultural emphasis distinguishes this group from the British object relations theorists.

39. **Chrzanowski G, Kasin E, Mitchell S:** Interpersonal psychoanalysis: its roots and its contemporary status. *Contemporary Psychoanalysis* 22:445–466, 1986

40. **Hoffman I:** The patient as interpreter of the analyst's experience. *Contemporary Psychoanalysis* 19:389–422, 1983

    In this article, transference and countertransference are viewed in terms of the interpersonal paradigm: the analyst's interpretations should be formulated to include the patient's "interpretations" of the analyst's countertransference.

41. *Mitchell S: *Relational Concepts in Psychoanalysis.* Cambridge, MA, Harvard University Press, 1988

    This is an attempt to formulate a relational model of psychoanalysis derived from an integration of object relations theory, self psychology, and interpersonal psychoanalysis.

42. **Sullivan HS:** *The Interpersonal Theory of Psychiatry.* New York, WW Norton, 1953

    In this book, intrapsychic phenomena and psychopathology are viewed as reflecting complex and dynamic interpersonal processes.

French Psychoanalysis: Jacques Lacan

The theory of Jacques Lacan attempts to integrate Freudian psychoanalysis, Levi-Strauss's structuralism, and deSaussure's linguistics. His central maxim, "the unconscious is structured like a language," employs an idea that 1) language is composed of signs and symbols that gain meaning only through their syntactical relationships (i.e., their relationship to one another) and 2) those syntactical relationships reflect enduring structures, or laws. In Lacan's conceptualization, intrapsychic phenomena like drives and symptoms are viewed as linguistic signs; concepts such as "condensation" and "displacement" become "metaphor" and "metonym." The task of the analyst-linguist is thus a hermeneutic one: to interpret a symbolic text in a search for meaning.

43. **Lacan J:** *Ecrits.* New York, WW Norton, 1977

44. *Leavy S:** The significance of Jacques Lacan. *Psychoanal Q* 46:201–219, 1977

45. **Muller J, Richardson W:** *Lacan and Language: A Reader's Guide to Ecrits.* New York, International Universities Press, 1982

    These papers provide a useful introduction to Lacan's central concepts.

5

Psychology: Cognition and Emotion

Jerome L. Singer, Ph.D.

I n the decade between 1960 and 1970, one can identify what may be termed a *paradigm shift* in psychology with respect to the conceptions of human functions and the organization of psychological processes. From 1910 to about 1960, under the influence of behaviorism and its emphasis on animal research as a basis for understanding human processes of learning and motivation, psychology was dominated by stimulus-response and drive-reduction models of behavior. During the 1960s, a confluence of theoretical analysis and research findings led to a shift from the more peripheralist concepts of organ-related drives to a more centralist view of humans as information-seeking and information-processing organisms with a much greater focus on the close tie between cognition and a differentiated emotional system in the person. Theoretical contributions by Ernest Schachtel, Robert W. White, and Silvan S. Tomkins may be cited among many others as anticipating or signaling this shift. The research on sensory deprivation stimulated by Donald O. Hebb, the studies of the sleep and dream cycles initiated by Kleitman and Dement, and the computer models of human thought developed by Newell and Simon all were influences on the changing perspective.

In effect, the current pervasive orientation of psychology increasingly emphasizes a systems approach and a biopsychosocial integration as a guiding schema. Humans are conceived as reflecting a series of differentiated but interacting systems of biological processes and information processing as well as affective functions, which are organized to relate to a surrounding milieu of physical objects and persons who themselves represent a broader culture or social system. Humans are viewed as seeking to organize complex novel stimulation into meaningful informational structures that can then be related to previously acquired knowledge and stored as new schemata "ticketed" for effective retrieval as necessary.

The emotions are closely tied to the novelty and complexity of information to be processed and are evoked specifically in relation to the degree of uncertainty or ambiguity in a stimulus field or to the extent that previous anticipations, "plans," or "scripts" are confirmed or disconfirmed by each new encounter with people or physical settings. The emphasis on information processing and the extensive research in cognitive psychology have demonstrated that attention and perception are not simply responses to a single stimulus but are processes occurring across time (at great but measurable speeds). Such processes have definable sequences and phases usually reflected in flowcharts. There are key points along the way in 1) how a search of a stimulus configuration is carried out; 2) how it is reflected on and encoded for storage (i.e., as a word meaning or as an episode or event, as a visual or auditory image or as an abstract class of events or objects); and 3) how it is mentally rehearsed in the form of memories, plans, daydreams, or fantasies after storage. Individual variations either genetically determined or overlearned through familial or sociocultural socialization (or some combination of both) may lead to different strategies of search and selection, encoding, retrieval, and rehearsal. These variations become crystallized as cognitive or personality styles and may also reflect persistent or situation-determined defensive maneuvers occasioned by threats to beliefs about the self.

A very large and impressive research literature has emerged in the area of cognition. There have been theoretical debates over the issue of whether thought is best reflected through computer analogies as a sequential process or (evoking new concepts that seek to model both the possibilities of new high-speed computers and the particular properties of complex neural networks widely distributed in the brain) whether a parallel distributed processing model is more useful.

A consequence of the cognitive-affective orientation is an increased interest in basic research on processes of mental representation, thinking, imagery, planning, and fantasizing. Organized belief systems such as those built around the self or the differentiation of the self from others are increasingly explored. Social psychologists are focusing their attention on how information about situations is stored and retrieved. Experimental evidence and clinical studies of brain-injured patients or intensive quantitative studies of patients in psychotherapy have revived interest in unconscious processes and on the relationship between conscious representations and highly automatized, but complex perceptual and cognitive operations that seem to function out of awareness. The following bibliography contains references that can provide basic scientific information on the cognitive-affective paradigm; the nature of cognition; the differentiated affect system; and the problems of storing, retrieving, and communicating information.

Shift From Drive to Cognitive-Affective Theories

The following readings highlight the shift in perspective and the emergence of a view of humans as more than drive-reducing organisms. All reflect a reappraisal of the classic psychoanalytic or drive-reduction learning theory models in the light of new findings on the motivating properties of human curiosity, competence, and the role of positive emotions of joy, excitement, and interest as well as negative emotions such as anxiety or anger. They also outline key issues reflecting a cognitive or cognitive-affective perspective.

1. *__Gardner H:__ *The Mind's New Science: A History of the Cognitive Revolution.* New York, Basic Books, 1985

   This book is a highly readable, general presentation of the emergence, research approaches, and implications of information processing and meaning-focused views of the human condition.

2. __Kreitler H, Kreitler S:__ *Cognitive Orientation and Behavior.* New York, Springer, 1976

   This book addresses broader aspects of cognition such as the role of meaningfulness and of one's cognitive orientation as a predictor of not only private attitude but of subsequent overt behavior.

3. *__McAdams DP:__ *The Person.* San Diego, CA, Harcourt Brace Jovanovich, 1990

4. *__Singer JL:__ *The Human Personality.* New York, Harcourt Brace Jovanovich, 1984

   These two personality textbooks highlight the cognitive-affective perspective and incorporate current research on cognition and emotion within a personality theory context.

5. *__Tomkins SS:__ *Affect, Imagery, Consciousness,* Vols. 1–3. New York, Springer, 1962, 1963, 1991

   The most ambitious and original attempt of the past 30 years at developing a new conception of personality, this work also reappraises drive theory, argues for the importance of understanding conscious thought, and proposes a revolutionary theory of emotion that has since found considerable empirical support in the research of Paul Ekman, Carroll Izard, Phoebe Ellsworth, Virginia Demos, and Gary Schwartz, among others.

6. **Tomkins SS:** The quest for primary motives: biography and autobiography of an idea. *J Pers Soc Psychol* 41:306–329, 1981

   This article formulates the concept of emotions as a basic organismic system characterized by 1) a distinct pattern of physiological representation in the brain and in peripheral autonomic or musculature processes, 2) a distinctive facial expression, and 3) a specific "felt" experience.

Modern Research in Cognitive Processes

The following references provide an up-to-date account of the nature of the information-processing sequence from initial attention through encoding and memory.

7. **Anderson JR:** *Cognitive Psychology and Its Implications,* 3rd Edition. New York, WH Freeman, 1991

8. *Neisser U:** *Cognition and Reality.* San Francisco, CA, WH Freeman, 1976

9. **Neisser A** (ed): *Memory Observed: Remembering in Natural Contexts.* New York, WH Freeman, 1982

10. **Schank R, Abelson R:** *Scripts, Plans, Goals and Understanding.* New York, Halsted, 1977

    Recent advances derived from studies of computer modeling and artificial intelligence have led to a formulation that human thought is organized not just into verbal phrases or fleeting images but into story-like scripts, some shared in common in a culture but many highly personalized because of unique experiences. The notion of personal scripts undoubtedly has important implications not only for research on memory and thought but also for the psychoanalytic concept of transference.

11. *Horowitz MJ** (ed): *Person Schemas and Maladaptive Interpersonal Styles.* Chicago, IL, University of Chicago Press, 1991

    This is an attempted integration of psychodynamic and clinical psychotherapeutic concepts and evidence with notions of schemata, scripts, and related research-derived structures drawn from cognitive studies. For example, Singer-Salovey's chapter presents research background for schemata and clinical phenomena like transference; Stinson and Palmer's chapter introduces parallel distributed processing models applied to clinical pathology.

12. **Witkin HA, Goodenough DR:** *Cognitive Styles: Essence and Origins.* New York, International Universities Press, 1981

   This book presents extensive research on a major cognitive style: field dependence and field independence.

Differentiated Emotions: Theory and Research

Although clinicians have always stressed the special role of emotions in human experience and in clinical intervention, there has been little development of a systematic theory of emotions in any of the psychotherapeutic theories of personality.

13. **Ekman P, Freisen W:** *Unmasking the Face.* Englewood Cliffs, NJ, Prentice-Hall, 1975

14. *Izard C: *The Psychology of Emotions.* New York, Plenum, 1991

15. **Mandler G:** *Mind and Body.* New York, WW Norton, 1984

   These books bring up to date important research and theory on the specific emotions. Izard's book is a basic text that reviews current knowledge on emotions from anger, sadness, and disgust to joy.

Imagery, Imagination, Consciousness, and the Self

The increased attention to conscious processes and to how humans represent the external social or physical environment that stems from a cognitive-affective perspective has led also to an increased interest in ongoing thought, to the study of images, fantasies, and day and night dreams. There has also been a considerable upsurge in research on self beliefs and schemata about self as these are manifested both consciously or outside of awareness. The phenomenon of hypnosis, long linked to neurotic trends, is now also being recognized as a basic human capacity or skill related to the absorption in imagery under conditions of self-attenuated consciousness. The following references document some of the major research findings relating to hypnosis, the stream of consciousness and imagery, and the studies of nocturnal dreaming derived from psychophysiological research in the sleep cycle. They point toward some of the clinical applications of the recent advances in understanding imaginative processes.

16. **Brown P:** *The Hypnotic Brain.* New Haven, CT, Yale University Press, 1991

    Brown provides a new and sophisticated review of the current status of thought concerning hypnotic phenomena set in a cognitive, social, and psychobiological context.

17. *****Ellman S, Antrobus JS** (eds): *The Mind in Sleep,* 2nd Edition. New York, Wiley Interscience, 1991

    The best single compendium of the current scientific knowledge and research on thought processes during sleep, this book provides basic reading for any modern understanding of dreams.

18. *****Higgins ET:** Self-discrepancy: a theory relating self and affect. *Psychol Rev* 94:319–340, 1987

    This is a seminal article opening up new avenues for systematic research linking cognition, emotion, and self schemata.

19. *****Kihlstrom JF:** The cognitive unconscious. *Science* 237:1445–1452, 1987

    This article is a concise but remarkably lucid and thorough statement of the nature of unconscious processes based on current cognitive and clinical neuropsychological research.

20. **Pope KS, Singer JL:** *The Stream of Consciousness.* New York, Plenum, 1978

21. **Singer JL, Pope KS:** *The Power of Human Imagination.* New York, Plenum, 1978

    These companion volumes include chapters reviewing the scientific literature on daydreaming, the stream of conscious, and related phenomena of ongoing thought. Singer and Pope address applications of these scientific findings in a variety of approaches to psychodynamic and to behavioral forms of psychotherapy.

22. *****Singer JL** (ed): *Repression and Dissociation: Implications for Personality, Psychopathology and Health.* Chicago, IL, University of Chicago Press, 1990

    This is an examination of the phenomena of selective, avoidant perceptual and memory processes and of repressor personality styles, bringing together leading psychodynamic and cognitive researchers.

Family

Ira D. Glick, M.D.
John F. Clarkin, Ph.D.

A rguably, the most important unit to influence our lives is the family. The issue has been studied extensively from many different fields, most prominently history, psychology, psychiatry, anthropology, sociology, and psychoanalysis, as well as game and communication theory.

In that context, the origins of humans may lie not (as commonly believed) in the development of a material culture, or as a result of bipedality, but in the development of the nuclear family. Of particular importance is the fact that throughout history, the structure of the nuclear family has altered to conform to the social mores of the times. This has caused particular roles and tasks of individual members of the family to change from one time period to another—an issue of major concern for women and men in the last two decades.

Family theory is distinguished from other developmental theories by its conceptual focus on the family system as a whole. In this view, major emphasis is placed on understanding individual behavior patterns as arising from, and inevitably feeding back onto, the complicated matrix of general family systems. Beneficial alterations in the larger marital and family unit will therefore have positive consequences for the individual family members, as well as for the larger systems. The major emphasis is placed on understanding and intervening in the family system's current patterns of interaction, with usually only a secondary interest in their origins and development.

Understanding family function is important then not only in understanding human development, but especially in our field as the basis for carrying-out marital and couples and family treatment (including alternative family forms such as single families and gay couples). "Family form" and "family function" are separate concepts—having a "conventional" family form (e.g., two parents and two children) does not imply high functionality; likewise an alternative form (e.g., single parent and a child) does not connote dysfunctionality. The model for understanding the family is different when one member has a diagnosable psychiatric disorder or has a member with a problem such as "aggression or delinquency," or a chronic medical or psychiatric illness. The treatment model is modified by cultural, ethnic, gender, social, and economic issues as well as whether the patient is in or out of the hospital.

Accordingly, these "essential" readings are grouped by our biases, which stress an integration of various theories and schools. We have organized this section by 1) general texts and overviews; 2) basic conceptual approaches that cover many different "schools" of therapy; 3) alternative family forms and the theory underlying their function; 4) stages of the family life cycle and their influence on therapy; 5) cultural, ethnic, and economic influences on family form, function, and role; and 6) specific psychopathology. Chapter 44 (Clarkin and Glick, this volume) details readings specifically targeted to family and marital therapy.

General Texts and Overviews

1. *Ackerman NW: *The Psychodynamics of Family Life.* New York, Basic Books, 1958

   This is the first comprehensive statement on modern family studies and treatment by the pioneer of family therapy in outpatient settings. Chapters 1 and 4 are essential.

2. **Bentovim A, Barnes G, Cooklin A:** *Family therapy.* London, Academic Press, 1982

   This excellent multiauthored textbook covers the field: the healthy family, the family in therapy, practical issues, life cycle, and family therapy in different settings (e.g., pediatric practice, in the psychiatric hospital system).

3. *Bowen M: *Family Therapy in Clinical Practice.* New York, Jason Aronson, 1978

This volume contains most of the seminal papers written by Murray Bowen, whose ideas on structure of family relations under stress have done much to shape the field.

4. **Glick ID, Clarkin JF, Kessler DR:** *Marital and family therapy,* 3rd Edition. Washington, DC, American Psychiatric Press, 1987

   This text has sections succinctly delineating the theoretical model underlining marital and family techniques and strategies. It also has sections on the functional and dysfunctional family, family evaluation, treatment, and guidelines.

5. *****Hoffman L:** *Foundation of Family Therapy: A Conceptual Framework for Systems Change.* New York, Basic Books, 1981

   Besides providing historical insight into the developments of systems thinking, this book is a tour de force on general systems theory and the cybernetic paradigm as applied to the family. It places such therapists as Minuchin, Bowen, Whitaker, Haley, Erikson, and Palazzoli in theoretical perspective.

6. **Minuchin S:** *Families and Family Therapy.* Cambridge, MA, Harvard Press, 1974

   This is an original classic detailing one therapist's view of theory and therapy.

7. **Simon R** (ed): *One on One: Conversations With the Shapers of Family Therapy.* New York, Guilford, 1992

   This book presents interviews and intimate glances with the stalwarts of family therapy, including Jay Haley, R. D. Laing, Salvadore Minuchin, Humberto Matyurana, Carl Whitaker, Cloe Madanes, Mara Selvini Palazzoli, Lynn Hoffman, and Virginia Satir. Pick and choose here as your interests lead you.

8. **Wynne LC, McDoniel SH, Weber TT** (eds): *Systems Consultation: A New Perspective for Family Therapy.* New York, Guilford, 1986

   This provided help in how to use the ideas of systems theory in practice with seriously ill patients. For once, there really is something new.

Conceptual Approaches

9. **Bertalanffy L von:** *General Systems Theory.* New York, Braziller, 1968

   This classic work considers "systems theory" in a broad context. The theoretical construct served as an inspiration for family systems' theoreticians and therapists.

10. **Boszormenyi-Nagy I, Spark GM:** *Invisible Loyalties: Reciprocity in Inter-generational Family Therapy.* New York, Harper & Row, 1973

    In the dynamic tradition, this volume explores the multigenerational family "justice" system in a convincing way.

11. *Dicks HV:** *Marital Tensions.* New York, Basic Books, 1967

    This relatively unknown work is a gem. Dicks illustrates that internalized representations of significant relationships from childhood shape the choice of marital partner and form the backup for interlocking patterns of marital and family pathology.

12. **Framo JL:** Symptoms from a family transactional viewpoint, in *Family Therapy in Transition.* Edited by Ackerman MW. New York, Little, Brown, 1970, pp. 125–171

    This is an early but seminal paper making a crucial theoretical link between family interaction patterns and the emergency of psychiatric symptoms.

13. **Lewis JM, Beavers WR, Gossett JT, Phillips VA:** *No Single Thread: Psychological Health in Family Systems.* New York, Brunner/Mazel, 1976

    Lewis et al. provide the best scientifically rigorous, as well as sensitive, research to assess the function and models of nonclinical families.

14. *Lidz T:** *The Family and Human Adaptation.* New York, International Universities Press, 1963

    These three lectures present data on the familial aspects of human adaptation, of personality structure, and of language and communication. Although somewhat dated, they are still very useful.

15. **McGoldrick M:** *Genograms in Family Assessment.* New York, WW Norton, 1985

    This definitive work on using genograms for assessment and treatment will help you organize your thinking when assessing a family.

16. **Murstein BI:** *Paths to Marriage.* Beverly Hills, CA, Sage, 1986

    Who chooses to marry whom and why? This book provides the best analysis (since your grandmother) of this basic question.

17. **Reiss D:** *The Family's Construction of Reality.* Cambridge, MA, Harvard University Press, 1981

    This book provides a very thoughtful look at how families function.

18. **Thomas L:** *Lives of a Cell.* New York, Bantam, 1974

    Not strictly about families or family therapy, this book contains essays about the nature of the world we live in, including how we get along with each other. Some believe this is necessary reading for all therapists.

19. **Walsh F:** *Normal Family Processes.* New York, Guilford, 1982

    This edited work is the best review to date. Noteworthy are the chapters on research contrasting normal and abnormal families (Beavers), the McMaster model of assessment (Epstein), families at risk (Wynne et al.), and a view of the family life cycle (McGoldrick and Carter).

20. **Watzlawick P, Beavin JH, Jackson DD:** *Pragmatics of Human Communications: A Study of Interactional Patterns, Pathologies, and Paradoxes.* New York, WW Norton, 1967

    This is a delightful and provocative view of human relationships seen with the concepts of homeostasis, positive and negative feedback, and paradoxical qualities of communication. These concepts are cleverly illustrated (e.g., an analysis of Albee's *Who's Afraid of Virginia Wolf*).

Alternative Families

21. **Bjorksten O:** *New Clinical Concepts in Marital Therapy.* Washington, DC, American Psychiatric Press, 1985

    This is a summary of new models to understand relationships and their effect on marital status and psychiatric morbidity and how to treat remarried families and unmarried couples.

22. **Sager CJ, Brown HS, Crohn H, Engel P, Rodstein E, Walker L:** *Treating the Remarried Family.* New York, Brunner/Mazel, 1983

    This is the best available summary of work with remarried families; it includes a section on prevention.

Stages and Life Cycle of the Family

23. *Carter B, McGoldrick M** (eds): The family life cycle and family therapy: an overview, in *The Family Life Cycle.* Edited by Carter B, McGoldrick M. New York, Gardner, 1980, pp. 3–20

    This chapter provides an excellent overview of life cycle issues as they affect the family.

24. **Imber-Black E:** Ritual themes in families and family therapy, in *Rituals in Families and Family Therapy*. Edited by Imber-Black E, Roberts J, Whiting R. New York, WW Norton, 1988, pp. 113–134

   This is a kind of "how-to-do it" family therapy text organized around family rituals as a way to understand and treat families, including use of rituals at various stages of the family life cycle.

25. **Pittman FS:** Family crises: expectable and unexpectable, in *Family Transitions: Continuity and Change Over the Life Cycle*. Edited by Falikov C. New York, Guilford, 1988, pp. 255–272

   Pittman is a very experienced and thoughtful clinician, who tells you everything you ever wanted to know about crises in the family, in a very readable way.

26. **Shapiro E:** Individual change and family development: individuation as a family process, in *Family Transitions: Continuity and Change Over the Life Cycle*. Edited by Falikov C. New York, Guilford, 1988, pp. 159–180

   Shapiro is an innovative thinker, who in this chapter details how individuation ought to be accomplished; the perspective is a "family" one, rather than an "analytic" one.

Cultural and Economic Aspects

27. **Falicove CJ** (ed): *Cultural Perspectives in Family Therapy*. Rockville, MD, Aspen System Corp, 1983

   This multiauthored book focuses on how ethnic and cultural factors influence individuals and families, including a chapter on becoming a "culturally conscious family therapist."

28. **McGoldrick M, Pearce K:** *Ethnicity and Family Therapy*. New York, Guilford, 1982

   Here collected in one place are chapters on the white Anglo-Saxon family, the Hispanic family, and so on; cultural and ethnic issues influence therapy.

29. **McGoldrick M, Anderson CM, Walsh F:** *Woman in Families: A Framework for Family Therapy*. New York, WW Norton, 1989

   This book provides indispensable information on gender issues serving as part of the foundation for the clinical practice of family therapy and the training of family therapists.

30. **Parsons T, Bales RF:** *Family Socialization and Interaction Process.* Glencoe, IL, Free Press, 1955

31. **Parsons T:** Social structure and the development of psychology and sociology. *Psychiatry* 21:321–340, 1958

    These two classics synthesize psychoanalytic theory of the personality of the individual and the sociological theory of the structure and functioning of social systems.

The Family and Specific Psychopathology

32. **Glick ID, Clarkin JF, Goldsmith SJ:** Combining medications with family psychotherapy, in *American Psychiatric Press Review of Psychiatry,* Vol. 12. Edited by Oldham JM, Riba MB, Tasman A. Washington, DC, American Psychiatric Press, 1993, pp. 585–610

    Here collected in one chapter is the literature from controlled studies bearing on the role of the family and specific psychopathology. There are sections on schizophrenia, mood disorder, anxiety disorder, substance abuse disorders, eating disorders, and borderline personality disorder. Causes, effects, and coping strategies are discussed.

Group Dynamics

Richard L. Munich, M.D.

G*roup dynamics* refers to processes inherent in the nature of groups: the vicissitudes of member-to-member interactions; the reciprocal relation between those interactions and between individual members and the group itself; and the relationship of these factors to the issues of group development and authority relations, structure, task, and goals. Group dynamics are active to a greater or lesser extent irrespective of the structure or work of any specific group, whether it be therapeutic, clinical-administrative, organizational, or primarily designed to study itself. Insofar as their services are most often delivered in the context of groups, a familiarity with group dynamics is important for mental health professionals. It may be of even greater relevance that, beginning with their families, clients continue to develop and exist within the framework of various group situations.

Selections for this bibliography have been made to emphasize the three most influential intellectual traditions in the development of group dynamics as a basic social science: individual psychology, social psychology, and sociology. Each of these traditions has its own theoretical assumptions and distinctive language. In an effort to understand group life, the psychologist examines the individual, the sociologist focuses on the cultural or structural aspects of the group itself, and the social psychologist studies the boundary between the social and the psychological and between members themselves. The disparity between their languages and the tension between points of view reflects the historical and theoretical roots of the study of group dynamics. These issues are represented graphically in Figure 1.

The struggle to formulate modes that organize experience in and of group dynamics are mainly aids in conceptualizing group process rather than prescriptions for action or thorough descriptions of what happens in groups. There is no substitute for experience in groups to learn about groups. Most of the first four groupings of annotations are considered core readings and refer to processes in small face-to-face groups that coincide with the majority of our work. The last group represents enduring examples of more practical and experiential applications of group dynamics and are recommended as useful supplements to the core.

Overview

1. **Cartwright D, Zander A** (eds): *Group Dynamics.* Evanston, IL, Row & Peterson, 1953 (available in 3rd Edition, 1968)

   This is an early collection of papers that helps set the stage for many modern developments.

2. *****Munich RL**: Group dynamics, in *Comprehensive Group Psychotherapy,* 3rd Edition. Edited by Kaplan HI, Sadock BJ. Baltimore, MD, Williams & Wilkins, 1993, pp. 21–32

   Munich provides a comprehensive account of the historical, psychological, sociological, and social-psychological roots and contributions to the study of group dynamics. Although the autonomy of each perspective is respected, an effort is made to integrate them.

Individual Psychology

3. *****Bion WR:** *Experience in Groups.* New York, Basic Books, 1961

   This classic work shows the development and describes the latent content of group process, labeled and known thereafter as the basic assumptions. The liberal use of the author's personal experiences as a leader of groups serves to intensify the impact as well as the import of the material, especially that relating to authority and leadership.

4. **Freud S:** Group psychology and the analysis of the ego (1921), *The Standard Edition of the Complete Psychological Works of Sigmund Freud,* Vol. 18. Translated and edited by Strachey J. London, Hogarth Press, 1955, pp. 67–133

   One of the earliest and most lucid accounts of the vicissitudes of the individual and the individual's mental activity within the context of a group, this was used by Freud to develop his concept of identification.

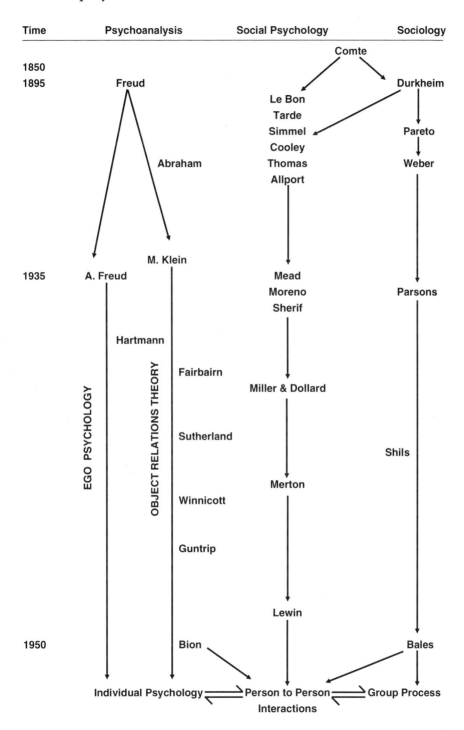

Figure 7–1. Intellectual and historical trends for group dynamics prior to 1950.

5. **Karterud S:** Two paradigms of group dynamics, in *The Difficult Patient in Group: Group Psychotherapy With Borderline and Narcissistic Disorders.* Edited by Roth BE, Stone WN, Kibel HD. Madison, CT, International Universities Press, 1989, pp. 45–65

   This is one of the few applications of the principles of self psychology to the field of group dynamics.

6. **Rioch MJ:** The work of Wilfred Bion on groups. *Psychiatry* 33:56–66, 1970

   Rioch provides a clear and concise exposition of Bion's work, which it takes further, elaborates, and relates more clearly to clinical phenomena. A useful companion to *Experience in Groups* (Bion 1961) above, which it does not replace.

7. *Slater PE: *Microcosm: Structural, Psychological and Religious Evolution in Groups.* New York, Wiley, 1966

   This is a detailed analysis of group development with an exposition of boundary formation, both of which relate emerging phenomena to primitive and enduring psychological and sociocultural themes. These important issues are abundantly documented with clinical material, especially with respect to the theme of group revolt.

8. *Turquet P: Threats to identify in the large group, in *The Large Group.* Edited by Kreeger L. Itasca, IL, Peacock, 1975, pp. 87–144

   The single most penetrating and illuminating account of the fate of the individual in the large group, this chapter gives specific, concrete notions about the complex machinations of ego boundary transformations vis-à-vis large group membership.

Social Psychology

9. *Bales RF, Slater PE: Role differentiation in small decision-making groups, in *Family, Socialization and Interaction Process.* Edited by Parsons T, Bales RF. New York, Free Press, 1955, pp. 259–306

   In this critically important study, the authors put a microscope on the step-by-step evolution of roles in a group, with special emphasis on that of the task and emotional leaders and the evolution of a common culture. This is also important as a demonstration of basic research strategies in social psychology.

10. **Gibbard GS, Hartmann JJ, Mann RD** (eds): *Analysis of Groups: Contributions to Theory, Research and Practice.* San Francisco, CA, Jossey-Bass, 1973

A useful collection of essays, some of which are classics, but which also pulls together various facets of group life derived from group psychotherapy, sensitivity training, and self-analytic classroom traditions. The essays on group development are especially useful.

11. **Heslin R, Dunphy D:** Three dimensions of member satisfaction in small groups. *Human Relations* 17:99–112, 1964

This article outlines how status consensus, progress toward group goals, and freedom to participate generate satisfaction in individuals in the group.

12. *Newton PM, Levinson DJ:** The work group within the organization: a socio-psychological approach. *Psychiatry* 36:115–142, 1973

In a brilliant exposition of a social system leading to a useful conceptualization of the interrelationship between task, social structure, social processes, and culture, the authors demonstrate how each perspective interacts with the other and enlarges our understanding of group life.

13. **Tuckman BW:** Developmental sequence in small groups. *Psychol Bull* 63:384–399, 1965

Tuckman reviews 50 articles to propose a two-dimensional view of group development—temporal and structural—and explains the origin of strains within the group. This view has been validated by subsequent and reliable studies.

Sociology

14. *Durkheim E:** *Suicide: A Study in Sociology (1897).* Translated by Spaulding JA, Simpson G. Glencoe, IL, Free Press, 1951

This classic work—which uses statistical analysis of social systems to account for anomic, egoistic, and altruistic forms of suicide—has been a major influence on subsequent sociological thought and group work.

15. **Edelson M:** Theory of groups, in *Sociotherapy and Psychotherapy.* Chicago, IL, University of Chicago, 1970, pp. 25–74

In a difficult but rewarding effort to conceptualize the lawfulness and regularity of group life, Edelson draws from general systems theory, Tavistock group relations theory, and Parson's theory of action to propose an interactive model of groups based on the framework of values that group members share.

16. **Mills T:** *The Sociology of Small Groups.* Englewood Cliffs, NJ, Prentice-Hall, 1967

   In an excellent account and example of model building in group theory from the point of view of the group itself, Mills provides a clear exposition of the evolution of thinking of the group as a miniature social system.

17. **Parsons T:** *The Structure of Social Action.* New York, Free Press, 1937

   This is an outstanding, abstract, and complex example of sociological theory building, which is at the foundation of modern sociology. Not for the faint of heart.

Applied Group Dynamics

18. **Goffman E:** *Asylums: Essays on the Social Situation of Mental Patients and Other Inmates.* Garden City, NY, Doubleday, 1961

   This biased collection of essays "on the social situation of mental patients and other inmates" moves from organization to individual. Although not explicit, the bias is vaguely antipsychiatric and antimedical, but in this it gathers some of its considerable strength.

19 **Golding W:** *Lord of the Flies.* New York, Putnam, 1964

   This fictional account of powerful group dynamics is, at this point, part of the popular culture. That the group is composed of children does not lessen the impact.

20. **Jaques E:** Social systems as a defense against persecutory and depressive anxiety, in *New Directions in Psychoanalysis.* Edited by Klein M, Heimann P, Money-Kyrle RE. New York, Basic Books, 1955, pp. 478–498

   This is an attempt to illustrate and define how the mechanisms of projective and introjective identification operate in linking individual and social behavior. More specifically, the author hypothesizes that a defense against psychotic anxiety is a crucial element in group cohesion.

21. **Kernberg O:** Toward an integrative theory of hospital treatment, in *Object Relations Theory and Clinical Psychoanalysis.* New York, Jason Aronson, 1976, pp. 241–275

   This is an extension of the author's well-known work on object relations into group and organizational dynamics. Kernberg was the first analyst to make a genuine effort to integrate administrative and clinical concerns in the theory of hospital psychiatry.

22. **Main TF:** The ailment. *Br J Med Psychol* 30:129–145, 1957

This article has probably helped more staff members out of jams with colleagues and patients than any other. The author shows the impact of individual psychopathology on a group's (ward staff) functioning.

23. **Menzies I:** A case-study in the functioning of social systems as a defense against anxiety, in *Group Relations Reader*. Edited by Coleman AD, Bexton WH. San Rafael, CA, Associates Printing and Publishing, 1975, pp. 281–312

This work is somewhat like that of Jaques (1955) above, but focusing on nursing staff in a general hospital. It considers the functional as well as dysfunctional aspects of the methods used by nursing staffs to alleviate anxiety.

24. **Munich RL:** Varieties of learning in an experiential group. *Int J Group Psychother* 43:345–361, 1993

This is a brief discussion of the British and American origins of experiential groups and the specific psychological, social-psychological, and "group-as-a-whole" learning that one might anticipate in such groups. There is a careful distinction made between group process learning, encounter, and psychotherapy groups.

25. **Rice AK:** *Learning for Leadership.* London, Tavistock, 1963

26. **Rice AK:** Selections, in *Group Relations Reader*. Edited by Coleman AD, Bexton WH. San Rafael, CA, Associates Printing and Publishing, 1975, pp. 71–158

Rice provides a full description of the rationale, method, and process of a group relations conference, established primarily to study authority relations in groups.

8

Social and Cultural Factors: Their Role in Mental Illness

Victor Lidz, Ph.D.

Human life is social life. Human individuals inevitably live in complex social environments, sharing an intricate symbolic culture with communities of others. The social nature of life affects the totality of the self or personality, including its most intimate and interior aspects. Even the individuality of human personalities must be understood as a result of social processes, as emerging from unique combinations of institutionally transmitted relational capacities, purposes, standards, and identities. Personality is in key respects an internalization of elements provided by the social and cultural life-world. Disciplined knowledge of culture and society, therefore, contributes an irreducible dimension to the understanding of personality and its functioning.

Proceeding within this framework of understanding, the contemporary social sciences have shed light on highly diverse phenomena relating to mental illness. Social and cultural factors at various levels of organization—for example, from general cultural premises; to values stressing specific kinds of activities, abilities, and social relationships; to the institutions of social class, law, community, and moral custom; to the interactive patterns of family life—have been implicated in the genesis of mental illness of several types. Moreover, mental illness is in all societies a source of social disturbances sufficient to call out specialized modes of social control. Everywhere there is a role of mental illness, and it articulates with roles of normality, with other modes of deviance, and with roles of treatment and informal socio-emotional support in ways that are affected by a wide range of social institutions. Hence, the social and personal consequences of mental illnesses, even of given diagnostic categories, differ from society to society in relation to broader differences among major institutions. Particular instances of mental illness should be viewed as in part normatively organized social processes, involving the role-related reactions of many independent actors, as well as being the "breakdown" of individual persons.

To convey the foregoing perspective on mental illness, readings have been assembled under several distinct headings. First, a core group of works represent the general analytic frameworks of sociology and anthropology as they bear on the sociocultural aspects of personality, individuality, and mental illness and its control. These readings set forth the conceptual schemes within which the remaining works take on sharper significance. A second section presents works that demonstrate, with respect to various societies, how fundamentally human personalities are shaped by the normative standards of particular cultures and social structures—and by the stresses generated in these structures. Along with the cross-cultural variability in human personality, these readings depict, even more fundamentally, the cultural and institutional makeup of personality under all circumstances, including the clinical encounter within our own society. The third section consists of leading studies that have explored variations in types and rates of mental illness in association with such factors as value-pattern, community integration, class structure, and family organization.

The fourth section brings together studies bearing on the role-relationships through which social control of mental illness is exercised by society at large. A major focus of these readings is the mental hospital, its historical origins, its legitimacy in terms of broader social values, its social organization, and the efforts to supplant it in recent decades. A final section is directed toward problems that are less well codified in the literature but that appear to have grown increasingly important in recent decades. Given the widely reported finding that only modest portions of personality disorders are effectively brought into psychiatric treatment, this section addresses the forms of social control that are active within the broader community, their strengths, vulnerabilities, and relations to psychiatric treatment.

The entire reading list emphasizes works that develop the implications of fundamental sociological and anthropological perspectives for understanding the phenomena of mental illness. An effort has also been made to include studies that provide linkage with the lists covering family, group dynamics, epidemiology, milieu therapy, and community psychiatry without overlapping them unduly. The reader should hold in mind that many works in those areas complement and extend the perspectives incorporated in the following list.

Sociocultural Theory

1. *Durkheim E: *Suicide: A Study in Sociology*. Glencoe, IL, Free Press, 1951 (original French edition, 1897)

   This work first presented the sociological method of treating rates of suicide—or by extension other forms of deviant conduct—as "social facts" indicative of basic conditions of society. Durkheim discusses anomie, egoism, and altruism as "pathological" conditions that can elevate rates of suicide or other types of deviance, including mental illness.

2. Evans-Pritchard EE: *Witchcraft, Oracles and Magic Among the Azande*. London, Oxford University Press, 1965

   A detailed analysis of the cultural beliefs and social institutions surrounding the practice and control of witchcraft, divination, and magic in an East African tribal society, this book discusses the kinds of motives and social situations that lead to use of witchcraft and magic and highlights the role of witch doctor and the grounds of popular faith in it.

3. Kleinman A: *Patients and Healers in the Context of Culture*. Berkeley, CA, University of California Press, 1980

   This work provides anthropological reportage and analysis of the processes and rationales through which people in the context of traditional Chinese culture experience and interpret medical and psychiatric symptoms while relating to family and friends, traditional healers, and physicians trained in Western medicine. Emphasis is on the cultural frameworks for the construction of illness and psychiatric diagnoses.

4. *Mead M: *Sex and Temperament in Three Primitive Societies*. New York, Morrow, 1935

   This comparative analysis of socialization and personality development among three New Guinea tribes emphasizes the variation in male and female roles and in relations between the sexes across cultures. It is a classic portrayal of the malleability of human personality under variation in cultural patterns.

5. Merton RK: Continuities in the theory of reference groups and social structure, in *Social Theory and Social Structure*. Edited by Merton RK. Glencoe, IL, Free Press, 1957, pp. 281–386 (available in 1969 Edition)

   A detailed and probing treatment of the kinds of relationships with social groups through which individuals take on standards for judging their own conduct and the conduct of others, this work is important for understanding the complexity of the group environments that affect personal orientation and conduct.

6. *Parsons T:* The Social System. New York, Free Press, 1951

    This treatise on basic concepts for the analysis of social interaction emphasizes that reciprocal normative expectations are an essential basis for stabilizing social relationships. Parsons argues that, because of the prominence of social interaction in all human life, the motivational structures of individual personalities must also be integrated through normative institutions. Chapter VI on socialization, Chapter VII on the genesis of deviant motivation and its social control, and Chapter X on the doctor-patient role-relationship are classics.

7. *Parsons T:* Social Structure and Personality. New York, Free Press, 1964

    This collection of essays integrates psychoanalysis with sociological theory, focusing on concepts of object relations and social structure. The integrated theory is applied to family relationships, processes of socialization, stages in the life cycle, Oedipal themes in culture, and institutions of social control, including medicine. Chapters 1 and 4, in treating the relationship between social institutions and stages of personality development, present core material.

8. **Parsons T:** An approach to psychological theory in terms of the theory of action, in *Psychology: A Study of a Science,* Vol. 3. Edited by Koch S. New York, McGraw-Hill, 1959, pp. 612–711

    This is an overview of Parsons' sociologically grounded approach to the understanding of personality systems in one lengthy essay.

9. **Parsons T, Bales RF, with the collaboration of Olds J, Zelditch M Jr, Slater PE:** *Family, Socialization, and Interaction Process.* Glencoe, IL, Free Press, 1955

    The social structure of the nuclear family is viewed as a template for the processes of socialization of children. The organization and dynamic mechanisms of the personality are then treated as motivational entities developed through interpersonal relationships centering in the family. Distortions or breakdowns in family functioning and their possible consequences for personal pathology are discussed. Chapters 3 and 4 are the most detailed exposition of Parsons' interdisciplinary treatment of the functioning of personality systems.

10. *Simmel G:* On Individuality and Social Forms: Selected Readings. Edited by Levine DN. Chicago, IL, University of Chicago Press, 1971

These insightful essays on the qualities of social relationships in modern societies consider exchange, authority, conflict, and sociable relations as elements of modern civilization. Modern individualism and rationalism, the complexity of modern social settings, and the stresses engendered by the loss of communal ties and the impersonality of modern urban life are also discussed. The component chapters may be read independently.

11. *Weber M: *From Max Weber: Essays in Sociology.* Edited by Gerth HH, Mills CW. New York, Oxford University Press, 1946

Parts III and IV present key materials from Weber's studies of religion and social institutions: the ways of life of American Puritans, Prussian Junkers, Indian Brahmins, and Confucian Mandarins. Weber treats variation in religious ethics, as embodied in the life-styles of leading status groups, as the key source of differences among civilizations regarding valued activities, modes of achievement, qualities of social relationships, and personal ideals and ambitions.

Culture, Social Order, and Personality in Comparative Perspective

12. **Bach-y-Rita G:** The Mexican American: religious and cultural influences, in *Mental Health and Hispanic Americans: Clinical Perspectives.* Edited by Becerra RM, Karno M, Escobar JI. New York, Harcourt Brace Jovanovich, 1982, pp. 29–40

This work is a succinct survey of religious, subcultural, and social class-related patterns of belief and personal conduct that psychotherapists must understand to establish therapeutic relationships with Hispanic American patients. Emphasis is on ideals of suffering in Hispanic Catholicism, the machismo complex, and the diffuseness of personal relationships.

13. *Bellah RN: Father and son in Christianity and Confucianism, in *Beyond Belief: Essays on Religion in a Post-Traditional World.* Edited by Bellah RN. New York, Harper & Row, 1970, pp. 76–99

Bellah reconsiders the relation between Confucianism and Chinese family patterns. In its ethic of filiality, Chinese civilization accentuates the motivational complex of the latency period rather than the Oedipal period emphasized in the West. The latency symbolism of filial piety is treated as a key to the general motivational patterns of Chinese society.

14. **Carstairs GM:** *The Twice-Born: A Study of a Community of High-Caste Hindus.* Bloomington, IN, Indiana University Press, 1957

    This is a psychoanalytic and ethnographic study of members of Brahmin, Rajput, and Bania caste groups in a North India town. Interviews and projective test materials are used along with selected autobiographies. Patterns of early socialization and their effects on the life course are highlighted. Emphasis is placed on explaining the general Indian motivational patterns of resignation, self-control, and serenity in interpersonal relations, but also their adaptation to the life circumstances of the different castes.

15. *Doi T:** *The Anatomy of Dependence.* San Francisco, CA, Kodansha International, 1973

    This book considers the sociopsychological pattern of amae (loved dependence or being indulged as a loved or admired person) as a basis of interpersonal relations in Japan, the elaborations of amae in various Japanese institutions (e.g., family, business firm, political agency), and the distortions of amae as a source of personal pathologies in Japan and as a feature of many Japanese social problems.

16. *Levy RI:** *Tahitians: Mind and Experience in the Society Islands.* Chicago, IL, University of Chicago Press, 1973

    Levy discusses the ethnography of psychological experience among Society islanders, patterns of thinking and feeling, styles of interpersonal relations, the nature of moral conduct, socialization, maturation in social roles, and the maintenance of personal integration in Tahitian culture and society.

17. **Parsons T:** Certain primary sources and patterns of aggression in the social structure of the Western world, in *Essays in Sociological Theory,* Revised Edition. Edited by Parsons T. New York, Free Press, 1954, pp. 298–322

    Parsons argues that the strongly activistic values of Western civilization, when frustrated, generate exceptionally aggressive patterns of reaction. Aggression is viewed as deeply seated in Western culture and the patterns of personal motivation that it values.

Social Structure and Rates of Mental Disorder

18. **Carstairs GM, Kapur RL:** *The Great Universe of Kota: Stress, Change and Mental Disorder in an Indian Village.* Berkeley, CA, University of California Press, 1976

This is a study of the rates of psychiatric symptoms and needs among three caste groups of a village in Southwest India. The data are based on a sample survey using a schedule adapted to Indian culture. The authors emphasize the high levels of psychiatric need, the relations between symptomatology and caste institutions, and the pathogenic stress of recent social change.

19. **DeVos G:** The relation of guilt toward parents to achievement and arranged marriage among the Japanese, in *Japanese Culture and Behavior; Selected Readings*, Revised Edition. Edited by Lebra TS, Lebra WP. Honolulu, HI, University of Hawaii Press, 1986, pp. 80–101

Using the Thematic Apperception Test, emotionally significant stories concerning issues of work and marriage were obtained from residents of an agricultural village. The stories show that underlying feelings of guilt, specifically diffuse worries over possible failure to honor parents and family, provide generalized motivation to achieve in occupational settings and follow traditional roles in family relationships.

20. *Dohrenwend BP:** The epidemiology of mental disorder, in *Handbook of Health, Health Care, and the Health Professions*. Edited by Mechanic D. New York, Free Press, 1983, pp. 157–194

Dohrenwend provides a critical review of the first two generations of research on the epidemiology of mental illness, with assessment of key findings and interpretations, and an overview of current agendas for further research.

21. **Hendin H:** *Suicide and Scandinavia*. New York, Grune & Stratton, 1964

This is a sociological as well as clinical psychiatric study. Suicide rates are elevated in Denmark by social patterns establishing strong dependency motives and in Sweden by frustration of institutionalized performance expectations and trouble in gaining emotional comfort from others. Rare suicides in Norway follow more traumatic life histories and guilt over antisocial behavior.

22. **Hollingshead AB, Redlich FC:** *Social Class and Mental Illness: A Community Study*. New York, Wiley, 1958

In an examination of the rates and types of mental illness in the population of New Haven as they vary by social class, the authors use a simple scheme of class analysis, showing the concentration of mental illness, especially the psychoses, at the bottom of the class structure. They also highlight the different kinds of psychiatric care and treatment provided to the higher and lower classes.

23. *Scheper-Hughes N: *Saints, Scholars and Schizophrenics: Mental Illness in Rural Ireland.* Berkeley, CA, University of California Press, 1979

This is an ethnographic study of the decline of the rural Irish way of life into a dispirited condition in which many community norms have lost their former moral authority. The author argues that, under these anomic conditions, the cultural standards of community and family life often produce an ascetic, affectively constricted personality structure. Emphasis is placed on the passivity, inferiority, and isolation with which many contemporary residents of rural Ireland, especially males, must often make stressful life-course decisions. The author concludes that the very high rate of schizophrenic withdrawal and depression in Ireland is deeply embedded in the general sociocultural pattern of the country's rural communities.

24. **Srole L, Langner TS, Michael ST, Fischer AK:** *Mental Health in the Metropolis: The Midtown Manhattan Study.* New York, McGraw-Hill, 1962 (also available from New York University Press, 1978)

In this psychiatric profile of the population of midtown Manhattan based on a large-scale interdisciplinary survey, the authors focus on socioeconomic status, as well as age groups, marital status, religious and national backgrounds, and length of city residence. They consider the large amounts of personal pathology that are not brought into psychiatric treatment.

The Mental Hospital and Medicalization of Mental Disorder

25. *Chrisman NJ, Kleinman A:** Popular health care, social networks, and cultural meanings: the orientation of medical anthropology, in *Handbook of Health, Health Care, and the Health Professions.* Edited by Mechanic D. New York, Free Press, 1983, pp. 569–590

This is a cross-cultural model of the processes by which people perceive illnesses and make decisions about needs for care by self, family, or informal groups in the community, by nonprofessional folk practitioners, and/or by trained professionals. The emphasis is on similarities and differences across cultures, and the authors show that the popular or community and nonprofessional folk sectors meet many routine needs even in modern societies, preventing the professional sector from being overwhelmed by high prevalence of less serious illnesses.

26. *Estroff SE: *Making It Crazy: An Ethnography of Psychiatric Clients in an American Community.* Berkeley, CA, University of California Press, 1981

In a participant-observer study of an outpatient program for chronically disturbed mental patients, Estroff discusses the patients' many discontents with the socio-psycho-physiological experience of participating in the program, including the difficulties of taking antipsychotic medications. The author emphasizes the disorganized and stigmatized life arrangements followed by most of the patients as well as the limitations of a program providing little social and emotional support.

27. **Foucault M:** *Madness and Civilization: A History of Insanity in the Age of Reason.* New York, Random House, 1965

This is a now classic work on the transformation of the social role of "the insane" that was brought about by the "Enlightenment" as a cultural movement. Under the influence of the Enlightenment, European society greatly elevated the ideals of "Reason." But the obverse of a new devotion to Reason was a perception of madness as a greater and more unitary threat to social order. Accordingly, special hospitals were established to confine the insane in separation from the general society, and professionals were given new moral authority to treat madness totalistically. This work examines the conceptions of and treatments for insanity devised under the rationalistic presuppositions of Enlightened culture.

28. **Fox RC:** The medicalization and demedicalization of American society, in *Essays in Medical Sociology: Journeys into the Field.* Edited by Fox RC. New York, Wiley, 1979, pp. 465–483

Fox examines the social dilemmas and public controversies that have emerged in the United States over the last generation concerning the boundaries of medical institutions. For example, are too many emotional problems or psychological shortcomings treated as medical issues? Should physicians determine when an ill person is permitted to die? Fox analyzes the popular and professional attention given to such boundary issues in terms of the ways in which they touch on deeply seated American values and focuses on the complex institutional mechanisms that define the boundaries of modern medicine.

29. **Munakata T:** Japanese attitudes toward mental illness and mental health care, in *Japanese Culture and Behavior: Selected Readings,* Revised Edition. Edited by Lebra TS, Lebra WP. Honolulu, HI, University of Hawaii Press, 1986, pp. 369–378

Munakata reviews key differences between Japan and Western countries with respect to care and treatment of psychiatric problems. Families care for most people with psychiatric illness, making for low rates of hospitalization. However, patients typically have long stays once hospitalized by families. Psychiatric hospitals are small and family-like, with patients and families tending to be dependent on "paternalistic" physicians.

30. **Murphy JM:** Psychiatric labeling in crosscultural perspective. *Science* 191:1019–1028, 1976

    Murphy juxtaposes recent work on invidious "labeling" as a factor in the social genesis of mental illness with cross-cultural research on the social roles of psychologically disturbed persons and emphasizes that all societies provide special roles for the "mentally ill."

31. *Rothman DJ:** *The Discovery of the Asylum: Social Order and Disorder in the New Republic.* Boston, MA, Little, Brown, 1971

    This work considers the related social movements in Jacksonian America through which prisons, insane asylums, almshouses, orphanages, and reformatories were founded as public responses to various forms of deviance; the anxiety raised in the public by insanity, crime, and economic dependence when seen as indications that the emerging social order was prone to demoralization, corruption, and breakdown; and the humanitarian program of asylum-based moral treatment for the insane and the forces that brought it into decline.

32. **Ruiz P:** The Hispanic patient: sociocultural perspectives, in *Mental Health and Hispanic Americans: Clinical Perspectives.* Edited by Becerra RM, Karno M, Escobar JI. New York, Harcourt Brace Jovanovich, 1982, pp. 17–28

    Ruiz discusses ways of establishing and strengthening the psychotherapeutic relationship with Hispanic patients and sensitivity to cultural categorizations of psychiatric symptoms, subcultural values as they may affect goals of treatment, ways of gaining support for therapy from families of patients, and styles of interpersonal communication by the therapist.

33. *Stanton AH, Schwartz JS:** *The Mental Hospital: A Study of Institutional Participation in Psychiatric Illness and Treatment.* New York, Basic Books, 1954

    In describing the ethnography of the disturbed ward at Chestnut Lodge, Stanton and Schwartz discuss the ongoing structure of role relationships in the hospital and its impact on patients' care and treatment; events in the social life of the ward that can affect the emotional states of all the patients, even producing epidemic-like waves of symptoms; and ways in which individual psychotherapy may be hindered or advanced by qualities of personal relationships on the ward.

Social Support, Social Control, and Social Breakdown in Contemporary American Communities

34. **Anderson E:** *A Place on the Corner: Identity and Rank Among Black Streetcorner Men.* Chicago, IL, University of Chicago Press, 1978

    Anderson describes the group of lower-class black men who frequent a bar in Chicago, including subgroups of employed "regular" citizens, street "hoodlums," and "wineheads." He presents the tactics of interaction by which members place one another in the status orders of their group and of metropolitan society generally and the relationships of caring and mutual support through which members assist one another in coping with personal problems and stresses.

35. *Blackwell B, Breakey W, Hammersley D, Hammond R, McMurray-Avila M, Seeger C:** Psychiatric and mental health services, in *Under the Safety Net: The Health and Social Welfare of the Homeless in the United States.* Edited by Brickner PW, Scharer LK, Conanen BA, Savarese M, Scanlan BC. New York, WW Norton, 1990, pp. 184–203

    In this overview of the problems confronting programs to provide psychiatric services to homeless people, the chronicity of the mental health problems, the difficulties in obtaining social service and support services for the homeless, the problems of gaining patient collaboration in treatment, and the complicated ways in which lack of basic services creates and exacerbates psychiatric conditions are considered.

36. **Dear MJ, Wolch JR:** *Landscapes of Despair: From Deinstitutionalization to Homelessness.* Princeton, NJ, Princeton University Press, 1987

    Dear and Wolch analyzes the concentration of homeless people in central city areas in the years since deinstitutionalization became a national policy. The homeless and the social service agencies attract each other to "service-dependent ghettos" in areas that were abandoned by businesses and middle-class residents during the economic changes of the past 30 years. Social and psychiatric problems have become geographically concentrated and thus overwhelm community institutions supporting social order and social control.

37. *Erikson KT:** *Everything in Its Path: Destruction of Community in the Buffalo Creek Flood.* New York, Simon & Schuster, 1976

    This book considers the loss of communal relationships and personal capacities to enter into them in the aftermath of a local disaster, the adverse factors in the history of the community that left people vulnerable to feelings of isolation and helplessness after the flood had disrupted life-routines and neighborhood relationships, and the personal pathologies suffered for years afterward.

38. **Kadushin C:** *Why People Go to Psychiatrists.* New York, Atherton, 1969

In a study of outpatients at 10 psychiatric clinics in New York that used questionnaires to examine how patients came to seek psychiatric treatment as a way of dealing with their personal problems, the research showed that a key role in placing patients in treatment is played by a large but loosely structured network of laypersons whose subculture favors psychiatric interpretations or understandings of personal difficulties. The volume also provides helpful advice to clinics about how to present their resources effectively to mentally troubled individuals.

39. **Wiseman JP:** *Stations of the Lost: The Treatment of Skid Row Alcoholics.* Chicago, IL, University of Chicago Press, 1970

Wiseman examines the life circumstances of alcoholic persons on "skid row" in a large West Coast city. Specific attention is given to the relationships of these persons with police, courts, jails, social workers, mental hospitals, and home missions. The author presents an important analysis of how "skid-rowers" undermine rehabilitative programs of various kinds, including psychiatric ones.

9

Psychiatric Epidemiology

Ewald Horwath, M.D.
Myrna M. Weissman, Ph.D.

E pidemiology is the study of the occurrence and distribution of specific disorders in populations. Epidemiologic studies can generate data on the prevalence and incidence of disorders, and on variations in these rates associated with demographic factors, time, comorbid illness, and other proposed risk factors. Such information can be used to test hypotheses about etiology, pathogenesis, and prevention and can generate new research ideas and insights to improve clinical care.

The scope of epidemiology in psychiatry has expanded markedly with the widespread use of specific diagnostic criteria, structured diagnostic instruments, sophisticated sampling techniques, and powerful statistical programs capable of rapid multivariable analyses. The works cited here are representative both of some of the classic studies and of these newer developments in psychiatric epidemiology.

Included are several overviews of the field, methodological reviews, and studies of children and adolescents. Variations in rates associated with genetic familial risk factors, cross-cultural factors, socioeconomic status, comorbid illness, birth cohort, and gender are examined. The implications of epidemiologic findings for preventive interventions, service utilization, impairment, and other public health issues are also examined.

Overviews

1. **Barrett JE, Rose RM** (eds): *Mental Disorders in the Community: Progress and Challenge.* New York, Guilford, 1986

   This volume presents the proceedings of the 75th Annual Meeting of the American Psychopathological Association, New York City, February 28—March 2, 1985. Included are data from the Epidemiologic Catchment Area study and the Lundby and Stirling County studies, a section on treatment and risk factors for schizophrenia, a review of methodological issues, and a discussion of the implications of epidemiologic findings for policy and program planning.

2. **Robins LN, Regier DA** (eds): *Psychiatric Disorders in America.* New York, Free Press, 1991

   This is a summary of some of the important descriptive epidemiology findings from the Epidemiologic Catchment Area study. Results are organized by psychiatric disorder, and the volume includes a brief description of the methods.

3. **Weissman MM, Myers JK, Ross CE** (eds): *Community Surveys of Psychiatric Disorders,* Vol. 4. New Brunswick, NJ, Rutgers University Press, 1986

   This volume reviews the methods and findings of various large community surveys of psychiatric disorders, including some classic studies, like the Midtown Manhattan and Stirling County studies, as well as more recent surveys, such as the Epidemiologic Catchment Area study and others. The volume also contains a section discussing conceptual problems in defining a case and descriptions of various screening and diagnostic instruments.

4. **Williams P, Wilkinson G, Rawnsley K** (eds): *The Scope of Epidemiological Psychiatry: Essays in Honour of Michael Shepherd.* London, Routledge, 1989

   This volume presents a wide range of interesting work organized as a tribute to Michael Shepherd at the time of his retirement from the Chair of Epidemiological Psychiatry at the University of London. It includes scholarly sections on scientific principles of epidemiologic and social inquiry in psychiatry, specific epidemiologic studies of mental disorders, the evaluation of treatment approaches and service organization, and a section on international and cross-cultural perspectives.

Methodological Issues

5. **Cohen P, Cohen J:** The clinician's illusion. *Arch Gen Psychiatry* 41:1178–1182, 1984

   The authors discuss one source of disagreement between clinicians and researchers regarding the long-term prognosis of certain disorders. Compared with population surveys, clinical samples tend to be biased toward cases of long duration. The statistical method of this bias is elucidated, and its consequences are explained.

6. **Eaton WW, Kessler LG** (eds): *Epidemiologic Field Methods in Psychiatry: The NIMH Epidemiologic Catchment Area Program.* Orlando, FL, Academic Press, 1985

   This is a detailed description of the methodology used in the Epidemiologic Catchment Area program. It includes sections on the history, objectives, study design, sampling method, field work, diagnostic and other survey instruments, and data analysis. Chapters are organized by methodological issues and include literature reviews of each area.

7. **Fleiss JL, Williams JB, Dubro AF:** The logistic regression analysis of psychiatric data. *J Psychiatr Res* 20:195–209, 1986

   This article provides a clear description of the application of logistic regression analysis to psychiatric data. The authors discuss the underlying principles of logistic regression and work through a detailed sample problem to demonstrate the practical application of this analytic method to categorical psychiatric data.

8. **Kleinbaum DG, Kupper LL, Morgenstern H:** *Epidemiologic Research: Principles and Quantitative Methods.* Belmont, CA, Lifetime Learning Publications (Wadsworth), 1982

   This excellent volume discusses principles and methods used in epidemiologic research studies. The focus is on quantitative issues, including study design, measurement, validity, and statistical analysis. Chapters 20 to 23, which present a detailed discussion of the theoretical and practical issues involved in logistic regression modeling, may be of particular interest to psychiatric investigators.

9. **Robins LN, Wing J, Wittchen HU, Helzer JE, Babor TF, Burke J, Farmer A, Jablenski A, Pickens R, Regier DA, Sartorius N, Towle LH:** The Composite International Diagnostic Interview: an epidemiologic instrument suitable for use in conjunction with different diagnostic systems and in different cultures. *Arch Gen Psychiatry* 45:1069–1077, 1988

This article discusses the design, development, and field testing of the Composite International Diagnostic Interview, a joint project of the World Health Organization and the U.S. Alcohol, Drug Abuse, and Mental Health Administration. One goal is to incorporate criteria from DSM-III-R and the *International Classification of Diseases,* 10th edition, into a reliable instrument suitable for use in many different populations and cultures.

10. **Wing JK, Bebbington P, Robins LN** (eds): *What Is a Case? The Problem of Definition in Psychiatric Community Surveys.* London, Grant McIntyre, 1981

One of the most difficult problems in psychiatric epidemiology has been that of case definition. This volume contains a stimulating and scholarly compendium of writings on this issue by some of the most respected and accomplished authors in the field. Topics covered include theoretical and conceptual problems, description and classification, reliability issues, episode definition, and measures of social functioning and role performance.

11. **Wittchen HU, Burke JD, Semler G, Pfister H, Von Cranach M, Zaudig M:** Recall and dating of psychiatric symptoms: test-retest reliability of time-related symptom questions in a standardized psychiatric interview. *Arch Gen Psychiatry* 46:437–443, 1989

This article reports on two independent test-retest reliability studies, using the Diagnostic Interview Schedule and the Composite International Diagnostic Interview Schedule. With two exceptions (anxiety disorders and alcohol abuse/dependence), the test-retest reliability of both instruments was high. Severe restrictions were found with regard to age at onset judgments of phobias, panic attacks, and depression.

Studies of Children

12. **Angold A:** Childhood and adolescent depression, I: epidemiological and aetiological aspects. *Br J Psychiatry* 152:601–617, 1988

Community studies of the prevalence of depressive symptoms and syndromes in child and adolescent populations over the past 50 years are reviewed. Methodological limitations are discussed; evidence for potential risk factors is considered; and specific future investigation is suggested.

13. **Bird HR, Canino G, Rubio-Stipec M, Gould MS, Ribera J, Sesman M, Woodbury M, Huerins-Goldman M, Pagan A, Sanchez-Lacay A,**

Moscoso M: Estimates of the prevalence of childhood maladjustment in a community survey in Puerto Rico: the use of combined measures. *Arch Gen Psychiatry* 45:1120–1126, 1988

Data are presented on an epidemiologic survey of children ages 4 through 16 years in Puerto Rico. The demographic correlates of maladjustment are examined, and prevalence rates are considered in light of the available mental health services. The authors conclude that these findings indicate a major public health problem for children on the island, particularly for children in families of low socioeconomic status, for whom rates of disorder are high, yet service availability is limited.

14. **Offord DR, Boyle MH, Szatmari P, Rae-Grant NI, Links PS, Cadman DT, Byles JA, Crawford JW, Blum HM, Byrne C, Thomas H, Woodward CA:** Ontario Child Health Study, II: six-month prevalence of disorder and rates of service utilization. *Arch Gen Psychiatry* 44:832–836, 1987

Data are presented on the 6-month prevalence of four child psychiatric disorders (conduct disorder, hyperactivity, emotional disorder, and somatization), and patterns of service utilization in different regions of Ontario are examined. More than half of the children had used ambulatory medical care over the previous 6 months, in contrast to a low utilization of mental health or social services. Implications for primary prevention and provision of child mental health services are discussed.

15. **Rutter M:** Isle of Wight revisited: twenty-five years of child psychiatric epidemiology, in *Annual Progress in Child Psychiatry and Child Development.* Edited by Chess S, Hertzig ME. New York, Brunner/Mazel, 1991, pp. 131–179

Child psychiatric epidemiology over the last 25 years is reviewed, using the Isle of Wight surveys of the 1960s as a starting point. Progress is reviewed in the study of preschool children, specific psychiatric disorders, risk factors, and therapeutic interventions. Methodological advances are discussed, and future challenges are considered.

16. **Shaffer D, Garland A, Gould M, Fisher P, Trautman P:** Preventing teenage suicide: a critical review. *J Am Acad Child Adolesc Psychiatry* 27:675–687, 1988

This article reviews the literature on risk factors for adolescent suicide and focuses on evidence for risks toward which preventive intervention could be directed. Evidence for the efficacy of a variety of interventions is reviewed.

Genetic Epidemiology

17. **Tsuang MT, Kendler KS, Lyons MJ** (eds): *Genetic Issues in Psychosocial Epidemiology.* New Brunswick, NJ, Rutgers University Press, 1991

    This volume provides a critical overview of methodological and theoretical issues, as well as a sampling of substantive findings, in the field of genetic epidemiology. The review of substantive findings includes sections on schizophrenia, depression and mania, anxiety disorders, obsessional disorders, and criminal behavior.

Cross-Cultural Studies

18. **Canino GJ, Bird HR, Shrout PE, Rubio-Stipec M, Bravo M, Martinez R, Sesman M, Guevara LM:** The prevalence of specific psychiatric disorders in Puerto Rico. *Arch Gen Psychiatry* 44:727–735, 1987

    A Spanish translation of the Diagnostic Interview Schedule was administered to 1,513 community respondents (ages 18–64 years) in Puerto Rico. Results showed that lifetime and 6-month prevalence rates for most psychiatric disorders were similar in Puerto Rico and at three mainland United States Epidemiologic Catchment Area sites. Severe cognitive impairment and somatization disorder had slightly higher rates in Puerto Rico.

19. **Jablensky A, Sartorius N:** Is schizophrenia universal? Berzelius Symposium XI: transcultural psychiatry. *Acta Psychiatr Scand* 344:65–70, 1988

    This article reviews cross-cultural studies of schizophrenia by the World Health Organization. Incidence rates are comparable in different populations and cultures, when similar methods are used. Differences between developed and developing countries in presentation and outcomes are discussed.

20. **Sartorius N, Jablensky A, Korten A, Ernberg G, Anker M, Cooper JE, Day R:** Early manifestations and first-contact incidence of schizophrenia in different cultures: a preliminary report on the initial evaluation phase of the WHO Collaborative Study on Determinants of Outcome of Severe Mental Disorders. *Psychol Med* 16:909–928, 1986

    Initial results of this World Health Organization collaborative study carried out at 12 centers in 10 countries show that schizophrenic patients in different cultures share many symptomatic features. Although symptomatic similarities outweigh differences, the 2-year course was more severe for schizophrenic patients in developed, industrialized countries than in developing countries.

Socioeconomic Status

21. **Dohrenwend BP, Levav I, Shrout PE, Schwartz S, Naveh G, Link BG, Skodol AE, Stueve A:** Socioeconomic status and psychiatric disorders: the causation-selection issue. *Science* 255:946–952, 1992

    A sample of about 5,000 Israel-born adults of European and North African background were selected from Israel's population register. Results of screening and psychiatric diagnosis indicated that the inverse relation between socioeconomic status and psychiatric disorder may be explained by social selection in schizophrenia. Social causation may play a more important role for depression in women and for antisocial personality and substance use disorders in men.

22. **Hollingshead AB, Redlich FC:** Class positions and types of mental illness, in *Social Class and Mental Illness: A Community Study.* Edited by Hollingshead AB, Redlich FC. New York, Wiley, 1958, pp. 220–250

    This chapter examines the relationship between social class and mental illness in a treated sample in New Haven, Connecticut, in 1955. More psychotic disorders were found in the lower social classes; more neurotic illnesses were found in the higher social classes.

Comorbidity

23. **Maser JD, Cloninger CR** (eds): *Comorbidity of Mood and Anxiety Disorders.* Washington, DC, American Psychiatric Press, 1990

    This volume has an excellent section that presents data regarding the comorbidity of mood and anxiety symptoms and disorders based on population-based studies in the United States; Zurich, Switzerland; Lundby, Sweden; and Atlantic, Canada (the Stirling County study). In addition to the epidemiologic evidence, the volume covers treated samples, family and genetic studies, biological studies, and theoretical and methodological issues.

24. **Regier DA, Farmer ME, Rae DS, Locke BZ, Keith SJ, Judd LL, Goodwin FK:** Comorbidity of mental disorders with alcohol and other drug abuse: results from the Epidemiologic Catchment Area (ECA) Study. *JAMA* 264:2511–2518, 1990

    The authors found evidence for significant comorbidity of alcohol, other drug, and mental disorders in the United States total community and institutional populations. Both alcohol and other drug abuse-dependence significantly increased the odds of having another mental disorder. For those with a mental disorder, the odds of having an addictive disorder were significantly greater, compared with those without a mental disorder. Comorbidity of mental and addictive disorders was higher in specialty mental health and addictive disorder clinics and highest in the prison population.

Cohort Effect

25. **Cross-National Collaborative Group:** The changing rate of major depression: cross-national comparisons. *JAMA* 268:3098–3105, 1992

    To estimate temporal trends in the rates of major depression, the Cross-National Collaborative Group examined data from approximately 39,000 subjects in nine population-based samples and 4,000 relatives in three family studies that were conducted independently in North America, Puerto Rico, Western Europe, the Middle East, Asia, and the Pacific Rim. The results indicate that, cross-nationally, more recent birth cohorts are at increased risk for major depression, although the magnitude of the increase varied by country. The authors conclude that further study of these variations and their association with demographic, economic, and social factors may provide clues to environmental factors that influence rates of major depression.

26. **Klerman GL, Lavori PW, Rice J, Reich T, Endicott J, Andreasen NC, Keller MB, Hirschfield RMA:** Birth-cohort trends in rates of major depressive disorder among relatives of patients with affective disorder. *Arch Gen Psychiatry* 42:689–695, 1985

    Using life-table and survival methods, the authors analyzed data from the National Institute of Mental Health Collaborative Program on the Psychobiology of Depression Clinical Study. The findings indicate a progressive increase in rates of depression in successive 20th-century birth cohorts and an earlier age at onset in each birth cohort. The female-to-male ratio of major depression also varied across time.

27. **Wickramaratne PJ, Weissman MM, Leaf PJ, Holford TR:** Age, period, and cohort effects on the risk of major depression: results from five United States communities. *J Clin Epidemiol* 42:333–343, 1989

    Results of this analysis of Epidemiologic Catchment Area data show a sharp increase in rates of major depression among both men and women in the birth cohort born during the years 1935–1945. Rates among females stabilized in those born since 1945; rates in men continued to rise among cohorts born in 1945–1955. Rates associated with period of onset continued to rise between 1960 and 1980 among both men and women of all ages studied.

Reviews of Other Risk Factor Studies

28. **Eaton WW:** Epidemiology of schizophrenia. *Epidemiol Rev* 7:105–126, 1985

    A review of prevalence, incidence, and risk factor studies of schizophrenia, this article also includes an excellent section on methodological recommendations for the epidemiologic study of schizophrenia.

29. **Weissman MM, Klerman GL:** Gender and depression, in *Women and Depression: A Lifespan Perspective*. Edited by Formanek R, Gurian A. New York, Springer, 1987, pp. 3–15

    Evidence is presented that the reported high rate of depression in females compared with males in clinic and community survey data is a real finding and not an artifact of reporting bias or increased help-seeking behavior in women. Possible explanations for the gender differences in rates of depression are discussed.

Implications of Epidemiologic Findings for Public Health

30. **Horwath E, Johnson J, Klerman GL, Weissman MM:** Depressive symptoms as relative and attributable risk factors for first onset major depression. *Arch Gen Psychiatry* 49:817–823, 1992

    Using longitudinal data from the Epidemiologic Catchment Area study, the authors estimated the relative and attributable risks of depressive symptoms in predicting first onset of major depression over 1 year. Persons with depressive symptoms, as compared with those without such symptoms, were 4.4 times more likely to develop an episode of major depression over 1 year. The attributable risk, a compound epidemiologic measure, which reflects both the relative risk (4.4) and the prevalence of the risk factor (24%), was greater than 50%. The authors conclude that the identification and treatment of depressive symptoms may have implications for the prevention of major depression.

31. **Johnson J, Weissman MM, Klerman GL:** Service utilization and social morbidity associated with depressive symptoms in the community. *JAMA* 267:1478–1483, 1992

    Estimates of population attributable risk indicated that physicians in the community actually provided services to more persons with depressive symptoms than to persons with formally defined conditions of depressive disorders. The authors conclude that subclinical depression, as a consequence of high prevalence, is a clinical and public health problem in need of further diagnostic and therapeutic attention.

32. **Kessler RC, McGonagle KA, Zhao S, Nelson CB, Hughes M, Eshleman S, Wittchen H-U, Kendler KS:** Lifetime and 12-month prevalence of DSM-III-R psychiatric disorders in the United States: results from the National Comorbidity Survey. *Arch Gen Psychiatry* 51:8–19, 1994

    The National Comorbidity Survey is the first to administer a structured psychiatric interview to a representative sample of the United States population. The results show a high prevalence of psychiatric disorders (almost 30% over previous 12 months) and a concentration of these disorders in roughly one-sixth of the population who have three or more comorbid disorders. As reported in the Epidemiologic Catchment Area study, the majority of people with psychiatric disorders failed to obtain treatment. From a public health perspective, these results suggest the need for a research focus on the causes of high comorbidity and barriers to professional help-seeking and increased clinical outreach to untreated persons with psychiatric disorders.

33. **Regier DA, Goldberg ID, Taube CA:** The de facto United States mental health services system. *Arch Gen Psychiatry* 35:685–693, 1978

    Based on United States population data, only 21% of those needing mental health care received it from a mental health professional; the remainder were treated by primary care physicians, general hospitals, or not at all.

34. **Wells KB, Stewart A, Hays RD, Burnam MA, Rogers W, Daniels M, Berry S, Greenfield S, Ware J:** The functioning and well-being of depressed patients: results from the Medical Outcomes Study. *JAMA* 262:914–919, 1989

    This study surveyed patients in general medical settings and found that depressed patients, including those with subclinical depression, suffered significant impairment and diminished sense of well-being, comparable in severity to other medical patients with chronic physical diseases.

History of Psychiatry

Nathan M. Kravis, M.D.
Leonard C. Groopman, M.D., Ph.D.

Burgeoning interest in the history of psychiatry has led to its emergence in the past decade as an important subdiscipline within history of medicine and within general history. The growth of this field has been marked by the founding of a new journal dedicated exclusively to it, the British-based *History of Psychiatry*, whose first volume appeared in 1990.

Such growth presents an embarrassment of riches and a problem of definition and selection. In our attempt to review and represent this expanding domain, we have elected to compose a sampling of scholarship in key areas of psychiatric history: dynamic psychiatry and psychoanalysis, biological and somatic psychiatry, institutional and forensic psychiatry, psychiatric nosology, and psychiatric historiography. These subdivisions are not meant to imply a neat compartmentalization of subject areas. In fact, there is considerable overlap, and many works could be situated under more than one of our categories. For example, Porter's (1987) *Mind Forg'd Manacles,* listed below under institutional and forensic psychiatry, might just as well have been included under biological and somatic psychiatry.

Our bibliography is also intended to reflect competing and complementary approaches to history, such as intellectual history, social and cultural history, and feminist history. It is not meant to provide exhaustive or even comprehensive coverage of this variegated and rapidly evolving field.

Furthermore, we have not included studies of non-Western psychiatry or psychiatrically pertinent studies of ancient Western medicine.

We have with one exception excluded recent editions of primary source material, although renewed interest in such works is further indication of the vitality of the field. A noteworthy recent example is *The Classics of Psychiatry and the Behavioral Sciences* series of reprints edited and introduced by Carlson and published by Gryphon Editions. We have made an exception for the new edition of Weyer's De Praestigiis Daemonum (Mora 1991), not only because it is the first English translation of this important text, but also because of its outstanding scholarly apparatus.

Dynamic Psychiatry and Psychoanalysis

1. **Crabtree A:** *From Mesmer to Freud: Magnetic Sleep and the Roots of Psychological Healing.* New Haven, CT, Yale University Press, 1993

   Crabtree covers some of the same territory as Gauld (1992) below, but focuses more narrowly on the evolution of psychotherapy. Consequently, of the two, this one will probably be of greater interest to most clinicians. Crabtree elucidates the indebtedness of psychoanalysis to the "alternate-consciousness paradigm" of 19th-century mesmeric and hypnotic therapeutics.

2. **Decker HS:** Freud in Germany: Revolution and Reaction in Science, 1893–1907. *Psychol Issues* (Monogr. No. 41):1–361, 1977

   In this ground-breaking study, which freshly examines Freud's relationship to his culture and his time, Decker challenges the psychoanalytic legend, originated by Freud and codified by Jones, of Freud's "splendid isolation." She carefully dismantles the myth of Freud's early psychoanalytic publications and ideas, meeting with a uniformly hostile reception. Decker offers instead a more sophisticated and balanced view of Freud's originality and of his place in the fin de siècle European Zeitgeist.

3. *****Ellenberger HF:** *The Discovery of the Unconscious: The History and Evolution of Dynamic Psychiatry.* New York, Basic Books, 1970

   Ellenberger's magnum opus remains the single best volume in this area. It is a massive tome whose richly referenced chapters are each scholarly essays that stand on their own. Each reflects Ellenberger's multilingual familiarity with primary source material, his encyclopedic command of the secondary literature, and his own historical insights derived from original research. The chapter on Janet is particularly outstanding. In many ways, this book marked the beginning of a new era of psychoanalytic historiography.

4. **Friedman L:** *The Anatomy of Psychotherapy.* Hillsdale, NJ, Analytic Press, 1988

   Although not an explicitly historical study, Friedman's book provides a cogent review of the development of modern psychoanalytic theory. With chapters devoted to Freud, George Klein, Schafer, Kohut, and other important theorists and theoretical trends, this book weaves together 20 years of thinking and writing by a leading psychoanalytic commentator.

5. **Gauld A:** *A History of Hypnotism.* Cambridge, England, Cambridge University Press, 1992

   This is a scholarly and readable survey of the mesmeric and hypnotic literature with an extensive reference list and an epilogue on contemporary views of hypnotic phenomena and multiple personality disorder.

6. **Harrington A:** *Medicine, Mind, and the Double Brain: A Study in Nineteenth-Century Thought.* Princeton, NJ, Princeton University Press, 1987

   This is an elegant and scholarly study of phrenology, hypnosis, early brain localization theory, and theories of mind and consciousness.

7. **Kravis NM:** James Braid's psychophysiology: a turning point in the history of dynamic psychiatry. *Am J Psychiatry* 145:1191–1206, 1988

   Through a detailed review of the works of James Braid (1795–1860), a central figure in the history of hypnotism, the author seeks to show how the 19th-century's golden era of hypnosis and hypnotic therapeutics led to important clinical and methodological advances that profoundly influenced the subsequent development of dynamic psychiatry. Questions about the psychology of suggestion and the nature of hypnotic influence that remain unresolved today are embedded in their historical context. This article includes an extensive list of references and a revised and updated Braid bibliography.

8. **Quen JM, Carlson ET** (eds): *American Psychoanalysis: Origins and Development.* New York, Brunner/Mazel, 1978

   This volume combines contributions by professional historians (e.g., John Burnham, Hannah Decker) and prominent psychoanalysts (e.g., Arnold Cooper, Robert Michels, George Pollock, Marianne Horney Eckardt) on the reception and growth of psychoanalysis in the United States, as well as reflections on its myriad institutional and theoretical schisms.

9. **Stepansky P** (ed): *Freud: Appraisals and Reappraisals: Contributions to Freud Studies,* Vol. 1. Hillsdale, NJ, Analytic Press, 1986

This first volume in an interdisciplinary series of Freud studies contains essays by Peter Swales, Edwin R. Wallace IV, and Barry Silverstein along with shorter contributions by Patrick Mahoney, Paul Stepansky, and John Gedo. It is a rich and varied example of post-Ellenbergian Freud scholarship. The lead essay by Swales concerns Freud's relationship with his patient Anna von Lieben. Since much of Swales' work has been privately printed, this volume provides a relatively accessible sample of his lively and sometimes controversial writing. Subsequent volumes in this series have not quite matched the standards of the first.

10.　*Sulloway FJ:* *Freud, Biologist of the Mind: Beyond the Psychoanalytic Legend.* New York, Basic Books, 1979

In a work that owes much to Ellenberger (1970) above but also contains a great deal of original research and interpretation, Sulloway casts a discerning eye over Freud's roots in 19th-century biological science and Darwinism. He critically reexamines psychoanalytic historiography and what he calls "the myth of the hero in psychoanalytic history." Along with Ellenberger, Sulloway sets a standard for meticulous scholarship in this often polemicized field. His book includes an extensive and valuable bibliography.

11.　**van der Kolk BA, van der Hart O:** Pierre Janet and the breakdown of adaptation in psychological trauma. *Am J Psychiatry* 146:1530–1540, 1989

Marking the centenary of Janet's 1889 *L'Automatisme Psychologique,* this excellent article places Janet in his well-deserved historical context as a major theorist of dissociation and psychological trauma. The authors highlight Janet's contribution to the contemporary study of memory, learning, posttraumatic stress disorder, and dissociative phenomena.

Biological and Somatic Psychiatry

12.　**Ackerknecht EH:** The history of the drug treatment of mental diseases. *Trans Stud Coll Physicians Phila* (series 5) 1:161–170, 1979

Ackerknecht describes some of the specific plant-derived agents used by the ancients as evacuants and sedatives. He notes that there were few changes in the principles of pharmacotherapy until the 16th century. Paracelsus (1493–1541) and his followers ushered in the era of chemically prepared drugs, mainly emetics, tonics, and sedatives. The use of emetics in the treatment of mental illness persisted well into the 19th century.

　　Psychopharmacology was again radically transformed by the introduction of bromides in the 1850s as sedatives and anticonvulsants. The development of chemical sedative-hypnotics in the second half of the 19th century brought with it the obsolescence of plant-derived drugs and the growth of the modern pharmaceutical industry. Ackerknecht's article concludes with a synopsis of the advent in the 1950s of most of the neuroleptics and thymoleptics now in use.

13. **Jackson SW:** The use of the passions in psychological healing. *J Hist Med Allied Sci* 45:150–175, 1990

Jackson delineates the principles that governed the use of drugs in the treatment of mental maladies for most of the past 2,500 years. Etiologic theories of humoral excess called for evacuative remedies, such as emetics, cathartics, and phlebotomy. Jackson explains how the Hippocratic notion that "opposites are cures for opposites" was elaborated by Aristotle, Galen, and Soranus. He traces the concepts of temperaments and passions in nosology and therapeutics from the ancients to the dawn of the 20th century.

14. **Tourney G:** History of biological psychiatry in America. *Am J Psychiatry* 126:29–42, 1969

Tourney describes how the second half of the 19th century brought a reaction in some quarters against moral therapy in favor of a strictly biological disease model. He elucidates the role of Wagner-Jauregg's malaria therapy for general paresis in stimulating interest in somatic therapies and concisely traces the subsequent rise of insulin coma therapy, convulsive therapies, and psychosurgery.

Institutional and Forensic Psychiatry

15. **Carlson ET, Dain N:** The psychotherapy that was moral treatment. *Am J Psychiatry* 117:519–524, 1960

The authors succinctly review the primary French, British, and American texts associated with the rise of moral treatment in the years 1750–1840. They show the emergence of talking therapy out of the gradual shift away from punitive methods of inpatient management toward methods that relied more on social coercion and milieu.

16. **Dain N:** *Clifford W. Beers: Advocate for the Insane.* Pittsburgh, PA, University of Pittsburgh Press, 1980

Through the life and writing of this celebrated former psychiatric patient turned social crusader, Dain describes the politics of mental health reform in America from the turn of the century to World War II. Thorough and detailed, it portrays the relationship of public and private interests, professional and lay forces, in the emergence of mental health advocacy.

17. **Goldstein J:** *Console and Classify: The French Psychiatric Profession in the Nineteenth Century.* Cambridge, England, Cambridge University Press, 1987

A sociological history of French psychiatric thought and professional politics from Pinel through Charcot. Medical-legal issues are given a central place in the history of the emergence of the French psychiatric profession. This work is always thought-provoking and challenging, even when the author has an axe to grind.

18. **Grob GN:** *Mental Illness and American Society: 1875–1940.* Princeton, NJ, Princeton University Press, 1983

Positioning himself between institutional psychiatry's apologists and its Marxist and social revisionists, an accomplished historian of American psychiatry carefully elucidates the complex interplay of forces that led to deinstitutionalization. Grob shows how the pursuit of cure came to clash with the provision of care as turn-of-the-century psychiatrists sought to redefine their expertise and professional turf while patient demographics and public policy shifted around them. This book is complemented by Grob's more recent volume, *The Inner World of American Psychiatry, 1890–1940* (New Brunswick, NJ, Rutgers University Press, 1985), a selection of unpublished correspondence by some of American psychiatry's leaders during a period of tremendous change within the profession and within society.

19. *Porter R:** *Mind-Forg'd Manacles: A History of Madness in England from the Restoration to the Regency.* Cambridge, MA, Harvard University Press, 1987

A creative synthesis of the vast literature on madness, confinement, and the nascent psychiatric profession in early modern England by probably the most prolific historian currently in the field. A chapter on historiographical issues helps orient the reader to the important theoretical debates. An exhaustive bibliography directs the reader toward further study.

20. **Rosenberg CS:** *The Trial of the Assassin Guiteau: Psychiatry and the Law in the Gilded Age.* Chicago, IL, University of Chicago Press, 1968

In reconstructing the events surrounding the assassination of President Garfield, the author creates a microcosm of late 19th-century American psychiatry: its cultural context, intellectual debates, and institutional conflicts. This is more than a study of forensic psychiatry.

21. *Scull A (ed): *Madhouses, Mad-Doctors, and Madmen: The Social History of Psychiatry in the Victorian Era.* Philadelphia, PA, University of Pennsylvania Press, 1981

This volume remains the best anthology in the social history of 19th-century Anglo-American psychiatry. Its 14 essays introduce the reader to historiographical debates around therapeutics, the asylum, the politics of the profession, and forensics.

22. **Smith R:** *Trial by Medicine: Insanity and Responsibility in Victorian Trials.* Edinburgh, Scotland, Edinburgh University Press, 1981

Smith describes the complex interweaving of medicine, law, and moral theory that comprised forensic psychiatry in Victorian England. This is, at times, a turgid work for a muddy area.

23. **Tomes N:** *A Generous Confidence: Thomas Story Kirkbride and the Art of Asylum-Keeping: 1840–1883.* Cambridge, England, Cambridge University Press, 1987

A rich and nuanced description of the religious, cultural, and economic roots of the 19th-century asylum, as well as of daily life within it. Tomes raises the often sterile debate surrounding the asylum to a high level of historical sophistication.

Psychiatric Nosology

24. **Brumberg J:** *Fasting Girls: The Emergence of Anorexia Nervosa as a Modern Disease.* Cambridge, MA, Harvard University Press, 1988

In this social constructionist account of the origins and meaning of a psychiatric disease, Brumberg provides a rich description of the significance of food in Victorian England and America and relates anorexia nervosa to social and cultural changes in the middle-class family. She discusses the general issues of the historicity of psychiatric diagnosis and the perils of retrospective psychiatric diagnosis.

25. **Foucault M:** *Madness and Civilization: A History of Insanity in the Age of Reason.* New York, Vintage, 1965

Ideologically strident and historically flawed, Foucault's brilliant book put the "problematic" of psychiatry on the historian's map. It is a classic in the field not only because of its daring breadth of vision but also because all subsequent writing about the birth of the asylum and modern psychiatric epistemology takes off from it.

26. **Gilman S:** *Seeing the Insane.* New York, Wiley, 1982

Gilman considers the iconography of madness from the 16th century to the present and the continuities and changes in how "the mad" were seen from the age of woodcut engravings to the photograph.

27. **Jackson SW:** *Melancholia and Depression: From Hippocratic Times to Modern Times.* New Haven, CT, Yale University Press, 1986

In an ambitious and wide-ranging volume, Jackson traces the 2,500-year history of medical writing about what has proven to be perhaps the most stable clinical entity in psychiatric nosology. Jackson skillfully leads the reader through centuries of clinical descriptions of the cardinal affective disorders, deftly shedding light on an impressive array of theories of etiology and treatment. Although not without its flaws, Jackson's book provides an invaluable guide and reference tool for students and researchers alike.

28. **Klerman GL, Vaillant GE, Spitzer RL, Michels R:** A debate on DSM-III. *Am J Psychiatry* 141:539–553, 1984

Four brilliant clinician-researchers and leaders of American psychiatry clash in this fascinating colloquy. Each invokes history and the philosophy of science in the arguments he makes concerning strategies and values in psychiatric nosology.

29. **Macdonald M:** *Mystical Bedlam: Madness, Anxiety, and Healing in Seventeenth Century England.* Cambridge, England, Cambridge University Press, 1981

Based on a cache of papers of an early 17th-century English healer, Macdonald explores the eclectic nature of healing in the age prior to the professionalization of psychiatry. This is probably the best work on the treatment of insanity in the 17th century.

30. **Mora G** (ed): *Witches, Devils, and Doctors in the Renaissance: Johann Weyer, De Praestigiis Daemonum.* Translated by Shea J. Binghamton, NY, Medieval & Renaissance Texts and Studies, 1991

In *De Praestigiis Daemonum,* the 16th-century court physician Johann Weyer argues with great vehemence and humanism against the persecution of witches. He pleads for a compassionate view of accused and self-professed witches as the deluded victims of disordered imagination and unbridled fantasy. These are seen by Weyer as symptoms of melancholia, to which women are said to be disproportionately susceptible. Shea's graceful translation, Mora's superb introductory essay, and the book's formidable scholarly apparatus mark it as the definitive English edition.

31. **Porter R:** *A Social History of Madness: The World Through the Eyes of the Insane.* New York, Weidenfeld & Nicholson, 1987

Porter seeks to capture the experience of madness through the writings and lives of well-known historical figures. Although at times tendentiously antipsychiatric, this survey from "the madman's" perspective is an essential complement to the histories of psychiatry written from the doctor's point of view.

32. **Schoeneman TJ:** Criticisms of the psychopathological interpretation of witch hunts: a review. *Am J Psychiatry* 139:1028–1032, 1982

This work incisively amplifies Spanos' (1978) refutation, below, of the psychopathological paradigm and further identifies methodological lapses by psychiatric historians.

33. **Spanos NP:** Witchcraft in histories of psychiatry: a critical analysis and an alternative conceptualization. *Psychol Bull* 85:417–439, 1978

Spanos' main thesis is that social learning theory explains the phenomena of the witchcraft era better than psychodynamic theories of psychopathology. He offers a scholarly and penetrating critique of the psychopathological interpretation of the Medieval and Renaissance European witchcraft craze favored by many psychiatric historians.

34. **Wilson M:** DSM-III and the transformation of American psychiatry: a history. *Am J Psychiatry* 150:399–410, 1993

Wilson places the decline of the psychosocial model and the rise of the neo-Kraepelinian descriptive psychiatry embodied in DSM-III in the context of intellectual, scientific, economic, and ideologic trends in the post-World War II American psychiatry. He bases his review in part on archival research and interviews with key figures. The author contends that advances in psychiatric research facilitated by the publication of DSM-III brought with them disadvantages, such as "reification of the discourse of descriptive psychiatry" and loss of the concept of the unconscious with consequent "narrowing of psychiatry's clinical gaze."

Psychiatric Historiography

35. Micale MS, Porter R (eds): *Discovering the History of Psychiatry.* New York, Oxford University Press, 1994

This invaluable volume of 21 essays by 22 scholars provides a broad and deep view of the discipline of the history of psychiatry. The volume emphasizes the multiplicity of voices and perspectives within the field and situates the history of psychiatry at the intersection of scholarship, public policy, and cultural criticism. The impact of individual scholars in shaping the field by setting its rhetorical agenda is given pride of place alongside the core themes and controversies around which historical writing about psychiatry has been organized in the last three decades. Specific national traditions in the history of psychiatry are examined, as is the burgeoning historiography of Freud and psychoanalysis.

II

Psychopathology

Nosology, Phenomenology, and Diagnosis

Nancy C. Andreasen, M.D., Ph.D.
Michael Flaum, M.D.

T he perceived importance of nosology, phenomenology, and diagnosis in psychiatry has fluctuated over time, along with changes in prevailing theories of etiology, treatment approaches, and the types of problems considered to be within the domain of the field.

Until the latter part of the 19th century, the primary purpose of psychiatric classification in the United States was to allow for census-like data collection that would assist in the planning and administration of large mental institutions. An international classification of mental diseases published in 1888 consisted of nine categories (mania, melancholia, monomania, dementia, general paralysis of the insane, epilepsy, toxic insanity, congenital mental deficiency, and moral insanity), all but the last of which were accepted as the official American nosology of the time. The conceptual basis for these categories varied in that some were defined by predominant symptom patterns, whereas others were defined by their presumed etiological mechanisms.

At about the same time, Emil Kraepelin began compiling meticulously detailed records of the various signs and symptoms he observed among patients in his clinic in Heidelberg, Germany. He would go on to follow this large sample longitudinally over the next several decades, believing that commonalities in their course and outcome would discriminate valid diagnostic categories. This approach, documented in a series of influential textbooks, led to the dichotomy of the major mental disorders into dementia praecox (later renamed schizophrenia by Bleuler) and manic-depressive insanity, a distinction that has been largely maintained in virtually all subsequent nosological systems. Kraepelin brought together a talented and diverse group of neuroscientists, including Alzheimer, Nissl, Brodmann, and others, in an attempt to elucidate the underlying pathophysiological processes of these disorders; for the most part, however, these goals proved to be unattainable at the time.

This inability to identify physical causes of mental disorders was coincident with, and perhaps, partly accounted for the great interest and enthusiasm with which psychological theories of mental illness were received during the middle part of the century, especially in the United States. World War II saw an increasing number of physicians entering psychiatry, and the apparent success of psychological approaches on a variety combat-related mental disorders fueled this enthusiasm. No longer was the focus on the nature or course of the prevailing symptom pattern, but rather on the effort to understand the dynamic between each individual and his or her unique set of environmental influences. Mental illness came to be perceived as part of a continuum with mental health. Symptom patterns were seen as clues to the timing or nature of the stressor(s), rather than as potential markers of specific disease processes. These ideas are reflected in the language of the first edition of the *Diagnostic and Statistical Manual* (DSM-I, published in 1952), in which the term *reaction* followed the name of most disorders. For example, an individual might be diagnosed as experiencing a "schizophrenic reaction," implying that an understanding of the disorder and its treatment would begin by determining environmental factors to which the person might be reacting. Further, prevailing treatment approaches of that era were largely nonspecific to any given diagnosis, and thus the importance of establishing diagnoses was of only marginal significance.

By the 1960s, however, several factors changed this situation, leading to a renewed interest in diagnostic practices in psychiatry. First, breakthroughs in psychopharmacology provided psychiatrists for the first time with a variety of safe and effective somatic therapies. Some of these, such as lithium for mania or tricyclics for depression, appeared to be relatively specific. Consequently, it became important to diagnose patients correctly, since diagnosis had clinically meaningful treatment implications. A second major factor was the recognition, through a series of studies, that diagnostic practices and concepts varied widely across geographic boundaries. For example, two large cross-national studies of diagnosis, the International Pilot Study of Schizophrenia and the United States/United Kingdom study, demonstrated that American psychiatrists tended substantially to over-diagnose schizophrenia in comparison with most of their international colleagues. Other studies revealed such differences even within countries as well as across temporal boundaries (i.e., patterns of diagnoses changed dramatically within a given institution over the span of one decade, without any evidence of a shift in the patient population). These problems in diagnostic reliability appeared to be primarily attributable to limitations in the existing nosology. It became apparent that without a more common and reliable psychiatric language, progress in research and clinical care would be severely impeded.

The goal of achieving high levels of diagnostic reliability was realized in the 1970s through the use of operationalized diagnostic criteria systems. In the United States, this began with the Washington University Criteria in 1972 and was followed by the Research Diagnostic Criteria in 1975. Originally intended for research purposes, the criterion-based method of diagnosis came into broad clinical use with the publication of DSM-III in 1980. The wide acceptance of DSM-III, and its impact on psychiatric practice not only in the United States but throughout much of the world, surpassed the expectations of almost everyone, including those involved in its development. Emphasis on making correct diagnoses was not just intellectually respectable again: it was seen as mandatory for doing good clinical work and good research.

There were some drawbacks to this phenomenon, however. The entrenchment of DSM-III, and later DSM-III-R in both clinical practice and psychiatric education made it easy to forget that these diagnostic categories reflected "tentative agreements to agree," based on the available knowledge of the time. The DSM manuals have been increasingly used as the main textbooks of psychiatry by medical students, nonpsychiatric medical colleagues, and even mental health clinicians. The symptoms listed in the various criteria sets are perceived as the "core" symptoms of the respective disorders, despite the fact that they may have been chosen on the basis of psychometric properties such as reliability or specificity, rather than on any evidence of their centrality to the disorder. In short, DSM-III and DSM-III-R constructs have tended to be reified, such that the syndromes they describe are easily mistaken for discrete diseases whose mechanisms are understood.

With the completion of DSM-IV, psychiatric nosology still remains at the syndromal level. However, many are optimistic that the mechanisms and causes of mental disorders will ultimately be revealed by combining increasingly sophisticated neuroscience technologies with careful phenomenological assessment. A variety of structured interview instruments and rating scales have been developed to enhance the reliability and validity of such phenomenological assessment, not only at the level of diagnosis, but of individual signs and symptoms as well. This allows for validity testing of different diagnostic constructs, against an increasing number of potential validators. Thus contemporary psychiatrists have returned to the methods of Kraepelin and his colleagues, but are now armed with more sophisticated methods.

The following references provide a selection of classic texts and articles that chronicle the development of this "neo-Kraepelinian revival" and stress the empirical approach to describing phenomenology and diagnosis in psychiatry.

Classic Historical Texts

1. **Bleuler E:** *Dementia Praecox or the Group of Schizophrenias.* Translated by Zinkin J. New York, International Universities Press, 1950

   In this classic contribution by Bleuler, he argues that schizophrenia or the splitting of the mental apparatus characterizes the syndrome or group of diseases that Kraepelin called dementia praecox.

2. **Fish FJ:** *Clinical Psychopathology: Signs and Symptoms in Psychiatry.* Briston, England, Wright, 1967

   In this excellent primer, Fish presents a coherent overview of the signs and symptoms of psychiatric disorder. The work reflects the mainstream views of British psychiatry in the 1960s.

3. **Jaspers KL:** *General Psychopathology.* Translated by Hoenig J, Hamilton MW. Manchester, England, Manchester University Press, 1963

   In this classic text, the author attempts to define, clarify, and systematize our knowledge of psychopathology from a phenomenological perspective. The text is most successful when it discusses discrete psychopathological phenomena, which can easily be located in this large text with the index and table of contents. The discussion of disease entities is more controversial, but has had a major influence on European psychiatry, principally through Kurt Schneider and Mayer-Gross.

4. **Kraepelin E:** *Manic-Depressive Insanity and Paranoia.* Edinburgh, Scotland, Livingstone, 1921 (also available from Salem, NH, Ayer Co, 1976)

   Now available in facsimile, this classic test is best understood as a work in progress that documents Kraepelin's continually evolving views. It is as relevant today as it was in 1920.

5. **Kraepelin E:** *Dementia Praecox and Paraphrenia.* Edited by Robertson GM. Huntington, NY, Krieger, 1971

   This classic contribution has become increasingly important during the past decade: it is Kraepelin's most developed view of his concept of dementia praecox. Of special interest is the precision and liveliness of the clinical phenomenology. No one, with the possible exception of Bleuler, has done it better.

6. **Leonhard K:** *The Classification of Endogenous Psychoses,* 5th Edition. Edited by Robins E. New York, Wiley, 1979

The author describes his classification derived from clinical observations and family studies. The book is of interest for its challenge of the historic classifications of Kraepelin and Bleuler. See especially his discussion of cycloid psychoses.

7. **Schneider K:** *Clinical Psychopathology.* Translated by Hamilton MW. New York, Grune & Stratton, 1959

This general textbook of psychopathology contains Schneider's description of his highly influential listing of "first-rank" symptoms of schizophrenia. Although not rich with clinical detail, it is interesting reading for its approach to the psychoses and personality disorders.

Diagnostic Criteria

8. **American Psychiatric Association:** *Diagnostic and Statistical Manual of Mental Disorders,* 3rd Edition. Washington, DC, American Psychiatric Association, 1980

DSM-III departed from previous editions by incorporating the methods of operationalized criteria to make psychiatric diagnoses. It produced a major change in American and international approaches to the collection of both clinical and research assessments and focused attention of the importance of accurate and reliable diagnosis.

9. **American Psychiatric Association:** *Diagnostic and Statistical Manual of Mental Disorders,* 3rd Edition, Revised. Washington, DC, American Psychiatric Association, 1987

This revision was intended to clarify ambiguities and inconsistencies in the classification, diagnostic criteria, and text of DSM-III, which had come to light during the intervening years. Although ultimately accepted by the majority of the psychiatric community, it was met with far less enthusiasm than its predecessor and set a tone of wariness and skepticism for subsequent revisions.

10. **American Psychiatric Association:** *Diagnostic and Statistical Manual of Mental Disorders,* 4th Edition. Washington, DC, American Psychiatric Association, 1994

This latest edition of the DSM represents the state of the art.

11. **Feighner JP, Robins E, Guze SB, Woodruff RA Jr, Winokur G, Munoz R:** Diagnostic criteria for use in psychiatric research. *Arch Gen Psychiatry* 26:57–63, 1972

This article presents a set of diagnostic criteria for 14 psychiatric disorders. This was the first system that employed the method of highly specific itemized criteria for psychiatric diagnosis and paved the way for the development of more inclusive systems, culminating in the publication of DSM-III.

12. **Frances A, Pincus HA, Widiger TA, Davis WW, First MB:** DSM-IV: Work in Progress. *Am J Psychiatry* 147:1439–1448, 1990

This article provides a conceptual overview of the rationale behind the development of DSM-IV. The authors outline the three stages of its empirical documentation: systematic literature reviews, analysis of unpublished data, and field trials. They also summarize the conceptual issues involved in revising nomenclature, such as the definition of mental disorder, the balance between multiple diagnosis and differential diagnosis, the use of categories versus dimensions, and the issues involved in the construction of criteria.

13. **Jampala VC, Sierles FS, Taylor MA:** The use of DSM-III in the United States: a case of not going by the book. *Compr Psychiatry* 29:39–47, 1988

In a random survey of 1,000 psychiatrists, most of whom endorsed the use of DSM-III, only a small minority were found to apply all aspects of the criteria with precision (using the diagnosis of mood disorders as an example). The authors conclude that the process by which clinicians actually make diagnoses differs from that required by diagnostic manuals and that diagnostic criteria should be simplified and limited to features that characterize the "gestalt" of the syndrome.

14. **Klerman GL, Vaillant GE, Spitzer RL, Michels R:** A debate on DSM-III. *Am J Psychiatry* 141:539–553, 1984

Although widely accepted, DSM-III was controversial. Here, the arguments are concisely and eloquently presented by leading proponents and opponents.

15. **Loranger AW:** The impact of DSM-III on diagnostic practice in a university hospital: a comparison of DSM-II and DSM-III in 10914 patients. *Arch Gen Psychiatry* 47:672–675, 1990

The author compared diagnostic patterns over the 5-year periods just before and after the adoption of DSM-III in his hospital. A marked reduction in the diagnosis of schizophrenia and a corresponding increase in the diagnosis of affective disorders was noted during the DSM-III years, along with a more than twofold increase in the diagnosis of personality disorders.

16. **Skodol AE, Spitzer RL** (eds): *An Annotated Biography of DSM-III.* Washington, DC, American Psychiatric Press, 1987

This volume has two components. Two introductory sections provide a general overview of the development of conceptualization of DSM-III, including topics such as nosology, diagnostic assessment, epidemiological perspectives, and education and training. A description of the rationale behind the development of various specific sections (e.g., childhood disorders, substance use disorders, schizophrenia and other psychotic disorders) is also provided in individual chapters. The second major component of the book consists of a listing of major articles that have used DSM approaches to study a broad range of topic areas. These key articles are accompanied by annotations that summarize the purpose of the article, its methods, and its results.

17. **Spitzer RL, Endicott J, Robins E:** Research Diagnostic Criteria: rationale and reliability. *Arch Gen Psychiatry* 35:773–782, 1978

The authors describe the initial reliability studies for their Research Diagnostic Criteria, which remains widely used in research and, along with the Washington University criteria, represents the seminal thinking that culminated in the creation of the DSM-III.

18. **Spitzer RL, Gibbon M, Skodol AE, Williams JBW, First MB:** *DSM-III-R Case Book.* Washington, DC, American Psychiatric Press, 1989

This volume was designed as an educational clinical tool that would complement the DSM criteria. It consists of a variety of case histories, submitted by clinicians throughout the United States and from international sites, accompanied by a discussion of differential diagnosis, a recommended DSM-III-R diagnosis, and information about follow-up.

19. **Tischler GL** (ed): *Diagnosis and Classification in Psychiatry: A Critical Appraisal of DSM-III.* New York, Cambridge University Press, 1987

This volume provides a comprehensive review of the utility and application of DSM-III. It includes a review of nosological principles; a description of the multiaxial approach; and a discussion of the clinical, educational, and administrative applications of DSM-III. A review of each of the major sections (e.g., personality disorders, anxiety and somatoform disorders, organic mental disorders, childhood disorders) is provided by senior investigators in each of the relevant content areas, with efforts to include both empirical and psychodynamic perspectives.

20. **World Health Organization:** *Classification of Mental and Behavioral Disorders (ICD-10): Clinical Descriptions and Diagnostic Guidelines.* Geneva, Switzerland, World Health Organization, 1992

Chapter 5 of the International Classification of Disease provides a description of a broad range of mental illnesses. The document includes both descriptions, designed for general clinical use, and specific criteria, designed primarily for research applications.

21. **Zimmerman M:** Why are we rushing to publish DSM-IV? *Arch Gen Psychiatry* 45:1135–1138, 1988

In this essay, the author argues that DSM-IV is being prepared prematurely, allowing for insufficient time for the accumulation of an adequate data base to guide its development, and resulting in unnecessary disruption to clinical and research practices.

Diagnostic Reliability

22. **Bartko JJ, Carpenter WT:** On the methods and theory of reliability. *J Nerv Ment Dis* 163:307–317, 1976

This is a readable yet relatively sophisticated discussion of reliability measures used in psychiatry, intended for a general psychiatric readership. It clarifies some of the common misperceptions in the area and explains appropriate reliability statistics suitable for different purposes.

23. **Grove WM, Andreasen NC, McDonald-Scott P, Keller MB, Shapiro RW:** Reliability studies of psychiatric diagnosis: theory and practice. *Arch Gen Psychiatry* 38:408–413, 1981

In this methodological article, the authors interpret trends in reliability studies of psychiatric diagnosis in the context of problems in research design and execution of such studies. The focus is on limitations of commonly used statistical techniques; alternative solutions are offered.

24. **Helzer JE, Robins LN, Taibleson M, Woodruff RA Jr, Reich T, Wish ED:** Reliability of psychiatric diagnosis, I: a methodological review. *Arch Gen Psychiatry* 34:129–133, 1977

25. **Helzer JE, Clayton PJ, Pambakian R, Reich T, Woodruff RA Jr, Reveley MA:** Reliability of psychiatric diagnosis, II: the test-retest reliability of psychiatric classification. *Arch Gen Psychiatry* 34:136–141, 1977

The authors present valuable insight on the problems of interrater reliability and recommend as correctives structured interviews, concise diagnostic criteria, and the creation of a residual diagnostic category, undiagnosed psychiatric illness. These two articles are essential reading for all those evaluating or designing psychiatric research. Reliability data for the Washington University criteria are provided.

26. **Kendell RE, Cooper JE, Gourlay AJ, Copeland JR, Sharpe L, Gurland BJ:** Diagnostic criteria of American and British psychiatrists. *Arch Gen Psychiatry* 25:123–130, 1971

This article presents the difference in diagnostic criteria for schizophrenia and manic depression in England and America as it existed in 1971. This study provided impetus for critical reevaluation of American diagnostic practices.

27. **Kreitman N, Sainsbury P, Morrissey J:** The reliability of psychiatric assessment: an analysis. *Journal of Mental Science* 107:887–908, 1961

This early study called attention to the problem of poor reliability in psychiatric assessment. This study initiated a series of subsequent studies that questioned agreement between clinicians, leading ultimately to the efforts to develop diagnostic criteria and structured interviews.

28. **Kuriansky JB, Deming WE, Gurland BJ:** On trends in the diagnosis of schizophrenia. *Am J Psychiatry* 131:402–408, 1974

This small but elegant study found that more than 80% of admissions to a New York psychiatric facility in the early 1950s were diagnosed with schizophrenia, as opposed to less than 40% in the same facility a decade earlier. Rediagnosis by research psychiatrists revealed no differences between the patient groups, demonstrating changes in the boundaries of diagnostic concepts over time.

29. **Shrout PE, Spitzer RL, Fleiss JL:** Quantification of agreement in psychiatric diagnosis revisited. *Arch Gen Psychiatry* 44:172–177, 1987

The authors review methodological issues and controversies concerning the use of the kappa statistic, arguing that it remains the statistic of choice for quantification of chance-corrected diagnostic agreement.

30. **Spitzer RL, Cohen J, Fleiss JL, Endicott J:** Quantification of agreement in psychiatric diagnosis. *Arch Gen Psychiatry* 17:83–87, 1967

In this seminal contribution, the authors summarized the significant problems in quantifying psychiatric diagnosis and recommended use of the weighted kappa to measure reliability and computer-assisted diagnosis.

31. **Spitzer RL, Endicott J, Robins E:** Clinical criteria for psychiatric diagnosis and DSM-III. *Am J Psychiatry* 132:1187–1192, 1975

The authors argue that criterion variance (the formal inclusion or exclusion of specific criteria) is the greatest source of unreliability in psychiatric diagnosis. Their view was accepted and is reflected in the structure of DSM-III.

32. **Ward CH, Beck AT, Mendelson M, Mock JD, Erbaugh JK:** The psychiatric nomenclature: reasons for diagnostic disagreement. *Arch Gen Psychiatry* 7:198–205, 1962

   The authors of this article undertook a study in diagnostic reliability and went on to determine and quantify causes of disagreement. The majority of disagreements were attributed to various limitations in the nosological system employed, which as the first DSM. This study was one of the first to demonstrate the need for more specific diagnostic guidelines.

Structured Interviews

33. **Andreasen NC, Flaum M, Arndt S:** The Comprehensive Assessment of Symptoms and History (CASH): an instrument for assessing diagnostic and psychopathology. *Arch Gen Psychiatry* 49:615–623, 1992

   The Comprehensive Assessment of Symptoms and History, a semi-structured interview, is designed to provide a flexible data base for research studies because the information base collected is broad. It is not wedded to a specific diagnostic system, but rather permits clinicians and investigators to make diagnoses using a wide range of systems, including Research Diagnostic Criteria, DSM-III, DSM-III-R, and the *International Classification of Diseases.* The interview is based on the rationale that because disorders in psychiatry are not at present defined at the etiological or pathophysiological level, diagnostic criteria are prone to ongoing revision as our knowledge base changes, and therefore an adaptable data base is required. Interrater reliability and test-retest reliability for this study have been documented to be acceptable to excellent.

34. **Carpenter WT Jr, Sacks MH, Strauss JS, Bartko JJ, Rayner J:** Evaluating signs and symptoms: comparison of structured interview and clinical approaches. *Br J Psychiatry* 128:397–403, 1976

   In this comparison of structured interviews with routine clinical assessment, it was found that the structured interview is generally acceptable in documenting symptoms but is inadequate in documenting signs.

35. **Endicott J, Spitzer RL:** A diagnostic interview: the Schedule for Affective Disorders and Schizophrenia. *Arch Gen Psychiatry* 35:837–844, 1978

   The authors describe a structured diagnostic interview designed to obtain detailed information about the current episode of illness and level of functioning during the week prior to evaluation. A lifetime version is also available for epidemiological work. The Schedule for Affective Disorders and Schizophrenia is currently one of the most widely used for psychiatric research in the United States. This interview forms the basis for making Research Diagnostic Criteria diagnoses.

36. **McGorry PD, Copolov DL, Singh BS:** Royal Park Multidiagnostic Instrument for Psychosis, part I: rationale and review. *Schizophr Bull* 16:501–515, 1990

The Royal Park Multidiagnostic Instrument for Psychosis is a semistructured interview designed to collect information concerning a broad range of signs and symptoms, which can then be applied to making diagnoses using a broad range of diagnostic systems. This interview is one of the most flexible diagnostic instruments currently available. Its reliability has also been carefully assessed.

37. **Robins LN, Helzer JE, Croughan J, Ratclaff KS:** National Institute of Mental Health Diagnostic Interview Schedule: its history, characteristics and validity. *Arch Gen Psychiatry* 38:381–389, 1981

The Diagnostic Interview Schedule was designed as a standard structured interview for making DSM-III diagnoses in large community samples. Its major virtues are ease and efficiency of use, accessibility to raters who do not have medical training, and well-developed psychometric properties. Its reliability and validity have been carefully assessed. It provided the nosological foundation for the Epidemiologic Catchment Area study, a major investigation of the incidence and prevalence of psychiatric disorders in the United States.

38. **Robins LN, Wing J, Wittchen HU, Helzer JE, Babor TF, Burke J, Farmer A, Jablenski A, Pickens R, Regier DA, Sartorius N, Towie LH:** The Composite International Diagnostic Interview. *Arch Gen Psychiatry* 45:1069–1077, 1988

This article introduces the Composite International Diagnostic Interview, which is an adapted version of the Diagnostic Interview Schedule, for use in international epidemiological studies. Like the Diagnostic Interview Schedule, it is fully structured and designed to be administered by lay interviewers. Coverage of signs and symptoms were substantially broadened to allow diagnoses to be generated from multiple diagnostic systems.

39. **Spitzer RL, Williams JBW, Gibbon M, First MB:** The Structured Clinical Interview for DSM-III-R (SCID), I: history, rationale, and description. *Arch Gen Psychiatry* 49:624–629, 1992

A technique for making diagnoses using a semistructured interview is described. The Structured Clinical Interview for DSM-III-R uses a decision tree approach, which permits the clinician to run through various modules and to skip out of sections. The major output from this instrument is the documentation of the presence or absence of a range of DSM-III-R diagnoses. Reliability of the instrument has been evaluated and has been found to be good to excellent.

40. **Stangl D, Pfohl B, Zimmerman M, Bowers W:** A Structured Interview for DSM-III Personality Disorder. *Arch Gen Psychiatry* 42:591–596, 1985

This article introduces the Structured Interview for DSM-III Personality Disorder, a semistructured interview designed to generate DSM-III Axis II diagnoses.

41. **Wing JK, Cooper JE, Sartorius N:** *Measurement and Classification of Psychiatric Symptoms.* Cambridge, Cambridge University Press, 1974

This volume describes the Present State Exam, a semistructured interview instrument developed in the 1960s at the Maudsley Hospital in England and used in several important studies of that era, including the United States/the United Kingdom study and the International Pilot Study of Schizophrenia. Strengths include broad symptom coverage and an accompanying system of generating diagnosis by a computer algorithm program (CATEGO). Limitations are that it covers symptoms only over the time frame of the past 1 month and that its administration requires a trained and experienced clinician.

42. **Wing JK, Babor T, Brugha T, Burke J, Cooper JE, Giel R, Jablenski A, Regier D, Sartorius N:** SCAN: Schedule for Clinical Assessment in Neuropsychiatry. *Arch Gen Psychiatry* 47:589–593, 1990

The Schedule for Clinical Assessment in Neuropsychiatry (SCAN), developed through a collaboration between the World Health Organization and investigators in Great Britain and the United States, grows out of earlier work that led to the development of the Present State Examination, which is included as one of the core schedules within the SCAN. In addition, however, the SCAN permits documentation concerning multiple episodes of illness that have occurred in the past. The SCAN was developed to facilitate the study of psychopathology across nations, regions, and cultures, with the goal of providing a basis for collaborative studies that will examine causes, risk factors, and outcomes of mental disorders. The SCAN and the Composite International Diagnostic Interview were designed as complimentary instruments: the former is less structured and requires an experienced professional interviewer, whereas the latter was designed for lay interviewers.

Rating Scales

43. **Andreasen NC:** Negative symptoms in schizophrenia: definition and reliability. *Arch Gen Psychiatry* 39:784–788, 1982

This article introduced the Scale for the Assessment of Negative Symptoms. Negative symptoms had been de-emphasized in the DSM-III criteria for schizophrenia partly because of concerns about an inability to assess them in a reliable manner. The development of this instrument was an important step leading to the resurgence of interest in negative symptoms over the past decade.

44. **Chapman LJ, Chapman JP:** Scales for rating psychotic and psychotic-like experiences as continua. *Schizophr Bull* 6:477–489, 1980

This article presents a rating scale that rates psychotic phenomena on a continuum of deviancy rather than as dichotomously deviant or non-deviant. The rating scale and the demonstration of its application challenge a prevailing view that psychotic symptoms are dichotomous events.

45. **Endicott J, Spitzer RL, Fleiss JL, Cohen J:** The Global Assessment Scale: a procedure for measuring overall severity of psychiatric disturbance. *Arch Gen Psychiatry* 33:766–771, 1976

This article provides a description of the Global Assessment Scale, a sensitive measure of overall severity of psychiatric illness, that has a wide application in psychiatric research, especially for patients in the community.

46. **Folstein MF, Folstein SE, McHugh P:** "Mini Mental State": a practical method for grading the cognitive state of patients for clinicians. *J Psychiatr Res* 12:189–198, 1975

The Mini Mental State Exam provides a standardized technique for rating the severity of cognitive dysfunctions in a broad range of disorders. It assesses various aspects of mental status, such as orientation, memory, and attention.

47. **Hamilton M:** A rating scale for depression. *J Neurol Neurosurg Psychiatry* 23:56–62, 1960

Hamilton presents a widely used objective rating scale for depression. Clinicians as well as researchers will find it a useful device to reduce the effects of idiosyncratic clinical assessment. Often used to monitor clinical change in psychopharmacological research, it is one of the oldest rating scales available, but still widely used.

48. **Overall JE, Gorham D:** Brief Psychiatric Rating Scale. *Psychol Rep* 10:799–812, 1962

The Brief Psychiatric Rating Scale is a widely used instrument that evaluates a range of symptoms, such as conceptual disorganization, anxiety, or depression. This scale was derived through factor analysis. It represents the first major effort to standardize clinical assessment, and it remains a central tool in clinical drug trials.

Approaches to the Development of Classification Systems

49. **Blashfield RK:** *The Classification of Psychopathology: Neo-Kraepelinian and Quantitative Approaches.* New York, Plenum, 1984

This book provides an overview of two very different conceptual frameworks by which diagnostic systems may be derived. The first half deals with issues related to classification systems based on clinically derived diagnoses (the neo-Kraepelininan approach). The second half discusses the use of multivariate statistical techniques (mainly factor analysis and cluster analysis) to derive classification systems de novo.

50. **Blashfield RK, Draguns JG:** Toward a taxonomy of psychopathology: the purpose of psychiatric classification. *Br J Psychiatry* 129:574–583, 1976

In this provocative article, the authors argue that any biological classification or diagnostic system must be viewed as a historically determined reconciliation of different and often conflicting perspectives such as clinical, social, political, theoretical, scientific, and statistical.

51. **Everitt BS, Gourlay AJ, Kendell RE:** An attempt at validation of traditional psychiatric syndromes by cluster analysis. *Br J Psychiatry* 119:399–412, 1971

The authors employed a cluster analysis statistical technique to data from a population of psychiatric patients and found that identifiable clusters could be obtained for chronic schizophrenia, but no significant clustering for depression, personality disorder, alcoholism, or neuroses could be found. This is a well-conceived study.

52. **Garside RE, Roth M:** Multivariate statistical methods and problems of classification in psychiatry. *Br J Psychiatry* 133:53–67, 1978

The authors argue that multivariate statistical methods are uniquely valuable in validating psychiatric diagnoses and classifications, but acknowledge that a general agreement as how best to utilize these techniques has not been achieved.

53. **Grob GN:** Origins of DSM-I: a study in appearance and reality. *Am J Psychiatry* 148:421–431, 1991

The author traces the history of psychiatric nosology in the United States from its origins in the early 19th century to the introduction of the first DSM in 1952. It is argued that nosologies, psychiatric or otherwise, reflect not only the current ideological framework of the field, but are the product of a variety of cultural and historical determinants as well.

54. **Kendell RE:** Psychiatric diagnoses: a study of how they are made. *Br J Psychiatry* 122:437–445, 1973

Raters trained at the same institution made consensually validated diagnoses with only 2 or 5 minutes of exposure to videotapes of psychotic patients. This finding suggests that diagnoses of psychotic patients are made in the first few minutes of an interview.

55. **Kendler KS:** Toward a scientific psychiatric nosology: strengths and limitations. *Arch Gen Psychiatry* 47:969–973, 1990

In this essay, the author discusses the advantages and disadvantages of applying the scientific method (e.g., hypothesis generating and hypothesis testing) to psychiatric nosology. He suggests that many nosological questions can and should be empirically investigated, whereas others are "fundamentally nonempirical," and that developers of nosology must be aware of which is which.

56. **Mezzich JE, Von Cranach M** (eds): *International Classification in Psychiatry: Unity and Diversity.* Cambridge, Cambridge University Press, 1988

This volume includes contributions from a large number of international experts in psychiatric nosology. The first two sections present classification systems in contemporary use in a variety of countries including China, Nigeria, Egypt, and Brazil, and cross-national differences in concepts of specific diagnostic syndromes. This is followed by descriptions of assessment techniques and other methodological issues in psychiatric classification, from an international perspective.

57. **Pfohl B, Andreasen NC:** Development of classification systems in psychiatry. *Compr Psychiatry* 19:197–207, 1978

The authors provide a rational approach to the development of new classification systems in psychiatry, including statistical and methodological options to be considered, selection of patients and variables, division of patients into groups, development of diagnostic criteria, and evaluation of the diagnostic system itself.

58. **Robins E, Guze SB:** Establishment of diagnostic validity in psychiatric illness: its application to schizophrenia. *Am J Psychiatry* 126:983–987, 1970

This widely quoted statement on the basic requirements for defining a psychiatric illness by the Washington University group is notable for its emphasis on family and outcome studies as methods for validating a diagnosis. The principles are illustrated by demonstrating that "good" prognosis schizophrenia and "poor" prognosis schizophrenia may be two different illnesses. This article has provided a strong basis for reevaluating classification systems during the 1970s and 1980s.

59. **Shepherd M:** Psychotropic drugs and taxonomic systems. *Psychol Med* 10:25–33, 1980

Shepherd presents a biological and molecular classification and opens to question the whole concept of classification and the different purpose classification serves.

60. **Zubin J:** Classification of the behavior disorders. *Annu Rev Psychol* 18:373–406, 1967

This is a general discussion of problems of psychiatric classification by a widely respected senior researcher in the field. It has an excellent discussion of Jaspers and the relationship between psychopathology and personality.

12

Schizophrenia

Rajiv Tandon, M.D.

D espite several recent advances in our understanding of the neurobiology of schizophrenia, there are as yet no external validating criteria to guide clinicians in its diagnosis. Consequently, there is no "laboratory test" for schizophrenia, which is still diagnosed on the basis of certain "typical clinical features." No single sign or symptom is pathognomonic for schizophrenia, however, and the symptoms of an individual patient often change over time. All current definitions of schizophrenia derive from the concepts of Emil Kraepelin (who emphasized chronicity and deterioration), Eugen Bleuler (who gave prominence to fundamental "negative" symptoms), and Kurt Schneider (who stressed characteristic "first-rank" psychotic or positive symptoms). These elements are emphasized to different extents in the various nosological systems. The introduction of DSM-III in America in 1980 significantly reduced diagnostic discrepancy between psychiatrists in America (where Bleulerian symptoms held sway until then) and the rest of the world (where Schneiderian symptoms and Kraepelinian deterioration were emphasized). ICD-9 (the current version of the *International Classification of Diseases*) gives a descriptive definition of schizophrenia. DSM-III-R provided an operational definition emphasizing positive symptoms, decline in psychosocial function, tendency toward chronicity (6-month criterion) and requiring exclusion of organicity and mood disorder. DSM-IV and ICD-10 are more similar; both provide operational criteria, stress positive symptoms, and mention negative symptoms.

Over the past decade, there has been a dramatic increase in our knowledge about the neurobiology of schizophrenia. Coincident with the emergence of new technologies in neuroscience (particularly various techniques of brain imaging and molecular biology), there has been a rapid increase in data about the neuroanatomical, neurochemical, and neurophysiologic correlates of the illness and heightened hope of identifying a specific genetic defect in schizophrenia. The introduction of clozapine into general practice in America and delineation of its unique clinical properties represents the most significant advance in the pharmacological treatment of schizophrenia since the advent of neuroleptics in the 1950s; it has also prompted a new look at the neurochemistry of schizophrenia and spurred efforts toward developing better antischizophrenic drugs. There have been notable improvements in psychosocial interventions in terms of psychoeducation, social skills training, and rehabilitation. The recent emergence of support and advocacy groups represents another important development.

In view of this promising state of affairs, there is tremendous optimism in the field and a sense that we are close to a breakthrough in our understanding of the nature of schizophrenia and the development of significantly better treatments. It is important to temper this optimism with caution and a sense of humility. Many rock-solid important findings of yesteryear are considered trivial or just plain wrong today. We should expect that some of today's seemingly certain findings will meet a similar fate tomorrow. Awareness of areas of disagreement is perhaps just as important as knowledge of "generally accepted facts." Similarly, an awareness of significant paradigms and theories of previous years (even though some may be discredited today) is important since many provided the basis for the advances of the past decade, and modern concepts are best understood against the background of their evolution.

Introduction to some of the classics, provision of an overview of current knowledge in various areas of schizophrenia, and an acquaintance with some topics of controversy in the field were the major guiding principles in this selection of core readings in schizophrenia. Other criteria in the selection of these core readings included 1) readings having a strong impact on the field (e.g., in terms of citation index, changing direction of research or practice); 2) seminal works or excellent recent comprehensive reviews; 3) works representative of major areas of current or past thought; 4) readings balanced in terms of coverage of various areas and different perspectives; and 5) written-well works easily available to most readers.

Clearly, in dealing with the voluminous literature in schizophrenia and the constraints of a limited bibliography, significant omissions will occur. This set of core readings should, however, acquaint the reader with some of the more important past and present issues and provide a reasonably inclusive framework for understanding contemporary and future approaches to clinical practice and research in schizophrenia. It is equally likely for readers to feel overwhelmed by what they consider "an impossibly long" and overexhaustive list of core readings. The following strategy may be useful. For an introduction to a given field, readers may want to start with a "core" overview or review paper; these listings are marked by an asterisk. For a more extensive review of an area, one can consult classic papers and papers highlighting a major area of controversy in that section. Articles pertaining to a particular major area of disagreement are grouped together; it is recommended that they be reviewed together to obtain a better awareness of the nature and relevance of the controversy. Certain topics relevant to schizophrenia are discussed in other chapters in this volume, particularly Chapter 9, "Psychiatric Epidemiology" (Horwath and Weissman); Chapter 11, "Nosology, Phenomenology, and Diagnosis" (Andreasen and Flaum); Chapter 20, "Chronically Mentally Ill Patients" (Cutler); and Chapter 36, "Psychopharmacology" (Salzman).

The books and articles selected in this bibliography are organized into the following sections: 1) reviews and overviews; 2) conceptual issues and models; 3) classification and phenomenology; 4) course; 5) heterogeneity and subtypes; 6) genetics; 7) epidemiology; 8) psychodynamic, family, and psychosocial issues; 9) neurochemistry; 10) structural and functional brain abnormalities; 11) neuropsychology and psychophysiology; 11) pharmacological treatment; and 12) psychological and psychosocial treatment. Virtually all topics contain one or more recent reviews, seminal papers and classics, and major areas of controversy (with representative papers grouped together).

Reviews and Overviews

1. **Nasrallah HA** (series ed): *Handbook of Schizophrenia*, Vols. 1–5. Amsterdam, Netherlands, Elsevier, 1986–1991

   This is an encyclopedic reference, not an overview or core reading material. It is by far the most comprehensive resource of information on schizophrenia. Readers may refer to this set of volumes for discussion of virtually any topic in schizophrenia. In addition to an in-depth coverage of various topics, there are excellent summary chapters on most topics as well. Uniformly good in quality, there are five multi-authored volumes in this series:

   - Volume 1: *The Neurology of Schizophrenia*. Edited by Nasrallah HA, Weinberger DR, 1986
   - Volume 2: *Neurochemistry and Neuropharmacology of Schizophrenia*. Edited by Henn FA, DeLisi LE, 1988
   - Volume 3: *Nosology, Epidemiology, and Genetics of Schizophrenia*. Edited by Tsuang MT, Simpson JC, 1988

- Volume 4: *Neurophysiology, Psychophysiology, and Information Processing.* Edited by Steinhauer SR, Gruzelier JH, Zubin J, 1991
- Volume 5: *Psychosocial Treatments of Schizophrenia.* Edited by Herz MI, Keith SJ, Docherty JP, 1990

2. **Wyatt RJ, Alexander RC, Egan MF, Kirch DG:** Schizophrenia, just the facts: what do we know, how well do we know it? *Schizophr Res* 1:3–18, 1988

   This is a succinct summary of the salient features of schizophrenia in terms of their reproducibility and significance for understanding the disorder.

Conceptual Issues and Models

3. **Carpenter WT Jr, Buchanan RW, Kirkpatrick B, Tamminga C, Wood F:** Strong inference, theory testing, and the neuroanatomy of schizophrenia. *Arch Gen Psychiatry* 50:825–831, 1993

   As we rapidly accumulate data about the phenomenology, course, etiology, pathophysiology, and treatment of schizophrenia, the need for a conceptual framework or models around which to organize (and thereby make sense of) this knowledge becomes paramount. Carpenter et al. clearly articulate the need to apply principles of strong inference and theory falsification to the study of schizophrenia. They further outline one method for hypothesis testing centered on behavioral anatomy and the reduction of schizophrenia syndrome heterogeneity.

4. **Crow TJ, Ball J, Bloom SR, Brown R, Bruton CJ, Colter N, Frith CD, Johnstone EC, Owens DGC, Roberts GW:** Schizophrenia as an anomaly of development of cerebral asymmetry. *Arch Gen Psychiatry* 46:1145–1150, 1989

   Crow et al. propose that schizophrenia is a disorder of the genetic mechanisms that control the development of cerebral asymmetry.

5. **Feinberg I:** Schizophrenia: caused by a fault in programmed synaptic elimination during adolescence. *J Psychiatr Res* 17:319–334, 1983

   Citing evidence from various fields, Feinberg proposes that schizophrenia may be due to a defect in the process of synaptic pruning (an important maturational process in adolescence).

6. **Murray RM, Lewis SW, Owen MJ, Foerster A:** The neuro-developmental origins of dementia praecox, in *Schizophrenia: The Major Issues.* Edited by McGuffin P, Bebbington P. London, Heinemann, 1988, pp. 90–107

Murray et al. present a neurodevelopmental perspective of schizophrenia and discuss the role of genetic and environmental factors in its etiology.

7. **Roth M:** Schizophrenia and the theories of Thomas Szasz. *Br J Psychiatry* 129:317–326, 1976

8. **Szasz TS:** Schizophrenia: the sacred symbol of psychiatry. *Br J Psychiatry* 129:308–316, 1976

Although Szasz's view of schizophrenia as a mythical construct developed by psychiatrists as part of society's attempt to label and control deviant behavior is much less influential today than it first was, his eloquent elaboration and Roth's brilliant critique of his theories are worthwhile reading.

9. **Weinberger DR:** Implications of normal brain development for the pathogenesis of schizophrenia. *Arch Gen Psychiatry* 44:660–669, 1987

In this article, Weinberger proposes an elegant neurodevelopmental model of schizophrenia. He suggests that the primary pathology in schizophrenia is a fixed brain lesion from early in life interacting with normal brain maturational events in adolescence and early adulthood.

10. **Zubin J, Steinhauer SR, Day R, van Kammen DP:** Schizophrenia at the crossroads: a blueprint for the 80s. *Compr Psychiatry* 26:217–240, 1985

Zubin et al. discuss schizophrenia from multiple perspectives and pose questions and approaches for future research. Zubin is one of this century's principal figures in schizophrenia research.

Classification and Phenomenology

11. **Andreasen NC, Flaum F:** Schizophrenia: the characteristic symptoms. *Schizophr Bull* 17:27–49, 1991

This article reviews the validity and descriptive value of the various signs and symptoms used to classify schizophrenia. The DSM-III-R definition of schizophrenia is compared with that proposed in ICD-10, and principles to guide the development of DSM-IV are suggested.

12. **Bleuler E:** *Dementia Praecox or the Group of Schizophrenias,* (1911). Edited By Zinkin J. New York, International Universities Press, 1950

13. **Kraepelin E:** *Dementia Praecox and Paraphrenia,* (1919). Edited by Robertson GM. New York, Krieger, 1971

These are the classic texts that shaped current thinking about schizophrenia. Their richness and thoroughness of clinical description is unparalleled. There is a wealth of information in these books, which are as relevant today as they were when they were originally published.

14. **Crow TJ:** The continuum of psychosis and its genetic origins. *Br J Psychiatry* 156:788–797, 1990

15. **Cloninger RC, Martin RL, Guze SB, Clayton PJ:** Diagnosis and prognosis in schizophrenia. *Arch Gen Psychiatry* 42:15–25, 1985

16. **Kendell RE, Brockington IF:** The identification of disease entities and the relationship between schizophrenic and affective psychoses. *Br J Psychiatry* 137:324–331, 1980

17. **Procci WR:** Schizoaffective psychosis: fact or fiction. *Arch Gen Psychiatry* 33:1167–1178, 1976

18. **Tsuang MT, Winokur G, Crowe RR:** Morbidity risks of schizophrenia and affective disorders among first degree relatives of patients with schizophrenia, mania, depression and surgical conditions. *Br J Psychiatry* 137:497–504, 1980

The precise demarcation between schizophrenia and mood disorders is still a matter of some debate; the two disorders have been found to be much less different (e.g., in terms of phenomenology, course, neurobiological abnormalities) than previously recognized. Although the overwhelming consensus among experts is still in favor of such a distinction, the precise boundaries are unclear. Cloninger et al. and Kendell and Brockington present unique studies that reached opposite conclusions regarding this issue (using novel methods for identifying a boundary between syndromes). Crow and Tsuang et al. address this question from a genetic standpoint. Procci's is a hallmark article on schizoaffective disorder. This issue is likely to attract greater attention in the next decade.

19. **David AS:** Insight and psychosis. *Br J Psychiatry* 156:798–808, 1990

This is a scholarly review of the concept of insight in psychosis from perspectives of phenomenology, clinical research, and experimental psychology; a scheme to standardize its assessment is proposed.

20. **Davison K:** Schizophrenia-like psychoses associated with organic cerebral disorders: a review. *Psychiatric Developments* 1:1–34, 1983

This is a comprehensive review of physical diseases that can mimic schizophrenia. The relationship of these organic cerebral disorders to "true schizophrenia" is discussed in clinical, genetic, and conceptual terms.

21. **Fish FJ:** *Clinical Psychopathology: Signs and Symptoms in Psychiatry*, 2nd Edition. Edited by Hamilton M. Bristol, John Wright, 1985

This is an excellent overview of the signs and symptoms of psychiatric disorder. The chapters on disorders of thought and perception are particularly relevant.

22. ***Mellor CS:** First rank symptoms of schizophrenia. *Br J Psychiatry* 117:15–23, 1970

This article provides a clear description of the Schneiderian "first-rank" symptoms with excellent clinical examples.

23. **Overall JE, Gorham DR:** The Brief Psychiatric Rating Scale. *Psychol Rep* 10:799–812, 1962

This article provides the original description of the most widely used scale for the clinical assessment of schizophrenia.

Course

24. **Bleuler M:** *The Schizophrenic Disorders.* New Haven, CT, Yale University Press, 1972

25. ***Ciompi L:** The natural history of schizophrenia in the long term. *Br J Psychiatry* 136:413–420, 1980

26. **Harding CM, Brooks GW, Ashikaga T, Strauss JS, Breier A:** The Vermont longitudinal study of persons with severe mental illness. *Am J Psychiatry* 144:718–735, 1987

Bleuler and Ciompi report on hallmark European follow-up studies that documented the heterogeneity of outcome in schizophrenia. The study of Harding et al. is a major American study that suggested a more favorable, long-term outcome for schizophrenia than previously believed.

27. ***Chapman J:** The early symptoms of schizophrenia. *Br J Psychiatry* 112:225–251, 1966

This is a classic study that provides a rich description of changes in mental function subjectively experienced by a group of schizophrenic patients in the prodromal phase of an acute psychotic episode.

28. Longitudinal perspectives on the pathophysiology of schizophrenia: examining the neurodevelopmental versus degenerative perspectives. *Schizophr Res* 5:183–210, 1991

    Although structural brain abnormalities in schizophrenia are fairly well documented, it is unclear as to when they occur in the course of the illness. Although there is clinical evidence for progression, histopathological data suggest an early developmental process; conceivably, there may be both developmental and degenerative components that may be related to different elements of schizophrenic psychopathology. This is a collection of 18 well-referenced succinct summaries on this issue with multiple different perspectives and lines of investigation by major authorities in the field.

29. **Docherty JP, Van Kammen DP, Siris SG, Marder SR:** Stages of onset of schizophrenic psychosis. *Am J Psychiatry* 135:420–426, 1978

    On the basis of a comprehensive literature review, the authors discuss the stages in the process of psychotic decompensation in schizophrenic patients.

Heterogeneity and Subtypes

30. **Andreasen NC:** Negative symptoms in schizophrenia. *Arch Gen Psychiatry* 39:784–794, 1982

31. **Carpenter WT Jr, Heinrichs D, Wagman A:** Deficit and nondeficit forms of schizophrenia: the concept. *Am J Psychiatry* 145:578–583, 1988

32. **Crow TJ:** Molecular pathology of schizophrenia: more than one disease process? *Br Med J* 280:66–68, 1980

    The positive-negative symptom dichotomy has been of considerable heuristic value in explaining the heterogeneity of schizophrenia. These are the original articles that present the three major conceptual approaches to this area.

33. **Greden JF, Tandon R** (eds): *Negative Schizophrenic Symptoms: Pathophysiology and Clinical Implications.* Washington, DC, American Psychiatric Press, 1991

    This is a comprehensive, well-referenced review of current understanding of the phenomenology, pathophysiology, etiology, treatment, and clinical implications of negative symptoms in schizophrenia. The introduction and the conclusion together provide a simple introduction to the area of negative symptoms.

34. **Liddle PF:** The symptoms of schizophrenia: a re-examination of the positive-negative symptom dichotomy. *Br J Psychiatry* 151:145–151, 1987

The author presents data that suggest that schizophrenic symptoms are better understood in terms of a trichotomy (reality distortion, psychomotor poverty, and disorganization) rather than a positive-negative symptom dichotomy. This formulation is attracting increasing interest and support.

35. **McGlashan TH, Fenton WS:** Classical subtypes of schizophrenia. *Schizophr Bull* 17:609–623, 1991

This is an excellent review of the validity of the classical subtypes of schizophrenia.

36. **Murray RM, O'Callaghan E, Castle DJ, Lewis SW:** A neuro-developmental approach to the classification of schizophrenia. *Schizophr Bull* 18:319–332, 1992

This is another elegant conceptual model that attempts to explain the heterogeneity of the disorder. Murray et al. suggest that schizophrenia consists of three distinct illnesses: 1) "congenital," early-onset, predominantly male, "Kraepelinian" schizophrenia; 2) adult-onset, predominantly female, affective-like schizophrenia; and 3) very late-onset degenerative paraphrenia.

37. **Strauss JS, Carpenter WT Jr, Bartko JJ:** The diagnosis and understanding of schizophrenia, III: speculations on the processes that underlie schizophrenic symptoms and signs. *Schizophr Bull* 11:61–75, 1974

In an attempt to relate phenomenology to the concept of schizophrenia, the authors suggest that schizophrenic symptoms can be understood in terms of three distinct processes: positive symptoms, negative symptoms, and disorder of interpersonal relationships.

Genetics

38. **Fish B, Marcus J, Hans SL, Auerbach JG, Perdue S:** Infants at risk for schizophrenia: sequelae of a genetic neurointegrative defect. *Arch Gen Psychiatry* 49:221–235, 1992

This is a review of the hypothesis that the schizophrenia genotype is manifested in infants by a neurointegrative defect called pandysmaturation.

39. *Gottesman II, McGuffin P, Farmer AE: Clinical genetics as clues to the "real" genetics of schizophrenia. *Schizophr Bull* 13:23–47, 1987

This is an excellent review of the genetics of schizophrenia, emphasizing the clinical and epidemiologic perspectives.

40. **Kallman FJ:** The genetic theory of schizophrenia. *Am J Psychiatry* 103:309–322, 1946

This is a classic early family history and twin study that provided strong evidence for a genetic basis for schizophrenia.

41. **Kendler KS, Diehl SR:** The genetics of schizophrenia: a current, genetic-epidemiologic perspective. *Schizophr Bull* 19:261–285, 1993

A concise summary of the current status of the genetics of schizophrenia, this article discusses the applicability and limitations of molecular genetic strategies to understanding schizophrenia in the context of the more traditional clinical-epidemiologic perspective.

42. **Kety SS, Rosenthal D, Wender P, Schulsinger F:** Studies based on a total sample of adopted individuals and their relatives: why they were necessary, what they demonstrated and failed to demonstrate. *Schizophr Bull* 2:413–428, 1976

This is an excellent summary of the landmark Danish adoption studies of schizophrenia provided by the investigators themselves.

43. *Owen MJ, McGuffin P:** DNA and classical genetic markers in schizophrenia. *Eur Arch Psychiatry Neurol Sci* 240:197–203, 1991

This is a succinct introduction to association and linkage studies in schizophrenia. In fact, the entire issue of the journal is devoted to the molecular genetics of schizophrenia.

Epidemiology

44. *Hafner H:** Epidemiology of schizophrenia, in *Search for the Causes of Schizophrenia,* Vol. 1. Edited by Hafner H, Gattaz WF, Janzarik W. Berlin, Germany, Springer-Verlag, 1987, pp. 47–74

Hafner provides an excellent summary of major epidemiologic findings in schizophrenia.

45. **Hare EH:** Schizophrenia as a recent disease. *Br J Psychiatry* 153:521–531, 1988

46. **Jeste DV, del Carmen R, Lohr JB, Wyatt RJ:** Did schizophrenia exist before the eighteenth century? *Compr Psychiatry* 26:493–503, 1985

In these two reviews, the authors present a historical perspective on the occurrence of schizophrenia. They reach opposite conclusions on the important question of whether schizophrenia is a unique disease of the 19th–20th century (Hare) or was also fairly common before then (Jeste et al.).

47. **Kirch DG:** Infection and autoimmunity as etiologic factors in schizophrenia: a review and reappraisal. *Schizophr Bull* 19:355–370, 1993

   This is a concise summary of current understanding of the possible role of infection and autoimmunity in causing schizophrenia.

48. **Mednick SA, Machon RA, Huttunen MO, Bonett D:** Adult schizophrenia following exposure to an influenza epidemic. *Arch Gen Psychiatry* 45:189–192, 1988

   In this important epidemiologic study, the authors observed an association between second-trimester prenatal exposure to influenza and increased risk of developing schizophrenia.

49. *Sartorius N, Jablensky A, Korten A, Ernberg G, Anker M, Cooper JE, Day R:** Early manifestations and first-contact incidence of schizophrenia in different cultures. *Psychol Med* 16:909–928, 1986

   Initial findings of an important cross-cultural study on the occurrence and natural history of schizophrenia are presented. Findings of the previous International Pilot Study of Schizophrenia are also summarized in the introduction.

Psychodynamic, Family, and Psychosocial Issues

50. **Brown GW, Birley JLT, Wing JK:** Influence of family life on the course of schizophrenic disorders: a replication. *Br J Psychiatry* 121:241–258, 1972

51. **Kavanagh DJ:** Recent developments in expressed emotion and schizophrenia. *Br J Psychiatry* 160:601–620, 1992

   Brown et al. provide an important original study, and Kavanagh provides a more recent review on the concept of expressed emotion and its relevance to the course of schizophrenia.

52. **Goldberg EM, Morrison SL:** Schizophrenia and social class. *Br J Psychiatry* 109:785–802, 1963

   This is a classic study explaining the observed association between low socioeconomic class and higher admission rates for schizophrenia.

53. **McGlashan TH:** Schizophrenia: psychodynamic theories, in *Comprehensive Textbook of Psychiatry/V*, 5th Edition, Vol. 1. Edited by Kaplan HI, Sadock BJ. Baltimore, MD, Williams & Wilkins, 1989, pp. 745–756

   An excellent summary of various psychodynamic theories of schizophrenia, this review presents the salient features and critically evaluates the various "psychogenic" models of schizophrenia, suggesting an appropriate role for psychodynamic factors in the understanding and treatment of this disorder.

54. **Turner WM, Tsuang MT:** Impact of substance abuse on the course and outcome of schizophrenia. *Schizophr Bull* 16:87–95, 1990

   Turner and Tsuang review the psychomimetic effects of various drugs and the impact of substance abuse on the course and long-term outcome of schizophrenia.

Neurochemistry

55. **Carlsson A:** The current status of the dopamine hypothesis. *Neuropsychopharmacology* 1:179–186, 1988

   This is a perspective on the status of the dopamine hypothesis of schizophrenia by one of its original proponents. This perspective is critiqued by Klein, Friedhoff, Meltzer, and Snyder, and this is followed by a response by Carlsson.

56. **Carlsson M, Carlsson A:** Schizophrenia: a subcortical neurotransmitter imbalance syndrome? *Schizophr Bull* 16:425–432, 1990

57. **Davis KL, Kahn RS, Ko G, Davidson M:** Dopamine in schizophrenia: a review and reconceptualization. *Am J Psychiatry* 148:1474–1486, 1991

58. **Meltzer HY:** The mechanism of action of novel antipsychotic drugs. *Schizophr Bull* 17:263–287, 1991

59. **Tandon R, Greden JF:** Cholinergic hyperactivity and negative schizophrenic symptoms: a model of cholinergic/dopaminergic interactions in schizophrenia. *Arch Gen Psychiatry* 46:745–753, 1989

60. **van Kammen DP, Peters J, Yao J, van Kammen WB, Neylan T, Shaw D, Linnoila M:** Norepinephrine in acute exacerbations of chronic schizophrenia. *Arch Gen Psychiatry* 47:161–168, 1990

   There has been a recent reappraisal of the role of the dopamine system in schizophrenia, with two broad approaches being adopted. The "modified dopamine hypothesis" postulates a co-occurrence of high and low dopamine activity in different brain regions and suggests that imbalance between these dopamine systems is the principal neurochemical abnormality in schizophrenia (elegantly summarized by Davis et al.). The other approach focuses on other neurotransmitters—serotonin (Meltzer), acetylcholine (Tandon and Greden), glutamate (Carlsson and Carlsson), and norepinephrine (van Kammen et al.)—in addition to dopamine and suggests that interactions and imbalance between dopamine and one of these other neurotransmitter systems is of primary pathophysiologic importance in schizophrenia.

61. **Farde L, Wiesel F-A, Stone-Elander S, Halldin C, Nordstrom A-L, Hall H, Sedvall G:** D_2 dopamine receptors in neuroleptic-naive schizophrenic patients. *Arch Gen Psychiatry* 47:213–219, 1990

62. **Wong DF, Wagner HN Jr, Tune LE, Dannals RF, Pearlson GD, Links JM, Tamminga CA, Broussolle EP, Ravert HT, Wilson AA, Toung JKT, Malat J, Williams JA, O'Tuama LA, Snyder SH, Kuhar MJ, Gjedde A:** Positron emission tomography reveals elevated D_2 dopamine receptors in drug-naive schizophrenics. *Science* 234:1558–1563, 1986

Positron-emission tomography has been used for in vivo neurotransmitter receptor imaging. These pivotal studies reach contradictory findings with regard to whether there is an increase in the number of dopamine D_2 receptors in the basal ganglia of schizophrenic patients.

63. **Meltzer HY, Stahl SM:** The dopamine hypothesis of schizophrenia: a review. *Schizophr Bull* 2:19–76, 1976

This is a comprehensive review of the "dopamine hypothesis" (schizophrenia due to increased dopaminergic activity) that has dominated biochemical and pharmacological thinking in schizophrenia for the past two decades.

Structural and Functional Brain Abnormalities

64. *Andreasen NC:* Brain imaging: applications in psychiatry. *Science* 239:1381–1388, 1988

Over the past decade, there have been tremendous advances in techniques of brain imaging: computed axial tomography, positron-emission tomography, single photon emission computed tomography, magnetic resonance imaging, and magnetic resonance spectroscopy. This article provides an excellent summary of these techniques and their application to schizophrenia.

65. *Bogerts B:** The neuropathology of schizophrenia, in *Search for the Causes of Schizophrenia.* Edited by Hafner H, Gattaz WF. Berlin, Germany, Springer-Verlag, 1991, pp. 229–241

This is a succinct summary of neuropathological findings in schizophrenia.

66. **Buchsbaum MS:** The frontal lobes, basal ganglia, and temporal lobes as sites for schizophrenia. *Schizophr Bull* 16:379–389, 1990

This is an excellent review of positron-emission tomography metabolic studies with fluorodeoxyglucose in schizophrenia.

67. *Goldman RS, Axelrod BN, Taylor SF:** Neuropsychological aspects of schizophrenia, in *Neuropsychological Assessment of Neuropsychiatric Disorders.* Edited by Grant I, Adams KM. London, Oxford University Press (in press)

This chapter is a succinct introduction to the neuropsychology of schizophrenia.

68. **Gur RE, Pearlson GD:** Neuroimaging in schizophrenia research. *Schizophr Bull* 19:337–353, 1993

This article is a recent summary of and attempt at integrating neuroimaging findings in schizophrenia.

69. **Ingvar DN, Franzen G:** Abnormalities of cerebral blood flow distribution in patients with chronic schizophrenia. *Acta Psychiatr Scand* 50:425–462, 1974

This is a classic study of cerebral blood flow in schizophrenia that first demonstrated hypofrontality.

70. **Johnstone EC, Crow TJ, Frith CD, Husband J, Kreel L:** Cerebral ventricular size and cognitive impairment in chronic schizophrenia. *Lancet* 1:924–926, 1976

The original computed tomography study that documented ventricular enlargement in the brains of schizophrenic patients, this article also references previous pneumo-encephalographic studies that had noted similar findings.

71. **Pettegrew JW, Keshavan MS, Panchalingam K, Strychor S, Kaplan DB, Tretta MG, Allen M:** Alterations in brain high-energy phosphate and membrane phospholipid metabolism in first-episode, drug-naive schizophrenics. *Arch Gen Psychiatry* 48:563–568, 1991

Magnetic resonance spectroscopy with H^1 and P^{31} isotopes have revealed altered membrane phospholipid composition and other metabolic abnormalities in the brains of schizophrenic patients. This is a major P^{31} magnetic resonance spectroscopy study of brains of first-episode, drug-naive schizophrenic patients.

72. **Sedvall G:** The current status of PET scanning with respect to schizophrenia. *Neuropsychopharmacology* 7:41–54, 1992

This is an excellent review of the current status of positron-emission tomography scanning (metabolic and receptor imaging) with respect to schizophrenia. This article is critiqued by Seeman, Murphy and Rapaport, Gur and Gur, Buchsbaum, and Wong; a response by Sedvall follows.

73. **Stevens JR:** An anatomy of schizophrenia? *Arch Gen Psychiatry* 29:177–189, 1973

A classic, this article was one of the first comprehensive attempts to construct a neurobiological substrate for schizophrenia.

74. **Suddath RL, Christison GW, Torrey EF, Casanova MF, Weinberger DR:** Anatomical abnormalities in the brains of monozygotic twins discordant for schizophrenia. *N Engl J Med* 322:789–794, 1990

This is a major magnetic resonance imaging study documenting structural brain abnormalities in schizophrenic patients in comparison to their unaffected monozygotic twin (an optimal control group).

75. **VanHorn JD, McManus IC:** Ventricular enlargement in schizophrenia: a meta-analysis of studies of the ventricle-brain ratio. *Br J Psychiatry* 160:687–697, 1992

This is a critical, well-referenced review of studies of ventricular enlargement in schizophrenia, using meta-analysis.

76. **Weinberger DR, Berman KF, Zec RF:** Physiological dysfunction of dorsolateral prefrontal cortex in schizophrenia. *Arch Gen Psychiatry* 43:114–124, 1986

This is the first in a series of cerebral blood flow activation studies from this group using the Wisconsin Card Sorting test, which suggested abnormal function of the dorsolateral prefrontal cortex in schizophrenia.

Neuropsychology and Psychophysiology

77. **Braff DL, Grillon C, Geyer M:** Gating and habituation of the startle reflex in schizophrenic patients. *Arch Gen Psychiatry* 49:206–215, 1992

This report argues for a theory of defective sensory filtering in schizophrenia and implicating dopaminergic dysfunction in this defect.

78. **Frith C, Done JD:** Towards a neuropsychology of schizophrenia. *Br J Psychiatry* 153:437–443, 1988

The authors propose a brain substrate for linking different neuropsychological deficits with positive and negative symptoms.

79. *Holzman PS:** Recent studies of psychophysiology in schizophrenia. *Schizophr Bull* 13:49–75, 1987

This is an excellent introductory review of psychophysiological and information-processing studies in schizophrenia.

80. **Holzman PS, Levy DL, Proctor LR:** Smooth pursuit eye movements, attention, and schizophrenia. *Arch Gen Psychiatry* 33:1415–1420, 1976

This article is one in a series of reports documenting dysfunction of smooth pursuit eye movements in schizophrenic patients and their relatives and discussing the relationship of this abnormality to attentional impairment and other cognitive abnormalities.

81. **Nuechterlein KH, Dawson ME:** Information processing and attentional functioning in the developmental course of schizophrenic disorders. *Schizophr Bull* 10:160–202, 1984

This is a selective review of deficits in information processing and attentional functioning in schizophrenia, emphasizing the concept of vulnerability and trait markers of the disorder.

82. **Strauss ME:** Relations of symptoms to cognitive deficits in schizophrenia. *Schizophr Bull* 19:215–231, 1993

Strauss evaluates the relationship between cognitive dysfunction and symptomatology in schizophrenia at various levels.

83. **Tandon R, Shipley JE, Taylor SF, Greden JF, Eiser A, DeQuardo J, Goodson J:** Electroencephalographic sleep abnormalities in schizophrenia. *Arch Gen Psychiatry* 49:185–194, 1992

Many rapid-eye-movement sleep abnormalities that were considered to be pathognomonic for major depression have been documented in schizophrenic patients as well. This is a comprehensive, well-referenced study of sleep abnormalities in schizophrenia and their relationship to previous neuroleptic treatment and positive and negative symptoms.

Pharmacological Treatment

84. **Baldessarini RJ, Cohen BM, Teicher M:** Significance of neuroleptic dose and plasma level in the pharmacological treatment of psychoses. *Arch Gen Psychiatry* 45:79–91, 1988

    This is a well-referenced study on the significance of neuroleptic dose and utility of neuroleptic plasma levels in the treatment of schizophrenia.

85. **Farde L, Nordstrom A-L, Wiesel F-A, Pauli S, Halldin C, Sedvall G:** Positron emission tomographic analysis of central D_1 and D_2 dopamine receptor occupancy in patients treated with classical neuroleptics and clozapine. *Arch Gen Psychiatry* 49:538–544, 1992

    Positron-emission tomography imaging of dopamine receptors is another strategy to study the biological effect of neuroleptics by evaluating changes in dopamine receptor occupancy. This is an elegant and well-referenced study in this area by one of the pioneering groups in this field. In this study, they evaluated D_1 and D_2 dopamine receptor occupancy in patients treated with typical and atypical neuroleptics in relationship to efficacy and side effects of these agents.

86. **Jeste DV, Caligiuri MP:** Tardive dyskinesia. *Schizophr Bull* 19:303–315, 1993

    This is an excellent summary of tardive dyskinesia, an important side effect of neuroleptic treatment of schizophrenia.

87. *****Kane JM, Marder SR:** Psychopharmacological treatment of schizophrenia. *Schizophr Bull* 19:287–302, 1993

    Kane and Marder provide a concise summary of state-of-the-art treatment in schizophrenia.

88. **Kane J, Honigfeld G, Singer J, Meltzer H, and the Clozaril Collaborative Study Group:** Clozapine for the treatment-resistant schizophrenic: a double-blind comparison with chlorpromazine. *Arch Gen Psychiatry* 45:789–796, 1988

    This is the report of a hallmark multicenter study on the efficacy and safety of clozapine in the treatment of treatment-refractory schizophrenic patients. The study design is as impressive as the findings.

89. **Lieberman J, Jody D, Geisler S, Alvir J, Loebel A, Szymanski S, Woerner M, Borenstein M:** Time course and biologic correlates of treatment response in first-episode schizophrenia. *Arch Gen Psychiatry* 0:369–376, 1993

In these data from a pivotal study of first-episode schizophrenia, Lieberman et al. describe the course and predictors (clinical and biological) of treatment response in the early phase of schizophrenic illness.

90. **Pickar D, Labarca R, Doran AR, Wolkowitz OM, Roy A, Breier A, Linnoila M, Paul SM:** Longitudinal measurement of plasma homovanillic acid levels in schizophrenic patients. *Arch Gen Psychiatry* 43:669–676, 1986

    Plasma homovanillic acid has been considered a marker of limbic dopaminergic activity and a biochemical correlate of psychosis in schizophrenic patients; basal levels and changes in plasma homovanillic acid with neuroleptic treatment have been considered to be an indicator of neuroleptic responsiveness and a marker of symptom change. This is one of the principal studies in this area.

91. *Safferman A, Lieberman JA, Kane JM, Szymanski S, Kinon B:** Update on the clinical efficacy and side effects of clozapine. *Schizophr Bull* 17:247–261, 1991

    This is an excellent review of the efficacy, side effects, and guidelines for clinical use of clozapine.

92. *Siris SG:** Adjunctive medications in the maintenance treatment of schizophrenia and its conceptual implications. *Br J Psychiatry* 163 (suppl 22):66–78, 1993

    This is a comprehensive overview of the use of adjunctive medications in schizophrenia.

Psychological and Psychosocial Treatment

93. **Arietti S:** Psychotherapy of schizophrenia. *Arch Gen Psychiatry* 6:112–122, 1962

    This is a concise formulation of some core principles of psychotherapy in schizophrenia.

94. **Attkisson C, Cook J, Karno M, Lehman A, McGlashan TH, Meltzer HY, O'Connor M, Richardson D, Rosenblatt A, Wells K, Williams J, Hohmann AA:** Clinical services research. *Schizophr Bull* 18:561–626, 1992

    In the past few years, there has been increasing recognition of the importance of outcomes assessment and evaluating the effectiveness of clinical interventions in clinical settings; these issues are likely to receive greater attention. This is a comprehensive introduction to this area.

95. **Bellack AS, Mueser KT:** Psychosocial treatment of schizophrenia. *Schizophr Bull* 19:317–336, 1989

This is a concise review of the application of various psychosocial techniques in the treatment of schizophrenia.

96. **Goldberg D:** Cost-effectiveness studies in the treatment of schizophrenia: a review. *Schizophr Bull* 17:453–459, 1991

This is an excellent introduction to the evaluation of the efficacy of various treatments of schizophrenia in terms of relative cost.

97. **Hogarty GE, Anderson C, Reiss D, Kornblith SJ, Greenwald DP, Javna CD, Madonia MJ:** Family psychoeducation, social skills training, and maintenance chemotherapy in the aftercare treatment of schizophrenia. *Arch Gen Psychiatry* 43:633–642, 1986

This study evaluates the efficacy of family psychoeducation, social skills training, and pharmacotherapy alone and together in the maintenance treatment of schizophrenic patients.

98. **Schwartz DP:** Schizophrenia: individual psychotherapy, in *Comprehensive Textbook of Psychiatry/V*, 5th Edition, Vol. 1. Edited by Kaplan HI, Sadock BJ. Baltimore, MD, Williams & Wilkins, 1989, pp. 806–815

This chapter is an excellent overview of individual psychotherapy in schizophrenia.

99. **Searles H:** *Collected Papers on Schizophrenia and Related Subjects.* New York, International Universities Press, 1965

This collection of papers provides a comprehensive and insightful description of the personal and interpersonal subjective experience of the schizophrenic patient and of his or her therapist and the relevance of these experiences to the process of treatment.

100. **Selzer MA, Sullivan TB, Carsky M, Terkelson KG:** *Working With the Person With Schizophrenia: The Treatment Alliance.* New York, New York University Press, 1989

This book provides an excellent, humane framework for the understanding and psychological and educational treatment of patients afflicted with schizophrenia.

13

Affective Disorders

J. Craig Nelson, M.D.

T he classification of affective disorders during the past three decades has been greatly influenced by research on response to various pharmacologic agents, in addition to distinctions based on family history and course of illness. Differences in treatment response directly relate to subtypes of psychotic depression, melancholia, atypical depression, and seasonal affective disorder. The effects of lithium in bipolar disorder generated interest in this disorder and the need to identify manic patients who might have been diagnosed as schizophrenic. Pharmacologic agents also provide a "pharmacologic bridge" that relates the action of the drugs to biological mechanisms in affective disorder. "Laboratory tests" have been proposed for use in identifying patients having a "biological depression." Interest in the description of depression led to extensive changes in classification, which are reflected in DSM-III, DSM-III-R, and DSM-IV. In this chapter, descriptive studies and biological studies that have preoccupied the field during the past decades have been emphasized.

Important historical works are first reviewed, particularly those that had an important and lasting impact. Next, papers presenting conceptual models of depression are reviewed. A few studies of stress and life events illustrate both their proposed relationship to depression and the methodological problems inherent in this area. Studies of diagnosis, classification, and description are presented. Information related to the DSM-III-R subtypes are included as well as syndromes such as atypical depression, which have a growing literature. Selected papers on the diagnosis and treatment of depression in medically ill patients are also listed. Examples of genetic studies of depression are presented. Laboratory tests that may have potential for diagnosis are reviewed. Finally, a number of papers dealing with the neurobiology of depression are presented. In selecting references, I have emphasized primary source articles that describe original findings, but also include a few papers that provide useful reviews of an area. This material should be helpful for trainees in psychiatry as well as other mental health professionals. Certain areas related to depression, such as epidemiology, suicide, bereavement, and pharmacologic treatment, are also discussed in other sections.

Early Papers

1. **Freud S:** Mourning and melancholia (1917), in *The Standard Edition of the Complete Psychological Works of Sigmund Freud,* Vol. 14. Translated and edited by Strachey J. London, Hogarth Press, 1957, pp. 239–258

   This paper is the source of the popularized "anger-turned-inward" theory of depression. Although subsequent empirical studies failed to support this hypothesis, the idea paved the way for psychological theories of depression.

2. **Gillespie RD:** The clinical differentiation of types of depression. *Guy's Hospital Report* 79:306–344, 1929

   Although Gillespie's work is not well known, his article of 1929 is surprisingly contemporary. Although others argued whether depression was the result of stress, Gillespie emphasized that some depressive syndromes run an autonomous course whereas others are responsive to psychosocial interventions.

3. **Kendell RE:** *The Classification of Depressive Illnesses.* New York, Oxford University Press, 1968

   The first chapter on the history of depressive classification is a very interesting account of diagnostic controversies of the first half of the century. His descriptions of the debates between the differing British "schools" are colorful and interesting to read.

4. **Kraepelin E:** *Manic-Depressive Insanity and Paranoia.* Edinburgh, Scotland, Livingstone, 1921

   Kraepelin's work of 1896 is a cornerstone of descriptive psychiatry of the past century. His distinction between manic-depressive disorder (or affective illness) and the nonaffective psychoses remains important to the present.

Conceptual Models

5. *Akiskal HS, McKinney WT Jr: Overview of recent research in depression: integration of ten conceptual models into a comprehensive clinical frame. *Arch Gen Psychiatry* 32:285–305, 1975

   This is a comprehensive review of conceptual models for depression. It is a very useful overview for trainees and a valuable reference for researchers.

6. Beck AT: *Depression: Clinical, Experimental and Theoretical Aspects.* New York, Harper & Row, 1967

   Negative attitudes and perceptions that distort the patient's experience are emphasized in Beck's theory of depression. These notions may be particularly important for understanding chronic characterologic depressions.

7. Bibring E: The mechanism of depression in affective disorders, in *Affective Disorders: Psychoanalytic Contributions to Their Study.* Edited by Greenacre P. New York, International Universities Press, 1953, pp. 13–48 (also available in 1961 edition)

   This chapter is one of the most important current psychodynamic explanations of depression. Bibring emphasizes an ego psychological model in which failure to meet standards and low self-esteem are central.

8. Seligman MEP, Beagley G: Learned helplessness in the rat. *Journal of Comparative and Physiological Psychology* 88:534–541, 1975

   Seligman and Beagley's animal studies add another dimension to behavioral theories about depression. They describe "learned helplessness" as an experimental animal model that may be relevant to understanding depression in human subjects.

9. *Siever LJ, Davis KL: Overview: toward a dysregulation hypothesis of depression. *Am J Psychiatry* 142:1017–1031, 1985

   This review and synthesis of biological mechanisms in depression shifts the focus from neurotransmitter deficits (e.g., too little norepinephrine) to a theory that focuses on regulatory mechanisms for neurotransmitter systems.

10. **Whybrow P, Parlatore A:** Melancholia, a model in madness: a discussion of recent psychobiologic research into depressive illness. *Int J Psychiatry Med* 4:351–378, 1973

    The authors describe a model of depression consistent with current notions of biological vulnerability. They distinguish between normal sadness and melancholia.

Stress and Life Events

11. *****Clayton PJ:** Bereavement, in *Handbook of Affective Disorders.* Edited by Paykel ES. Edinburgh, Scotland, Churchill Livingstone, 1982, pp. 403–415

    This chapter is included here because bereavement is one form of "reactive" depression. Bereaved patients frequently experience depressive symptoms in response to a common life event.

12. **Garmany G:** Depressive states: their aetiology and treatment. *Br Med J* 2:341–344, 1958

    This was one of the first empirical studies to examine the presence or absence of stress prior to the onset of depression. In a large patient sample, stress commonly preceded both reactive and endogenous depressions.

13. **Paykel ES, Myers JK, Dienelt M, Klerman GL, Lindenthal JJ, Pepper MP:** Life events and depression: a controlled study. *Arch Gen Psychiatry* 21:753–760, 1969

    This is an interesting study of the relationship of stress and depression that also reviews the methodological issues in a study of this kind (e.g., the effect of depression on the patient's description of prior events).

Epidemiology

14. **Myers JK, Weissman MM, Tischler GL, Holzer CE, Leaf PJ, Orvaschel H, Anthony JC, Boyd JH, Burke JD, Kramer M, Stoltzman R:** Six month prevalence of psychiatric disorders in three communities: 1980–1982. *Arch Gen Psychiatry* 41:959–970, 1984

15. **Regier DA, Myers JK, Kramer M, Robins LN, Blazer DG, Hough RL, Eaton WW, Locke BZ:** The NIMH Epidemiologic Catchment Area program: historical context, major objectives, and study population characteristics. *Arch Gen Psychiatry* 41:934–941, 1984

16. **Robins LN, Helzer JE, Weissman MM, Orvaschel H, Gruenberg E, Burke JD, Regier DA:** Lifetime prevalence of specific psychiatric disorders in three sites. *Arch Gen Psychiatry* 41:949–958, 1984

These reports describe the methods and findings of the Epidemiologic Catchment Area study of psychiatric disorders in five United States communities. This project provides the best estimates of the prevalence of depression and bipolar disorder using current diagnostic criteria.

Major Depression

17. **Coryell W, Endicott J, Keller M:** Outcome of patients with chronic affective disorder: a five year follow-up. *Am J Psychiatry* 147:1627–1633, 1990

In a report from the National Institute of Mental Health Collaborative Study on the Psychobiology of Depression, Coryell et al. describe the 5-year course of illness in patients with major depression and examine factors that predict long-term outcome.

18. **Elkin I, Shea T, Watkins JT, Imber SD, Sotsky SM, Collins JF, Glass DR, Pilkonis PA, Leber WR, Docherty JP, Fiester SJ, Parloff MB:** NIMH treatment of depression collaborative research program: general effectiveness of treatments. *Arch Gen Psychiatry* 46:971–982, 1989

This report describes the results of the collaborative study of depression. It presents a comparison of the effects of imipramine, psychological treatments, and placebo in major depression. The results not only have specific implications for the treatments studied but also have broader implications for the classification of depression.

19. **Keller MB, Shapiro RW, Lavori PW, Wolfe N:** Recovery in major depressive disorder. *Arch Gen Psychiatry* 39:905–910, 1982

20. **Keller MB, Shapiro RW, Lavori PW, Wolfe N:** Relapse in major depressive disorder. *Arch Gen Psychiatry* 39:911–915, 1982

These two reports by Keller et al. describe rates of recovery and relapse in depressed patients in the National Institute of Mental Health Collaborative Study on the Psychobiology of Depression. Clinical factors associated with recovery and relapse are examined.

21. **Kendell RE:** The classification of depressions: a review of contemporary confusion. *Br J Psychiatry* 129:15–28, 1976

Kendell reviews a variety of concepts and models that have been generated to explain severe depressive illness. He concludes that endogenous depression is a distinct entity but that nonendogenous depression is a heterogeneous grouping.

22. *Klein DF: Endogenomorphic depression: a conceptual and terminologic revision. *Arch Gen Psychiatry* 31:447–454, 1974

    Klein reiterates the view that endogenous depression is characterized by the nature of the syndrome once developed rather than the presence or absence of precipitating stress. The loss of the ability to experience pleasure is a central feature. He also predicts differences in drug and placebo response for acute situational depressions, endogenous depressions, and chronic dysphorias.

23. *Nelson JC, Charney DS: The symptoms of major depressive illness. *Am J Psychiatry* 138:1–13, 1981

    Nelson and Charney review previous studies of the endogenous-nonendogenous distinction and use this review as a basis for deriving symptoms characteristic of endogenous depression.

24. Rosenthal SH: The involutional depressive syndrome. *Am J Psychiatry* 124:21–35, 1968

    The diagnosis of involutional melancholia has been discarded. This is a comprehensive review of involutional melancholia and the evidence suggesting that it does not constitute a distinct entity.

25. *Zimmerman M, Spitzer R: Melancholia: from DSM-III to DSM-III-R. *Am J Psychiatry* 146:20–28, 1989

    This review examines empirical studies of the melancholic distinction. It finds insufficient evidence for classification of this syndrome as a distinct subtype.

Psychotic Depression

26. *Charney DS, Nelson JC: Delusional and nondelusional unipolar depression: further evidence for distinct subtypes. *Am J Psychiatry* 138:328–333, 1981

27. *Glassman AH, Roose SP: Delusional depression a distinct clinical entity? *Arch Gen Psychiatry* 38:424–427, 1981

    These descriptive studies of psychotic depression support the view that this syndrome constitutes a distinct entity.

28. **Coryell W, Tsuang MT:** Primary unipolar depression and the prognostic importance of delusions. *Arch Gen Psychiatry* 39:1181–1184, 1982

    This interesting retrospective study examined psychotic and nonpsychotic depressive patients over a 40-year period, finding that psychotic depressive patients did less well 1 year after the episode but had a long-term course similar to nonpsychotic depressive patients.

29. **Glassman AH, Kantor SJ, Shostak M:** Depressive delusions, and drug response. *Am J Psychiatry* 132:716–719, 1975

    This brief article argues that delusional or psychotic depressed patients respond less well to tricyclic antidepressants than nonpsychotic patients. The article stimulated considerable research and is in part responsible for the DSM-III distinction of psychotic depression.

30. **Kettering RL, Harrow M, Grossman L, Meltzer HY:** The prognostic relevance of delusions in depression: a follow-up study. *Am J Psychiatry* 144:1154–1160, 1987

    This prospective follow-up of depressed patients validates prior findings of an increased recurrence of delusions in patients initially psychotic. Recurrence of delusions was independent of severity.

31. *Schatzberg AF, Rothschild AJ:** Psychotic (delusional) major depression: should it be included as a distinct syndrome in DSM-IV? *Am J Psychiatry* 149:733–745, 1992

    The authors provide a review of this literature, concluding that psychotic depression is a distinct type of depression.

32. *Spiker DG, Weiss JC, Dealy RS, Griffin SJ, Hanin I, Neil JF, Perel JM, Rossi AJ, Soloff PH:** The pharmacological treatment of delusional depression. *Am J Psychiatry* 142:430–436, 1985

    This prospective study validates Glassman et al.'s (1975) report of decreased response to tricyclics alone in psychotic depression and validates the effectiveness of combined neuroleptic-tricyclic treatment in this disorder.

Primary-Secondary Depression

33. **Andreasen NC, Winokur G:** Secondary depression: familial, clinical, and research perspectives. *Am J Psychiatry* 136:62–66, 1979

    This is a useful review of the concept of secondary depression.

34. **Woodruff RA Jr, Murphy GE, Herjanic M:** The natural history of affective disorders, I: symptoms of 72 patients at the time of index hospital admission. *J Psychiatr Res* 5:255–263, 1967

This is one of the earliest articles describing the distinction between primary and secondary depression. Patients with "primary affective disorder" are distinguished from patients with depressions associated with other psychiatric syndromes.

Atypical and Anxious Depression

35. *Davidson JR, Miller RD, Turnbull CD, Sullivan JL:** Atypical depression. *Arch Gen Psychiatry* 39:527–534, 1982

A very helpful review of the literature on atypical depression, this article describes different uses of the term and summarizes the current status of this disorder.

36. *Klerman GL, Endicott J, Spitzer RL, Hirschfeld MA:** Neurotic depressions: a systematic analysis of multiple criteria and meanings. *Am J Psychiatry* 136:57–61, 1979

This article describes the current status of neurotic depression and systematically reviews the various meanings of the term.

37. **Liebowitz MR, Quitkin FM, Stewart JW, McGrath PJ, Harrison W, Rabkin J, Tricamo E, Markowitz JS, Klein DF:** Phenelzine v imipramine in atypical depression. *Arch Gen Psychiatry* 41:669–677, 1984

38. **Liebowitz MR, Quitkin FM, Stewart JW, McGrath PJ, Harrison W, Markowitz JS, Rabkin J, Tricamo E, Goetz DM, Klein DF:** Antidepressant specificity in atypical depression. *Arch Gen Psychiatry* 45:129–137, 1988

These two articles describe the Columbia University group's definition of atypical depression. They demonstrate this subtype of depression is more responsive to monoamine oxidase inhibitors than tricyclic antidepressants.

39. **Robinson DS, Nies A, Ravaris CL, Lamborn KR:** The MAOI, phenelzine, in the treatment of depressive-anxiety states. *Arch Gen Psychiatry* 29:407–413, 1973

This article describes patients responsive to monoamine oxidase inhibitors.

40. **West ED, Dally PJ:** Effects of iproniazid in depressive syndromes. *Br Med J* 1:1491–1494, 1959

This is one of the earliest articles describing atypical depression and the particular usefulness of monoamine oxidase inhibitors for its treatment.

Seasonal Affective Disorder

41. **Blehar MC, Rosenthal NE:** Seasonal affective disorders and phototherapy. *Arch Gen Psychiatry* 46:469–474, 1989

    This article reviews the proceedings of a National Institute of Mental Health workshop on seasonal affective disorder and presents a review of research findings.

42. **Wehr TA, Rosenthal NE:** Seasonality and affective illness. *Am J Psychiatry* 146:829–839, 1989

    This article reviews the concept of seasonal affective disorder.

Dysthymic Disorder

43. *__*Akiskal HS:__ Dysthymic disorder: psychopathology of proposed chronic depressive subtypes. *Am J Psychiatry* 140:11–20, 1983

    Akiskal discusses current concepts of "characterologic depression" and makes the distinction between depressions associated with personality disorder and those associated with affective disorder that has become chronic.

44. **Keller MB, Shapiro RW:** "Double depression": superimposition of acute depressive episodes on chronic depressive disorders. *Am J Psychiatry* 139:438–442, 1982

    This is a useful discussion of the concept of "double depression."

45. *__*Kocsis JH, Frances AJ:__ A critical discussion of DSM-III dysthymic disorder. *Am J Psychiatry* 144:1534–1542, 1987

    Kocsis and Frances provide a critical discussion of dysthymic disorder.

Depression in Medically Ill Patients

46. **Clark DC, Cavanaugh SV, Gibbons RD:** The core symptoms of depression in medical and psychiatric patients. *J Nerv Ment Dis* 171:705–713, 1983

The authors empirically derive symptoms useful for the diagnosis of depression in medically ill patients. In these patients, some depressive symptoms (e.g., anorexia, anergia) may be associated with medical illness and are of limited use.

47. **Popkin MK, Callies AL, Mackenzie TB:** The outcome of antidepressant use in the medically ill. *Arch Gen Psychiatry* 42:1160–1163, 1985

This study describes the hazards of antidepressant treatment in medically ill patients.

48. *Rodin G, Voshart K:** Depression in the medically ill: an overview. *Am J Psychiatry* 143:696–705, 1986

This is a good review of the subject.

Bipolar Disorder

49. **Akiskal HS, Walker P, Puzantian VR, King D, Rosenthal TL, Dranon M:** Bipolar outcome in the course of depressive illness: phenomenologic, familial, and pharmacologic predictors. *J Affect Disord* 5:115–128, 1983

Predictors of bipolar outcome in depression are reported and discussed in this article. These predictors include early onset, psychotic features, and antidepressant-induced mania.

50. **Bauer MS, Whybrow PC, Winokur A:** Rapid cycling bipolar affective disorder, I: association with grade I hypothyroidism. *Arch Gen Psychiatry* 47:427–432, 1990

An association of rapid cycling and hypothyroidism is reported in this article. The complicated interaction of gender, hypothyroidism, and effects of lithium on thyroid indices is explored.

51. **Bunney WE Jr, Murphy DL, Goodwin FK, Borge GF:** The "switch process" in manic depressive illness, 1: a systematic study of sequential behavioral changes. *Arch Gen Psychiatry* 27:295–302, 1972

The "switch process" is an important concept that has become part of the psychiatric vocabulary and has stimulated further research.

52. **Carlson GA, Goodwin FK:** The stages of mania: a longitudinal analysis of the manic episode. *Arch Gen Psychiatry* 28:221–228, 1973

This interesting description of the progression of symptoms during an acute manic episode is one of the few reports in the literature that not only details symptom differences between patients but emphasizes how symptoms may differ with respect to stage of the illness.

53. **Dunner DL, Fleve RR:** Clinical factors in lithium carbonate prophylaxis failure. *Arch Gen Psychiatry* 30:229–233, 1974

Poor response to lithium prophylaxis helped to identify a group of rapid cycling patients. This article provided the stimulus for continued efforts to describe and understand this intractable group of patients.

54. *Krauthammer C, Klerman GL:** Secondary mania. *Arch Gen Psychiatry* 35:1333–1339, 1978

The authors provide a useful review of other causes of mania.

55. **Leonhard K:** *Aufteilung der endogenen Psychosen*, 2nd Edition. Berlin, Germany, Akademie Verlag, 1959

This seminal work describes the distinction between unipolar and bipolar depressive illnesses.

56. **Lipkin KM, Dyrud J, Meyer GG:** The many faces of mania: therapeutic trial of lithium carbonate. *Arch Gen Psychiatry* 22:262–267, 1970

This article persuasively argues that manic patients may present with paranoid psychotic symptoms that may be mistaken for schizophrenia. Cases are presented.

57. **McElroy SL, Keck PE, Pope HG, Hudson JI, Faedda GL, Swann AC:** Clinical and research implications of the diagnosis of dysphoric or mixed mania or hypomania. *Am J Psychiatry* 149:1633–1644, 1992

The syndrome of mania "mixed" with depressive or dysphoric symptoms has received increased attention. This review examines clinical aspects of this syndrome and discusses whether it constitutes a distinct affective state. Preliminary operational criteria are proposed.

58. **Perris C:** A study of bipolar (manic-depressive) and unipolar recurrent depressive psychoses. *Acta Psychiatr Scand* 42, suppl 194, 1966

Perris examines a series of variables in unipolar and bipolar patients. The comprehensive monograph provided support for the unipolar-bipolar distinction.

59. *Pope HG Jr, Lipinski JF, Cohen BM, Axelrod DT:** Schizoaffective disorder: an invalid diagnosis: a comparison of schizoaffective disorder, schizophrenia, and affective disorder. Am J Psychiatry 137:921–927, 1980

The authors review the concept of schizoaffective disorder. Patients with schizoaffective, manic type disorder appear to have a family history, response to lithium, and course similar to bipolar patients.

60. **Strober M, Carlson G:** Bipolar illness in adolescents with major depression. *Arch Gen Psychiatry* 39:549–555, 1982

This prospective follow-up study examines the clinical, genetic, and pharmacologic predictors of bipolar disorder in 60 adolescents presenting with major depression. The predictive value of rapid onset, motor retardation, and psychotic features; family history of affective disorder or bipolar disorder; and drug-induced mania are discussed.

61. **Taylor MA, Abrams R:** The phenomenology of mania: a new look at some old patients. *Arch Gen Psychiatry* 29:520–522, 1973

This study demonstrated that many patients receiving the diagnosis of "schizophrenia" in fact had symptoms and other characteristics suggestive of bipolar illness.

62. **Wehr TA, Sack DA, Rosenthal NE, Cowdry RW:** Rapid cycling affective disorder: contributing factors and treatment responses in 51 patients. *Am J Psychiatry* 145:179–184, 1988

This article, from the Clinical Psychobiology Branch at the National Institute of Mental Health, examines the clinical, genetic, and treatment characteristics of 51 rapid cycling patients.

63. **Young RC, Klerman GL:** Mania in late life: focus on age at onset. *Am J Psychiatry* 149:867–876, 1992

This review examines the prevalence and age at onset of mania in elderly patients. The relationship of late onset to family history, course, and treatment response is explored.

Genetic Studies

64. *Gershon ES, Hamovit J, Guroff JJ, Dibble E, Leckman JF, Sceery W, Targum SD, Nurnberger JI, Goldin LR, Bunney WE:** A family study of schizoaffective bipolar I, bipolar II, unipolar, and normal control probands. *Arch Gen Psychiatry* 39:1157–1167, 1982

65. **Weissman MM, Kidd KK, Prusoff BA:** Variability in rates of affective disorders in relatives of depressed and normal probands. *Arch Gen Psychiatry* 39:1397–1403, 1982

In these articles, data from two of the largest, most carefully designed genetic studies are presented. There is clear support for the heritability of affective illness. The authors propose a continuum of genetic vulnerability, such that bipolar illness is manifested when vulnerability is most severe and unipolar illness manifested when it is less severe.

66. **Leckman JF, Weissman MM, Prusoff BA:** Subtypes of depression. *Arch Gen Psychiatry* 41:833–838, 1984

   Leckman et al. found, as others have, that psychotic depression was not associated with a family history of schizophrenia. This study was unusual in finding an increased risk of psychotic depression in relatives of psychotic depressed probands.

Biological Markers

67. *The APA Task Force on Laboratory Tests in Psychiatry:** The dexamethasone suppression test: an overview of its current status in psychiatry. *Am J Psychiatry* 144:1253–1262, 1987

68. *Arana GW, Baldessarini RJ, Ornsteen M:** The dexamethasone suppression test for diagnosis and prognosis in psychiatry. *Arch Gen Psychiatry* 42:1193–1204, 1985

   These two reviews examine the evidence supporting the value of the dexamethasone suppression test as a diagnostic marker for depression.

69. **Carroll BJ:** The dexamethasone suppression tests for melancholia. *Br J Psychiatry* 140:292–304, 1982

70. **Carroll BJ, Feinberg M, Greden JF, Tarika J, Albala AA, Haskett RF, James NM, Kronfol Z, Lohr N, Steiner M, Vigne JP, Young E:** A specific laboratory test for the diagnosis of melancholia: standardization, validation and clinical utility. *Arch Gen Psychiatry* 38:15–22, 1981

   These two articles propose that the dexamethasone suppression test is a useful diagnostic laboratory test for endogenous depression. These articles review the research leading to the standardization of the test and its present uses and limitations.

71. **Gillin JC, Duncan W, Pettigrew KD, Frankel BL, Snyder F:** Successful separation of depressed, normal, and insomniac patients by EEG sleep data. *Arch Gen Psychiatry* 36:85–90, 1979

72. **Reynolds CF III, Kupfer DJ:** Sleep research in affective illness: state of the art circa 1987. *Sleep* 10:199–215, 1987

These two articles describe sleep electroencephalogram abnormalities in depression and the use of this technique for diagnosis.

73. **Kupfer D:** REM latency:a biological marker for primary depressive illness. *Biol Psychiatry* 11:159–174, 1976

    This article describes the association of reduced rapid-eye-movement latency and endogenous depression.

74. *****Loosen PI, Prange AJ:** Serum thyrotropin response to thyrotropin-releasing hormone in psychiatric patients: a review. *Am J Psychiatry* 139:405–416, 1982

    There is extensive evidence that the serum thyrotropin (thyroid-stimulating hormone) response to thyrotropin-releasing hormone is blunted in a subgroup of depressed patients. This article is an excellent review of those studies.

Neurobiology

75. **Asberg M, Traskman L, Thoren P:** 5-HIAA in the cerebrospinal fluid: a biochemical suicide predictor? *Arch Gen Psychiatry* 33:1193–1197, 1976

76. **Traskman L, Asberg M, Bertilsson L, Sjostrand L:** Monoamine metabolite in CSF and suicidal behavior. *Arch Gen Psychiatry* 38:631–636, 1981

    These two articles provide evidence for an association between a low concentration of cerebrospinal fluid 5-hydroxyindoleacetic acid (5-HIAA) and suicidal behavior. These data are consistent with the hypothesis that altered brain serotonin function is of etiologic significance in depression.

77. **Banerjee SP, Kung LS, Riggi SJ, Chanda SK:** Development of beta-adrenergic receptor subsensitivity by antidepressants. *Nature* 268:455–456, 1977

78. **Vetulani J, Stawarz RJ, Dingell JV, Sulser F:** A possible common mechanism of action of antidepressant treatments. *Naunyn Schmiedebergs Arch Pharmacol* 293:109–114, 1976

    These two articles propose that down-regulation of beta-receptors may be the mechanism by which antidepressants exert their beneficial action and implicates adrenergic dysfunction in depression.

79. **Blier P, de Montigny C, Chaput Y:** Modifications of the serotonin system by antidepressant treatments: implications for the therapeutic response in major depression. *J Clin Psychopharmacol* 7:24S–35S, 1987

80. **Murphy DL, Campell IC, Costa JL:** The brain serotonergic system in the affective disorders. *Progr Neuropsychopharmacol* 2:5–31, 1978

81. **van Praag HM:** Central monoamines and the pathogenesis of depression, in *Handbook of Biological Psychiatry, Part IV: Brain Mechanisms and Abnormal Behavior—Chemistry.* Edited by van Praag HM, Lader MH, Rafaelsen OJ, Sachar EJ. New York, Marcel Dekker, 1981, pp. 159–205

These three papers are informative reviews of the role of abnormal serotonin function in the genesis of depressive illness. Studies comparing the levels of the serotonin metabolite, 5-hydroxyindoleacetic acid (5-HIAA) in the cerebrospinal fluid of depressed patients and healthy subjects are discussed as are the actions of antidepressant drugs on the serotonin system.

82. **Brunello N, Baraccia ML, Chuang D-M, Costa E:** Down-regulation of beta-adrenergic receptors following repeated injections of desmethylimipramine: permissive role of serotonergic axons. *Neuropharmacology* 21:1145–1149, 1982

83. **Sulser F:** Serotonin-norepinephrine receptor interactions in the brain: implications for the pharmacology and pathophysiology of affective disorders. *J Clin Psychiatry* 48:12–18, 1987

These two articles describe the interaction of the serotonin system with the norepinephrine system. They suggest a permissive role of serotonin in modulating noradrenergic function.

84. *Charney DS, Menkes DB, Heninger GR:** Receptor sensitivity and the mechanism of action of antidepressant treatment: implications for the etiology and therapy of depression. *Arch Gen Psychiatry* 38:1160–1180, 1981

85. **Heninger G, Charney DS:** Mechanism of action of antidepressant treatments: implications for the etiology and treatment of depressive disorders, in *Psychopharmacology: The Third Generation of Progress.* Edited by Meltzer HY. New York, Raven, 1987, pp. 535–544

These papers provide extensive reviews of the catecholamine and indolamine hypotheses of depression in light of research on the effect of antidepressant treatment on monoamine receptor sensitivity. Etiologic models of depressive illness are presented.

86. **Checkley SA:** Neuroendocrine tests of monamine function in man: a review of basic theory and its application to the study of depressive illness. *Psychol Med* 10:35–53, 1980

This is an excellent review of the findings of neuroendocrine studies designed to evaluate the monoamine deficiency hypothesis of depressive illness.

87. **Delgado P, Charney DS, Price LH, Aghajanian GK, Landis H, Heninger GR:** Serotonin function and the mechanism of antidepressant action: reversal of antidepressant-induced remission by rapid depletion of plasma tryptophan. *Arch Gen Psychiatry* 47:411–418, 1990

This report provides compelling evidence for the role of serotonin in mediating antidepressant action and presumably in the pathogenesis of depression.

88. **Maas JW:** Biogenic amines and depression. *Arch Gen Psychiatry* 32:1357–1361, 1975

89. **Schildkraut JJ:** Current status of the catecholamine hypothesis of affective disorders, in *Psychopharmacology: A Generation of Progress.* Edited by Lipton MA, DiMascio A, Killam KF. New York, Raven, 1978, pp. 1223–1234

These papers review the evidence supporting the hypothesis that decreased catecholamine function exists in at least a subgroup of depressed patients. Particular attention is directed toward studies of catecholamine metabolite levels in depressed patients.

90. **Maas JW, Kocsis JH, Bowden CL, Davis JM, Redmond DE, Hanin I, Robins E:** Pre-treatment neurotransmitter metabolites and response to imipramine or amitriptyline treatment. *Psychol Med* 12:37–43, 1982

Previous studies suggested that low levels of urinary 3-methoxy-4-hydroxyphenylglycol (MHPG) predict a positive response to imipramine and high MHPG levels a positive response to amitriptyline. However, this large-scale collaborative study found that, although low urinary MHPG predicted response to imipramine, there was not a relationship between pretreatment MHPG and response to amitriptyline.

General References

91. **Goodwin FK, Jamison KR:** *Manic Depressive Illness.* New York, Oxford University Press, 1990

Goodwin and Jamison have written an extraordinarily comprehensive review of bipolar disorder. All aspects of the disorder are reviewed.

Clinicians will find this work it useful for diagnosis and treatment of bipolar patients. Researchers will find its extensive review of the literature (about 3,900 references) a helpful resource.

92. Paykel ES (ed): *Handbook of Affective Disorders,* 2nd Edition. New York, Guilford, 1992

This is a useful general reference on affective disorder written by an international group of contributors selected for their expertise. It includes sections on description, etiology, somatic treatments, psychosocial treatments, and special issues (e.g., bereavement, suicide). It might be particularly helpful for psychiatric residents or clinicians wishing a review.

93. Willner P: *Depression: A Psychobiological Synthesis.* New York, Wiley, 1985

This is a relatively concise volume, but is an impressive undertaking by one individual. It is well researched, with approximately 2,700 references. What is relatively unique is Willner's attempt to link biological findings with behavioral correlates. This is a particularly worthwhile source for information on different areas of biological research in depression (e.g., animal models of depression, neurotransmitter findings, neuroanatomic data) and the relationships of these areas to each other.

Unusual Psychoses and Culture-Bound Syndromes

Ruth E. Levine, M.D.
Albert C. Gaw, M.D.

D espite the numerous categories in the diagnostic nomenclature, a number of seemingly rare, exotic, and difficult to classify syndromes are cast in the area of "psychotic disorder not otherwise specified." DSM-IV includes in this category disorders with "psychotic symptomatology . . . about which there is inadequate information to make a specific diagnosis or . . . there is contradictory information, or disorders with psychotic symptoms that do not meet criteria for any specific psychotic disorder" (p. 315). In DSM-III-R, this category was known as "atypical psychosis," a term used to describe a variety of syndromes that generally fell into three categories: culture-bound syndromes, unusual syndromes, and other psychotic syndromes defying easy classification.

The first category, culture-bound syndromes, is now described extensively in an appendix of DSM-IV. These unusual forms of psychopathology, so influenced by their indigenous culture as to be considered "culture-bound," include a wide variety of phenomena encompassing both psychotic and nonpsychotic syndromes. With some exceptions, most of these disorders originate in non-Western societies, making the influence of culture highly visible. Some of the better known examples include:

- *Koro.* A fear that one's genitals are retracting into one's body and that full retraction will eventuate in death, this is seen primarily in South China and Singapore. It can occur in epidemics.
- *Amok.* A syndrome of homicidal frenzy preceded by brooding and ending in exhaustion and amnesia, this is seen primarily in Southeast Asia.
- *Ataque de nervios.* This disorder is found in Latin American countries, otherwise known as "Puerto Rican syndrome." The symptoms include shaking, palpitations, flushing, and numbness, and are often accompanied by shouting or striking out and followed by falling, convulsive body movements, or amnesia.

Literally hundreds of disorders have been described as culture-bound. Most are recognized, expected, and, to some degree, sanctioned by their respective societies in response to certain culturally defined precipitants. Others are not discrete disorders but illnesses, defined by attribution to a culturally defined culprit such as witchcraft or spirits. Although some of these disorders are rare, others are common in their respective cultures.

One must be careful to consider culture before defining a presentation as psychotic. Traditional Western psychiatry has insufficiently regarded the influence of culture on psychopathology. As psychiatric researchers become more sophisticated, the influences of both familiar and exotic cultures will become more apparent. For practical reasons, clinicians should be aware of these issues. Increases in worldwide travel and immigration are significantly influencing the demographics of patient populations. The modern psychiatrist will need to recognize that even common syndromes can become confusing in a patient from an unfamiliar culture. Cultural sensitivity is already becoming an important component of effective diagnosis and treatment.

The second category is that of unusual syndromes. Some syndromes are related to common psychiatric disorders, yet contain distinctive and exotic symptoms sufficient to warrant unique designation. Others consist of one unusual feature, but lack sufficient criteria to fit into an existing category. Most of these disorders are fairly rare. Examples include:

- *Capgras syndrome.* This is the delusion that doubles of significant others, or of oneself, exist.
- *Erotomania.* Also known as Clerembault's syndrome, this is the delusional belief that a stranger, often a prominent person, is in love with the patient from afar.
- *Induced psychotic disorder.* Also known as folie a deux, this is a phenomena whereby two or more members of an intimate relationship share a delusion or delusions.
- *Autoscopy.* This is a condition consisting of delusions or hallucinations of the self. The hallucinations are most commonly visual.

The third category is that of other psychotic syndromes defying easy classification. This category is probably the most variable, changing as different syndromes become controversial. It is also a fairly large category, including any seemingly psychotic disorder that defies easy classification. Examples include:

- *Epileptic psychosis.* This is a heterogenous group of phenomena, including temporal lobe epilepsy. Although these probably belong in the organic psychoses, they are often placed in the atypical category.
- *Nonresponsive psychosis.* This is another heterogenous spectrum of disorders defined by their atypical responsiveness or unresponsiveness to conventional therapies.
- *Postpartum psychosis.* This disorder is defined by its association to the postpartum period. Although an episode is supposed to be unrelated to an organic disorder, a mood disorder, or another psychosis, frequently it is the precursor to more common disorders.

Syndromes are deemed difficult to classify because of some controversy regarding characterization, such as the case with epileptic psychosis. An ongoing debate regarding the nature of epileptic psychosis bridges the gap between psychiatry and neurology. Several "unusual syndromes" demonstrate symptoms suggestive of neurological lesions. Some of the most important research in the field is being conducted in this area, and it is work of which psychiatrists should be aware.

The suggested readings are primarily current critical reviews, which emphasize the controversy these syndromes evoke. A few classic descriptions also are included; others can be obtained from references cited in the reviews.

Culture-Bound Syndromes

1. **Bernstein RL, Gaw AC:** Koro: proposed classification for DSM-IV. *Am J Psychiatry* 147:1670–1674, 1990

   Although rarely seen in the West, koro has been described in East Asia in epidemic proportions. This article reviews past attempts to characterize and classify koro and proposes a means of DSM-IV classification that could be used for other culture-specific disorders.

2. **Gaw AC, Bernstein RL:** Classification of Amok in DSM-IV. *Hosp Community Psychiatry* 43:789–793, 1992

   This is a review of the syndrome of amok, with the suggestion it be included in the DSM-III-R category of intermittent explosive disorder.

Included is a discussion of a means of defining disorders as "culture-specific."

3. *Guarnaccia PJ, De La Cancela V, Carrillo E:** The multiple meanings of ataques de nervios in the Latino community. *Med Anthropol* 11:47–62, 1989

Like many other culture-specific phenomenon, ataques de nervios is recognized by the Latin American community as a common expression of anger or distress occurring in response to grief, shock, or family conflict. The authors quite eloquently review the social contributions to this phenomenon. One comes away from this discussion with a better understanding that applying a simple Western diagnosis, such as panic or dissociative disorder, can be inadequate and a disservice to the patient.

4. *Lin TY:** Neurasthenia revisited: its place in modern psychiatry. *Cult Med Psychiatry* 13:105–129, 1989

Largely abandoned in the West, the concept of neurasthenia is a mainstay in Eastern psychiatry. In this elegant review, Lin describes how the role of history and culture of East Asia contributed to the firm establishment of this diagnostic entity. Although not a "culture-specific" syndrome, neurasthenia demonstrates the relevance of culture in defining psychopathology.

5. **Simons RC, Hughes CC** (eds): *The Culture Bound Syndromes: Folk Illnesses of Psychiatric and Anthropologic Interest.* Dordrecht, Holland, D Reidle Publishing, 1985

This is a comprehensive review with possibly the best discussion to date of the issues regarding modern classification. The appendix contains an excellent glossary of culture-bound and folk psychiatric syndromes.

6. *Simons RC, Hughes CC:** Culture-bound syndromes, in *Culture, Ethnicity, and Mental Illness.* Edited by Gaw AC. Washington, DC, American Psychiatric Press, 1993, pp. 75–99

This concise, well-written chapter makes many of the points found in the book. Describes several of the more common syndromes, with recommendations regarding classification. Included are Western syndromes not ordinarily considered "culture-bound." Essential reading for students of cross-cultural psychiatry.

Unusual Syndromes

7. **Berson RJ:** Capgras' syndrome. *Am J Psychiatry* 140:969–978, 1983

   Benson reviews 133 cases of Capgras' syndrome and provides a nice outline of the history, phenomenology, and controversy regarding this syndrome. Although acknowledging the contributions of organic conditions, Benson argues as to the importance of psychodynamic factors.

8. *Enoch MD, Trethowan WH: *Uncommon Psychiatric Syndromes.* Cambridge, England, Butterworth-Heineman, 1991

   In this excellent overview, Enock provides detailed reviews of many unusual syndromes, with case illustrations. In addition to coverage of several classic syndromes, there are also chapters on Ekbom's syndrome (delusional parasitosis) and possession states.

9. **Fahy T, Wessely S, David A:** Werewolves, vampires and cannibals. *Med Sci Law* 28:145–150, 1988

   This fascinating discussion of these unusual phenomenon demonstrates the overlap between delusion, superstition, and myth.

10. *Friedmann CTH, Faguet RA (eds): *Extraordinary Disorders of Human Behavior.* New York, Plenum, 1982

    This comprehensive volume includes detailed reviews of most of the unusual psychoses, as well as some other exotic psychiatric syndromes. This is probably the best place to start for an overall review of the topic.

11. *Sacks MH: Folie a deux. *Compr Psychiatry* 229:270–277, 1988

    In this concise and well-organized review, Sacks suggests that the phenomenon of induced psychotic disorder may be more common than most clinicians realize. Included is discussion of epidemiology, clinical subtypes, and treatment.

12. *Segal JH: Erotomania revisited: from Kraepelin to DSM-III-R. *Am J Psychiatry* 146:1261–1266, 1989

    This well-written review includes history, theories of etiology, course, and treatment of erotomania—also a nice discussion of Kraepelin's concept of paranoia, of which erotomania was considered a subtype. Segal, quite convincingly, demonstrates the similarities between the DSM-III-R category of delusional disorder and Kraepelin's formulation.

13. *Weinstein EA, Burnham DL: Reduplication and the syndrome of Capgras. *Psychiatry* 54:78–88, 1991

Although Benson emphasizes the psychodynamic meanings in Capgras syndrome, Weinstein and Burnham focus on the neurological applications of this fascinating phenomenon. They compare and contrast features of reduplication found in neurological patients with Capgras and the other delusional misidentification syndromes.

14. **Whitlock FA:** The Ganser syndrome. *Br J Psychiatry* 113:19–29, 1967

This is a critical analysis of Ganser syndrome, an unusual syndrome sometimes found in prisoners, marked by disturbances of consciousness, amnesia, hallucinations, and peculiar verbal responses to questions. Whitlock discusses the controversy regarding the nature of this syndrome and argues that it is a transient psychotic disorder.

Psychotic Syndromes Defying Easy Classification

15. **Cutting J:** Relationship between cycloid psychosis and atypical affective psychosis. *Psychopathology* 23:212–219, 1990

In this analysis of 73 inpatients with cycloid psychosis, Cutting convincingly argues that the syndrome be considered an atypical variety of affective psychosis.

16. **Kumar R:** *Postpartum Psychosis. Baillieres Clin Obstet Gynaecol* 3:823–838, 1989

This comprehensive discussion of postpartum psychosis has an excellent bibliography.

17. *McKenna PJ, Kane JM, Parrish K: Psychotic syndromes in epilepsy. *Am J Psychiatry* 142:895–904, 1985

In this critical review of the controversial relationship between epilepsy and psychoses, McKenna et al. argue for a significant association between epilepsy and both brief and persistent psychotic states. Included is a discussion of temporal lobe epilepsy and epileptic psychoses, with an exploration of etiological factors.

18. **Neppe VM, Tucker GJ:** Atypical, unusual and cultural psychoses, in *Comprehensive Textbook of Psychiatry/V*, 5th Edition, Vol. 1. Edited by Kaplan HI, Sadock BJ. Baltimore, MD, Williams & Wilkins, 1989, pp. 842–852

This concise review has particularly good discussions of the issues involved in cultural psychoses and epileptic psychoses.

15

Anxiety Disorders, Phobias, and Obsessive-Compulsive Disorder

Daphne Simeon, M.D.
Eric Hollander, M.D.

The anxiety disorders have emerged in epidemiologic studies as the most common of all psychiatric disorders and may result in marked subjective distress, functional impairment, and even an increased mortality risk. Anxiety is the common symptom in these disorders and may be experienced directly, as in panic and generalized anxiety, or may be bound to specific situations, thoughts, or behaviors, as with phobias, obsessions, and compulsions.

A historical overview of the anxiety disorders may lead to a deeper understanding of the field, and so a number of historically important papers have been referenced. However, in the last two decades, rapid and significant advances in the nosology of anxiety disorders have been made. These advances have stemmed from new developments in pharmacological and psychological treatment responses; biological determinants; family, twin, and epidemiologic studies; and early genetic investigations, along with improved methodology and more rigorous research standards. Major advances have included the pharmacological dissection and delineation of panic and generalized anxiety as distinct syndromes; the identification of specific patterns of familial risk for the various anxiety disorders; and the elucidation of serotonergic dysfunction associated with obsessive-compulsive disorder and more recently with an extended group of related disorders. Furthermore, the systematic study of specific syndromes, the emergence of new classes of medications, and the expansion and refinement of cognitive-behavioral treatment techniques have led to highly effective treatments for conditions previously considered chronic and refractory such as agoraphobia and obsessive-compulsive disorder. Studies have demonstrated the often greater efficacy of combined pharmacological and psychotherapeutic (cognitive-behavioral) treatment. Such findings continue to emphasize the importance of being open-minded and broadly trained in the face of heightened specialization that characterizes modern psychiatry. Although psychodynamic psychotherapy alone is no longer the treatment of choice for panic attacks, phobias, and obsessions and compulsions, basic knowledge of psychodynamic principles remains invaluable in the treatment of personality traits and deeper conflicts that can be intimately intertwined with and may limit the benefits to be derived from more target-focused treatments. It has now been shown, for example, that the presence of underlying personality disorder may be of great prognostic significance in the overall outcome of Axis I anxiety disorders.

Therefore, in choosing the references for this chapter, we have attempted to integrate major historical papers and landmark advances from all psychiatric disciplines with rigorously designed research studies and informative, state-of-the-art chapters or books in the anxiety disorders. The references designated as core (*) have been selected as the most essential and should be useful both for beginning students and as key articles.

General

1. *Beck AT, Emery G, Greenberg RL:** Anxiety Disorders and Phobias: a Cognitive Perspective.* New York, Basic Books, 1985

   By one of the leaders in the field of cognitive therapy, this is a thorough and readily applicable guide to the cognitive structures and restructuring techniques for generalized anxiety, panic, simple phobia, agoraphobia, and social phobia.

2. *Bowlby J:** Attachment and Loss, Vol. 2: Separation: Anxiety and Anger.* New York, Basic Books, 1973

   Bowlby presents his highly influential model of an inborn primary instinct for attachment, whereby anxiety and phobias constitute the response to insecure attachment and threatened separation.

3. *Gray J: *The Neuropsychology of Anxiety.* Oxford, England, Clarendon Press/Oxford University Press, 1982

By one of the major neuropsychological theorists of anxiety, this book elaborates the structure and function of the septohippocampal system and its relationship to anxiety.

4. *Hollander E, Simeon D, Liebowitz MR, Gorman JM: Anxiety disorders, in *The American Psychiatric Press Textbook of Psychiatry* 2nd Edition. Edited by Hales RE, Yudofsky SC, Talbott JA. Washington, DC, American Psychiatric Press, 1994, pp. 495–563

This chapter is a well-balanced, thorough, and up-to-date presentation of the various anxiety disorders.

5. Klein DF (ed): *Anxiety.* New York, Karger, 1987

With an introduction attempting to elucidate the origins of anxiety, Klein provides a succinct overview of generalized anxiety, panic, agoraphobia, social phobia, and simple phobia.

6. Klein RG, Last CG: *Anxiety Disorders in Children.* Newbury Park, CA, Sage, 1989

For the general clinician, this is a concise and enjoyable overview of the classification, assessment, and treatment of childhood anxiety disorders.

7. *MacKinnon RA, Michels R: The obsessive patient, in *The Psychiatric Interview in Clinical Practice.* Philadelphia, PA, WB Saunders, 1971, pp. 89–109; **MacKinnon RA, Michels R:** The phobic patient, in *The Psychiatric Interview in Clinical Practice.* Philadelphia, PA, WB Saunders, 1971, pp. 147–173

Although more applicable to the personality type rather than the Axis I disorder, this is basic reading for students of psychiatry on the psychopathology, psychodynamics, and treatment principles with obsessive or phobic patients.

8. *Marks IM: *Fears, Phobias, and Rituals: Panic, Anxiety, and Their Disorders.* New York, Oxford University Press, 1987

In this comprehensive synthesis by one of the leaders of behavioral psychology, Marks discusses the nature of fear and anxiety and the development of fear-related clinical syndromes and cogently summarizes treatment principles and findings, behavioral and other.

9. *Maser JD, Cloninger CR (eds): *Comorbidity of Mood and Anxiety Disorders.* Washington, DC, American Psychiatric Press, 1990

In this most comprehensive and up-to-date volume on comorbidity of anxiety and mood disorders, Maser and Cloninger review comorbidity findings from epidemiologic, clinical, family, and biological studies and present a variety of theoretical models that attempt to understand the relationship between anxiety and depression.

10. *Roth M, Noyes R, Burrows GD** (eds): *Handbook of Anxiety, Vol. 4: The Treatment of Anxiety.* New York, Elsevier, 1990

This is a well-written, state-of-the-art collection of papers on the pharmacotherapy and psychotherapy of all the anxiety disorders.

Panic and Generalized Anxiety Disorders

General/Diagnosis/Phenomenology

11. **Faravelli C, Pallanti S:** Recent life events and panic disorder. *Am J Psychiatry* 146:622–626, 1989

The findings of this study support that the number and severity of recent life events may precipitate the onset of panic disorder, especially events related to loss.

12. *Klein DF:** Delineation of two drug-responsive anxiety syndromes. *Psychopharmacologia* 5:397–408, 1964

This is an early landmark article that demonstrated that imipramine treats panic but not anticipatory anxiety or phobic avoidance. Two syndromes were delineated: a group with childhood separation anxiety postulated to have a biological dysfunction of an innate separation anxiety regulatory mechanism leading to the development of panic under separation or loss, and a group with unremarkable developmental history.

13. **Lelliott P, Marks I, McNamee G, Tobena A:** Onset of panic disorder with agoraphobia. *Arch Gen Psychiatry* 46:1000–1004, 1989

The authors present an integrated model of the development of panic with agoraphobia, combining biological, learning, and evolutionary factors.

14. **Noyes R Jr, Reich JH, Suelzer M, Christiansen J:** Personality traits associated with panic disorder: change associated with treatment. *Compr Psychiatry* 32:283–294, 1991

This personality follow-up of panic patients who received treatment for 3 years suggests that initial avoidant and dependent traits were to a large extent state dependent.

15. **Rapee RM:** Panic disorder. *International Review of Psychiatry* 3:141–149, 1991

    This article is a review of panic disorder, covering diagnosis, etiologies, and pharmacological and behavioral treatments.

16. *Raskin M, Peeke HV, Dickman W, Pinsker H:** Panic and generalized anxiety disorder. *Arch Gen Psychiatry* 39:687–689, 1982

    This interesting study compares the developmental and psychiatric histories of patients with panic versus generalized anxiety, in support of the distinctness of the two disorders.

Epidemiology and Comorbidity

17. **Coryell W, Endicott J, Andreasen NC, Keller MB, Clayton PJ, Hirschfeld RM, Scheftner WA, Winokur G:** Depression and panic attacks: the significance of overlap as reflected in follow-up and family study data. *Am J Psychiatry* 145:293–300, 1988

    The findings here show that panic complicating depression predicts a worst outcome for the depression. Also, an anxiety-depression continuum with a common underlying diathesis is not supported by the data.

18. *Johnson J, Weissman MM, Klerman GL:** Panic disorder, comorbidity, and suicide attempts. *Arch Gen Psychiatry* 47:805–808, 1990

    The authors estimates the lifetime rate of suicide attempts in persons with uncomplicated panic disorder at 7%, comparable to a 7.9% rate for uncomplicated major depression, and in contrast to a 1% rate for people without psychiatric disorder.

19. **Leckman JF, Weissman MM, Merikangas KR, Pauls DL, Prusoff BA:** Panic disorder and major depression. *Arch Gen Psychiatry* 40:1055–1060, 1983

    The findings of this family study suggest that panic and depression may share a partial underlying diathesis.

20. **Regier DA, Boyd JH, Burke JD, Rae DS, Myers JK, Kramer M, Robins LN, George LK, Karno M, Locke BZ:** One-month prevalence of mental disorders in the United States: based on five Epidemiologic Catchment Area sites. *Arch Gen Psychiatry* 45:977–986, 1988

This article discusses the largest epidemiologic study of psychiatric disorders to date for the United States, demonstrating that anxiety disorders (phobia, panic, obsessive-compulsive) are the most prevalent of all major groups of disorders, phobia being the single most common disorder, with interesting comparisons to international epidemiologic data.

21. **Torgersen S:** Comorbidity of major depression and anxiety disorders in twin pairs. *Am J Psychiatry* 147:1199–1202, 1990

   In this twin study, Torgersen found that pure anxiety and panic were unrelated to major depression, whereas mixed anxiety with depression was more related to major depression without anxiety.

Biology

22. **Abelson JL, Glitz D, Cameron OG, Lee MA, Bronzo M, Curtis GC:** Blunted growth hormone response to clonidine in patients with generalized anxiety disorder. *Arch Gen Psychiatry* 48:157–162, 1991

   This neuroendocrine finding supports a role for the noradrenergic system in generalized anxiety disorder; the presence of this finding in other disorders also characterized by anxiety is discussed.

23. *****Ballenger JC** (ed): *Neurobiology of Panic Disorder.* New York, Wiley-Liss, 1990

   This book is a compilation of animal, genetic, and neurobiological models regarding the biology of panic by a number of prominent researchers in the field.

24. **Bradwejn J, Kossycki D, Shriqui C:** Enhanced sensitivity to cholecystokinin tetrapeptide in panic disorder: clinical and behavioral findings. *Arch Gen Psychiatry* 48:603–610, 1991

   This comparison of panic disorder patients with healthy volunteers suggests that enhanced sensitivity to the brain neuropeptide cholecystokinin may be implicated in the neurobiology of panic attacks.

25. *****Gorman JM, Fyer MR, Goetz R, Askanazi J, Liebowitz MR, Fyer AJ, Kinney J, Klein DF:** Ventilatory physiology of patients with panic disorder. *Arch Gen Psychiatry* 45:31–39, 1988

   Based on the experimental findings here, it is proposed that both CO_2 and lactate-induced panic may be mediated by brain-stem CO_2 receptor hypersensitivity leading to an exaggerated ventilatory response.

26. **Gorman JM, Liebowitz MR, Fyer AJ, Stein T:** A neuroanatomical hypothesis for panic disorder. *Am J Psychiatry* 146:148–161, 1989

This review article on the biology of panic disorder attempts to integrate the three behavioral components (panic attacks, anticipatory anxiety, and phobic avoidance) via a tripartite neuroanatomical model.

27. *Liebowitz MR, Gorman JM, Fyer AJ, Levitt M, Dillon D, Levy G, Appleby IL, Anderson S, Palij M, Davies SO, Klein DF:** Lactate provocation of panic attacks, II: biochemical and physiological findings. *Arch Gen Psychiatry* 42:709–719, 1985

Three broad biological theories of the mechanism of panic (altered chemistry, central nervous system vulnerability, and nonspecific stress vulnerability) are cogently presented. The data here suggest that central noradrenergic activation may be the mechanism involved.

28. **Mason ST, Fibiger HC:** Anxiety: the locus ceruleus disconnection. *Life Sci* 25:2141–2147, 1979

Mason and Fibiger argue against the locus ceruleus model of panic, presenting evidence that this brain region mediates arousal and not anxiety.

29. **Nutt DJ, Glue P, Lawson C, Wilson S:** Flumazenil provocation of panic attacks. *Arch Gen Psychiatry* 47:917–925, 1990

The use of the benzodiazepine receptor antagonist flumazenil suggests that people with panic disorder may have an altered benzodiazepine receptor set point that renders them in a chronic state of lowered gamma-aminobutyric acid (GABA) inhibition.

Psychodynamics

30. **Freud S:** On the grounds for detaching a particular syndrome from neurasthenia under the description "anxiety neurosis" (1895), in *The Standard Edition of the Complete Psychological Works of Sigmund Freud,* Vol. 3. Translated and edited by Strachey J. London, Hogarth Press, 1962, pp. 90–115

This is Freud's earlier formulation regarding the genesis of anxiety, conceptualized as the direct physical transformation of undischarged instinctual drives without mediation of the psychic apparatus.

31. *Freud S:** Inhibitions, symptoms, and anxiety (1926), in *The Standard Edition of the Complete Psychological Works of Sigmund Freud,* Vol. 20. Translated and edited by Strachey J. London, Hogarth Press, 1962, pp. 87–172

This is a later paper where anxiety is conceptualized as a signal of intrapsychic conflict in accordance with structural theory. In response to signal anxiety, inhibitions and neurotic symptoms develop that allow only partial gratification of instinctual wishes.

32. **Klein M:** A contribution to the theory of anxiety and guilt. *Int J Psychoanal* 29:114–123, 1948

    In opposition to Freud's emphasis on sexual instincts in the generation of anxiety, Klein conceptualized aggression toward the loved object as the primary factor in the causation of anxiety.

33. *Michels R, Frances A, Shear MK:* Psychodynamic models of anxiety, in *Anxiety and the Anxiety Disorders.* Edited by Tuma AH, Maser JD. Hillsdale, NJ, Lawrence Erlbaum Associates, 1985, pp. 595–618

    This is a very informative overview of the psychodynamic formulations of anxiety from Freud to the present, also comparing and contrasting these to other theories.

Genetics

34. *Crowe RR, Noyes R, Pauls DL, Slymen D:* A family study of panic disorder. *Arch Gen Psychiatry* 40:1065–1069, 1983

    In this major pedigree study of panic disorder, Crowe et al. found panic to have a significant familial component, without an increased familial risk for other psychiatric disorders, including generalized anxiety disorder.

35. **Kendler KS, Neale MC, Kessler RC, Heath AC, Eaves LJ:** Generalized anxiety disorder in women: a population-based twin study. *Arch Gen Psychiatry* 49:267–272, 1992

    This study shows that the familial aspect of generalized anxiety disorder is almost entirely genetic and not environmental, with a modest heritability of about 30%.

36. **Torgersen S:** Genetic factors in anxiety disorders. *Arch Gen Psychiatry* 40:1085–1089, 1983

    Based on the comparison of monozygotic and dizygotic twins, a genetic component was identified for panic and agoraphobia but not for generalized anxiety. Obsessive-compulsive disorder and social phobia are also discussed.

Treatment

37. *Ballenger JC, Burrows GD, DuPont RL Jr, Lesser IM, Noyes R Jr, Pecknold JC, Rifkin A, Swinson RP:** Alprazolam in panic disorder and agoraphobia: results from a multicenter trial, I: efficacy in short-term treatment. *Arch Gen Psychiatry* 45:413–422, 1988

    This article presents a large, multicenter treatment study documenting the efficacy of alprazolam in the treatment not only of panic attacks, but also anticipatory anxiety, phobic avoidance, and overall disability.

38. *Barlow DH, Craske MG, Carny JA, Klosko JS:** Behavioral treatment of panic disorder. *Behavior Therapy* 20:261–282, 1989

    Barlow et al. report on a long-term treatment outcome study for panic attacks without agoraphobia, comparing relaxation therapy, interoceptive exposure plus cognitive restructuring, or a combination of the two techniques.

39. *Beck AT, Sokol L, Clark DA, Berchick R, Wright F:** A crossover study of focused cognitive therapy for panic disorder. *Am J Psychiatry* 149:778–783, 1992

    This study demonstrated the marked superiority of focused cognitive therapy over brief supportive therapy in the acute treatment of panic, with very high maintenance of response at 1-year follow-up.

40. **Clark DM, Salkovskis PM, Chalkley AJ:** Respiratory control as a treatment for panic attacks. *J Behav Ther Exp Psychiatry* 16:23–30, 1985

    This study demonstrated that pure breathing retraining without other interventions significantly reduced panic attacks over a 2-week period.

41. **Hoehn-Saric R, McLeod DR, Zimmerli WD:** Differential effects of alprazolam and imipramine in generalized anxiety disorder: somatic versus psychic symptoms. *J Clin Psychiatry* 49:293–301, 1988

    Hoehn-Saric et al. found a similar early efficacy for alprazolam and imipramine, with alprazolam acting more on somatic symptoms and imipramine more on psychic symptoms of negative affects and cognitions.

42. **Mavissakalian M:** Differential effects of imipramine and behavior therapy on panic disorder with agoraphobia. *Psychopharmacol Bull* 25:27–29, 1989

    This brief review article summarizes studies on the efficacy of behavioral therapy with or without imipramine and examines whether these two treatments have a differential effect on the panic versus the phobic component.

43. *Sheehan DV, Ballenger J, Jacobsen G:** Treatment of endogenous anxiety with phobic, hysterical and hypochondriacal symptoms. *Arch Gen Psychiatry* 37:51–59, 1980

   This article presents a large placebo-controlled study that established a similar efficacy for imipramine and phenelzine in the treatment of panic attacks.

44. **Tesar GE, Rosenbaum JF, Pollack MH, Otto MW, Sachs GS, Herman JB, Cohen LS, Spier SA:** Double-blind, placebo-controlled comparison of clonazepam and alprazolam for panic disorder. *J Clin Psychiatry* 52:69–76, 1991

   This controlled study showed similar efficacy for two high-potency benzodiazepines—clonazepam and alprazolam—in the acute treatment of panic attacks, phobic avoidance, and overall disability.

45. **Welkowitz LA, Papp LA, Cloitre M, Liebowitz MR, Martin LY, Gorman JM:** Cognitive-behavior therapy for panic disorder delivered by psychopharmacologically oriented clinicians. *J Nerv Ment Dis* 179:473–477, 1991

   This is a highly applicable article emphasizing the utility and effectiveness of basic cognitive-behavioral training for psychopharmacologically oriented clinicians.

Course and Outcome

46. **Allgulander C, Lavori PW:** Excess mortality among 3302 patients with "pure" anxiety neurosis. *Arch Gen Psychiatry* 48:599–602, 1991

   This article reports on a large retrospective survey from Sweden in support of the emerging finding that panic may be associated with an increased suicide risk, in the absence of comorbid diagnoses.

47. *Mavissakalian M, Perel JM:** Clinical experiments in maintenance and discontinuation of imipramine therapy in panic disorder with agoraphobia. *Arch Gen Psychiatry* 49:318–323, 1992

   Probably the most thorough study on this topic, this article documents the success of half-dose imipramine in preventing relapse during a 1-year maintenance, as opposed to a very high panic relapse rate if medication is discontinued after 6 months of acute treatment.

48. **Nagy LM, Krystal JH, Woods SW, Charney DS:** Clinical and medication outcome after short-term alprazolam and behavioral group treatment in panic disorder: 2.5-year naturalistic follow-up study. *Arch Gen Psychiatry* 46:993–999, 1989

Like other follow-up studies, this study also shows overall good maintenance of acute treatment gains at follow-up, less so if complicated by histories of depression.

49. *Noyes R Jr, Reich J, Christiansen J, Suelzer M, Pfohl B, Coryell WA:** Outcome of panic disorder: relationship to diagnostic subtypes and comorbidity. *Arch Gen Psychiatry* 47:809–818, 1990

In a 3-year follow-up of people with panic disorder, Noyes et al. present an overall good outcome in two-thirds of patients. Symptoms remained worse in patients who initially had depression or marked phobic avoidance, whereas comorbid personality disorder and not panic was the major predictor of later social maladjustment.

Phobic Disorders

General/Diagnosis/Phenomenology

50. **Franklin JA:** Agoraphobia. *International Review of Psychiatry* 3:151–162, 1991

This is a concise review of the diagnosis, etiology, course, treatment, and prognosis of agoraphobia.

51. **Himle JA, Crystal D, Curtis GC, Fluent TE:** Mode of onset of simple phobia subtypes: further evidence of heterogeneity. *Psychol Res* 36:37–43, 1991

This is an interesting phenomenological study that found different patterns of onset in four different types of simple phobia. Implications are discussed.

52. **Marks I:** Blood-injury phobia: a review. *Am J Psychiatry* 145:1207–1213, 1988

Marks presents an in-depth review of the origins and treatment of a phobia, which can have a significant impact on the utilization of needed medical care.

53. **Schneier FR:** Social phobia. *Psychiatric Annals* 21:349–353, 1991

This is a review article outlining epidemiology, treatment approaches, and models of neurochemical dysfunction.

Epidemiology and Comorbidity

54. *Schneier FR, Johnson J, Hornig CD, Liebowitz MR, Weissman MM: Social phobia: comorbidity and morbidity in an epidemiological sample. *Arch Gen Psychiatry* 49:282–288, 1992

This is the most comprehensive epidemiologic study of social phobia, addressing prevalence, demographics, associated impairment, and comorbidity with other psychiatric disorders.

55. **Stein MB, Tancer ME, Gelernter CS, Vittone BJ, Uhde TW:** Major depression in patients with social phobia. *Am J Psychiatry* 147:637–639, 1990

A significantly lower rate of major depression was found in patients with social phobia compared with panic disorder, and the authors speculate that this may be related to the greater unpredictability and helplessness generated by the latter disorder.

Psychodynamics

56. *Deutsch H: Section II: Phobia, in *Neuroses and Character Types: Clinical Psychoanalytic Studies.* New York, International Universities Press, 1965, pp. 74–116

Lucid clinical descriptions of two cases of simple phobias (a cat phobia and a hen phobia) and of agoraphobia are presented, illustrating the complex interplay of pre-Oedipal and Oedipal dynamics in the genesis of phobic symptoms.

57. *Freud S: Analysis of a phobia in a five-year-old boy (1909), in *The Standard Edition of the Complete Psychological Works of Sigmund Freud,* Vol. 10. Translated and edited by Strachey J. London, Hogarth Press, 1962, pp. 5–149

This is the classic case of Little Hans, a 5-year-old boy who developed a fear of horses stemming from Oedipal conflict.

58. *Nemiah JC: A psychoanalytic view of phobias. *Am J Psychoanal* 41:115–120, 1981

This article is an attempt to integrate psychodynamic, biological, and learning theories in the understanding of the development of phobias.

Genetics

59. **Fyer AJ, Mannuzza S, Gallops MS, Martin LY, Aaronson C, Gorman JM, Liebowitz MR, Klein DF:** Familial transmission of simple phobias and fears: a preliminary report. *Arch Gen Psychiatry* 47:252–256, 1990

This is an interesting family study that showed a strong component of familial transmission for simple phobias, without an increased risk for other phobic or anxiety disorders, supporting the conceptualization of simple phobias as a distinct entity.

60. **Kendler KS, Neale MC, Kessler RC, Heath AC, Eaves LJ:** The genetic epidemiology of phobias in women: the interrelationship of agoraphobia, social phobia, situational phobia, and simple phobia. *Arch Gen Psychiatry* 49:273–281, 1992

Kendler et al. examines, via the study of twins, the relative contribution of genetic and environmental factors as well as the type of environmental events to the different types of phobias.

Treatment

61. *Gelernter CS, Uhde TW, Cimbolic P, Arnkoff DB, Vittone BJ, Tancer ME, Bartko JJ:** Cognitive-behavioral and pharmacological treatments of social phobia: a controlled study. *Arch Gen Psychiatry* 48:938–945, 1991

Interestingly, all treatment modes resulted in significant improvement in this study. The implications of this are discussed.

62. **Klein DF, Zitrin CM, Woerner MG, Ross DC:** Treatment of phobias, II: behavior therapy and supportive psychotherapy: are there any specific ingredients? *Arch Gen Psychiatry* 40:139–145, 1983

This is an interesting interpretation of the finding that phobic patients did equally well with supportive or behavioral therapy: therapy-generated hopeful expectation is the common nonspecific active ingredient that then leads to change-generating in vivo exposure.

63. *Klein DF, Ross DC, Cohen PC:** Panic and avoidance in agoraphobia: application of path analysis to treatment studies. *Arch Gen Psychiatry* 44:377–385, 1987

Klein et al. make the important point that the treatment course of panic attacks and phobic avoidance may not parallel each other. They compare the differential effect on these two components of imipramine and exposure therapy.

64. *Liebowitz MR, Schneier F, Campeas R, Hollander E, Hatterer J, Fyer A, Gorman J, Papp L, Davies S, Gully R, Klein DF:** Phenelzine vs atenolol in social phobia: a placebo-controlled comparison. *Arch Gen Psychiatry* 49:290–300, 1992

This study confirms the superiority of phenelzine in treating social phobia, with about two-thirds of patients responding to this drug. Atenolol was not significantly superior to placebo.

65. *Mattick RP, Andrews G, Hadzi PD, Christensen H:** Treatment of panic and agoraphobia: an integrative review. *J Nerv Ment Dis* 178:567–576, 1990

This is an extensive review and meta-analysis of 51 treatment studies, pharmacological and cognitive-behavioral, of panic and agoraphobia.

66. *Telch MJ, Agras WS, Taylor CB, Roth WT, Gallen CC:** Combined pharmacological and behavioral treatment for agoraphobia. *Behav Res Ther* 23:325–335, 1985

This is a well-designed 26-week study that found combined imipramine and exposure to be significantly superior to either treatment alone for panic with agoraphobia. The implications are discussed.

67. **Versiani M, Mundim FD, Nardi AE, Liebowitz MR:** Tranylcypromine in social phobia. *J Clin Psychopharmacol* 8:279–283, 1988

This open 1-year trial found significant clinical improvement in about 80% of patients taking tranylcypromine.

68. *Zitrin CM, Klein DF, Woerner MG:** Treatment of agoraphobia with group exposure in vivo and imipramine. *Arch Gen Psychiatry* 37:63–72, 1980

This is another study that supports that combined imipramine and behavioral therapy is superior to behavioral therapy alone for panic, agoraphobia, and global change.

69. *Zitrin CM, Klein DF, Woerner MG, Ross DC:** Treatment of phobias, I: comparison of imipramine hydrochloride and placebo. *Arch Gen Psychiatry* 40:125–138, 1983

This is the largest-scale controlled study demonstrating the efficacy of imipramine in the treatment of panic (with or without agoraphobia) but not in the treatment of simple phobias.

Course and Outcome

70. **Mavissakalian M, Michelson L:** Two-year follow-up of exposure and imipramine treatment of agoraphobia. *Am J Psychiatry* 143:1106–1112, 1986

    This is a systematic follow-up study showing that initial marked responders to imipramine and exposure therapy tend to maintain their gains in the long term.

Obsessive-Compulsive Disorders

General/Diagnosis/Phenomenology

71. *Goodman WK, Price LH, Rasmussen SA, Mazure C, Fleischmann RL, Hill CL, Heninger GR, Charney DS:** The Yale-Brown Obsessive Compulsive Scale, I: development, use, and reliability. *Arch Gen Psychiatry* 46:1006–1011, 1989

    This article describes the development of the Yale-Brown Obsessive Compulsive Scale, a much-needed scale for quantifying obsessive and compulsive symptoms that has since greatly facilitated research studies of obsessive-compulsive disorder.

72. *Hollander E:** Serotonergic drugs and the treatment of disorders related to obsessive-compulsive disorder, in *Current Treatments of Obsessive-Compulsive Disorder.* Edited by Pato M, Zohar J. Washington, DC, American Psychiatric Press, 1991, pp. 173–191

    This is an interesting chapter speculating on the existence of a group of obsessive-compulsive, disorder-related disorders, which includes body dysmorphic disorder, trichotillomania, depersonalization, anorexia nervosa, and Tourette's syndrome.

73. *Hollander E** (ed): *Obsessive-Compulsive Related Disorders.* Washington, DC, American Psychiatric Press, 1993

    This is the first book to describe the close relationship between obsessive-compulsive disorder and a spectrum of clinical syndromes related in phenomenology, associated features, family history, etiology, and response to behavioral and medication treatments. Body dysmorphic disorder, depersonalization disorder, trichotillomania, anorexia nervosa, Tourette's syndrome, pathological gambling, and the impulsive and delusional spectrums are discussed.

74. *Rapoport JL (ed): *Obsessive-Compulsive Disorder in Children and Adolescents.* Washington, DC, American Psychiatric Press, 1989

Now the classic text for childhood obsessive-compulsive disorder, this is enjoyable reading illustrated with clinical cases. Rapoport outlines comprehensive evaluation procedures and treatment principles and presents a variety of theoretical models for understanding childhood obsessive-compulsive disorder.

Epidemiology and Comorbidity

75. **Karno M, Golding JM, Sorenson SB, Burnam MA:** The epidemiology of obsessive-compulsive disorder in five US communities. *Arch Gen Psychiatry* 45:1094–1099, 1988

From the Epidemiologic Catchment Area study, this is a detailed report that shed new light on the epidemiology of obsessive-compulsive disorder, highlighting its primary nature as a psychiatric disorder and a lifetime prevalence of 1.9%—3.3%, up to 60 times greater than that previously estimated from clinical samples.

Biology

76. *Baxter LR Jr, Phelps ME, Mazziotta JC, Guze BH, Schwartz JM, Selin CE:** Local cerebral glucose metabolic rates in obsessive-compulsive disorder: a comparison with rates in unipolar depression and normal controls. *Arch Gen Psychiatry* 44:211–218, 1987

This imaging study suggests basal ganglia involvement in obsessive-compulsive disorder.

77. **Charney DS, Goodman WK, Price LH, Woods SW, Rasmussen SA, Heninger GR:** Serotonin function in obsessive-compulsive disorder: a comparison of the effects of tryptophan and m-chlorophenylpiperazine in patients and healthy subjects. *Arch Gen Psychiatry* 45:177–185, 1988

This neuroendocrine challenge study lends only partial support to the serotonergic dysfunction hypothesis of obsessive-compulsive disorder.

78. *Hollander E, Schiffman E, Cohen B, Rivera-Stein MA, Rosen W, Gorman JM, Fyer AJ, Papp L, Liebowitz MR:** Signs of central nervous system dysfunction in obsessive-compulsive disorder. *Arch Gen Psychiatry* 47:27–32, 1990

The findings here support that there may be at least a subgroup of patients with obsessive-compulsive disorder who have an underlying structural brain abnormality.

79. *Hollander E, DeCaria CM, Nitescu A, Gully R, Suckow RF, Cooper TB, Gorman JM, Klein DF, Liebowitz MR: Serotonergic function in obsessive-compulsive disorder: behavioral and neuroendocrine responses to oral m-chlorophenylpiperazine and fenfluramine in patients and healthy volunteers. *Arch Gen Psychiatry* 49:21–28, 1992

This article elaborates the complexities of serotonergic involvement in obsessive-compulsive disorder as it attempts to clarify the specific receptors, brain areas, and regulatory mechanisms that may be dysfunctional.

80. Pitman RK: Animal models of compulsive behavior. *Biol Psychiatry* 26:189–198, 1989

Various animal models of compulsive behavior, mostly mediated by dopaminergic basal ganglia dysfunction, are presented.

81. Swedo SE, Schapiro MB, Grady CL, Cheslow DL, Leonard HL, Kumar A, Friedland R, Rapoport SI, Rapoport JL: Cerebral glucose metabolism in childhood-onset obsessive-compulsive disorder. *Arch Gen Psychiatry* 46:518–523, 1989

This is a positron-emission tomography study, suggesting, similarly to Baxter et al. (1987), that frontal-limbic-basal ganglia dysfunction may be involved in obsessive-compulsive disorder.

82. *Swedo SE, Leonard HL, Kruesi MJ, Rettew DC, Listwak SJ, Berrettini W, Stipetic M, Hamburger S, Gold PW, Potter WZ, Rapoport JL: Cerebrospinal fluid neurochemistry in children and adolescents with obsessive-compulsive disorder. *Arch Gen Psychiatry* 49:29–36, 1992

Swedo et al. present evidence that not only the serotonergic system, but also vasopressin and oxytocin, via their effects on attention and memory, may be involved in compulsive rituals.

83. Thoren P, Asberg M, Bertilsson L, Mellstrom B, Sjoqvist F, Traskman L: Clomipramine treatment of obsessive-compulsive disorder, II: biochemical aspects. *Arch Gen Psychiatry* 37:1289–1294, 1980

This is one of the earlier neurochemical studies of obsessive-compulsive disorder. The findings support a serotonergic dysfunction hypothesis as pretreatment elevated cerebrospinal fluid (CSF) 5-hydroxyindoleacetic acid (5-HIAA) and posttreatment reduction of CSF 5-HIAA were related to clomipramine responsivity.

84. Zohar J, Insel TR, Zohar-Kadouch RC, Hill JL, Murphy DL: Serotonergic responsivity in obsessive-compulsive disorder: effects of chronic clomipramine treatment. *Arch Gen Psychiatry* 45:167–172, 1988

This study demonstrates serotonergic hyporesponsivity in obsessive-compulsive disorder patients treated with clomipramine, supporting the biological theory that obsessive-compulsive psychopathology may be related to excess serotonergic tone.

85. *Zohar J, Insel TR, Rasmussen SA (eds): *The Psychobiology of Obsessive Compulsive Disorder.* New York, Springer, 1991

This is a collection of papers integrating the psychobiology of obsessive-compulsive disorder, including sections on genetics, brain imaging, neuropsychology, and neurochemistry.

Psychodynamics

86. **Esman AH:** Psychoanalysis and general psychiatry: obsessive-compulsive disorder as paradigm. *J Am Psychoanal Assoc* 37:319–336, 1989

Implications of biological treatments for psychoanalytic theory and research are discussed in this article.

87. *Freud S:** Notes upon a case of obsessional neurosis (1909), in *The Standard Edition of the Complete Psychological Works of Sigmund Freud,* Vol. 10. Edited and translated by Strachey J. London, Hogarth Press, 1962, pp. 155–249

This is the case of the Rat Man, the first in-depth psychoanalytic study of obsessional neurosis.

Treatment

88. **Beech HR, Vaughan M:** *Behavioural Treatment of Obsessional States.* New York, Wiley, 1978

Beech and Vaughan provide a thorough guide to a variety of behavioral treatment approaches for obsessive-compulsive disorder.

89. *The Clomipramine Collaborative Study Group:** Clomipramine in the treatment of patients with obsessive-compulsive disorder. *Arch Gen Psychiatry* 48:730–738, 1991

This is a multicenter treatment study of patients with obsessive-compulsive disorder that definitively documents the success of clomipramine, which resulted in an approximately 40% reduction of symptoms by 10 weeks.

90. **Flament MF, Rapoport JL, Berg CJ, Sceery W, Kilts C, Mellstrom B, Linnoila M:** Clomipramine treatment of childhood obsessive-compul-

sive disorder: a double-blind controlled study. *Arch Gen Psychiatry* 42:977–983, 1985

This is the first systematic study to document the efficacy of clomipramine in the treatment of children with obsessive-compulsive disorder.

91. *Goodman WK, McDougle CJ: Serotonin reuptake inhibitors in the treatment of obsessive-compulsive disorder. *Annals of Clinical Psychiatry* 2:173–181, 1990

This is a concise summary for clinicians of the medication treatment of obsessive-compulsive disorder, including strategies for treatment-refractory patients.

92. Goodman WK, Price LH, Delgado PL, Palumbo J, Krystal JH, Nagy LM, Rasmussen SA, Heninger GR, Charney DS: Specificity of serotonin reuptake inhibitors in the treatment of obsessive-compulsive disorder: comparison of fluvoxamine and desipramine. *Arch Gen Psychiatry* 47:577–585, 1990

The superiority of fluvoxamine over desipramine supports serotonergic as opposed to noradrenergic dysfunction in obsessive-compulsive disorder.

93. *Jenike MA, Baer L, Minichiello WE: *Obsessive-Compulsive Disorders: Theory and Management,* 2nd Edition. Chicago, IL, Chicago Year Book Medical Publishers, 1990

This book is highly recommended for a comprehensive overview of obsessive-compulsive disorder, including presentation, etiology, and integrated treatment (pharmacological, behavioral, cognitive, psychodynamic). It includes useful appendixes with information for patients and with the most popular rating instruments.

94. Jenike MA, Baer L, Summergrad P, Minichiello WE, Holland A, Seymour R: Sertraline in obsessive-compulsive disorder: a double-blind comparison with placebo. *Am J Psychiatry* 147:923–928, 1990 (erratum: 147:1393, 1990)

Although the interpretation of this finding is considered controversial, this is so far the only published obsessive-compulsive disorder trial of the Food and Drug Administration approved serotonin reuptake blocker sertraline. It failed to show efficacy at 200 mg/day.

95. *Jenike MA, Baer L, Ballantine HT, Martuza RL, Tynes S, Giriunas I, Buttolph ML, Cassem NH: Cingulotomy for refractory obsessive-compulsive disorder: a long-term follow-up of 33 patients. *Arch Gen Psychiatry* 48:548–555, 1991

Although retrospective, this series applies rigorous criteria and suggests that surgical cingulotomy may be of substantial benefit to at least one-third of patients with refractory obsessive-compulsive disorder.

96. **Leonard HL, Swedo SE, Rapoport JL, Koby EV, Lenane MC, Cheslow DL, Hamburger SD:** Treatment of obsessive-compulsive disorder with clomipramine and desipramine in children and adolescents: a double-blind crossover comparison. *Arch Gen Psychiatry* 46:1088–1092, 1989

    Leonard et al. showed that clomipramine's antiobsessional effect in adults also holds for children and adolescents.

97. **Marks IM:** Review of behavioral psychotherapy, I: obsessive-compulsive disorders. *Am J Psychiatry* 138:584–592, 1981

    This is a good review of the principles and efficacy of in vivo exposure therapy alone for the acute and long-term treatment of compulsions.

98. *****Pato MT, Zohar J** (eds): *Current Treatments of Obsessive-Compulsive Disorder.* Washington, DC, American Psychiatric Press, 1991

    This is a short, easy-to-read book on the pharmacological, behavioral, and family treatment of obsessive-compulsive disorder in adults and in children.

99. **Pigott TA, Pato MT, Bernstein SE, Grover GN, Hill JL, Tolliver TJ, Murphy DL:** Controlled comparisons of clomipramine and fluoxetine in the treatment of obsessive-compulsive disorder. *Arch Gen Psychiatry* 47:926–932, 1990

    This crossover design study shows that fluoxetine may be of comparable efficacy to clomipramine in treating obsessive-compulsive disorder.

100. **Salzman L:** *Treatment of the Obsessive Personality.* New York, Jason Aronson, 1980

    This is a classic volume on the psychodynamic psychotherapy of the obsessional personality and of obsessive and compulsive symptoms.

Course and Prognosis

101. **Leonard HL, Swedo SE, Lenane MC, Rettew DC, Cheslow DL, Hamburger SD, Rapoport JL:** A double-blind desipramine substitution during long-term clomipramine treatment in children and adolescents with obsessive-compulsive disorder. *Arch Gen Psychiatry* 48:922–927, 1991

In this controlled study, Leonard et al. point out the need for long-term medication maintenance in obsessive-compulsive disorder to prevent relapse.

102. **Pato MT, Zohar-Kadouch R, Zohar J, Murphy DL:** Return of symptoms after discontinuation of clomipramine in patients with obsessive-compulsive disorder. *Am J Psychiatry* 145:1521–1525, 1988

This prospective study shows that the great majority of obsessive-compulsive disorder patients experience relapse within a few weeks of medication discontinuation, suggesting that prolonged maintenance may be indicated in obsessive-compulsive disorder.

Personality Disorders

Katharine A. Phillips, M.D.
John G. Gunderson, M.D.

T he personality disorders have been the focus of intense interest among mental health professionals in recent decades. Controversies about their diagnosis, classification, etiology, and
treatment abound in the literature, and the revision of their diagnostic
criteria in each succeeding version of DSM continues to prompt much
debate and research.

DSM-IV contains 10 personality disorders and a "personality disorder
not otherwise specified" category on Axis II, several personality disorders in
the appendix for "Criteria Sets and Axes Needing Further Study," and a new
category for "personality change disorders." Although the references presented in this chapter are organized according to this classification system,
it is important to note some of its limitations.

First, it is a diagnostic system in flux. Only a few personality disorders
have been included in every version of DSM, whereas other personality
disorders (e.g., avoidant personality disorder) have been added to more
recent versions, and one (passive-aggressive personality disorder) was omitted from DSM-IV. Some personality disorders (e.g., borderline personality
disorder) have been empirically well validated, whereas the existence of
some others (e.g., avoidant personality disorder and depressive personality
disorder) remains the subject of some debate. One category (narcissistic
personality disorder) is found in DSM-IV but is not represented among the

otherwise similar types of personality disorder found in ICD-10.

Second, many patients with a personality disorder have traits that do not fit neatly into only one diagnostic category but are instead characteristic of more than one disorder. Or they may have problematic personality traits that are not represented by any of the DSM categories.

Finally, the DSM categories describe personality traits that exist in individuals without personality disorders as well as those with full-blown disorders. The disorders whose traits are best conceptualized as existing on a continuum with persons without a disorder, we subgroup as trait types, and we include some references that familiarize the reader with personality traits rather than personality disorders. Other disorders exist as part of a spectrum with traditional forms of Axis I psychopathology, which we subgroup as spectrum types of personality disorder. A final subgroup, called self types, include severe disorders characterized by instability, fragility, or extreme social deviance.

Also included is a set of general references on the personality disorders, some of which address specific topics and others of which give general overviews of the field. These references may serve as starting points for subsequent readings on individual disorders.

The references listed present basic information on clinical presentation, diagnosis, etiology, psychodynamics, and treatment. They include classic earlier works as well as more recent publications.

Personality Disorders: General

1. **Akiskal HS, Akiskal K:** Cyclothymic, hyperthymic, and depressive temperaments as subaffective variants of mood disorders, in *American Psychiatric Press Review of Psychiatry*, Vol. 11. Edited by Tasman A, Riba MB. Washington, DC, American Psychiatric Press, 1992, pp. 43–62

   This is an erudite overview of the history and types of affective temperaments. It reviews evidence suggesting that they are basic forms of personality that can underlie different personality disorders when they match poorly with one's social environment.

2. **Blatt SJ, Zuroff DC:** Interpersonal relatedness and self-definition: two prototypes for depression. *Clinical Psychology Review* 12:527–562, 1992

   The idea of two basic forms of personality grew out of the senior author's extensive experience with psychological measures of object relations. One form, organized around interpersonal needs and fears, consists of preoccupation with separation and attachment issues. The other is organized around self-definition where self-esteem is measured by achievements, distinctiveness, and autonomy. The authors suggest that these types underlie symptom-based affective disorders and help explain differences in therapeutic response and course.

3. **Cloninger CR:** A systematic method for clinical description and classification of personality variants: a proposal. *Arch Gen Psychiatry* 44:573–588, 1987

The author proposes a distinctive new theory for the classification of both normal and abnormal personality variants. Three underlying dimensions of personality are defined in terms of the stimulus-response characteristics of novelty seeking, harm avoidance, and reward dependence. Their possible underlying genetic and neurophysiological bases are discussed.

4. *Gunderson JG, Phillips KA:** Personality disorders, in *Comprehensive Textbook of Psychiatry/VI*, 6th Edition. Edited by Kaplan HI, Sadock BJ. Baltimore, MD, Williams & Wilkins (in press)

This is an up-to-date and comprehensive overview of the issues relating to all personality disorders (e.g., their significance, definition, classification models, and assessment) along with a description of each specific type of disorder's history, epidemiology, etiology, diagnosis and clinical features, and treatment. Prototypic cases are also included.

5. **Kernberg OF:** *Severe Personality Disorders: Psychotherapeutic Strategies.* New Haven, CT, Yale University Press, 1984

This seminal book focuses on the diagnosis and treatment of severe cases of borderline and narcissistic pathology. Its approach is largely clinical, and it provides a broad array of specific psychotherapeutic techniques. The author also discusses developments in ego psychology and object relations theory, with an elaboration on the theoretical issues of ego weakness, identity diffusion, and severe superego pathology.

6. *Millon T:** *Disorders of Personality—DSM III: Axis II.* New York, Wiley, 1981

Although Millon presents a controversial formulation of the personality disorders with the use of three dimensions—active-passive, subject-object, and pleasure-pain—this book is a brilliant and scholarly summary of past and present thinking. It is an excellent companion to all the other readings in this section.

7. **Reich W** (ed): On the technique of character analysis, in *Character Analysis,* 3rd Edition. New York, Simon & Schuster, 1949, pp. 39–113

This book provides an excellent introduction to the psychological treatment of the personality disorders, specifically emphasizing the need for persistent and repeated analysis of resistance.

8. **Rutter M:** Temperament, personality, and personality disorder. *Br J Psychiatry* 150:443–458, 1987

This thought-provoking overview usefully examines past and current conceptualizations of temperament, personality, and personality disorder and their relationship to one another. Drawing on a wide range of research findings, Rutter points out various strengths and weaknesses of these conceptualizations and offers his own well-informed view on this topic.

9. **Shapiro D:** *Neurotic Styles.* New York, Basic Books, 1965

This book contains excellent descriptions of the basic cognitive styles of various personality types. Of particular interest are chapters on hysterical, paranoid, and obsessive-compulsive styles.

10. *Siever LJ, Davis KL:** A psychobiological perspective on the personality disorders. *Am J Psychiatry* 148:1647–1658, 1991

This is an excellent overview of current thinking about genetic and biological substrates of personality—a topic of increasing interest in the field. Siever and Davis propose, and review the evidence for, a psychobiological model that spans Axis I and II disorders and is based on dimensions of cognitive and perceptual organization, impulsivity and aggression, affective instability, and anxiety and inhibition.

Axis II Personality Disorders

Spectrum Types

11. **Siever LJ:** Schizophrenia spectrum personality disorders, in *American Psychiatric Press Review of Psychiatry*, Vol. 11. Edited by Tasman A, Riba MB. Washington, DC, American Psychiatric Press, 1992, pp. 25–42

This chapter documents how similarities in phenomenology are reflections of a common biogenetic disposition for the schizotypal, paranoid, and schizoid types of personality disorder. These overlaps probably will set the stage for future developments in their definition and classification.

Paranoid

12. **Meissner WW:** *Psychotherapy and the Paranoid Process.* Northvale, NJ, Jason Aronson, 1986

    Meissner's wide-ranging scholarship and psychoanalytic orientation combine to offer readers a comprehensive and clinically relevant account of paranoid phenomena.

Schizoid

13. **Guntrip HJ:** The schizoid problem, in *Psychoanalytic Theory, Therapy, and the Self.* Edited by Guntrip H. New York, Basic Books, 1971, pp. 145–173

    This is an eloquent description of the hidden self and the internal life that Guntrip has discovered lie behind the manifest phenomena of schizoid persons. This chapter is probably not specific to such patients but describes an aspect of other severely disturbed personalities as well.

Schizotypal

14. **Meehl PE:** Schizotaxia, schizotypy, schizophrenia. *Am Psychol* 17:827–838, 1962

    This article attempted to link certain clinical phenomena associated with schizotypal personality to a genetic predisposition to schizophrenia. It provided an impetus for continued studies and remains an area of high interest and controversy.

Self Types

Antisocial

15. *Cleckley H: *The Mask of Sanity,* 4th Edition. St. Louis, MO, CV Mosby, 1964

    This book contains the classic description of the "psychopathic personality," along with a pioneering effort to distinguish antisocial personality as a psychiatric diagnosis distinct from criminality.

16. **Glueck S, Glueck E:** *Delinquents and Non-Delinquents in Perspective.* Cambridge, MA, Harvard University Press, 1968

    This book presents the findings of a controlled study of juvenile delinquents with a comprehensive analysis of the social, psychological, and physical factors contributing to antisocial behavior.

17. **Robins LN:** *Deviant Children Grow Up: A Sociological and Psychiatric Study of Sociopathic Personality.* Baltimore, MD, Williams & Wilkins, 1966

In this report of a prospective 30-year follow-up study, Robins analyzes the social and psychological factors that are predictive of adult antisocial behavior and further refines the definition of antisocial personality disorder. Possible implications for treatment are outlined. Chapter 13 provides a concise summary of the study findings.

18. **Vaillant GE:** Sociopathy as a human process. *Arch Gen Psychiatry* 32:178–183, 1975

This article provides an important psychodynamic perspective on the apparent intractability of antisocial personality disorder in the community and the possibilities for treatment when acting-out behavior of sociopathic individuals is strictly curtailed in a hospital or prison setting.

19. **Widiger TA, Corbitt EM, Millon T:** Antisocial personality disorder, in *American Psychiatric Press Review of Psychiatry,* Vol 11. Edited by Tasman A, Riba MB. Washington, DC, American Psychiatric Press, 1992, pp. 63–79

This up-to-date compilation of evidence about the etiology and psychopathology of antisocial personality disorder gives particular attention to its descriptive characteristics and to questions of differential diagnosis.

Borderline

20. **Gunderson JG:** *Borderline Personality Disorder.* Washington, DC, American Psychiatric Press, 1984

This tightly written synthesis of the clinical and research literature offers clinicians insights into the dynamic basis for the descriptive characteristics of borderline personality disorder. This understanding is then applied to individual, hospital, and family therapies and the management of crises involving rage and suicide.

21. **Gunderson JG, Zanarini MC:** Pathogenesis of borderline personality, in *American Psychiatric Press Review of Psychiatry,* Vol 8. Edited by Tasman A, Hales RE, Frances AJ. Washington, DC, American Psychiatric Press, 1989, pp. 25–48

This chapter documents the shifting focus from disturbed mothering, to schizophrenia, to affective disorder, to trauma in the ongoing search for underlying pathogenic forces that cause borderline personality disorder to develop.

22. *Kernberg O: Borderline personality organization. *J Am Psychoanal Assoc* 15:641–685, 1967

    This seminal psychoanalytic article describes and organizes the intrapsychic characteristics of borderline and other severely disturbed patients.

23. **Masterson JF:** *Treatment of the Borderline Adolescent: A Developmental Approach.* New York, Wiley, 1972

    This book encouraged more enthusiasm for ambitious treatments of borderline patients by illustrating principles of treatment and the potential for adaptive changes in the basic psychopathology of these patients.

Narcissistic

24. **Akhtar S, Thomson JA:** Overview: narcissistic personality disorder. *Am J Psychiatry* 139:12–20, 1982

    This article reviews major contributions and persisting controversies about narcissistic personality disorder.

25. **Cooper AM, Ronningstam E:** Narcissistic personality disorder, in *American Psychiatric Press Review of Psychiatry*, Vol 11. Edited by Tasman A, Riba MB. Washington, DC, American Psychiatric Press, 1992, pp. 80–97

    A thoughtful melding of psychoanalytic perspectives and emerging empirical findings, this chapter is broadly informative even as it raises questions about the validity of the DSM-based definition.

26. *Kohut H: The psychoanalytic treatment of narcissistic personality disorders: outline of a systematic approach. *Psychoanal Study Child* 23:86–113, 1968

    This article outlines a treatment approach that reflects the author's original and seminal ideas about the origins of narcissism and its forms of expression in the transference.

Trait Types

Histrionic

27. **Breuer J, Freud S:** *Studies on hysteria (1893–1895)*, in *The Standard Edition of the Complete Psychological Works of Sigmund Freud*, Vol. 2. Translated and edited by Strachey J. London, Hogarth Press, 1955

    This pioneering work describes Freud and Breuer's early understanding of the mechanism by which hysterical symptoms develop, along with methods of treatment that were the forerunners of psychoanalysis. Of particular importance are Chapter I ("Preliminary Communication") and Chapter IV ("The Psychotherapy of Hysteria"). The case reports are both lively and informative.

28. **Chodoff P:** The diagnosis of hysteria: an overview. *Am J Psychiatry* 131:1073–1078, 1974

Chodoff describes three major conditions labeled as *hysterical:* Briquet's hysteria, conversion symptoms, and hysterical personality disorder. He differentiates among these uses of the term *hysteria* and points to areas in which greater precision in diagnostic labeling is indicated.

29. **Pfohl B:** Histrionic personality disorder: a review of available data and recommendations for DSM-IV. *Journal of Personality Disorders* 5:150–166, 1991

This article examines the major issues considered for histrionic personality disorder's revision for DSM-IV, such as whether the DSM-III-R criteria are congruent with the descriptive literature and are biased or prejudicial in any way, the criteria's reliability and validity, and the disorder's distinctiveness from other disorders. In so doing, it usefully incorporates a broad range of references from the empirical literature on histrionic personality disorder.

Avoidant

30. **Kagan J:** Temperamental influences on the preservation of styles of social behavior. *McLean Hospital Journal* 14:23–34, 1989

This summary of Kagan's pioneering work documents the relative stability of socially inhibited and uninhibited temperaments in children and describes their physiological correlates. He then expresses wariness about extrapolating from such childhood temperaments to adult personality disorders.

31. **Millon T:** Avoidant personality disorder: a review of data on DSM-III-R descriptors. *Journal of Personality Disorders* 5:353–362, 1991

This is a useful review by a major proponent of the avoidant personality disorder construct. This article discusses some of the issues considered in this disorder's revision for DSM-IV, including the question of whether it has adequate empirical support, what prototypal traits characterize the disorder's essential features, and whether avoidant personality disorder can be distinguished from other disorders such as Axis I social phobia.

Dependent

32. **Hirschfeld RMA, Shea MT, Weise R:** Dependent personality disorder: perspectives for DSM-IV. *Journal of Personality Disorders* 5:150–166, 1991

   This article reviews the major issues considered in dependent personality disorder's revision for DSM-IV, including the extent to which this disorder overlaps conceptually and empirically with other personality disorders, the performance of individual criteria, and the question of whether its use involves gender bias.

33. **Livesley WJ, Schroeder ML, Jackson DN:** Dependent personality disorder and attachment problems. *Journal of Personality Disorders* 4:232–240, 1990

   This interesting article examines the underlying dimensions of dependent personality disorder—dependency and pathological attachment—and concludes that they are relatively distinct from each other. Various implications of this finding are discussed.

Obsessive-Compulsive

34. **Abraham K:** Contributions to the theory of the anal character. *Int J Psychoanal* 4:400–418, 1923

   In the colorful and broad-ranging style of early psychoanalytic writing, this article develops Freud's observation of the connection between early anal developmental issues and their role in formation of the obsessive-compulsive adult.

35. *Freud A: Obsessional neurosis: a summary of psychoanalytic views as presented at the Congress (24th Int'l Congress). *Int J Psychoanal* 47:116–122, 1966

   This article represents an effort to synthesize and update the expanding psychoanalytic views of obsessional patients. It draws attention to the enduring characterological forms of obsessionality and attempts to integrate a more ego-centered psychology with earlier theories.

36. **Pfohl B, Blum N:** Obsessive-compulsive personality disorder: a review of available data and recommendations for DSM-IV. *Journal of Personality Disorders* 5:363–375, 1991

   This article reviews the major issues considered in this personality disorder's revision for DSM-IV. These issues include the criteria's validity and congruence with the descriptive literature and whether obsessive-compulsive disorder is distinct from other personality disorders and from Axis I disorders—in particular, obsessive-compulsive disorder.

Other Personality Disorders

Depressive

37. **Phillips KA, Gunderson JG, Hirschfeld RMA, Smith LE:** A review of the depressive personality. *Am J Psychiatry* 147:830–837, 1990

   This article reviews the extensive historical literature on this personality type, including descriptions by Kraepelin, Schneider, and Kernberg. It also identifies and explores the issues and controversies relevant to this disorder's inclusion in DSM-IV's appendix as a personality disorder that may be linked to Axis I depressive disorder.

Self-Defeating

38. **Fiester SJ:** Self-defeating personality disorder: a review of data and recommendations for DSM-IV. *Journal of Personality Disorders* 5:150–166, 1991

   This article reviews the major issues and controversies that led to this disorder's consideration for inclusion in DSM-IV. These issues include its reliability and validity, possible sex bias, whether its inclusion in DSM-III-R had any harmful consequences for women, and its clinical utility.

39. **Kernberg OF:** Clinical dimensions of masochism. *J Am Psychoanal Assoc* 36:1005–1028, 1988

   This useful psychoanalytic article presents a classification of masochistic psychopathology and its diagnostic, treatment, and prognostic implications. It also describes and elaborates on relations among a wide variety of masochistic phenomena, including "normal" masochism, the depressive-masochistic personality, sadomasochistic personality, and extreme forms of self-destructiveness.

17

Neuropsychiatric Syndromes

Richard C. Haaser, M.D.
Hillel Grossman, M.D.
Eric D. Caine, M.D.

Aneuropsychiatrist treats patients suffering from brain diseases that cause mental and behavioral disorders. One might say that this field represents at once a neurology of the mind and a psychiatry of the brain. The neuropsychiatrist attempts to understand the behavior as partly determined by neuroanatomy, neurophysiology, and neurochemistry, as well as by social, psychological, and genetic factors. We see the brain as the locus of interaction for these forces and behavior as a final common pathway for their expression.

Broadly speaking, there are three types of brain-mediated disorders that come to the attention of the neuropsychiatrist. The first reflects fundamental genetic defects or abnormalities acquired in utero or during the first years of life that profoundly affect a person's basic brain development. These influence the unfolding or emergence of behavioral traits and intellectual abilities, and how the growing child experiences the surrounding environment. The second occurs when normally developed adults suffer in mid-life conditions that disrupt (usually in an acute fashion) homeostatic function. Lastly, we encounter patients with neurodegenerative diseases that gradually and progressively erode established cognitive psychological and interpersonal skills. These disorders most often result from the selective disruption of discrete (although widespread) neurochemical systems.

205

Some of the papers that are discussed in this chapter are old by the usual standards of medical literature reviews. The neuropsychiatric perspective on behavior is not newly arrived. Earlier workers, even in the 19th century, attempted to understand aberrant behavior as potentially produced by various etiologies working through the brain. We strive to elude reductionism, either biological or psychological. We assert that mental and behavioral disorders have unique meanings, which cannot be left solely to biology, and a structure imposed by cerebral pathophysiology, which is often neglected by psychology. Since neuropsychiatry is concerned with the meaning of abnormal behavior, as well as its mechanisms of expression, the old dichotomy between "functional" and "organic" pathology has little utility.

Indeed, the diagnosis "organic mental disorder" is not used in DSM-IV. Although it was invoked originally to imply "structural pathology" that caused psychopathological symptoms, in contrast to the "physiological disruption" of so-called functional illness, *organic* came to mean biologically linked, whereas *functional* evolved to imply psychological. Organic disorders often were defined solely by the presence of identifiable brain alteration or by detection of systemic disease.

Coexistence is not sufficient to establish causal linkage, however, and the absence of an established etiology does not prove that psychological disturbances are paramount. Where an etiology has been defined, DSM-IV designates the specific mental disorder that is "due to" a defined or specific general medical condition; idiopathic disorders are recorded as "primary" psychiatric disorders. These changes are designated as they have been for many years by syndromic labels such as major depression, panic disorder, or obsessive-compulsive disorder; they underscore the need for clinicians to undertake a judicious process of clinical reasoning when considering the pathobiological causes for their patients' symptoms and signs.

In practical terms, the neuropsychiatrist approaches the patient both through sections of the neurological examination, emphasizing the appraisal of mental state and behavioral features, and the psychiatric evaluation, defining personal history and subjective experience as well as formal mental status. When the central nervous system is disrupted, it manifests disease symptoms through a limited number of functional systems, including mentation, sensation, and behavior. Symptoms and signs of disordered central nervous system function can be grouped into six domains or behavioral "pathways," each of which has some neurophysiological and neuroanatomic implications: 1) arousal, attention, and concentration; 2) mood and affect; 3) perception (both internal and external, ideational, and physical); 4) personality (e.g., "He's changed; he's not the same person he used to be."); 5) intellectual functioning (e.g., language, memory); and 6) motoric behavior.

In this chapter, we present a sample of articles and books that are especially relevant to neuropsychiatry. Initially, we consider references that broadly address the interface between psychiatry and neurology, or provide a useful perspective on disordered behavior. Following sections on major references and useful journals, citations are then arranged according to the six "pathways" through which we approach our patients in assessment and therapy.

Overview

1. **Caine ED, Joynt RJ:** Neuropsychiatry . . . Again. *Arch Neurol* 43:325–327, 1986

   A brief neuropsychiatric manifesto, this editorial offers one view of what constitutes modern neuropsychiatry and defines its differences from behavioral neurology and neuropsychology, as well as the parent fields of psychiatry and neurology. It describes the origins of the field and offers recommendations for future directions.

2. *McHugh PR, Slavney PR:* *The Perspectives of Psychiatry,* 2nd Edition. Baltimore, MD, Johns Hopkins University Press, 1986

   This 150-page book succinctly outlines four approaches that psychiatrists utilize when evaluating patients, describing the logic particular to each approach or perspective. This book is must reading for any student of psychiatry. For the neuropsychiatrist, the methods recommended provide a most useful framework for integrating disease manifestations within a life-course, psychologically sensitive view of illness as a personal and social process.

3. **Reynolds EH:** Structure and function in neurology and psychiatry. *Br J Psychiatry* 157:481–490, 1990

   This essay traces the history of neuroses and concepts of brain-behavior relationships and argues eloquently that dichotomies between "functional" and organic are superficial and inaccurate. Reynolds presents an approach that focuses on brain function rather than lesion localization and emphasizes the need for understanding the influence of psychological and social factors on brain function.

Reference Materials

4. **Andreasen NC** (ed): *Brain Imaging: Applications in Psychiatry.* Washington, DC, American Psychiatric Press, 1989

   This book is a successful attempt by a leader in the field of psychiatric neuroimaging to present for the novice the range of current imaging work being done. It includes contributions by experts in positron-emission tomography, single photon emission computed tomography, magnetic resonance imaging, and imaging using brain-evoked potentials. Each chapter explains the technology and summarizes relevant research. Its primary findings may become dated, however.

5. *Cummings JL: *Clinical Neuropsychiatry*. Needham Heights, MA, Allyn & Bacon, 1985

This is a concise review of the field of clinical neuropsychiatry by a behavioral neurologist. Particular strengths of this book include numerous, well-illustrated examples of bedside cognitive examination techniques and an introduction nicely summarizing the foundation beliefs of neuropsychiatry. The reader will appreciate the coherence of form and thought inherent in a book written by a single expert author.

6. **Garber HJ, Weilburg JB, Buonanno FS, Manschreck TC, New PF:** Use of magnetic resonance imaging in psychiatry. *Am J Psychiatry* 145:164–171, 1988

7. **Weinberger DR:** Brain disease and psychiatric illness: when should a psychiatrist order a CAT scan? *Am J Psychiatry* 141:1521–1527, 1984

Weinberger reviews brain diseases associated frequently with disturbances in behavior, mood, movement, cognition, or personality and provides criteria for ordering a computed tomography scan. Garber et al. expand this discussion further, considering the use of magnetic resonance imaging and defining when computed tomography might be preferable. They provide illustrative case histories as well.

8. **Goetz CG, Cohen MM:** Neurotoxic agents, in *Clinical Neurology*. Edited by Joynt RJ. Philadelphia, PA, JB Lippincott, 1989

This chapter presents a succinct, thoroughly detailed source of information about toxic syndromes. It reviews the effects of metals, solvents, pesticides, animal and plant toxins, and medications. Its reference list includes 630 citations.

9. **Hales RE, Yudofsky S** (eds): *American Psychiatric Press Textbook of Neuropsychiatry*, 2nd Edition. Washington, DC, American Psychiatric Press, 1992

This multiauthored book presents an overall review of neuropsychiatry. Strengths include thoughtful organization and the contributors' expertise. Beginning with a section devoted to basic principles of neuroscience, the text then reviews neuropsychiatric assessment. A discussion of symptom complexes follows; consideration of neuropsychiatric syndromes is organized by specific physical etiologies. The book concludes with a chapter reviewing treatment issues.

10. **Lezak MD:** *Neuropsychological Assessment.* New York, Oxford University Press, 1983

One might consider this text the encyclopedia of clinical neuropsychological testing, especially useful for physicians and students. (Neuropsychologists might want more depth.) It contains an extensive index that allows the reader to refer to specific tests and their uses. It also provides a review of cognitive processes and their central nervous system substrates, although much has been learned since it was written.

11. *Lishman WA:** *Organic Psychiatry: The Psychological Consequences of Cerebral Disorder,* 2nd Edition. Oxford, England, Blackwell, 1988 (distributed in the United States by JB Lippincott, Philadelphia, PA)

This volume remains the single most comprehensive description of neuropsychiatric syndromes gathered under one cover. A truly impressive, single-author work, it provides an especially cohesive view of complex disorders. Chapters are organized around specifically defined etiologies and describe the varied resultant behavioral syndromes. The book includes an extensive 71-page list of references.

12. **Mesulam M-M:** *Principles of Behavioral Neurology.* Philadelphia, PA, FA Davis, 1985

Presenting a specific way of thinking about brain-behavior relationships, Mesulam conceives of brain systems as interacting networks, not discrete entities working in isolation. He has become an especially original thinker in this rapidly evolving field, with a remarkable ability to integrate his complex understanding of neurobiology with astute clinical observation. The book offers a picture of the brain's structural organization as it pertains to behavior and describes techniques for clinical assessment at the bedside.

13. *Strub RL, Black FW:** *The Mental Status Examination in Neurology.* Philadelphia, PA, FA Davis, 1985

This brief, inexpensive paperback describes bedside cognitive examination and provides a succinct discussion using a localizationist view of intellectual functions. The book pays little attention to behavioral phenomenology or psychopathology, such as mood disturbance or disordered thought content; thus it alone cannot suffice as a text for learning mental status assessment in neuropsychiatry. It goes beyond Taylor's (1982) book, however, in its introduction to neuropsychology.

14. **Taylor MA:** *The Neuropsychiatric Mental Status Examination: A Phenom-enologic Program Text.* Jamaica, NY, Spectrum, 1982

An excellent introduction for medical students and beginning resi-dents, this programmed text for the mental status examination pays better attention to psychiatric phenomenology than Strub and Black (1985) above. Cognitive testing techniques are introduced.

15. **Woods SW, Pearsall HR, Seibyl JP, Hoffer PB:** Single-photon emission computed tomography in neuropsychiatric disorders, in *Year Book of Nuclear Medicine.* Edited by Hoffer PB. St. Louis, MO, Mosby Year Book, 1991, pp. xiii–xlvii

Woods et al. review the state of single photon emission computed tomography imaging in psychiatric research. They discuss some of the methodological difficulties in utilizing this exciting tool for studying brain function.

Journals

The past decade has seen a dramatic change in the content of major medical journals. Brain-behavior and behavior-brain relationships are now common topics for discussion. The neuropsychiatric perspective has be-come a central organizing theme for many published articles. Neuropsychi-atry is back in fashion!

Thus, journals such as *Archives of General Psychiatry, American Journal of Psychiatry, British Journal of Psychiatry, Archives of Neurology,* and *Neurology* often present relevant reports. *Brain* has long published such work, and during the past 4 years, two new journals (*Journal of Neuropsychiatry and Clinical Neuroscience* and *Neuropsychiatry, Neuropsychology, and Behavioral Neu-rology*) have appeared. *Psychological Medicine,* the *Journal of Neurology, Neuro-surgery, and Psychiatry,* and the *Journal of Nervous and Mental Disease* have sat astride the border zone of the disciplines for many years. As well, several new journals devoted to geriatric psychiatry address neuropsychiatric issues arising in the elderly.

Given this plethora of journals, one might wonder whether there will be a sufficient number of high-quality manuscripts to fill the available pages.

Disorders of Arousal

Intact arousal, attention, and concentration are prerequisites for the ade-quate performance of the mental status examination. These disorders are warnings that the central nervous system has sustained some physical insult requiring immediate and direct evaluation. The neuroanatomy of this system is perhaps better known than any other section of the mental status.

16. Drugs that cause psychiatric symptoms. *Med Lett Drugs Ther* 31:113–118, 1989

> This is the most recent edition of a very useful article listing those drugs common to medical and surgical practice that have been reported to cause psychiatric symptoms. Although limited in detail, it easily proves its worth, particularly for those performing consultations.

17. **Engel GL, Romano J:** Delirium: a syndrome of cerebral insufficiency. *J Chronic Dis* 9:260–277, 1959

> More than three decades ago this article placed the challenge of the toxic and metabolic encephalopathies before psychiatry. With an argument that remains cogent today, Engel and Romano distinguish delirium, a potentially reversible syndrome of cerebral dysfunction, from dementia and the major functional psychiatric disorders with which it is often intermingled. The relevance of electroencephalographic testing in patients with behavior disorders is well described.

18. **Lipowski ZJ:** *Delirium: Acute Confusional States.* New York, Oxford University Press, 1990

> This monograph is composed of two sections, the first encompassing epidemiology, clinical features, psychopathology, and pathogenesis of delirium, and the second examining specific etiologies. Particularly interesting is Lipowski's historical review of delirium as a concept in Western medicine.

19. *Plum F, Posner C:* *The Diagnosis of Stupor and Coma,* 3rd Edition. Philadelphia, PA, FA Davis, 1980

> This is "the source" for those seeking a neuroanatomic perspective for understanding disorders of arousal. Case examples abound. Bibliographies are thorough and accompany each chapter.

Disorders of Mood and Emotion

There is a complex interaction between feeling states and the brain. Mood disturbances may be generated by some neuropathological lesions and neurodegenerative diseases; dementing syndromes may be mimicked by mood disorders. Investigators and clinicians debate the neuroanatomic substrates that subserve emotional expression.

20. **Caine ED, Shoulson I:** Psychiatric syndromes in Huntington's disease. *Am J Psychiatry* 140:728–733, 1983

Among individuals with the autosomal-dominant, reliably defined disease of Huntington's, one encounters a range of symptoms that nearly covers the waterfront of descriptive psychiatric diagnosis, including affective disorders, anxiety states, personality changes, and schizophrenic-like psychoses. Some patients remain symptom-free. The implications of this finding for psychiatric diagnostic schemes based on phenomenology are discussed.

21. *Papez JW:** A proposed mechanism of emotion. *Archives of Neurological Psychiatry* 38:725–743, 1937

In this classic article, Papez puts forward the hypothesis that there is a neuroanatomy of the emotions. He describes the limbic system and its neuroanatomic connections and proposes that emotional tone can be understood in terms of neurophysiologic outflow from this system to the cortex. This hypothesis has stood the test of time and still has no clearer statement than in this original article.

22. **Sackheim HA, Greenberg MS, Weiman AL, Gur RC, Hungerbuhler JP, Geschwind N:** Hemispheric asymmetry in the expression of positive and negative emotions: neurologic evidence. *Arch Neurol* 39:210–218, 1982

In this retrospective study, Sackheim et al. review 122 case descriptions of the syndrome of emotional lability in structural brain disease. They discern a functional asymmetry in the regulation of emotional experience by the two sides of the brain. When the lesions are in the dominant hemisphere, pathological weeping is far more common; when in the nondominant hemisphere, pathological laughing occurs more often. The potential relevance of this finding to our understanding of the process of emotional expression in persons without this disorder is discussed.

23. **Starkstein SE, Bryer JB, Berthier ML, Cohen B, Price TR, Robinson RG:** Depression after stroke: the importance of cerebral hemisphere asymmetries. *Journal of Neuropsychiatry and Clinical Neuroscience* 3:276–285, 1991

This is a recent publication in a 10-year series of articles by Starkstein and colleagues that link depression to stroke. It illustrates the evolution in the thinking of these pioneers in the systematic study of psychopathological syndromes arising from focal brain lesions.

24. **Williams D:** The structure of emotions reflected in epileptic experiences. *Brain* 79:29–67, 1956

Williams carefully interviewed 100 persons with epilepsy who felt that emotional changes were included in their ictal experiences. This report did much to further the idea that emotional experience, too, had cerebral representation within the brain.

Disorders of Perception

Included in this category are those diseases and conditions that manifest with hallucinations in any of the sensory domains, as well as delusions or other ideational disturbances. There have been two approaches to understanding these disorders: brain-to-behavior (i.e., looking for psychopathology in patients with known brain disease) and behavior-to-brain (i.e., searching for brain abnormalities in patients with known psychopathology).

25. **Barta PE, Pearlson GD, Powers RE, Richards SS, Tune LE:** Auditory hallucinations and smaller superior temporal gyral volume in schizophrenia. *Am J Psychiatry* 147:1457–1462, 1990

Barta et al. describe their findings of an anatomic abnormality detected by magnetic resonance imaging in the primary auditory association cortex that correlates with the extent of severity of auditory hallucinations in schizophrenic patients. This article is of research interest, given the attempt to develop correlations between specific symptoms and brain dysfunction utilizing the behavior-to-brain approach.

26. **Benson DF, Stuss DT:** Frontal lobe influences on delusions: a clinical perspective. *Schizophr Bull* 16:403–411, 1990

Benson and Stuss, utilizing case histories, attempt to understand delusions as a manifestation of the disturbance of frontal lobe function and the loss of ability for censoring and analyzing thoughts prior to their expression.

27. **Cummings JL:** Organic delusions: phenomenology, anatomical correlations and review. *Br J Psychiatry* 146:184–197, 1985

Cummings attempts to determine predisposing factors, natural history, response to therapy, and anatomic correlates of delusional syndromes. He provides an extensive review of literature extending back as far as 1930, as well as results of a small-scale prospective study of delusional conditions due to specific disease processes. The author suggests some distinguishing factors for categorizing and localizing various secondary delusions.

28. *Davison K, Bagley CR:** Schizophrenia-like psychoses associated with organic disorders of the central nervous system: a review of the literature. *Br J Psychiatry* (Special Publ No 4):113–184, 1969

Perhaps the diagnostic nomenclature of this article is dated, but this comprehensive appraisal of the pre-1969 literature describes those brain diseases specifically associated with psychotic symptoms. It is a classic article that organizes its review based on disease categories such as epilepsy, trauma, and tumor, and ultimately emphasizes the nonspecificity of psychotic symptoms.

29. **Gur RE, Resnick SM, Alavi A, Gur RC, Caroff S, Dann R, Silver FL, Saykin AJ, Chawluk JB, Kushner M, Reivich M:** Regional brain function in schizophrenia, I: a positron emission tomography study. *Arch Gen Psychiatry* 44:119–125, 1987

One of many studies utilizing positron-emission tomography technology to study the major idiopathic psychiatric syndromes, this article illustrates both how positron-emission tomography work is done and how it can challenge previous psychiatric theory. This study did not find evidence in the schizophrenic patients for "hypofrontality" as has been hypothesized.

30. *Penfield W, Perot P:** The brain's record of auditory and visual experience: a final summary and discussion. *Brain* 86:596–695, 1963

In this classic study of electrical stimulation of the cerebral cortex in epileptic patients undergoing surgical resection, Penfield and Perot report eliciting an impressive array of perceptual disturbances, including auditory and visual hallucinations or illusions, isolated emotions, and other abnormal experiences such as deja vu and jamais vu. Anatomic drawings detail the locations stimulated and the responses detected.

31. **Stevens JR:** Abnormal reinnervation as a basis for schizophrenia: a hypothesis. *Arch Gen Psychiatry* 49:238–243, 1992

Aberrant neuronal regeneration and "miswiring" of neurons projecting from limbic structures has been demonstrated in both epilepsy and Alzheimer's disease. The author reviews the evidence for similar aberrant synaptic reorganization in schizophrenia and presents an intriguing hypothesis regarding how this reorganization may explain the age at onset and the variation in symptoms and course seen in schizophrenia.

32. **Trimble MR:** First rank symptoms of Schneider: a new perspective? *Br J Psychiatry* 156:195–200, 1990

In this article, a noted neuropsychiatrist and epileptologist reviews the literature of psychotic disorders in epilepsy. Although the diagnostic category of schizophrenia in epilepsy does not localize to any particular anatomic focus, he concludes that specific psychotic symptoms (Schneiderian first-rank symptoms) do point to an abnormality of the temporal-limbic structures of the dominant hemisphere. This is a compelling and fascinating presentation.

33. *Weinberger DR:* Implications of normal brain development for the pathogenesis of schizophrenia. *Arch Gen Psychiatry* 44:660–669, 1987

Weinberger integrates what is known about the clinical history of schizophrenia with findings arising from family studies and neuroimaging and neurophysiological research into an eloquent tour de force. He offers a tantalizing and cohesive theory that accounts for both the symptoms and the life course of schizophrenia. It is a "must read."

Disorders of Personality

Personality is defined as the enduring traits and behavioral style that uniquely characterize and distinguish a person. Neuropsychiatry is interested in both how individual uniqueness and variation develop in personality as well as how injury to particular brain areas can abolish these qualities and create monolithic, acquired personality syndromes.

34. *Bigelow HJ:* Dr. Harlow's case of recovery from the passage of an iron bar through the head. *Am J Med Sci* (New Series) 20:2–22, 1850

This 19th century case describes the change in personality that occurred to a railroad worker after sustaining a frontal lobe injury. Dr. Harlow's detailing of the behavior, affect, and cognitive style of the injured worker, Phineas Gage, remains a classic description of frontal lobe personality changes.

35. *Chapman LF, Wolff HG:* The cerebral hemispheres and the highest integrative functions of man. *Arch Neurol* 1:357–424, 1959

This lengthy report of psychological assessments in 60 persons who had undergone focal brain extirpations for lesions such as tumor propounds a nonlocalizationist point of view. The authors describe a spectrum of behavioral dysfunction, beginning with mild personality change and ending in global dementia. The alterations are related to the number of grams of brain tissue removed, rather than the anatomic site involved. Research since this report has focused almost exclusively on attempts to localize specific anatomic lesions with specific behavioral syndromes. This alternative view should be kept in mind.

36. **Kagan J, Reznick JS, Snidman N:** Biological bases of childhood shyness. *Science* 240:167–171, 1988

Kagan et al. have studied temperament or inborn biological propensities. This article reports on longitudinal studies of toddlers who were extremely shy and restrained in unfamiliar context and developed into quiet, cautious, and socially avoidant children. This was contrasted to toddlers who were unrestrained and spontaneous when exposed to unfamiliar settings, who later developed into talkative and socially interactive children. Physiological parameters implied greater sympathetic reactivity among the restrained, inhibited children. The authors integrate their data into a measured theory of the biological basis of childhood shyness that can serve as a paradigm for understanding the biological substrate for development of other personality traits.

37. *Stuss DT, Benson DF: *Frontal Lobes*. New York, Raven, 1986

This brief textbook provides a broad-ranging review of frontal lobe anatomy and function covering basic sciences, primate research, and clinical information. There is an extensive chapter on personality change associated with frontal lobe injury.

38. **Waxman SG, Geschwind N:** The interictal behavior syndrome of temporal lobe epilepsy. *Arch Gen Psychiatry* 32:1580–1586, 1975

The authors describe personality style and behavioral tendencies thought unique to patients with temporal lobe epilepsy. Eloquent theories of temporal lobe function and personality development have been elaborated based on this syndrome, although subsequent research has been unable to verify the specificity of these traits for temporal lobe or any other form of epilepsy.

Disorders of Cognition

It is difficult to discuss cognition in isolation from the other neuropsychiatric disorders. Practically, cognitive disorders frequently present with noncognitive symptoms; mood and psychotic disorders are often accompanied by evidence of cognitive impairment. From a theoretical perspective we have already referenced articles that attempt to understand psychotic symptoms as cognitive disturbances involving disruption of associative processes. Knowledge of normal brain function has become increasingly important for the clinician treating patients with neuropsychiatric diseases.

39. **Cummings JL** (ed): *Subcortical Dementia*. New York, Oxford University Press, 1991

The still controversial concept of subcortical dementia has expanded previous views regarding the clinical phenomenology and neurobiology of cognitive disorders. This well-edited, multiauthored text offers essays on a broad range of topics pertinent to subcortical function in a variety of neuropsychiatric syndromes.

40. *Cummings JL, Benson DF: *Dementia: A Clinical Approach*, 2nd Edition. Boston, MA, Butterworth-Heinemann, 1992

This textbook emphasizes breadth over depth. Virtually any condition that can cause cognitive impairment is discussed, with a primary emphasis on clinical features. An extensive bibliography points the reader in search of greater detail toward appropriate sources.

41. **Kertesz A** (ed): *Localization in Neuropsychology*. New York, Academic Press, 1983

This multiauthored text provides a thoughtful presentation of the evidence tying specific neurobehavioral syndromes to focal brain regions. With 8 of 21 chapters devoted to aphasia in its various forms, it is especially useful as a resource for those clinicians wishing to know more about language disorders.

42. **Luria AR:** *Higher Cortical Functions in Man*, 2nd Revision. New York, Basic Books, 1980

Perhaps no one has studied individuals with focal lesions of the central nervous system in as great depth as Luria. He developed his own tools for cognitive assessment and applied them imaginatively to his subjects. Testing procedures are set forth in detail along with his theories of brain function. Speech disorders, disorders of complex sensation, memory disorders, and disorders of conceptual reasoning are among the neuropsychological problems considered. Some of his theories about the neurological underpinnings of such syndromes run counter to established ideas in the West, making Luria's work valuable as a counterpoint. It is exciting to experience this man's thinking.

43. **Weintraub S, Mesulam MM:** Developmental learning disabilities of the right hemisphere: emotional, interpersonal, and cognitive components. *Arch Neurol* 40:463–468, 1983

This short fascinating article describes the cognitive, behavioral, and personality limitations in 14 patients with developmental right-hemispheric abnormality. Although such a syndrome has not been verified as a distinct entity, the article serves to emphasize the need to consider a neurodevelopmental perspective when assessing cognitive impairment and calls attention to nonverbal learning disabilities.

Disorders of Movement

The movement disorders, perhaps more than any other area of interest in neuropsychiatry, reveal the complex interplay of neurological and psychiatric symptomatology. The apparent similarity between symptoms such as psychomotor retardation in major depression and the mild bradykinesia of early Parkinson's disease points toward new avenues for research.

44. **Joseph AB, Young RR:** *Movement Disorders in Neurology and Neuropsychiatry.* Boston, MA, Blackwell Scientific Publications, 1992

   This new volume is a comprehensive textbook of developmental, acquired, and iatrogenic movement disorders. Its 95 chapters discuss the expected disorders (e.g., Parkinson's disease, tardive dyskinesia) as well as topics such as wandering demented patients and bruxism. Joseph and Young rightly emphasize that the boundary zone between the study of movement disorders and psychiatry is ill-defined, porous, and ever changing.

45. **Rogers D, Lees AJ, Smith E, Trimble M, Stern GM:** Bradyphrenia in Parkinson's disease and psychomotor retardation in depressive illness: an experimental study. *Brain* 110:761–776, 1987

   This neuropsychological study demonstrates the commonality of bradyphrenia in Parkinson's disease and psychomotor retardation as seen in major depression. It illustrates the great potential for neuropsychiatric research to develop theories for idiopathic psychiatric symptoms utilizing neurological diseases having known neuropathological substrates.

Treatment of Neuropsychiatric Disorders

The systematic treatment of neuropsychiatric syndromes is in its infancy. Controlled treatment trials are few, and most work examines the application of established psychiatric treatments to the neuropsychiatric analogues of idiopathic psychiatric syndromes. Interventions involve both direct and symptomatic therapies. Although there are as yet few means available for directly reversing or retarding the course of a brain disease, the search continues. In clinical settings the initial focus is most often on symptomatic treatments, with the aim of ameliorating specific symptoms (e.g., aggression) or syndromes (e.g., major depression). Rehabilitation aims at maximizing existing capacities.

Somatic Therapies

46. **Davis KL, Thal LJ, Gamzu ER, Davis CS, Woolson RF, Gracon SI, Drachman DA, Schneider LS, Whitehouse PJ, Hoover TM, Morris JC, Kawas CH, Knopman DS, Earl NL, Kumar V, Doody RS and the Tacrine Collaborative Study Group:** A double-blind, placebo-controlled multicenter study of tacrine for Alzheimer's disease. *N Engl J Med* 327:1253–1259, 1992 (see accompanying editorial by **Growdon JH:** Treatment for Alzheimer's disease. *N Engl J Med* 327:1306–1308, 1992)

47. **Farlow M, Gracon SI, Hershey LA, Lewis KW, Sadowsky CH, Dolan-Ureno J:** A controlled trial of tacrine in Alzheimer's disease. *JAMA* 268:2523–2529, 1992 (see accompanying editorial by **Small GW:** Tacrine for treating Alzheimer's disease. *JAMA* 268:2564–2565, 1992)

Alzheimer's disease has been the focus of two decades of research looking for a direct treatment that would retard or reverse the degenerative process. Tacrine hydrochloride, a cholinesterase inhibitor, has been both the most promising and disappointing agent yet investigated. These two multicenter studies present results that are modest, at best, and are subject to differing interpretations, perhaps depending on one's level of scientific enthusiasm or skepticism: Read both articles as well as the accompanying editorials for a view of complex methods seeking small effects and the medical scientific version about "beauty" and those who behold it.

48. **Douyon R, Serby M, Klutchko B, Rotrosen J:** ECT and Parkinson's disease revisited: a "naturalistic" study. *Am J Psychiatry* 146:1451–1455, 1989 (see accompanying editorial by **Abrams R:** ECT for Parkinson's disease. *Am J Psychiatry* 146:1391–1393, 1989)

49. **Schaerf FW, Miller RR, Lipsey JR, McPherson RW:** ECT for major depression in four patients infected with human immunodeficiency virus. *Am J Psychiatry* 146:782–784, 1989

These studies point to the efficacy of electroconvulsive therapy in depression associated with Parkinson's disease and human immunodeficiency virus infection. Interestingly, in the patients with Parkinson's disease, there were improvements in both mood and bradykinesia associated with the treatment. This calls attention to the overlap of motor and mood symptoms in subcortical disease.

50. **Lipsey JR, Robinson RG, Pearlson GD, Rao K, Price TR:** Nortriptyline treatment of post-stroke depression: a double-blind treatment trial. *Lancet* 1:297–300, 1984

In general, medications that work for idiopathic psychiatric syndromes are similarly effective in neuropsychiatric disorders having the same manifestations, as seen when using standard treatments for depression among stroke patients.

51. **Robinson RG, Parikh RM, Lipsey JR, Starkstein SE, Price TR:** Pathological laughing and crying following stroke: validation of a measurement scale and a double-blind treatment study. *Am J Psychiatry* 150:286–293, 1993

Pathological laughing and crying, also known as affective incontinence or pseudobulbar affect, represents the extremes of emotional dyscontrol. This well-designed study provides a means of quantifying and treating such symptoms.

52. **Ruedrich SL, Grush L, Wilson J:** Beta adrenergic blocking medications for aggressive or self-injurious mentally retarded persons. *Am J Ment Retard* 95:110–119, 1990

53. **Schneider LS, Sobin PB:** Non-neuroleptic medications in the management of agitation in Alzheimer's disease and other dementia: a selective review. *International Journal of Geriatric Psychiatry* 6:691–708, 1991

Aggressive or violent behavior is probably the most difficult management problem in patients with brain damage of any etiology. The state of the art is unfortunately quite primitive, with most studies involving small numbers, no control subjects, or no reliable quantification of the disruptive behavior. The clinician must often borrow from treatment literature regarding one population (e.g., dementia) and creatively apply the result to another population (e.g., head trauma or mental retardation).

54. **Shoulson I:** Neuroprotective clinical strategies for Parkinson's disease. *Ann Neurol* 32 (suppl):S143–145, 1992

L-Deprenyl has been demonstrated to delay the need for pharmacologic treatment of motor symptoms in Parkinson's disease. Although it is not yet known whether L-deprenyl treatment can delay or prevent the affective and cognitive symptoms of Parkinson's disease, such neuroprotective strategies serve as paradigms for further research in the direct treatment of degenerative brain disease.

Rehabilitation

55. **Berrol S:** Issues in cognitive rehabilitation. *Arch Neurol* 47:219–220, 1990; **Volpe BT, McDowell FH:** The efficacy of cognitive rehabilitation

in patients with traumatic brain injury. *Arch Neurol* 47:220–222, 1990; **Levin HS:** Cognitive rehabilitation: unproved but promising. *Arch Neurol* 47:223–224, 1990; **Hachinski V:** Cognitive Rehabilitation. *Arch Neurol* 47:1185–1188, 1990

Cognitive rehabilitation aims to restore or compensate for acquired intellectual deficits with the ultimate goal of increasing functional capacity. This journal symposium highlights the potential and limits of cognitive rehabilitation as well as the controversy in assessing the current state of the art. To quote Hachinski: "Without therapeutic enthusiasm there would be no innovation and without skepticism there would be no proof. Cognitive rehabilitation deserves further evaluation."

56. **Glisky EL, Schacter DL:** Extending the limits of complex learning in organic amnesia: computer training in a vocational domain. *Neuropsychologia* 27:107–120, 1989

This article is one in a series of reports detailing testing and performance of a "famous" patient, H.D. H.D. clearly demonstrates improved memory after being subjected to weeks and months of intensive training by well-known academic neuropsychologists. Whether one can generalize from this patient and her unique retraining to other brain-damaged patients and the general field of cognitive rehabilitation is unclear.

57. **Wilson BA:** *Rehabilitation of Memory.* New York, Guilford, 1987

The author, who is a psychologist working in a rehabilitation center, gives us a realistic, pragmatic approach to assisting people with memory impairments. In each chapter, she presents in sequence a particular clinical problem of memory or a theory of rehabilitation, then a specific case example. She follows with a blow-by-blow account of the application of theory-based techniques to patient care and clinical outcome. The reader will appreciate the honest description of success and failure, and the way she reflects her case material and outcome data back on the original theory.

Conclusions

Neuropsychiatry is a burgeoning field, yet one must also recognize the very significant gaps in our understanding of behavior-brain relationships and their varied manifestations in the disorders we seek to treat. The first involves issues of *sensitivity* and *specificity*. No clinician or investigator can say with certainty what percentage of patients with a focal lesion will develop a discrete behavioral syndrome. (For example, of 100 patients with a left frontal lobe tumor, how many will develop a frontal lobe syndrome?) Conversely, we do not yet know the correlation between clearly defined clinical syndromes and specific central nervous system substrates. (For example, how often do patients with "frontal lobe syndrome" have frontal lobe lesions, or lesions at other sites within the brain?)

Our understanding of the natural history of these disorders also is relatively primitive. How does a disorder with an acute onset (e.g., stroke, missile wound) differ in its effects from a gradually evolving process (e.g., tumor)? We have sparse data regarding the natural history of many of these disorders once they have begun. As well, the study of brain-behavior relationships is highly dependent on the type of subject population one chooses: Predictable or "lawful" brain-behavior and behavior-brain relationships may vary greatly, depending on whether one is evaluating subjects with acute focal lesions (e.g., infarctions), patients with evolving neurodegenerative disorders affecting widespread neurochemical systems, or healthy control subjects participating in experimental paradigms. Infarctions, for example, reflect vascular anatomy primarily, whereas neurodegenerative diseases often select specific neurochemical systems that ramify widely through the brain.

There are few well-designed controlled studies to evaluate the effectiveness of treatments applied to patients with neuropsychiatric disorders. Cognitive rehabilitation has boomed during recent years as a health care industry for patients with behavioral and cognitive disorders arising from head trauma and other acute disease processes. Despite the allocation of substantial resources for care, specific therapeutic effects remain uncertain. No doubt, there are individuals who will benefit from such treatment, but who are they? Psychopharmacology has been used liberally among neuropsychiatric patient populations, but without clear guidelines derived from double-blind, placebo-controlled trials. Medications pass in and out of favor. Too often, pharmacotherapy has been used as a less-expensive substitute for thoughtful environmental and psychological approaches, with nonspecific effects such as sedation as the primary index of response. Thus, although the field has made great advances in the understanding of case description and pathobiology, and has utilized evermore sophisticated technology, its approach to therapeutic intervention has remained empiric and unsophisticated. Patients, and no doubt their families, will benefit from future efforts that strive to address these deficiencies.

HIV and AIDS

Francine Cournos, M.D.
Ewald Horwath, M.D.

The literature on the human immunodeficiency virus (HIV) and acquired immunodeficiency syndrome (AIDS) is vast, and tens of thousands of abstracts, articles, books, and book chapters have now been published on these topics. HIV infection is important to the practice of psychiatry for the following reasons:

- HIV infection and related opportunistic diseases affect the central nervous system and create neuropsychiatric syndromes that psychiatrists should be able to recognize.
- Receiving a diagnosis of HIV infection or illness can produce a range of psychiatric symptoms and disorders that require intervention.
- The spread of HIV is best contained, at present, by promoting behavioral change. Among the medical specialties, psychiatry is the best equipped to develop effective risk-reduction interventions.
- Patients with serious psychiatric illnesses have elevated HIV seroprevalence rates and engage in behavior that poses the risk of acquiring or transmitting HIV infection.

However, it is not possible to achieve an adequate understanding of these areas without a solid knowledge of the relevant medical facts. This bibliography, therefore, covers the areas of medical findings and treatment and the epidemiology of the disease. The literature on HIV/AIDS changes daily. To avoid creating a bibliography that would rapidly become outdated, we have concentrated on landmark articles and on publications that are periodically updated.

Overviews: Historical, Medical, Psychiatric, and Research Perspectives

1. *AIDS Summary: A Practical Synopsis of the International Conference.* Richmond, VA, Philadelphia Sciences Group (annual)

   This volume is published annually after the yearly International AIDS Conference. It offers succinct, integrated summaries of recent research on the broad spectrum of topics covered in the meeting.

2. *The Journal of NIH Research* Vol. 4, No. 7, 1992

   This issue is largely focused on HIV/AIDS and nicely summarizes many topics of current interest. Included in this issue are discussions of the following: HIV-1 vaccines, activities of the Gay Men's Health Crisis and ACT UP, the controversial case of HIV transmission from a dentist to five of his patients, projected worldwide estimates for HIV infection, discovery of the HIV-1 receptor, and a diagram of the HIV-1 life cycle.

3. **MMWR* (Morbidity and Mortality Weekly Report), Centers for Disease Control and Prevention

   These reports provide some of the most useful and up-to-date summary data on such topics as epidemiology, prevention, treatment, and concerns of health care workers. The following are of particular interest.

   - *MMWR* 30 (No. 21, pp. 250–252, 1981) is of historical interest as the first published report of what later became known as the HIV epidemic. It contains a description of several cases of pneumocystic pneumonia in Los Angeles, California.
   - *MMWR* 38 (No. S–6, pp. 1–37, 1989) offers guidelines for the prevention of transmission of HIV and hepatitis B, as well as other blood-borne pathogens in health care settings.
   - *MMWR* 39 (No. RR-1, pp. 1–14, 1990) describes the management of occupational exposure to HIV, including the postexposure use of zidovudine (AZT).
   - *MMWR* 41 (No. RR-17, pp. 1–19, 1992) contains the 1993 revised classification system for HIV infection and expanded surveillance case definition for AIDS among adolescents and adults.

4. *Ostrow DG: *Psychiatric Aspects of Human Immunodeficiency Virus Infection.* Kalamazoo, MI, Upjohn Company, 1990

This pamphlet provides an excellent review of the literature emphasizing psychiatric aspects of HIV and includes sections on epidemiology, natural history and classification of HIV disease, psychological reactions to HIV infection and illness, neuropsychiatric complications, and HIV-related guidelines issued by The American Psychiatric Association.

5. *A Psychiatrist's Guide to AIDS and HIV Disease: AIDS Primer.* Washington, DC, American Psychiatric Association AIDS Education Project, 1990

Prominent psychiatrists in the field succinctly review all areas of AIDS/HIV for mental health professionals. Topics include immunology, classification, neuropsychiatric syndromes, psychological reactions, prevention, testing, guidelines, and legal and ethical concerns.

6. **Shilts R:** *And The Band Played On.* New York, St. Martin's Press, 1987

In this widely read popular book, Shilts, a reporter for the *San Francisco Chronicle*, describes the history of the AIDS epidemic in the United States from 1980 to 1985. The narrative is detailed and provocative and includes the history of the medical discoveries and the responses of health professionals, scientists, politicians, reporters, and infected individuals who suffered and died in the early phases of the epidemic.

7. **Tasman A, Goldfinger SM, Kaufmann CA** (eds): *American Psychiatric Association Review of Psychiatry,* Vol. 9 (Chapters 28–32). Washington, DC, American Psychiatric Press, 1990

These chapters contain a complete overview of HIV/AIDS through 1989, written for psychiatrists. Topics include historical perspective; pathophysiology; staging; opportunistic infections; neuropsychiatric complications; psychiatric diagnosis, psychotherapy, and pharmacotherapy; special populations; psychosocial issues; and legal and ethical issues.

8. **Wallack JJ, Snyder S, Bialer PA, Gelfand JL, Poisson E:** An AIDS bibliography for the general psychiatrist. *Psychosomatics* 32:243–254, 1991

This is a bibliography of 158 articles, chapters, and books selected for their relevance to the general psychiatrist. Of particular note are the sections on the needs of special populations, including the elderly, hemophiliac persons, women, children, health care workers, intravenous drug users, homosexual men, and members of minority groups.

Medical Findings and Developments

9. **Friedland GH, Saltzman BR, Rogers MF, Kahl PA, Lesser ML, Mayers MM, Klein RS:** Lack of transmission of HTLV-III/LAV infection to household contacts of patients with AIDS or AIDS-related complex with oral candidiasis. *N Engl J Med* 314:344–349, 1986

   This landmark study helped quell fears about transmission of HIV through casual contact by demonstrating the safety of nonsexual close contact with infected individuals.

10. **Rothenberg R, Woelfel M, Stoneburner R, Milberg J, Parker R, Truman B:** Survival with the acquired immunodeficiency syndrome: experience with 5,833 cases in New York City. *N Engl J Med* 317:1297–1302, 1987

    The first report on survival among a large sample of patients in the United States with AIDS, this article establishes that white homosexual men presenting with Kaposi's sarcoma only have the most favorable survival rate. Factors that shorten survival, including opportunistic infections, older age, female sex, and being black or Hispanic, are also addressed.

11. **Volberding PA, Lagakos SW, Koch MA, Pettinelli C, Myers MW, Booth DK, Balfour HH, Reichman RC, Bartlett JA, Hirsch MS, Murphy RL, Hardy WD, Soeiro R, Fischl MS, Bartlett JG, Merrigan TC, Hyslop NE, Richman DD, Valentine FT, Corey L, and the AIDS Clinical Trials Group of the National Institute of Allergy and Infectious Diseases:** Zidovudine in asymptomatic human immunodeficiency virus infection: a controlled trial in persons with fewer than 500 CD4-positive cells per cubic millimeter. *N Engl J Med* 322:941–949, 1990

    The results of this randomized, double-blind trial indicated that zidovudine therapy could delay the onset of AIDS when it was administered to asymptomatic HIV-infected patients with fewer than 500 $CD4^+$ cells per cubic millimeter. The design of the study did not permit determination of whether zidovudine treatment would result in improved longevity or other long-term benefits.

    (See also *MMWR* references above.)

Epidemiology and Risk Behavior

12. **Chu SY, Buehler JW, Berkelman RL:** Impact of the human immunodeficiency virus epidemic on mortality in women of reproductive age, United States. *JAMA* 264:225–229, 1990

This study uses national mortality data from 1980 to 1988 to demonstrate the rapid rise of HIV/AIDS as a cause of death among women of reproductive age. The trend is particularly pronounced among black women ages 15–44, and in certain states HIV/AIDS has become the leading cause of death for this subgroup.

13. **Connor E:** Advances in early diagnosis of perinatal HIV infection. *JAMA* 266:3474–3475, 1991

    This article provides a brief review of mother-infant HIV transmission and the complexity of establishing an HIV diagnosis in newborns.

14. **Des Jarlais DC, Friedman SR:** HIV infection and intravenous drug use: critical issues in transmission dynamics, infection outcomes, and prevention. *Rev Infect Dis* 10:151–158, 1988

    This article reviews the seroprevalence of HIV antibodies among intravenous drug users, discusses heterosexual transmission from intravenous drug users to their partners, and reviews prevention efforts with this population.

15. **Martin JL, Dean L, Garcia M, Paul W:** The impact of AIDS on a gay community: changes in sexual behavior, substance use, and mental health. *Am J Community Psychol* 17:269–293, 1989

    This is a good summary of the prevalence of HIV infection among gay men, the successful reduction of sexual and drug use risk behaviors in this population, and the impact of the HIV epidemic on the psychological well-being of gay men.

Health Care Workers' Risk

16. **Chamberland ME, Conley LJ, Bush TJ, Ciesielski CA, Hammett TA, Jaffe HW:** Healthcare workers with AIDS: National Surveillance Update. *JAMA* 266:3459–3462, 1991

    This article reviews 5,425 reported cases of AIDS in United States health care workers, concluding that most health care workers acquired their infection through a nonoccupational route.

17. **Henderson DK, Gerberding JL:** Prophylactic zidovudine after occupational exposure to the human immunodeficiency virus: an interim analysis. *J Infect Dis* 160:321–327, 1989

    This article reviews the risk to health care workers of acquiring HIV following parenteral exposure, the animal model evidence that zidovudine (AZT) may be helpful for postexposure chemoprophylaxis, and the issues involved in implementing a chemoprophylaxis program for health care workers.

(See also *MMWR* references above.)

Neuropsychiatric Complications

18. **Brew B, Sidtis JJ, Price R:** The nervous system: pathophysiology and clinical manifestations, in *The Epidemiology of AIDS.* Edited by Kaslow RA, Francis DP. New York, Oxford University Press, 1989, pp. 68–83

    This chapter offers an excellent review of the range of central nervous system manifestations of HIV-related illness, including the direct effect of HIV as well as opportunistic infections and neoplasms.

19. **Johns DR, Tierney M, Felsenstein D:** Alteration in the natural history of neurosyphilis by concurrent infection with the human immunodeficiency virus. *N Engl J Med* 316:1569–1572, 1987

    This early report on four cases of neurosyphilis in young homosexual HIV-positive men suggests that HIV infection may alter the natural course of syphilis, resulting in rapid progression from primary syphilis to central nervous system involvement.

20. **McArthur JC, Cohen BA, Selnes OA, Kumar AJ, Cooper K, McArthur JH, Soucy G, Cornblath DR, Chmiel JS, Wang M-C, Starkey DL, Ginzburg H, Ostrow DG, Johnson RT, Phair JP, Polk BF:** Low prevalence of neurological and neuropsychological abnormalities in otherwise healthy HIV-1-infected individuals: results from the Multicenter AIDS Cohort Study. *Ann Neurol* 26:601–611, 1989

    After some earlier studies had raised concerns about a possible high prevalence of early neurological and neuropsychological impairments in individuals with HIV-1 infection, this large, well-designed, multicenter study, comparing otherwise healthy homosexual and bisexual men who were HIV positive with those who were negative, indicated that such early abnormalities were of similar low prevalence in the two groups.

21. **Musher DM, Hamill RJ, Baughn RE:** Effect of human immunodeficiency virus (HIV) infection on the course of syphilis and the response to treatment. *Ann Intern Med* 113:872–881, 1990

    Reviewing 40 cases, this article extends the work of Johns et al. (1987) above by demonstrating that concurrent HIV infection alters the course of syphilis, with more rapid progression to neurosyphilis and less complete response to penicillin. Recommendations for more intensive medical treatment are included.

22. **Navia BA, Price RW:** The acquired immunodeficiency syndrome dementia complex as the presenting or sole manifestation of human immunodeficiency virus infection. *Arch Neurol* 44:65–69, 1987

This report on 29 patients played a significant role in bringing attention to the AIDS dementia complex as a source of cognitive, motor, and behavioral dysfunction in some HIV-infected patients who had not yet developed major systemic opportunistic infections or neoplasms.

23. *****Perry SW:** Organic mental disorders caused by HIV: update on early diagnosis and treatment. *Am J Psychiatry* 147:696–710, 1990

This article provides a thorough review of the literature through mid-1989 of the cognitive, emotional, and behavioral manifestations of HIV-induced organic mental disorders followed by a brief discussion of treatment strategies.

24. **Schmitt FA, Bigley JW, McKinnis R, Logue PE, Evans RW, Drucker JL, and the AZT Collaborative Group:** Neuropsychological outcome of zidovudine (AZT) treatment of patients with AIDS and AIDS-related complex. *N Engl J Med* 319:1573–1578, 1988

This double-blind, placebo-controlled study of 281 patients with AIDS or AIDS-related complex shows that patients with HIV-associated cognitive abnormalities may show improved cognition after treatment with zidovudine.

Psychiatric Disorders Associated With HIV

25. **Atkinson JH, Grant I, Kennedy CJ, Richman DD, Specter SA, McCutchan A:** Prevalence of psychiatric disorders among men infected with human immunodeficiency virus: a controlled study. *Arch Gen Psychiatry* 45:859–864, 1988

This study suggests that there may be a higher prevalence of anxiety disorder and major depressive illness in homosexual men when compared with sociodemographically matched heterosexual men and that the psychiatric morbidity may have preceded the onset of the AIDS epidemic.

26. **Dew MA, Ragni MV, Nimorwicz P:** Infection with human immunodeficiency virus and vulnerability to psychiatric distress: a study of men with hemophilia. *Arch Gen Psychiatry* 47:737–744, 1990

This study looks at psychiatric symptoms among HIV-seropositive and HIV-seronegative men with hemophilia. Results show that the combination of being HIV positive and having psychosocial liabilities is associated with being highly symptomatic.

27. **Fernandez F, Holmes VF, Levy JK, Ruiz P:** Consultation-liaison psychiatry and HIV-related disorders. *Hosp Community Psychiatry* 40:146–153, 1989

   The authors describe neuropsychiatric, psychosocial, and ethical-legal problems associated with HIV infection that are commonly encountered in the consultation-liaison setting.

28. **Marzuk PM, Tierney H, Tardiff K, Gross EM, Morgan EB, Hsu MA, Mann JJ:** Increased risk of suicide in persons with AIDS. *JAMA* 259:1333–1337, 1988

   This was the first published study to demonstrate a substantially increased risk for suicide among homosexual and bisexual men with AIDS.

29. **Rabkin JG, Harrison WM:** Effect of imipramine on depression and immune status in a sample of men with HIV infection. *Am J Psychiatry* 147:495–497, 1990

   The results of this study provide evidence of the safety and efficacy of imipramine in treating major depression in HIV-infected men. A placebo-controlled study investigating efficacy and effects on CD4 counts and other measures of immune competence is in progress.

30. **Rabkin JG, Williams JBW, Neugebauer R, Remien RH, Goetz R:** Maintenance of hope in HIV-spectrum homosexual men. *Am J Psychiatry* 147:1322–1326, 1990

   This study of 208 homosexual men who volunteered as research subjects found high levels of hope and low levels of current syndromal disorder or depressive symptoms among both HIV-positive and HIV-negative participants.

31. **Tross S, Hirsch DA:** Psychological distress and neuropsychological complications of HIV infection and AIDS. *Am Psychol* 43:929–934, 1988

   This article is a useful review of the various sources of psychological distress, including disease progression, social discrimination, bereavement, pressure for lifestyle change, and neurological impairment, faced by people with HIV infection, AIDS-related complex, or AIDS.

(See also Ostrow 1990; *A Psychiatrist's Guide to AIDS and HIV Disease: AIDS Primer* 1990; Tasman et al. 1990—all above.)

HIV Counseling and Risk Reduction

32. *Higgins DL, Galavotti C, O'Reilly KR, Schnell DJ, Moore M, Rugg DL, Johnson R:** Evidence for the effects of HIV antibody counseling and testing on risk behaviors. *JAMA* 266:2419–2429, 1991

    This article reviews 66 studies on the behavioral effects of HIV antibody counseling and testing, providing results on diverse populations, including homosexual men, intravenous drug users, and pregnant women.

33. **Perry SW, Markowitz JC:** Counseling for HIV testing. *Hosp Community Psychiatry* 39:731–739, 1988

    This article provides a summary of the early literature on HIV counseling, epidemiological data providing guidelines for selection of people at risk, interpretation of HIV antibody tests, the basics of pre- and posttest counseling, and case examples.

34. **Perry S, Fishman B, Jacobsberg L, Young J, Frances A:** Effectiveness of psychoeducational interventions in reducing emotional distress after human immunodeficiency virus antibody testing. *Arch Gen Psychiatry* 48:143–147, 1991

    This study compares three interventions intended to reduce distress after voluntary HIV antibody testing.

35. **Rotherham-Borus MJ, Koopman C, Haignere C, Davies M:** Reducing HIV sexual risk behaviors among runaway adolescents. *JAMA* 266:1237–1241, 1991

    This study demonstrates the efficacy of an HIV/AIDS risk-reduction intervention program with runaway adolescents and likely has implications for other groups of patients, such as those with severe mental illness, who tend to have similar risk behaviors and unstable life situations.

HIV and Severe Mental Illness

36. **Carmen E, Brady SM:** AIDS risk and prevention for the chronic mentally ill. *Hosp Community Psychiatry* 41:652–657, 1990

Carmen and Brady were the first to publish a description of an HIV prevention program for chronic mentally ill persons. In the absence of definitive research data concerning the efficacy of any intervention with this population, it remains a seminal article on the topic.

37. **Cournos F, Empfield M, Horwath E, Kramer M:** The management of HIV infection in state psychiatric hospitals. *Hosp Community Psychiatry* 40:153–157, 1989

    This article provides an overview of basic issues in the management of HIV-infected patients in state hospitals, including admission criteria, infection control, testing and confidentiality, medical care, restraint and seclusion, sexual behavior, education and training, and discharge of patients.

38. **Cournos F, Empfield M, Horwath E, McKinnon K, Meyer I, Schrage H, Curry C, Agosin B:** HIV seroprevalence among patients admitted to two psychiatric hospitals. *Am J Psychiatry* 148:1225–1230, 1991

    This article was one of the first published anonymous seroprevalence studies of hospitalized psychiatric patients demonstrating an elevated rate of HIV infection (5.5%) among newly admitted psychiatric patients with severe mental illness. This finding was confirmed by subsequent reports.

39. **Kelly JA, Murphy DA, Bahr GR, Brasfield TL, Davis DR, Hauth AC, Morgan MG, Stevenson LY, Eilers MK:** AIDS/HIV risk behavior among the chronic mentally ill. *Am J Psychiatry* 149:886–889, 1992

    This study of 60 severely mentally ill patients attending an inner-city clinic demonstrated high rates of sexual and drug use HIV risk behavior in this population.

40. **Sacks MH, Perry S, Graver R, Shindledecker R, Hall S:** Self-reported HIV-related risk behaviors in acute psychiatric inpatients: a pilot study. *Hosp Community Psychiatry* 41:1253–1255, 1990

    This was one of the first studies of HIV risk behavior among newly admitted psychiatric inpatients. Based on self-report, about half of the study patients had some risk behavior, and one-fifth of them were at high risk for HIV infection.

Legal and Ethical Issues

41. **Reamer FG** (ed): *AIDS and Ethics.* New York, Columbia University Press, 1991

A group of prominent scholars cover the range of legal and ethical issues associated with HIV infection and AIDS.

(See also *AIDS Summary* annual; Ostrow 1990; *A Psychiatrist's Guide to AIDS and HIV Disease* 1990; Tasman et al. 1990; Wallack et al. 1991—all above.)

Mental Retardation

Mark Fleisher, M.D.
Fred D. Strider, Ph.D.

The great strides that have been made in the study of mental illness have been facilitated in part by the study of developmental disabilities. Because of the explosion of new knowledge in these areas, we have tried to select the most useful current information and review articles wherever possible. The central themes of this chapter are similar to those of the original core readings because, as clinicians and researchers in mental retardation and mental illness, we need to have an understanding of both the historical dimensions of the syndrome as well as the broader issues that have divided and united patient, parent, and caregiver. It can be said that everything is history and that even the most current material will need to be viewed from its context. This is especially true in the early readings selected here as they must be understood for their historical value as well as for what they might yet teach us about the value of life and illness and how our feelings change over time. It was not that long ago when language we would not use today was the correct scientific terminology. No doubt, one day, the correctness of using the term *mentally retarded* will provoke feelings similar to how we feel today about yesterday's classification of individuals as *idiots* or *morons*. What has changed is our acceptance of the biological factors of mental illness and that those same illnesses can affect mentally retarded individuals in a similar or more devastating fashion.

We focus on the clinical aspects of genetic breakthroughs because the advances of genetics become the advances of diagnosis and treatment of persons with developmental disabilities and mental illness. The realization that mental illness responds to active pharmacological intervention and that there is no reason to believe that because someone has a damaged central nervous system that produces difficulties in life and in learning that they are not at risk for similar illness has produced a wealth of new ideas and research. The allied issues of training, advocacy, and social-political consequences from historical, transitional, and contemporary points of view remain pertinent as our moral and political compass. Science, morality, and public policy must work for the common good.

Overview and History

1. **Balthazar EE, Stevens HA:** *The Emotionally Disturbed Mentally Retarded: A Historical and Contemporary Perspective.* Englewood Cliffs, NJ, Prentice-Hall, 1975

   This work represents a worthwhile overview of both historical and diagnostic issues involving mental retardation and mental illness as concurrent entities in the same individual.

2. **Campbell M, Malone R:** Mental retardation and psychiatric disorders. *Hosp Community Psychiatry* 42:374–379, 1991

   This article offers a thorough overview of the current level of understanding within mentally retarded and mentally ill persons. The authors offer several suggestions for future work in the field.

3. **Itard J:** *The Wild Boy of Aveyron.* Translated by Humphrey G, Humphrey M. New York, Appleton-Century-Crofts, 1962

   This work is historically significant for its description of the effects of therapy on the syndrome of mental retardation. This work deals with basic psychological and specialized educational needs and introduces mental retardation into the arena of psychiatry. It provides an interesting historical perspective.

4. **Kanner L:** *A History of the Care and Study of the Mentally Retarded.* Springfield, IL, Charles C Thomas, 1964

   This work provides a comprehensive overview and history of the treatment of mentally retarded individuals.

5. **Menolascino FJ** (ed): *Psychiatric Approaches to Mental Retardation.* New York, Basic Books, 1970

This edited volume is currently and historically significant as a source for its variety of points of view on the transformation of thinking in the area of concurrent mental retardation and mental illness. By casting a wide net and using several respected voices, this book represents a broad view of the topic.

Genetic Aspects

6. **Bellugi U, Bihrle A, Jernigan T, Trauner D, Doherty S:** Neuropsychological, neurological, and neuroanatomical profile of Williams syndrome. *Am J Med Genet Suppl* 6:115–125, 1990

   Bellugi et al. set a standard in describing genetic disorders that should be the ideal where possible. A specific disorder is studied from several specific facets to delineate its presentation more fully.

7. **Berg J, Gosse G:** Specific mental retardation disorders and problem behaviors. *International Review of Psychiatry* 2:53–60, 1990

   Five disorders and their genetic etiology are discussed. This is a very useful review for tuberous sclerosis, phenylketonuria, Lesch-Nyhan syndrome, Rett's syndrome, and Prader-Willi syndrome.

8. **Dykens EM, Hodapp RM, Leckman JF:** Adaptive and maladaptive functioning of institutionalized and noninstitutionalized fragile X males. *J Am Acad Child Adolesc Psychiatry* 28:427–430, 1989

   Fragile X males were studied in various settings and measured a variety of scales. The findings are significant for the treatment and intervention of this population.

9. *Kaplan P, Mazur A, Field M, Berlin JA, Berry GT, Heidenreich R, Yudkoff M, Segal S:** Intellectual outcome in children with Maple Syrup Urine disease. *J Pediatr* 119:46–50, 1991

   This article reports important findings on the treatment and diagnosis of a genetic disorder. The method to prevent mental retardation due to a specific disorder is outlined.

10. **Meyers BA, Pueschel SM:** Psychiatric disorders in persons with Down syndrome. *J Nerv Ment Dis* 179:609–613, 1991

    Almost 500 individuals diagnosed as trisomic and mentally ill were the subjects of this study. Subjects older than age 20 and subjects younger than age 20 are included. Pertinent data were obtained for behavioral problems, signs of dementia, and mental illness. Various aspects of medical illnesses are also examined.

11. **Oberle I, Rousseau F, Heitz D, Kretz C, Devys D, Hanauer A, Boue J, Bertheas MF, Mandel JL:** Instability of a 550-base pair DNA segment and abnormal methylation in fragile X syndrome. *Science* 252:1097–1102, 1991

This is a rather technical article detailing specific abnormalities that lead to the phenotypic expressions found in fragile X syndrome.

12. *****Reiss AL, Freund L:** Neuropsychiatric aspects of the fragile-X syndrome. *Brain Dysfunction* 3:9–22, 1990

This is a very good review article that discusses behavioral phenotypes for males and females for an extremely important genetic disorder. There is currently a large amount of work on fragile X syndrome, and further readings of high quality are available and recommended for those interested.

13. **Smith I, Beasley MG, Ades AE:** Intelligence and quality of dietary treatment in phenylketonuria. *Arch Dis Child* 65:472–478, 1990

The relationship between good dietary control of phenylketonuria and the rise or fall in IQ is explored. As in many disorders, early onset and significant treatment can prevent developmental difficulties.

Diagnostic Aspects

14. **Borthwick-Duffy S, Eyman R:** Who are the dually diagnosed? *Am J Ment Retard* 94:586–595, 1990

More than 78,000 individuals with mental retardation were reviewed for traits associated with mental illness, which are discussed from a variety of interpretable perspectives.

15. **Dosen A:** Diagnosis and treatment of mental illness in mentally retarded children: a developmental model. *Child Psychiatry Hum Dev* 20:73–84, 1989

This important article attempts to provide a useful overview from a developmental perspective into the study of the dually diagnosed child. Practical clinical applications are also discussed.

16. **Glue P:** Rapid cycling affective disorders in the mentally retarded. *Biol Psychiatry* 26:250–256, 1989

Whether or not mentally retarded individuals can be diagnosed with the full range of mental illnesses continues to be discussed, and the validity is often a function of the level of retardation. This article clearly describes affective disorders in this special population.

17. *Reid A: Schizophrenia in mental retardation: clinical features. *Research in Developmental Disabilities* 10:241–249, 1989

Symptomatic, diagnostic, and clinical features of schizophrenia in mentally retarded individuals are discussed. Differential diagnosis and treatment approaches are also addressed.

18. **Singh NN, Sood A, Sonenklar N, Ellis CR:** Assessment and diagnosis of mental illness in persons with mental retardation. *Behav Modif* 15:419–433, 1991

Models for methods and measurements to assess and diagnose individuals are presented but only for depression and schizophrenia. Many research suggestions are offered to expand on the authors' paradigms.

Treatment Aspects

19. **Barrett RP, Feinstein C, Hole WT:** Effects of naloxone and naltrexone on self-injury: a double-blind, placebo-controlled analysis. *Am J Ment Retard* 93:644–651, 1989

This report demonstrates naltrexone's ability to extinguish self-injury in autistic and mentally retarded individuals. The results are discussed from a pharmacological and behavioristic point of view.

20. *Clarke DJ: Antilibidinal drugs and mental retardation: a review. *Med Sci Law* 29:2:136–146, 1989

Clarke reviews the topic of mental retardation and the use of antilibidinal medications for the purpose of controlling severely inappropriate sexual behaviors. The topic is reviewed from the aspect of the law, pharmacology, and behavioristic necessity.

21. **Gedye A:** Dietary increase in serotonin reduces self-injurious behaviour in a Down's syndrome adult. *J Ment Defic Res* 34:195–203, 1990

This is a brief report that lends support to the serotonin theory of self-injurious behavior.

22. **Hurley AD:** Individual psychotherapy with mentally retarded individuals: a review and call for research. *Res Dev Disabil* 10:261–275, 1989

Psychotherapy for mentally retarded individuals is reviewed from a variety of perspectives. This is an important contribution because the therapy it advances broadens the range of interventions available for populations with special needs.

23. **Langee HA:** Retrospective study of mentally retarded patients with behavioral disorders who were treated with carbamazepine. *Am J Ment Retard* 93:640–643, 1989

This retrospective study of 76 patients concludes that, for a subgroup with behavior disorders, carbamazepine can be useful and, at the time of the report, was underutilized.

24. *Lazarus A, Jaffe R, Dubin W:** Electroconvulsive therapy and major depression in Down's syndrome. *J Clin Psychiatry* 51:422–425, 1990

The authors report the usefulness of electroconvulsive therapy for major depressive disorder in mentally retarded individuals. Included in this group were those that were poor responders to traditional antidepressants.

25. *Markowitz P:** Fluoxetine treatment of self-injurious behavior in mentally retarded patients. *J Clin Psychopharmacol* 10:299–300, 1990

This anecdotal report of the author's use of fluoxetine to treat self-injury in retarded individuals will certainly focus attention on serotonin availability and its role in some cases of self-abuse. Because a psychiatric diagnosis was made in only one case, however, much is left to speculation. Positive effects may be related to organicity, impulsivity, or affective disorder.

26. *Spreat S, Behar D, Reneski B, Miazzo P:** Lithium carbonate for aggression in mentally retarded persons. *Compr Psychiatry* 30:505–511, 1989

In a retrospective study, 38 patients with violence, aggression, and hyperactivity were studied for responsiveness to lithium. It was found that nearly two of three showed a significant reduction in target signs.

27. **Szymanski L, Tanguay PE** (eds): *Emotional Disorders of Mentally Retarded Persons.* Baltimore, MD, University Park Press, 1980

This volume continues to be a worthwhile overview of issues affecting developmental aspects of child psychiatry as it interfaces with elements of mental retardation. Many important topics are included, although the psychopharmacology section is somewhat dated.

Training, Advocacy, Education, and Social Aspects

28. **Braddock D, Fujiura G:** Politics, public policy, and the development of community mental retardation services in the United States. *Am J Ment Retard* 95:369–387, 1991

    Data culled from the various states from 1977 to 1988 are analyzed, and implications for community planning are discussed.

29. **Donaldson JY, Menolascino FJ:** Past, current and future roles of child psychiatry in mental retardation. *Journal of the American Academy of Child Psychiatry* 16:38–52, 1977

    This remains an important article for viewing the treatment approaches to disabled individuals as a team concept that must involve a variety of fields.

30. **Hardy RE, Cull JG** (eds): *Mental Retardation and Physical Disability.* Springfield, IL, Charles C Thomas, 1974

    This work focuses on the many physical disabilities that concurrently challenge the mentally retarded individual and their caregivers.

31. **Hawkins BA, Eklund SJ:** Planning processes and outcomes for an aging population with developmental disabilities. *Ment Retard* 28:35–40, 1991

    The authors identify needs and planning strategies for an often over-looked segment of the population: aging mentally retarded persons.

32. **Menolascino FJ, Fleisher MH:** Training psychiatric residents in the diagnosis and treatment of mental illness in mentally retarded persons. *Hosp Community Psychiatry* 43:500–503, 1992

    The issues of the serious shortage of psychiatrists trained in the areas of treatment and diagnosis of mentally retarded and mentally ill individuals are addressed. Guidelines for training programs are offered.

33. **Reiss S, Levitan GW, McNally RJ:** Emotionally disturbed mentally retarded people. *Am Psychol* 37:361–367, 1982

    The mental health needs of retarded individuals and programs to match those needs are reviewed for this article. The point of view is multidisciplinarian and continues to be a reference for those involved in program issues.

34. **Schaefer GB, Bodensteiner JB:** Evaluation of the child with idiopathic mental retardation. *Pediatr Clin North Am* 39:4:929–943, 1992

This review chapter is unusually well written and referenced and provides a fine starting point for the study of the relationship between
genetics and mental retardation. Although no review chapter can be
all-inclusive, the authors' approach is from varied perspectives. The
strength of this work is also to be found in its accessibility. It is written
with technical precision without being overly complex and will be of
real value to the clinician. The 81 references will also become a useful
starting point to pursue the reader's interests.

35. **Schalock RL, Keith K, Hoffman K, Karan O:** Quality of life: its measure-
    ment and use. *Ment Retard* 27:25–31, 1989

    The authors have constructed a very able instrument to determine the
    effectiveness of programs or the environments of individuals with men-
    tal retardation.

36. **Williams W, Spruill J:** The criminal justice/mental health system and
    the mentally retarded, mentally ill defendant. *Soc Sci Med* 25:1027–1032,
    1987

    This article reviews the studied differences in processing and disposi-
    tion between retarded and nonretarded defendants incompetent to
    stand trial.

37. **Wolfensberger W, Nirje B:** *The Principles of Normalization in Human
    Services.* Toronto, Canada, National Institute on Mental Retardation,
    1972

    Normalization within the home community remains the ideal standard
    of care in this country toward which nearly all programs aim. This idea
    is at the core of most of the writing on services for mentally retarded
    and mentally ill persons.

20

Chronically Mentally Ill Patients

David L. Cutler, M.D.

Since 1984, when the last edition of this publication was compiled, there has been a significant change in the plight of the "deinstitutionalized chronically mentally ill." Indeed, deinstitutionalization is not nearly as much of an issue in the 1990s as are some of the results of having chronically mentally ill persons "at large" in the community: homelessness, dual diagnosis, coercive treatment (both inpatient and outpatient), the rise of the family movement, and the consumer movement. New methodologies, such as case management and psychosocial rehabilitation, have revolutionized public psychiatry as it relates to chronically mentally ill persons. Moreover, the very term *chronically mentally ill* is now rapidly losing favor or, one might say, becoming "politically incorrect" (Bachrach 1992). "Severe and persistent mental illness," or "serious mental illness," or "recovering mental patient," or just plain "mental health consumer" are more current examples of society's attempts to destigmatize by renaming. Of course, as they say, a rose by any other name is still a rose, and long-term mental illness continues to be persistent and have similar (although some might argue, in the "age of clozapine," somewhat less devastating) consequences to those unlucky young and old who suffer from it.

In the 1980s the concept of "dual diagnosis" became increasingly im-

243

portant. By this concept I refer not only to those persons with mental illness and drug abuse problems, but also to those persons with mental illness and developmental disabilities or mental illness and physical problems, and one might even add mental illness and social problems (such as homelessness). Here there is a growing literature that simply did not exist 10 years ago.

Nevertheless, despite some of the disastrous implications of deinstitutionalization, there is considerable good news to be found in the journals. Whereas important early writings tended to describe innovative but not necessarily reproducible model programs that disseminate poorly from one model community to another, some of the new clinical literature looks at client-centered concepts such as strengths, psychosocial rehabilitation, and "culture broker" network builders for helping people learn, do, and use the things they want to as opposed to what professionals think they ought to. There is also material that describes mainstream housing and psychosocial rehabilitation for the long-term patient and many new articles considering consumer-oriented, -operated, and -controlled treatment and projects.

Although not much is written about the linkage, some of this new psychosocial vitality is, to some considerable extent, connected to and dependent on a burgeoning of new, more effective biological treatments for schizophrenia and bipolar disorder. Many "deinstitutionalized" patients in the past did not have opportunities to take clozapine for their schizophrenia or carbamazepine for their bipolar disorder. As a result of some of these psychopharmacological discoveries, both positive and negative symptoms have been reduced enough to make some previously very regressed individuals accessible to modern psychiatric rehabilitation methodologies. State hospitals are continuing to get smaller, and community mental health centers are continuing to fine tune their service systems to focus on the most severely disabled individuals in their catchment areas.

Finally, something should be said here for the economics of chronic illness. The 1984 edition of this volume provided very little material regarding funding sources and funding streams and their impact on mental health systems. In the past several years, there has been an expanding interest in the concept of "managed care," which is supposed to ensure that funding heads for the right patients and is spent in an efficient and effective manner. Each day, to a greater extent, managed-care forces impact on the treatment of chronically mentally ill persons, and the effects of this cannot be ignored.

I try to include these various issues in appropriate topical areas; included here are classic older articles as well as important newer ones. Categories are as follows: reviews and overviews, advocacy, case management, consumer movement, deinstitutionalization, epidemiology, housing, mental health treatment systems, mental illness through the life cycle, policy and funding, psychosocial rehabilitation, and social networks.

Reviews and Overviews

1. *Bachrach LL:** Overview: model programs for chronic mental patients. *Am J Psychiatry* 137:1023–1031, 1980

   This classic article looks at the most successful model community programs from the 1970s. It extracts basic principles associated with their success. It is perhaps Bachrach's most important article. A key point is her conclusion that model programs are very difficult to disseminate.

2. **Bachrach LL:** What we know about homelessness among mentally ill persons: an analytic review and commentary. *Hosp Community Psychiatry* 43:453–464, 1992

   This article summarizes the very extensive literature on the homeless mentally ill population. It is a result of the work of the American Psychiatric Association Task Force on the Needs of the Homeless Mentally Ill Population.

3. *Braun P, Kochansky G, Shapiro R, Greenberg S, Gudeman JE, Johnson S, Shore MF:** Overview: deinstitutionalization of psychiatric patients: a critical review of outcome studies. *Am J Psychiatry* 138:736–749, 1981

   This overview is also one of the critical articles reviewing the model programs of the 1960s and 1970s. It basically concludes that a variety of alternatives, both inpatient and outpatient, result in similar results. In essence, Braun et al. propose that if follow-up is available, deinstitutionalization can be effective. On the other hand, they admit that there was insufficient comparative data at that time to evaluate the relative efficacy of various community-based models, such as sheltered workplaces, halfway houses, and group homes. This is a very important article for its time.

Advocacy

4. **Bachrach LL:** The "chronic patient" in search of a title? *Hosp Community Psychiatry* 43:867–868, 1992

   This article reflects the confusion and controversy regarding the term *chronic mentally ill.* Bachrach expresses her frustration over deinstitutionalization semantics. What advantages are there to the term *chronic?* What do consumers think? What do families think? Should we develop new, less stigmatizing terminology? Should she change the name of her column? See what you think.

5. **Geller JL:** Clinical encounters with outpatient coercion at the CMHC: questions of implementation and efficacy. *Community Ment Health J* 28:81–94, 1992

This article addresses the legal, clinical, and resource issues in the course of outpatient treatment and the need to utilize coercive techniques to treat uncooperative patients successfully. It is an important strategy for difficult, yet also potentially very treatable, individuals.

Case Management

6. **Anthony WA, Cohen M, Farkas M, Cohen BF:** Chronical care update: the chronically mentally ill: case management—more than a response to a dysfunctional system. *Community Ment Health J* 26:219–228, 1988

This article by the Boston University Center for Psychosocial Rehabilitation describes a model for case management with the ultimate goal of responding to client goals by appropriately linking clients to meaningful services and providing an anchoring therapeutic relationship. This type of case management forms the basis for the client-centered approach to psychosocial rehabilitation advocated by the Boston University Center.

7. *****Chamberlain R, Rapp CA:** A decade of case management: a methodological review of outcome research. *Community Ment Health J* 27:171–188, 1991

Case management has become a panacea for chronic mentally ill patients over the past 15 years. Does it work? What does the literature say? This is a comparison of the major studies to date and the models on which they are based. It helps to sort the wheat from the chaff.

8. *****Solomon P:** The efficacy of case management services for severely mentally disabled clients. *Community Ment Health J* 28:163–180, 1992

Here is an even more comprehensive review of the literature on case management as a core service for long-term patients. The article summarizes the studies to date regarding various outcome measures of four models of case management. It concludes that case management is effective in reducing hospital recidivism and also in improving quality of life, but that more rigorous research is needed as to its efficacy.

Consumer Movement

9. **Chamberlain J, Rogers JA, Sneed CS:** Consumers, families, and community support systems. *Psychosocial Rehabilitation Journal* 12:93–106, 1989

This article lays out the philosophy of the consumer movement and its current state of the art. It strongly supports the notion of self-help and the idea of user-run programs. It discusses the role of self-help vis-à-vis community support systems and includes the perspective of families as well.

10. **Mowbray CT, Chamberlain P, Reed C:** Consumer-run mental health services: results from five demonstration projects. *Community Ment Health J* 24:151–156, 1988

The authors describe five demonstration projects funded by the Michigan Department of Mental Health to promote self-help initiatives for psychiatric patients. The five projects included a rural program matching volunteers with clients, a rural program employing ex-patient advocates to visit clients in the hospital, a project designed to develop natural support networks around chronically mentally ill people, a day-break drop-in center to a suburban area providing a social club, and a suburban for-profit consumer-owned and -operated janitorial service. All the projects are described as successful, and their results have had an impact on planning in the state of Michigan for consumer-operated projects.

11. **Nikkel RE, Smith G, Edwards D:** A consumer-operated case management project. *Hosp Community Psychiatry* 43:577–579, 1992

This report describes a community support and intensive community treatment service operated entirely by ex-patients or recovering patients. The project was modeled after the famous PACT program in Madison, Wisconsin, and is funded by the state of Oregon. Case-management teams go into the state hospital, find severely mentally ill individuals who might be placeable, and bring them to the community, where they are provided intensive support and on-site psychiatric treatment. This article describes perhaps the most intensive and radical consumer-operated project in existence; yet the project works very closely with the state and county mental health programs to ensure its success.

12. **Solomon P, Draine J:** Satisfaction with mental health treatment and randomized trial of consumer case management. *J Nerv Ment Dis* 182:179–184, 1994

This article is the first in a series of papers describing the effects of hiring consumers to be case managers for persons with severe mental illness. In this study, the consumer case managers needed to have a major mental disorder as defined in DSM-III-R, at least one prior psychiatric hospitalization in either a public or private institution, and a minimum of 14 days of psychiatric hospitalization or at least five psychiatric emergency service contacts over a 1-year period, as well as regular contact with a mental health provider for treatment of the mental illness. Patients were recruited to the consumer case-management team and also to another team utilizing the same model but with nonconsumers as case managers. Between the two teams, 96 persons were recruited, and 91 were followed up after a year. The study showed that regardless of consumer or nonconsumer, the capacity of the case manager to provide empathic support made a great deal of difference in terms of patient satisfaction with the treatment. In this study, each team was under a different agency and had different re-sources available. Consequently, not much can be said about overall satisfaction with treatment since the treatment was quite different. Similar studies are being designed and carried out in other parts of the country, which will have the two teams within the same agency and should shed further light on whether the empathic edge that consumer case managers have can have an overall effect on treatment satisfaction.

This is a very important early study in an area that is quite contro-versial. It will become a milestone in the literature with regard to the treatment of severely mentally ill consumers by other consumers with major mental illness backgrounds.

Deinstitutionalization

13. **Bassuk EL** (ed): The mental health needs of homeless persons. *New Dir Ment Health Ser*, Vol. 30, 1986

Bassuk provides an excellent overview of the problems of homeless mentally ill persons and their families. In particular, she studies the effects of homelessness on various populations throughout the life cycle. The first chapter recapitulates an earlier article by Bassuk analyz-ing the relationship between the implementation of deinstitutionaliza-tion and the increasing phenomena of large numbers of severely mentally ill adults among the homeless.

14. **Bigelow DA, Cutler DL, Moore LJ, McComb P, Leung P:** Characteristics of state hospital patients who are hard to place. *Hosp Community Psychi-atry* 39:181–186, 1988

This article describes a group of chronic patients still institutionalized after the deinstitutionalization era and suggests residential options tailored to the needs of these difficult, hard-to-place patients. Many of these patients have become more placeable due to treatment with clozapine. However, most communities still have not developed adequate residential spectrums for these individuals who continue to be in need of supportive housing.

15. **Drake RE, Wallach MA:** Mental patients' attraction to the hospital: correlates of living preference. *Community Ment Health J* 28:5–12, 1992

A study of 187 aftercare patients of an urban state hospital, this article points out that patients who are attracted to hospitals can be identified and can also be expected to get admitted more frequently than other patients. The authors point out that the provision of decent affordable housing for these long-term mentally disabled would help to solve the problem.

16. *Goldman HH, Gattozzi AA, Taube CA:** Defining and counting the chronically mentally ill. *Hosp Community Psychiatry* 32:21–27, 1981

This is a key article on the epidemiology of chronic mental illness. Who are these chronically mentally ill persons? What are they like? How many of them are there? The article estimates there are 1.7–3 million in the country. There are more now, but this was a good look at the late 1970s and early 1980s.

17. *Minkoff K:** Beyond deinstitutionalization: a new ideology for post-institutional care. *Hosp Community Psychiatry* 38:945–950, 1987

This article provides principles for a new, more practical array of therapeutic interventions, necessary in the postinstitutional era. These principles, in essence, recognize the patient as an individual who, along with family and community-based treatment, can address their own struggle in the community with clinical and social help from practitioners and agencies.

18. *Stein L, Test MA:** Alternative to mental hospital treatment, I: conceptual model, treatment program, and clinical evaluation. *Arch Gen Psychiatry* 37:392–397, 1980; **Weisbrod BA, Test MA, Stein LI:** Alternative to mental hospital treatment, II: economic benefit-cost analysis. *Arch Gen Psychiatry* 37:400–405, 1980; **Test MA, Stein LI:** Alternative to mental hospital treatment, III: social cost. *Arch Gen Psychiatry* 37:409–412, 1980

These articles provide perhaps **the** most important model program evaluation. In the first article, Stein and Test describe the program they developed in Madison, Wisconsin, for intensive community treatment. This article and its two companions provide the reader with a description of how the famous Madison model works, how effective the project was, and the social and economic costs and benefits.

19. **Talbott JA:** Deinstitutionalization: avoiding the disasters of the past. *Hosp Community Psychiatry* 30:621–624, 1979

Talbott's classic article is still relevant today. He describes the problems of deinstitutionalized patients and prescribes Talbott's "Ten Commandments for Community Psychiatry."

Epidemiology

20. **Bassuk E, Gershon ES:** Deinstitutionalization and mental health services. *Sci Am* 238:46–53, 1978

This is a classic early article that links deinstitutionalization with the appearance of chronically mentally ill persons in the homeless population. It points out problems with the community mental health movement and potential consequences if these problems are not addressed. Of course, they still have not been addressed.

21. **Davies MA, Bromet EJ, Schulz SC, Dunn LO, Morgenstern M:** Community adjustment of chronic schizophrenic patients in urban and rural settings. *Hosp Community Psychiatry* 40:824–830, 1989

Early studies suggested that social disorganization causes or exacerbates mental illness. The authors of this article compare urban and rural patients with schizophrenia and conclude that those living in rural communities adjust better than those in the urban areas.

22. **Minkoff K:** A map of chronic mental patients, in *The Chronic Mental Patient: Problems, Solutions, and Recommendations for a Public Policy*. Edited by Talbott JA. Washington, DC, American Psychiatric Association, 1978, pp. 11–37

Minkoff's article continues to be a basic epidemiological reference comprehensively covering patients from the hospital to the community focusing on both the history and the developmental evolution of chronically mentally ill persons. This is a very important seminal piece of work.

Housing

23. **Cutler DL:** Community residential options for the chronically mentally ill. *Community Ment Health J* 22:61–73, 1986

This article reviews the literature on community housing up to the mid-1980s. It describes several levels of care for a range of hard-to-place patients. It introduces the notion of semi-independent living and illustrates how one state has approached the housing spectrum.

24. **Fairweather GW, Sanders DH, Maynard H, Cressler DL, Bleck DS:** *Community Life for the Mentally Ill: An Alternative to Institutional Care.* Chicago, IL, Aldine, 1969

Can chronically disabled persons actually live together and support one another outside the range of professionals? Fairweather et al. think they can and, in this seminal work, tell how they do it. Numerous projects are based on this model.

25. *Goering P, Durbin J, Foster R, Boyles S, Babiak T, Lincee B:** Social networks of residents in supportive housing. *Community Ment Health J* 28:199–214, 1992

This is a great article on the nature of supportive housing. What makes housing supportive? Networks do. What is the right size and function of those networks? This study turns up some interesting findings and gives us a glimpse as to how to manage natural support networks around chronic patients.

26. *Gudeman JE, Shore MF:** Beyond deinstitutionalization: a new class of facilities for the mentally ill. *N Engl J Med* 311:832–836, 1984

This is an important article focusing on new designs for facilities that meet the specific needs of chronic mentally ill patients. This article is a very thoughtful look at difficult-to-place chronic patients.

27. **Hogan MF, Carling PJ:** Normal housing: a key element of a supported housing approach for people with psychiatric disabilities. *Community Ment Health J* 28:215–226, 1992

Finding adequate housing is a key problem for chronic patients. What is the supported housing approach? How can consumers make their own choices? Can there be community housing for difficult patients? The authors propose criteria for community mental health centers to plan for those services.

Mental Health Treatment Systems

28. **Cutler DL** (ed): Effective aftercare for the 1980s. *New Dir Ment Health Ser,* Vol. 19, 1983

This monograph proposes a range of services necessary to maintain long-term patients in the community. It advocates for a services and

natural support network to be built around each consumer and analyzes some of the barriers and fragmentation problems that interfere
with the development of these systems. There are chapters on building
natural networks, developing productive activities, establishing "therapeutic relationships," and developing treatment plans. It continues to
be a good manual for community mental health professionals and is of
value today.

29. *Lamb HR: *Community Survival for Long-Term Patients.* San Francisco,
CA, Jossey-Bass, 1976

This book still must be thought of as the basic text for the treatment of
chronically mentally ill persons. In addition to an excellent chapter
describing guiding principles in the treatment of these individuals,
Lamb's chapter on individual psychotherapy continues to be a state-of-
the-art contribution to understanding long-term therapeutic relationships with long-term patients.

30. *Lamb HR: *Treating the Long Term Mentally Ill.* San Francisco, CA, Jossey-
Bass, 1982

This follow-up to Lamb's (1976) classic above, *Community Survival for
Long-Term Patients,* builds on the previous book but in many ways goes
much further. It provides a section on societal reaction to chronically
mentally ill persons in the community, an overview on appropriate
housing, special chapters on young adult chronic patients, and families
of the mentally ill as well as individualized treatment including psychotherapy and case management. It even provides the reader with a guide
to benefits and problems with the Social Security supplemental security
income system. This is a major contribution to the literature and still
clearly relevant.

31. **Minkoff K:** Resistance of mental health professionals to working with
the chronic mentally ill. *New Dir Ment Health Serv* 33:3–20, 1987

Minkoff looks at the resistance of mental health professionals themselves to working with chronic mentally ill patients and offers some
recommendations as to how training programs can address the issue
early so that professionals may be more oriented toward working with
the population.

32. *Drake RE, McLaughlin P, Pepper B, Minkoff K** (eds): Dual diagnosis
of major mental illness and substance disorders. *New Dir Ment Health
Serv* 50:3–12, 1991

This very comprehensive monograph contains articles by the editors
and others on the assessment of dual-diagnosis disorders. There are

also several interesting perspectives regarding integrated treatment. This is a very important handbook for those working with this population.

33. **Pepper B, Ryglewicz H** (eds): The young adult chronic patient. *New Dir Ment Health Serv*, Vol. 14, 1982

This is a basic handbook on the uninstitutionalized young chronic mentally ill patient, the person who frequently does not believe that he or she has a mental illness, but needs treatment anyway. Liberalized commitment laws, deinstitutionalization, and modern psychopharmacological methods have resulted in large numbers of young severely mentally ill persons who have never seen the inside of a state hospital. Who are they, what are they like, where do they live, and how do they respond to stress? The answers to these questions and several others can be found in this 14-chapter basic volume on young adult chronic patients.

34. **Pepper B, Ryglewicz H** (eds): Advances in treating the young adult chronic patient. *New Dir Ment Health Serv* 21:5–15, 1984

Although basically an update on the earlier work by Pepper and Ryglewicz (1982) above, this monograph contains many useful concepts and programmatic models valuable to a practitioner working in this area. Included are numerous chapters on case management, working with families, and increasing medication compliance, as well as innovative, imaginative approaches for working with disillusioned young people.

35. **Stein LI, Test MA** (eds): *Alternatives to Mental Hospital Treatment.* New York, Plenum, 1978

This book may not have been a bestseller, but it should have been. Although hard to find, this book is full of innovations in the care of long-term patients such as the Madison, Wisconsin, PACT model; the Southwest Denver, Colorado, Project; and Fountain House. You cannot miss with these ideas.

36. **Talbott JA:** *The Chronic Mentally Ill: Treatment, Programs, Systems.* New York, Human Sciences Press, 1981

A comprehensive approach to treatment, programming, special populations, and model service systems, this book includes chapters from a wide range of state-of-the-art professionals in clinical research and administrative aspects delivering service to chronically mentally ill persons.

Mental Illness Through the Life Cycle

37. *Baker F, Jodrey D, Intagliata J:** Social support and quality of life in community support clients. *Community Ment Health J* 28:397–412, 1992

The authors have conducted an assessment of 729 severely mentally ill adults enrolled in state-supported community support services with an eye toward the relationship between quality of life and social support. They found a strong correlation between satisfaction in various life domains and the availability and adequacy of social support. This is a key article linking these two major research areas regarding the well-being of chronically mentally ill patients.

38. **Sheets JL, Prevost JL, Rihman J:** Young adult chronic patients: three hypothesized subgroups. *Hosp Community Psychiatry* 33:197–203, 1982

This article presents a convenient, although somewhat simplistic and overly concrete, trichotomy of long-term psychiatric patients who are low energy–low demand, high energy–high demand, and high functioning–high aspiration. The authors hypothesize that each of the three groups requires a different kind of programming. There are numerous important insights in this clinically useful article. The classification system, even though it fails to work for many patients, can be applied to understand various individuals at points in the developmental course of dealing with their illness.

39. *Straus J, Hafez H, Liberman P, Harding C:** The course of psychiatric disorder, III: longitudinal principles. *Am J Psychiatry* 142:289–296, 1985

This article is truly a landmark contribution to the understanding of the developmental processes of chronic mental illness. It describes the existential phases and stages that individuals with long-term mental illness experience. In particular, it reveals how prolonged these phases can be and how dramatic and unpredictable the changes between them may appear. It also describes the reactions of immediate supporters to the illness. This is a very important seminal article, which should be read by all clinicians working in the field.

Policy and Funding

40. **Aviram U:** Community care of the seriously mentally ill: continuing problems and current issues. *Community Ment Health J* 26:69–88, 1990

It is refreshing to read an exceptionally analytic and critical outsider's view on how mental health in America works and does not work. This article points out how serious disastrous problems (such as homelessness and poverty) for severely mentally ill persons creates havoc in trying to provide services. In particular, the author notes the ambivalent ideological, economic, and political contradictions that make it so difficult to define problems and develop rational approaches. His critique includes a look at the failings of the so-called medical model and the impossibility of the case-management situation. This is a sobering article that forces us to take a critical look at the way we see things and do business.

41. *Cutler DL, Bigelow D, McFarland B: The cost of fragmented mental health financing: is it worth it? *Community Ment Health J* 28:121–134, 1992

In an era where cost cutting seems to be the key planning principle, zealous efforts of "managed care" appear to be eroding the basic support for core services. Performance, contracting, managed care, and health maintenance organizations form a complex hodgepodge that can change over night in a given mental health system. Fragmented funding mechanisms frequently result in fragmented treatment to a population that requires long-term continuity of care.

42. McFarland BH: Health maintenance organizations and persons with severe mental illness. *Community Mental Health J* 30:221–242, 1994

The big question in the new age is how well managed care entities captivated models and other new health reform schemes affect the care of chronically mentally ill persons. There is plenty of evidence that existing mental health programs will be expected to compete, like other private entities, for the same dollars that they used to be guaranteed from the states and the federal government to serve chronically mentally ill persons. Medicaid programs are already being contracted to health maintenance organizations (HMOs). This article looks at the capacity of the HMO model to serve persons with severe mental illness. It points out a number of the problems inherent in this new atmosphere, including the potential for low bidding, underreimbursement, and potential collapse of certain providers and also the possibility of success. It warrants that community mental health providers are going to need to understand this new atmosphere to be able to compete successfully for the dollars that they are already getting and then to be successful as well at delivering the service. This is a very important article that makes some sense out of what most clinicians are finding a very confusing financial puzzle. If you want to know what is coming— better yet, if you want to know what is already here in many places— read this article.

43. **Paulson RI:** People and garbage are not the same: issues in contracting for public mental health services. *Community Ment Health J* 24:91–102, 1988

    Paulson describes mechanisms used to provide financial remuneration for community mental health centers that serve chronically mentally ill persons. He points out that many of these funding mechanisms create special dilemmas in providing adequate treatment for chronically mentally ill persons. He suggests a cautionary note in the movement toward privatization and that such a movement may well not be a panacea.

44. **Schefler R, Grogan C, Couple B, Penner S:** Specialized mental health plans for persons with severe mental illness under managed competition. *Journal of Hospital and Community Psychiatry* 44:937–942, 1993

    In utilizing comprehensive principles of health maintenance organizations, the authors propose the development of mental health maintenance organizations that are designed to serve persons with severe mental illness. They propose mechanisms for reimbursement either through health insurance purchasing cooperatives on a capitated risk adjustment basis or on a contracting basis through the general health plan. In each of these models, the region's health insurance purchasing cooperative would provide oversight as well as gatekeeping for referrals into this mental health maintenance organization. The plans are designed to ensure that persons with severe mental illness are not inappropriately shifted to state hospitals or denied services in other manners. It would integrate the health maintenance with the mental health maintenance's function. Of course, it would also be also be structured to provide funding incentives that would produce cost-effective outcomes.

    This article provides a nice outline for how the successful funding schemes would work under managed competition to provide services for severely mentally ill persons effectively and efficiently without screening them out altogether. Let us hope they are right.

45. **Talbott JA:** The chronic mentally ill: what do we now know, and why aren't we implementing what we know?, in *The Chronic Mental Patient/II*. Edited by Menninger WW, Hannah G. Washington, DC, American Psychiatric Press, 1987, pp. 1–29

    This particular chapter is perhaps the most important in this book. It reviews the results of successful programs and describes why we have failed so miserably at being able to disseminate these successful programs.

Psychosocial Rehabilitation

46. **Anthony WA, Liberman RP:** The practice of psychiatric rehabilitation: historical, conceptual, and research based. *Schizophr Bull* 12:542–559, 1986

   This excellent overview of the field of psychiatric rehabilitation takes into account the historical context and the current most popular models. It comes from a position of severe, persistent mental illness as a psychiatric disability, making the assumption that skills training can be extremely effective in overcoming social and living skill problems and maintaining an adequate quality of life. This article is an excellent overview and basic theoretical framework for those consumers and staff who want to understand the philosophy and methodology of psychosocial or psychiatric rehabilitation.

47. **Liberman RP:** *Social Skills Training for Psychiatric Patients.* New York, Pergamon, 1989

   This is a handbook that provides the ABCs of psychosocial rehabilitation, including assessment, training, and overcoming resistance. In addition, the appendixes are extremely important, providing checklists and instruments to measure assertiveness and interactiveness as well as distress. The materials in this handbook could be used by community mental health centers, case-management teams, and by day-treatment programs to provide detailed programming in psychosocial rehabilitation for chronically mentally ill persons. It is a simple, straightforward, very useful guidebook and represents the state-of-the-art in psychosocial rehabilitation for chronically mentally ill persons.

48. **Rapp CA, Winterstein R:** The strengths model of case management: results from those demonstrations. *Psychosocial Rehabilitation Journal* 13:23–32, 1989

   This article outlines what is one of the more popular theories in the field regarding case management. The model suggests that it is important not only to evaluate the psychiatric and social disabilities in the chronic patient, but also the strengths of the patient and the patient's network. In fact, treatment planning should center on enhancing the strengths and talents of the individual as opposed to focusing on deficits.

49. *****Rapp CA, Gowdy E, Sullivan WP, Winters DR:** Client outcome reporting: the status method. *Community Ment Health J* 24:118–133, 1988

   This article describes the development of a method that provides a measurement of community integration and quality of life in the community. It focuses on living arrangements and vocational independence as measures of community survival status. The method is useful for community mental health workers in determining whether or not they have their chronically mentally ill deinstitutionalized clients adequately embedded in the community.

50. *Talbott JA (ed): *The Chronic Mental Patient: Five Years Later.* New York, Grune & Stratton, 1984

This book, second in a series by Talbott (1981) above, looks at the "explosion of information" concerning the chronically mentally ill population since the report of the President's Commission on Mental Health. It also includes state-of-the-art chapters by extremely well-known authorities. However, it focuses somewhat differently than the previous volume in that it covers research and education, treatment and rehabilitation, community treatment, and systems issues. It is a somewhat more sophisticated piece of work than the earlier book.

Social Networks

51. *Cutler DL:** Clinical care update: chronically mentally ill. *Community Ment Health J* 21:3–13, 1985

Cutler summarizes the various natural network elements necessary to be in place to ensure that a chronically mentally ill person can survive in the community. He advocates a support system to guide mental health workers and planners in building supports that include consumers, families, and natural helpers around each chronically disabled individual.

52. **Hanson JC, Rapp CA:** Families perceptions of community mental health programs for their relatives with a severe mental illness. *Community Ment Health J* 28:181–198, 1992

This article points out that despite considerable controversy, families continue to provide a major share of the care of people with severe and persistent mental illness. Unfortunately, there is considerable distance between the families' perception of the needs for their relatives and the community mental health system's capacity to provide such services. The article reports the results of a study of family perspectives and their local mental health services across a midwestern state's mental health system.

53. **Hatfield AB** (ed): Families of the mentally ill: meeting the challenges. *New Dir Ment Health Serv,* Vol. 34, 1987

This edited volume is really a comprehensive description of the family movement and its attitude toward chronically mentally ill persons and the treatment systems that serve them. It contains important perspectives from professionals, family members themselves, and consumers. This is an important volume for those wishing to understand the plight of families of chronically mentally ill persons.

54. **Solomon P, Beck S, Gordon B:** Family members' perspectives on psychiatric hospitalization and discharge. *Community Ment Health J* 24:108–117, 1988

The authors describe a comprehensive look at the attitudes of family toward the treatment that mentally ill relatives have gotten. Their study shows that there was considerable anxiety regarding the family burden of soon-to-be-discharged patients and suggests families need to be better informed regarding the capabilities of their mentally ill relatives and provided with support to enable them to manage.

55. *Wasylenki D, James S, Clark C, Lewis J, Goering P, Gillies L:* Clinical issues in social network therapy for clients with schizophrenia. *Community Ment Health J* 28:427–440, 1992

The authors describe methodology for intervening with the fragmented social network surrounding clients with schizophrenia. They present examples of clinical issues that occur in social-network–oriented interventions that address those issues. The article is an important addition to the literature in understanding and working with support systems around severely mentally ill individuals. It links research with direct social network clinical intervention and as such provides a basis for reconceptualizing case-management functions.

21

Sleep, Sleep Disorders, and Dreaming

Daniel J. Buysse, M.D.
Charles F. Reynolds III, M.D.
David J. Kupfer, M.D.

leep and its disorders have long intrigued psychiatric clinicians and researchers. This interest stems from several sources, including 1) the recognition that sleep is often disturbed during the course of psychiatric disorders; 2) the notion that disturbed sleep can lead to psychiatric or psychological symptoms; 3) neurobiological studies suggesting common regulatory mechanisms for sleep and mood; 4) theories suggesting that dreams provide insights into subconscious thought; and 5) the presence of behavioral and physiological disorders that arise exclusively, or predominantly, during sleep.

The history of the study of sleep shows a general movement from psychological theories to the neurobiology and clinical disorders of sleep. Early psychiatric interest in sleep focused on the role of dreaming. Although Freud sought to approach dreaming and other unconscious thought from a neurobiological perspective, psychodynamic views of sleep and dreaming remain as almost pure theoretical constructs. The electroencephalographic work of Loomis, Kleitman, and Aserinsky heralded the advent of the physiological study of sleep, with the recognition of different sleep "stages" cycling periodically throughout a sleep period. A great deal of work in normative aspects of human sleep as well as anatomical and physiological research in animal sleep followed in the 1960s and 1970s. Investigators also turned their attention to the physiological study of sleep pathologies, including narcolepsy and sleep apnea. Clinical sleep disorders medicine continues to grow, with the American Board of Sleep Medicine seeking to gain recognition from the American Board of Medical Specialties. In terms of psychiatric sleep research, early work focused on schizophrenia and alcohol dependence, until the identification of electroencephalographic (EEG) sleep findings as possible "markers" of depressive disorders. From the mid-1970s to the mid-1990s, psychiatric sleep research expanded rapidly and has moved from descriptive cross-sectional studies to studies using longitudinal designs, pharmacological and physiological "probes," mathematical modeling, and metabolic brain-imaging techniques. In a relative sense, dream research has languished, although a small number of investigators continue to explore dreaming in areas such as posttraumatic stress disorder and major life changes (e.g., divorce).

The study of sleep and the treatment of sleep disorders involve multidisciplinary efforts. Investigators from the fields of basic neuroscience, neurology, psychiatry, psychology, and pulmonary medicine continue to make active contributions to the field.

This chapter includes three main sections: 1) general references on sleep and its disorders, 2) basic and applied science aspects of sleep, and 3) specific references for clinical sleep disorders. Given that most readers will be approaching this chapter from the perspective of general clinical psychiatry, we have given more emphasis to psychiatric aspects of sleep. We have not addressed in detail psychoanalytic theories of sleep and dreaming. This reflects a general trend in sleep research over the past 20–25 years and is not meant to minimize psychoanalytic contributions to the field. Beyond the summary of psychoanalytic theory contained in some of our listed references, the reader can find a more detailed discussion of this topic elsewhere in this volume (Edelson, Chapter 3; Levine, Chapter 38).

We have emphasized reviews and overviews rather than primary works, because much of sleep medicine falls outside the usual purview of clinical psychiatry. Of course, the interested reader will be able to access more of the primary works through the more general references. We have also included several texts as general references. These contain chapters on most of the subsequent topics listed. In the section on clinical sleep disorders, we have followed the outline of the DSM-IV section on sleep disorders. Finally, we have tried to emphasize more recent works, again with the assumption that earlier works will be accessible through later ones.

General References

1. *Hauri PJ: *Sleep Disorders,* (Current Concepts series). Kalamazoo, MI, Upjohn Company, 1992

This slim (48-page) monograph, now in its second edition, includes a wealth of basic and clinical information regarding sleep and its disorders. It provides an excellent overview, complemented by brief case histories and clear illustrations.

2. *Hobson JA: *Sleep.* New York, Scientific American Library, 1989

   This beautifully written and illustrated book covers a wide variety of topics including phenomenology, neurobiology, evolutionary aspects, and dreaming. Its conversational tone is well suited to lay readers and students as well as physicians.

3. **Horne J:** *Why We Sleep: The Functions of Sleep in Humans and Other Mammals.* Oxford, England, Oxford University Press, 1988

   This book takes an informal but scholarly approach to the question of sleep function. It draws a wide variety of both human and animal studies into a thought-provoking discussion. Horne's review of sleep deprivation and its effects on psychological and physiological functioning is particularly engaging.

4. *Kryger MH, Roth T, Dement WC** (eds): *Principles and Practice of Sleep Medicine,* 2nd Edition. Philadelphia, PA, WB Saunders, 1993

   This multiauthored volume is the first comprehensive textbook of sleep and its disorders. Its chapters address basic sleep physiology and clinical sleep disorders.

5. **Thorpy MJ** (ed): *Handbook of Sleep Disorders.* New York, Marcel Dekker, 1990

   This is another multiauthored compendium, which contains a brief section on basic aspects and a more detailed discussion of clinical sleep disorders. It is written primarily for neurologists, but will be readily accessible to psychiatrists as well.

Anatomy, Physiology, Monitoring, and Normal Sleep

Neuroanatomy and Neurophysiology

6. **Hobson JA:** Sleep and dreaming. *J Neurosci* 10:371–382, 1990

   Despite its brevity, this article reviews central aspects of the neuroanatomy, neurophysiology, and neurochemistry of sleep and discusses their clinical relevance for several specific disorders, including depression.

7. *Jones BE: Basic mechanisms of sleep-wake states, in *Principles and Practice of Sleep Medicine*. Edited by Kryger MH, Roth T, Dement WC. Philadelphia, PA, WB Saunders, 1989, pp. 121–138

Brain mechanisms underlying sleep and wakefulness are difficult to elucidate, because they involve redundant and overlapping systems. Although this chapter is not easy reading, it does provide a reasonably brief and well-organized overview of the area.

8. **Siegel JM:** Mechanisms of sleep control. *J Clin Neurophysiol* 7:49–65, 1990

This article focuses on the mechanisms underlying rapid eye movement (REM) sleep, but it also presents a brief discussion of non–rapid eye movement (NREM) sleep mechanisms.

Pharmacology of Sleep

9. *Gaillard J-M, Nicholson AN, Pascoe PA: Neurotransmitter systems, in *Principles and Practice of Sleep Medicine*. Edited by Kryger MH, Roth T, Dement WC. Philadelphia, PA, WB Saunders, 1989, pp. 202–212

The pharmacology of sleep can be as difficult as its neuroanatomy. This chapter reviews effects of the "classic" neurotransmitters and their effects on sleep in a comprehensible fashion. It does not discuss gamma-aminobutyric acid (GABA) or benzodiazepines.

10. *Greenblatt DJ: Benzodiazepine hypnotics: sorting the pharmacological facts. *J Clin Psychiatry* 52 (suppl):4–10, 1991

This brief review (similar to lengthier discussions by the same author) gives a synopsis of pharmacological principles applied to benzodiazepines. The information has direct practical significance in the clinical use of hypnotics.

11. **Jouvet M:** The role of monoamines and acetylcholine-containing neurons in the regulation of the sleep-waking cycle. *Ergebnisse der Physiologie, Biologischen Chemie und Experimentellen Pharmakologie* 64:166–307, 1972

This is a classic reference describing the role of neurotransmitters on sleep and wake states. Although some information is dated (e.g., the discussion of serotonin), it still is a benchmark work in the pharmacology of sleep.

12. *Mendelson WB: Pharmacological treatment of insomnia, in *Human Sleep: Research and Clinical Care*. Edited by Mendelson WB. New York, Plenum Medical, 1987, pp. 81–105

This chapter reviews evidence for the efficacy of hypnotic drugs, their residual effects, and special topics such as the effect of benzodiazepines on respiration and use of benzodiazepines in the elderly. For the interested reader, the same volume also includes a chapter on general sleep pharmacology, which reviews much of the earlier work in the field.

Physiological Monitoring of Human Sleep

13. *Carskadon MA, Rechtschaffen A: Monitoring and staging human sleep, in *Principles and Practice of Sleep Medicine.* Edited by Kryger MH, Roth T, Dement WC. Philadelphia, PA, WB Saunders, 1989, pp. 665–683

    This chapter discusses the essentials of polysomnographic sleep recordings. It provides more detail than most nonsleep specialists require, but serves as an excellent introduction to those who wish to learn about human sleep.

Normal Human Sleep

14. *Aserinsky E, Kleitman N: Regularly occurring periods of eye motility, and concomitant phenomena, during sleep. *Science* 118:273–274, 1953

    The classic article first described cycles of rapid eye movement (REM) and non–rapid eye movement (NREM) sleep across the night in human subjects as well as the association between REM and dreaming. This 2-page report arguably formed the basis for modern sleep research and sleep disorders medicine.

15. Bliwise DL: Sleep in normal aging and dementia. *Sleep* 16:40–81, 1993

    This is a comprehensive and scholarly summary of sleep in aging, with more than 700 references.

16. *Carskadon MA, Dement WC: Normal human sleep: an overview, in *Principles and Practice of Sleep Medicine.* Edited by Kryger MH, Roth T, Dement WC. Philadelphia, PA, WB Saunders, 1989, pp. 3–13

    This short chapter discusses the essential features of polysomnographically defined human sleep, as well as the major factors that influence its expression, such as age, drugs, and circadian timing.

17. Dahl RE: Child and adolescent sleep disorders, in *Child and Adolescent Neurology for the Psychiatrist.* Edited by Kaufmann DM. Baltimore, MD, Williams & Wilkins, 1992, pp. 169–194

This chapter gives an overview of age-related changes in sleep during childhood and adolescence, as well as the common behavioral, neurological, and medical sleep disorders affecting this age group.

18. *Dement WC, Kleitman N:** Cyclic variations in EEG during sleep and their relation to eye movements, body motility, and dreaming. *Electroencephalogr Clin Neurophysiol* 9:673–690, 1957

The second "classic" article at the foundation of sleep medicine, this article describes in great detail the association between rapid eye movement (REM) sleep and dreaming mental activity. It also refines the description of cyclic alternations between REM and non–rapid eye movement (NREM) sleep.

19. *Moore-Ede MC, Sulzman FM, Fuller CA:** Circadian timing of physiological systems, in *The Clocks That Time Us.* Cambridge, MA, Harvard University Press, 1982, pp. 201–294

This chapter elucidates the role of the circadian system in the expression of sleep and wakefulness, drawing on both animal and human studies. A subsequent chapter in the book discusses sleep disorders associated with circadian dysfunction. Interested readers will find that the entire book provides a fascinating overview of circadian rhythms.

20. **Orem J, Keeling J:** A compendium of physiology in sleep, in *Physiology in Sleep.* Edited by Orem J, Barnes CD. New York, Academic Press, 1980, pp. 315–335

This chapter summarizes more lengthy presentations in the same volume, but it includes sufficient detail (and references) to give an excellent overview of physiology during sleep.

21. *Prinz PN, Vitiello MV, Raskind MA, Thorpy MJ:** Geriatrics: sleep disorders and aging. *N Engl J Med* 323:520–526, 1990

This succinct review discusses "normal" age-related changes in sleep in the elderly and provides an outline for assessing and treating their more common sleep disorders.

22. **Williams RL, Karacan I, Hursch CJ:** *Electroencephalography (EEG) of Human Sleep: Clinical Applications.* New York, Wiley, 1974

This classic work is the standard reference for normal human sleep, from infancy through old age.

Dreaming

23. **Cartwright R:** A network model of dreams, in *Sleep and Cognition*. Edited by Bootzin RR, Kihlstrom JF, Schacter DL. Washington, DC, American Psychological Association, 1990

    Cartwright's work exemplifies the consolidation of physiological and psychological sleep research. This brief summary describes the psychophysiological study of sleep and dreams during mood-disturbing events and proposes a model of memory "networks" activated during rapid eye movement sleep.

24. **Foulkes D:** *A Grammar of Dreams*. New York, Basic Books, 1978

    Early sections of Foulkes' work review and summarize the contributions of Freud, "ego psychology," structuralism, linguistics, and cognitive psychology. The second half proposes an empirical research technique for analyzing dream content. The former sections are of general interest, whereas the latter is appealing mainly to those with a research interest in dreams.

25. *Hirshkowitz M, Howell JW:** Advances and methodology in the study of dreaming, in *Sleep Disorders; Diagnosis and Treatment*. Edited by Williams RL, Karacan I, Moore CA. New York, Wiley, 1988, pp. 215–242

    This chapter serves as a useful primer on dream theory and methodology. It briefly reviews the history of dream studies; influences of factors such as sex, age, and stress; and the phenomenon of lucid dreaming. A detailed bibliography is included.

26. **Hobson JA:** *The Dreaming Brain*. New York, Basic Books, 1988

    After reviewing previous dream research, the author presents his "activation-synthesis" hypothesis of dreaming, based on neurobiological studies of sleep. The hypothesis directly challenges many assumptions of psychoanalytic dream interpretation, particularly regarding the source of dreams and the transparency of their content.

Nosology of Sleep Disorders

27. *American Psychiatric Association:** *Diagnostic and Statistical Manual of Mental Disorders*, 4th Edition. Washington, DC, American Psychiatric Association, 1994

    DSM-IV includes a more comprehensive list of sleep disorders than DSM-III-R, and these are organized differently. The text for each disorder gives a more complete description of core and associated clinical features.

28. **Diagnostic Classification Steering Committee (Thorpy MJ, Chairman):** *International Classification of Sleep Disorders: Diagnostic and Coding Manual.* Rochester, MN, American Sleep Disorders Association, 1990

This book contains 84 specific sleep-wake disorders, far more than DSM-IV or ICD-9, which most psychiatrists will use. Nevertheless, this book contains concise descriptions of both common and uncommon sleep disorders, which may prove useful in evaluating specific patients with unusual sleep-wake complaints.

Primary Sleep Disorders

Primary Insomnia

29. **Hauri P, Fisher J:** Persistent psychophysiological (learned) insomnia. *Sleep* 9:38–53, 1986

This carefully reported study distinguishes the clinical and polysomnographic features of "learned" insomnia from the insomnia of dysthymic disorder. The introduction also gives a clear description of the conditioning and physiological factors underlying psychophysiological insomnia.

30. *Reynolds CF III, Kupfer DJ, Buysse DJ, Coble PA, Yeager A:* Subtyping DSM-III-R primary insomnia: a literature review by the DSM-IV Work Group on Sleep Disorders. *Am J Psychiatry* 148:432–438, 1991

One of the ongoing debates in sleep medicine concerns the desirability and validity of "narrow" versus "broad" diagnostic categories, particularly with regard to insomnia. This article reviews the evidence for distinct subtypes of insomnia related to behavioral and conditioning factors and concludes that there is insufficient evidence to warrant subtyping at this time.

31. *Spielman AJ, Caruso LS, Glovinsky PB:* A behavioral perspective on insomnia treatment. *Psychiatr Clin North Am* 10:541–553, 1987

This brief chapter summarizes the techniques of the most commonly employed behavioral treatments of insomnia. The reference list includes many of the important primary studies, for more detailed discussion of specific techniques.

Primary Hypersomnia

32. **Billiard M:** Other hypersomnias, in *Handbook of Sleep Disorders.* Edited by Thorpy MJ. New York, Marcel Dekker, 1990, pp. 353–371

Primary hypersomnia, or the group of disorders that fall under this designation, have not received a great deal of attention in clinical or research studies. This brief chapter presents the clinical features and variants of these disorders.

Narcolepsy

33. *Aldrich MS:** Narcolepsy. *N Engl J Med* 323:389–394, 1990

This succinct review discusses the epidemiology, genetics, clinical features, and treatment of the "classic" sleep disorder of narcolepsy.

34. **Rechtschaffen A, Wolpert EA, Dement WC, Mitchell SA, Fisher C:** Nocturnal sleep of narcoleptics. *Electroencephalogr Clin Neurophysiol* 15:599–609, 1963

This article was the first to describe sleep-onset rapid eye movement (REM) in patients with narcolepsy and to suggest that accessory symptoms of narcolepsy (e.g., sleep paralysis and sleep-related hallucinations) may be dissociated phenomena of REM sleep. The findings pioneered more intensive investigations of sleep patterns in sleep disorders.

Breathing-Related Sleep Disorders

35. **Sanders MH:** The management of sleep-disordered breathing, in *Cardiorespiratory Disorders During Sleep.* Edited by Martin RJ. Mount Kisco, NY, Futura Publishing, 1990, pp. 141–187

This is a clearly described overview of treatments for sleep apnea, including risk-factor modification, position training, medications, continuous positive airway pressure, and surgery. Although it focuses more heavily on obstructive sleep apnea, it also discusses treatment of central sleep apnea. The reference list is comprehensive.

36. *Westbrook PR:** Sleep disorders and upper airway obstruction in adults. *Otolaryngol Clin North Am* 23:727–743, 1990

This review discusses epidemiology, pathophysiology, clinical features, and treatment of sleep apnea in a clear, concise format.

Circadian Rhythm Sleep Disorders

37. *Wagner DR: Circadian rhythm sleep disorders, in *Handbook of Sleep Disorders*. Edited by Thorpy MJ. New York, Marcel Dekker, 1990, pp. 493–527

    This chapter provides general background, followed by specific details about the clinical features, presumed pathophysiology, and treatment of circadian rhythm sleep disorders.

38. Weitzman ED, Czeisler CA, Coleman RM, Spielman AJ, Zimmerman JC, Dement W, Richardson G, Pollack CP: Delayed sleep phase syndrome: a chronobiological disorder with sleep-onset insomnia. *Arch Gen Psychiatry* 38:737–746, 1981

    This classic article describes the clinical features, presumed pathophysiology, and recommended treatment of one of the most common circadian rhythm sleep disturbances. The principles discussed have implications for other circadian rhythms sleep disturbances as well.

Restless Legs Syndrome and Periodic Limb Movements

39. Lugaresi E, Cirignotta F, Coccagna G, Montagna P: Nocturnal myoclonus and restless legs syndrome, in *Advances in Neurology, Vol. 43: Myoclonus*. Edited by Fahn S, Marsden CD, Van Woert MH. New York, Raven, 1986, pp. 295–307

    This review focuses on the clinical and polysomnographic features of these two related disorders and displays representative polysomnographic examples. It gives only brief mention to treatments.

40. Montplaisir J, Lapierre O, Warnes H, Pellitier G: The treatment of the restless legs syndrome with or without periodic limb movements. *Sleep* 15:391–395, 1992

    This article gives a brief overview of treatments for restless legs syndrome. Previous treatment studies are briefly reviewed, and specific recommendations presented.

Nightmare Disorder

41. Hartmann E: *The Nightmare: The Psychology and Biology of Terrifying Dreams*. New York, Basic Books, 1984

    This informally written and engaging book describes the clinical and laboratory phenomenology, history, and biological underpinnings of nightmares. Hartmann also presents a theory of nightmare sufferers as being characterized by "thin" ego boundaries.

Sleep Terror and Sleepwalking Disorders

42. **Broughton RJ:** Sleep disorders: disorders of arousal. *Science* 159:1070–1078, 1968

    In this classic article, Broughton presents the clinical features of common non–rapid eye movement (NREM) sleep parasomnias, including sleepwalking, and introduces the first evidence that they represent partial arousals from slow-wave sleep.

43. **Kales JD, Kales A, Soldatos CR, Cadwell AB, Charney DS, Martin ED:** Night terrors: clinical characteristics and personality patterns. *Arch Gen Psychiatry* 37:1413–1417, 1980

    This in-depth study of adults with sleep (night) terror disorder describes their clinical and psychological characteristics. It advances the conclusion that adults with sleep terrors tend to inhibit outward, waking expressions of anger.

44. *Thorpy MJ:** Disorders of arousal, in *Handbook of Sleep Disorders*. Edited by Thorpy MJ. New York, Marcel Dekker, 1990, pp. 531–549

    This chapter reviews sleep terror disorder and other related parasomnias associated with partial arousal, such as sleepwalking and confusional arousals. It includes descriptions of clinical and polysomnographic features and treatment approaches.

Parasomnias Not Otherwise Specified

45. **Mahowald MW, Ettinger MG:** Things that go bump in the night: the parasomnias revisited. *J Clin Neurophysiol* 7:119–143, 1990

    The authors catalog both common and uncommon parasomnias, including terse clinical descriptions and treatment recommendations. The reference list is comprehensive.

46. *Schenck CH, Bundlie SR, Ettinger MG, Mahowald MW:** Chronic behavioral disorders of human REM sleep: a new category of parasomnia. *Sleep* 9:293–308, 1986

    This is a "classic" article that describes a parasomnia marked by the loss of usual muscle atonia during rapid eye movement (REM) sleep. The clinical manifestations are related to basic science findings regarding the regulation of REM sleep.

Sleep Disorders (Insomnia and Hypersomnia) Related to Another Mental Disorder

Depressive Disorders

47. *Benca RM, Obermeyer WH, Thisted RA, Gillin JC:** Sleep and psychiatric disorders: a meta-analysis. *Arch Gen Psychiatry* 49:651–668, 1992

    This comprehensive analysis reviewed 177 studies with 7,151 patients to identify consistent electroencephalographic sleep characteristics for specific psychiatric disorders, including affective disorders. In addition to its main conclusions (that no single sleep variable could be considered specific for any disorder, but that certain *patterns* are observed), this article provides a comprehensive bibliography of the field.

48. *Kupfer DJ:** REM latency: a psychobiologic marker for primary depressive disease. *Biol Psychiatry* 11:159–174, 1976

    This article summarizes early research on electroencephalographic sleep in depression, focusing on rapid eye movement sleep latency. It presages subsequent questions in the study of sleep and depression, such as the sensitivity and specificity of findings, episodic versus persistent features, and relation to other biological measures.

49. *McCarley RW:** REM sleep and depression: common neurobiological control mechanisms. *Am J Psychiatry* 139:565–570, 1982

    This is a classic article that ties together neurobiological studies of rapid eye movement (REM) sleep and the sleep characteristics of depression. The author reviews the influential "reciprocal interaction model" of sleep regulation of REM and non–rapid eye movement (NREM) sleep.

50. **Reynolds CF III, Kupfer DJ:** Sleep research in affective illness: state of the art circa 1987. *Sleep* 10:199–215, 1987

    This review summarizes advances in the "second wave" of depression: sleep research occurring during the late 1970s through the late 1980s. It also addresses theoretical models and future directions.

51. **Vogel GW, Thurmond A, Gibbons P, Gibbons P, Sloan K, Walker M:** REM sleep reduction effects on depression syndromes. *Arch Gen Psychiatry* 32:765–777, 1975

    This classic article describes the therapeutic effects of selective rapid eye movement (REM) sleep deprivation in patients with endogenous depression. These findings stand at the center of literature supporting a link between REM sleep regulation and mood regulation in depression.

52. *Wehr TA: Effects of wakefulness and sleep on depression and mania, in *Sleep and Biological Rhythms: Basic Mechanisms and Applications to Psychiatry.* Edited by Montplaisir J, Godbout R. New York, Oxford University Press, 1990, pp. 42–86

One of the leading authorities on sleep and biological rhythm changes in affective disorders reviews the effects of sleep deprivation and other sleep-wake manipulations on mood. The author goes considerably beyond a mere recitation of the findings to discuss clinical and theoretical implications of sleep-mood interactions. The chapter is well written and thought provoking.

Schizophrenia

53. **Ganguli R, Reynolds CF III, Kupfer DJ:** Electroencephalographic sleep in young, never-medicated schizophrenics. *Arch Gen Psychiatry* 44:36–44, 1987

This article presents evidence *supporting* the relative specificity of short rapid eye movement latency in affective disorders relative to schizophrenia, as well as evidence for differences in slow-wave sleep patterns across the night.

54. *Keshavan MS, Reynolds CF III, Kupfer DJ:** Electroencephalographic sleep in schizophrenia: a critical review. *Compr Psychiatry* 30:34–47, 1990

This review considers both early and more recent investigations of sleep in schizophrenia and examines their implications for theoretical models and future investigations.

55. **Zarcone VP Jr, Benson KL, Berger PA:** Abnormal rapid eye movement latencies in schizophrenia. *Arch Gen Psychiatry* 44:45–48, 1987

One of several investigations of sleep in schizophrenia, this report challenges the specificity of short rapid eye movement latency for affective disorders.

Panic Disorder

56. **Hauri PJ, Friedman M, Ravaris CL:** Sleep in patients with spontaneous panic attacks. *Sleep* 12:323–327, 1989

This article gives a detailed clinical and polysomnographic description of panic attacks arising during sleep.

57. *Mellman TA, Uhde TW:** Electroencephalographic sleep in panic disorder. *Arch Gen Psychiatry* 46:178–184, 1989

This is a comprehensive description of polysomnographic features in patients with panic disorder, comparing those with and without sleep-related attacks and control subjects without the disorder.

Dementia

58. *Prinz PN, Peskind ER, Vitaliano PR, Raskind MA, Eisdorfer C, Zemcuznikov N, Gerber CJ:** Changes in the sleep and waking EEGs of nondemented and demented elderly subjects. *J Am Geriatr Soc* 30:86–93, 1982

    This is one of the first articles to describe sleep electroencephalographic patterns in patients with dementia. The investigators identified not only reductions in stage 3/4 sleep and rapid eye movement, but also the appearance of polyphasic sleep-wake patterns in patients with dementia.

59. **Reynolds CF III, Kupfer DJ, Houck PR, Hoch CC, Stack JA, Berman SR, Zimmer B:** Reliable discrimination of elderly depressed and demented patients by electroencephalographic sleep data. *Arch Gen Psychiatry* 45:258–264, 1988

    The investigators report correct identification of 80% of patients with dementia and depression, using multivariate analysis of electroencephalographic sleep data.

Alcoholism

60. *Gillin JC, Smith TL, Irwin M, Kripke DF, Schuckit M:** EEG sleep studies in "pure" primary alcoholism during subacute withdrawal: relationships to normal controls, age, and other clinical variables. *Biol Psychiatry* 27:477–488, 1990

    This study summarizes the important findings in the "first generation" of sleep-alcohol research (conducted during the 1960s and 1970s) and presents more recent polysomnographic and clinical data.

Secondary Sleep Disorders Due to Medical or Neurological Conditions

61. **Lugaresi E, Cirignotta F, Mondini S, Montagna P, Zucconi M:** Sleep in clinical neurology, in *Sleep Disorders; Diagnosis and Treatment.* Edited by Williams RL, Karacan I, Moore CA. New York, Wiley, 1988, pp. 245–263

The authors review sleep findings in various neurological disorders, including epilepsy and headaches. Although the discussion of each disorder is brief, the references are comprehensive.

62. **Wooten V:** Medical causes of insomnia, in *Principles and Practice of Sleep Medicine*. Edited by Kryger MH, Roth T, Dement WC. Philadelphia, PA, WB Saunders, 1989, pp. 456–475

Although medical disorders frequently are associated with sleep disturbance, there is limited information regarding specific sleep disturbances caused by specific disorders. This chapter summarizes available information regarding a wide variety of medical conditions.

Substance-Induced Sleep Disorders

63. *****Buysse DJ:** Drugs affecting sleep, sleepiness, and performance, in *Sleep, Sleepiness, and Performance*. Edited by Monk TH. Chichester, England, Wiley, 1991, pp. 249–306

The author reviews in detail the sleep effects of seven major classes of drugs and briefly summarizes the effects of other drugs. The chapter includes a detailed reference list.

64. **Kay DC, Samiuddin Z:** Sleep disorders associated with drug abuse and drugs of abuse, in *Sleep Disorders: Diagnosis and Treatment*. Edited by Williams RL, Karacan I, Moore CA. New York, Wiley, 1988, pp. 315–371

This chapter comprehensively reviews studies of sedative-hypnotics, opioids, stimulants, and hallucinogens. After a detailed catalog of available studies, the authors summarize each class of drugs' major effects on sleep and raise methodological and design issues in drug studies.

22

Sexual Disorders

Helen Singer Kaplan, M.D., Ph.D.

The Kinsey reports on the sexual behaviors of American men and women that were published in 1948 and 1953 broke the silence about sex that had prevailed in the Western world for millennia and ushered in the modern era of sexology. Although the work of Kinsey and his group has recently been the subject of criticisms, the two volumes of the Kinsey report remain classics in the field.

The next major breakthrough was made by Masters and Johnson, who found, as a result of extensive clinical research, that disabling sexual disorders frequently result from "minor" and consciously perceived causes, such as performance anxieties, socially induced sexual guilt, poor communications with the partner, and inadequate sexual techniques. Masters and Johnson supported these contentions by demonstrating that the majority of patients with functional sexual problems respond to a brief (2-week) intensive course of behaviorally oriented sex therapy. Masters and Johnson published the results of their studies in 1970. Their landmark book, *Human Sexual Inadequacy* (see Kaplan, Chapter 49, this volume) caused some consternation in psychoanalytic circles because these findings ran directly contrary to the traditional view, that sexual disorders such as impotence and "frigidity" are always the product of serious unconscious and deeply buried sexual conflicts that derive from painful childhood experience and that require lengthy insight-promoting therapies.

Initially, Masters and Johnson focused exclusively on the genital aspects of sexual function and dysfunction and did not concern themselves with

277

sexual motivation. This omission was corrected, and further clarity was brought to the field by the recognition that deficient sexual desire constitutes an important sexual disorder, on par with impotence or anorgasmia. In the book, *Disorders of Sexual Desire and Other New Concepts and Techniques in Sex Therapy* (Kaplan 1979), desire disorders were given their due, and the human sexual response was reconceptualized as comprising three physiologically discrete phases: sexual desire, excitement, and orgasm; the sexual disorders were defined as specific impairments of any one of these three phases.

This new paradigm facilitated the development of specific and more effective treatments for desire disorders, as well for the genital phase dysfunctions, and became the basis for the classification system that was incorporated into the official nomenclature of the American Psychiatric Association (DSM-III) in 1980.

In addition to these basic texts on sexuality and sexual disorders, the bibliography also includes readings on specific disorders, as well as on topics of special interest including sexual physiology and medicine, women's sexuality, gender, perversion, and sexual issues in autoimmune deficiency syndrome (AIDS).

Sexology occupies the interface between medicine and psychology, and clinicians in this field need to keep abreast of developments in both disciplines. The biological aspects of sexuality have recently been the subject of intensive and productive research, and the references in the bibliography are intended to provide a representative sampling of the new research and of the emerging concepts in this area.

I have also attempted to find a representative selection of references that reflect the growing recognition, long overdue, that women's medical needs differ from those of men, especially in the gender dimorphic area of sexual health.

The literature abounds with fascinating and creative work on gender development, gender identity, and sexual orientation. To avoid overloading the bibliography on this topic, only a few of the most important examples have been selected from a wide array of excellent publications in this area.

In a similar vein, no bibliography on sexual disorders would be complete without readings on the sexual perversions or paraphilias, which have held a major fascination for sexologists since Kraft von Ebbing (1906/1965) below published his *Psychopathia Sexualis* in the 19th century. Although innumerable publications on this topic are available, only the most important works by the most influential authors have been included in the bibliography.

Sex and sexual desire cannot be meaningfully discussed without considering love and romantic relationships. Because of the diversity and the extremely uneven quality of the publications on these subjects—much of this is in the popular literature—it was difficult to select basic or definitive references in this area, and the bibliography on these topics should be considered a sampler and not in any sense comprehensive.

Because there is considerable overlap between the content of the literature on sexual disorders and on sex therapy, the reader is referred to Chapter 49 on "Sex Therapy," which contains further references pertinent to the sexual disorders.

Basic Texts

1. *American Psychiatric Association: *Diagnostic and Statistical Manual of Mental Disorders*, 4th Edition. Washington, DC, American Psychiatric Association, 1994

   The classification system used in the DSMs are based on the triphasic concept of human sexuality and sexual disorders, which divides sexual disorders into impairments of desire, excitement, and orgasm. The descriptions of the clinical features and diagnostic criteria for the various sexual syndromes are accurate, clear, and concise and underscore the similarities between male and female sexual function and dysfunction. This manual belongs in the library of every clinician who treats patients with sexual disorders.

2. *Kaplan HS: *Disorders of Sexual Desire and Other New Concepts and Techniques in Sex Therapy*. New York, Brunner/Mazel, 1979

   Loss of interest in sex and the development of aversion to sexual stimulation are now recognized as being among the most prevalent sexual complaints encountered in clinical practice. This book presents the first description of clinical desire disorders and discusses the pathogenesis of hypoactive sexual desire from a pluralistic, multicausal perspective. The author also proposes a brief, integrated behavioral-psychodynamic treatment approach that has been found helpful in treating these difficult patients. Case studies of treatment successes and failures illustrate the didactic material.

   Also in this book, the sexual disorders are recategorized as impairments of the desire, excitement, and orgasm phases, and the different treatment requirements of each syndrome are described.

3. **Kinsey AC, Pomeroy WB, Martin CE:** *Sexual Behavior in the Human Male.* Philadelphia, PA, WB Saunders, 1948

4. **Kinsey AC, Pomeroy WB, Martin CE, Gebhardt PH:** *Sexual Behavior in the Human Female.* Philadelphia, PA, WB Saunders, 1953

   No one would suggest that these two compendium volumes, which are filled with statistics and tables, should be read from cover to cover. However, they are invaluable reference books that belong in the library of every clinician who treats patients with sexual disorders.

The books, which are based on more than 18,000 interviews, are a veritable font of highly detailed information on every conceivable aspect of human sexual behavior (e.g., number of orgasms, masturbation, childhood sexuality, sexuality in old age).

Kinsey's work was a major breakthrough that did much to legitimize sexual research, and it is sincerely hoped that the recent criticism, alleging sampling errors and sexual misconduct, will prove unfounded.

5. *Masters WH, Johnson V: *The Human Sexual Response.* Boston, MA, Little Brown, 1966

This ground-breaking volume was based on 10 years of painstaking scientific laboratory studies and observations of more than 14,000 sexual acts. The resulting descriptions of male and female genital functioning provided the foundation for modern sex therapy. The reader is also referred to Masters and Johnson's (1970) second book in this series, *Human Sexual Inadequacy* (see Kaplan, Chapter 49, this volume).

Biological Aspects

6. Crenshaw TL, Goldberg JP, Stern PC: Pharmacologic Modification of Psychosexual Dysfunction. *J Sex Marital Ther* 13:239–252, 1987

One of the first controlled investigations of the sexually stimulating effects of a nonsteroidal substance, bupropion on physically normal, nondepressed patients with psychogenic sexual dysfunctions, this study heralds the future availability of drugs with true clinical "aphrodisiac" effects.

7. Davidson JM, Meyer LS: Endocrine factors in sexual psychophysiology, in *Patterns of Sexual Arousal: Psychophysiological Processes and Clinical Applications.* Edited by Rosen RC, Beck JG. New York, Guilford, 1988, pp. 158–186

This superb review provides a clearly written, concise summary of studies on testosterone and male sexuality. The omission of a comparable review of androgen deficiency in women is unfortunate.

8. Pedersen CA, Caldwell JD, Jirikowski GF, Insel TR: *Oxytosin in Maternal, Sexual and Social Behaviors.* New York, Academy of Science, 1992

The functions of oxytocin and vasopressin in reproductive behavior have long been a mystery. Recent evidence suggests that these hormones may play a significant role in mammalian bonding, and this volume is a compendium of the best studies in this emerging field.

9. **Rosen RC, Beck JG** (eds): *Patterns of Sexual Arousal: Psychophysiological Processes and Clinical Applications.* New York, Guilford, 1988

    This volume presents a scholarly review of contemporary theories and data on normal and pathological human sexual psychophysiology. There are chapters reviewing the data on the physiology of normal male and female genital functioning and on the genital phase disorders (erectile and orgasm dysfunctions). The authors' failure to include studies on the neurophysiology of the human sex drive or sexual desire is a shortcoming of this book.

10. **Schiavi RC, White D:** Androgens and male sexual functioning: a review of human studies. *J Sex Marital Ther* 2:214–228, 1976

    This scholarly article, although in need of some revision, remains the best review of this complex topic.

Male Disorders

11. **Lue T** (ed): *World Book of Impotence Research.* London, Smith-Gordon & Co, 1992

    This is a compendium of brief, clear, concise articles by a multidisciplinary international group of experts in erectile disorders on the latest assessment and treatment techniques.

12. **Kaplan HS:** The post-ejaculatory pain syndrome. *J Sex Marital Ther* 18:91–103, 1993

    The author reviews the clinical features and concepts of pathogenesis of a variety of ejaculatory disorders (retarded ejaculation, partially retarded ejaculation, anesthetic ejaculation, postejaculatory pain, and premature ejaculation) and describes, for the first time in the literature, the syndrome of psychogenic postejaculatory pain. This disorder is discussed within the context of a spectrum of ejaculatory impairments, which range from the most complete, retarded ejaculation to the least severe, inadequate ejaculatory control. A therapeutic strategy is proposed.
    The reader is also referred to Kaplan (Chapter 49, this volume), which contains further references to publications on impotence and ejaculatory disorders.

13. **Rosen RC, Leiblum SR** (eds): *Erectile Disorders: Assessment and Treatment.* New York, Guilford, 1992

    This newest in a series of volumes of multiauthored collections of writings about specific sexual disorders is uneven. The strongest chapters are on the biological aspects of impotence. The chapters by Segraves on "Aging and Drug Effects on Sexuality," by Schiavi on "Laboratory Methods for Evaluating Erectile Dysfunctions," and by Davidson and Rosen on "Hormonal Determinants of Erectile Dysfunction" are excellent. However the chapters on the psychological aspects of impotence and its treatments are disappointing, with the exception of Leiblum and Rosen's interesting piece on "Couples' Therapy," which describes the authors' innovative systems-oriented approach.

Female Sexuality

14. **Hite S:** *The Hite Report*, New York, McMillan, 1976

Although this survey was not conducted by a professional in the field of human sexuality, Hite's book is nevertheless a valuable source of detailed information about the sexual functioning and preferences of American women. By asking specific and detailed questions about clitoral stimulation and vaginal penetration, the author obtained important data on how females reach orgasm. This information had not been elicited previously by more male-oriented researchers, such as Kinsey and Hunt.

15. **Kaplan HS:** A neglected issues: the sexual side effects in the treatment of breast cancer. *J Sex Marital Ther* 18:3–19, 1992

The use of adjuvant chemotherapy and hormonal therapy constitutes a significant advance in the management of early breast cancer. Because adjuvants can sometimes delay or prevent recurrence of the disease, increasing numbers of women are undergoing these treatments. However, cytotoxic chemotherapeutic agents and, to a lesser degree, antiestrogens can interfere with the synthesis, secretion, or the bioavailability of sex hormones, and thus produce serious sexual impairments. This article describes the sexual side effects of adjuvant and other treatments for breast cancer and suggests potential remedies.

16. **Kirkpatrick M** (ed): *Women's Sexual Development: Explorations of Inner Space.* New York, Plenum, 1980

17. **Kirkpatrick M** (ed): *Women's Sexual Experience: Explorations of the Dark Continent.* New York, Plenum, 1982

These books are the best of a series of multiauthored volumes entitled, "Women in Context: Development and Stresses," all edited by Kirkpatrick. Both books are comprised of interesting but uneven collections of chapters representing diverse points of view on contemporary issues of female sexual development in the first volume, and controversies about female sexual experience and responsiveness in the other. In both volumes, the chapters come from many sources—academicians, researchers, psychoanalysts, sexologists, gynecologists, historians, and sociologists—who cover a wide range of topics on female sexuality.

18. **Ladas AK, Whipple B, Perry JG:** *The G Spot and Other Recent Discoveries About Human Sexuality.* New York, Holt Rhinehart & Winston, 1982

Although it is not yet clear whether or not the G spot is a valid or common anatomic and physiological entity, experts in sexuality should be knowledgeable about this much-discussed topic, which is clearly described in this seminal book.

19. **Notman MT, Nadelson CC** (eds): *Women and Men: New Perspectives and Gender Differences.* Washington, DC, American Psychiatric Press, 1991

This is an uneven but important collection of brief chapters on some of the gender dimorphic issues that are just now emerging into the consciousness of the profession. I particularly liked McEwen's chapter on "Sex Differences in the Brain: What Are They and How Do They Arise?"; this chapter contains a concise, clear summary of the new neurophysiologic data on male and female brain differences.

20. **Schucket E, Levinson NA:** *Female Psychology: An Annotated Psychoanalytic Bibliography.* Hillsdale, NJ, Analytic Press, 1992

Perhaps it is not de rigueur to include an annotated bibliography in an annotated bibliography, but this is such a unique reference work that it could not be omitted. Chapters 18 and 19 on the female sexual disorders, gender-identity disorders, paraphillias and ego-dystonic homosexualities contain comprehensive lists of references, thoughtfully annotated on psychoanalytic works on these topics.

21. **Sherwin BB, Gelfan MM, Bender W:** Androgen enhances the sexual motivation of women: a prospective cross-over study of sex steroid administration in the surgical menopause. *Psychosom Med* 47:339–351, 1985

This article presents the results of Sherwin et al.'s pioneering studies on the vital role that androgens play in female sexuality and on the benefits, in terms of restoring libido, of androgen replacement for postmenopausal women.

Love, Perversion, and Gender

22. **Fogel GI, Myers WA** (eds): *Perversions and Near Perversions in Clinical Practice.* New Haven, CT, Yale University Press, 1991

This is an interesting, albeit uneven compendium by some leading contemporary psychoanalysts on the ever-intriguing topic of sexual perversions. High points include Cooper's thoughtful comments on the unconscious core of perversions and Stoller's refreshing views on this topic. Kernberg's thought-provoking contribution on aggression and love is also excellent. L. Kaplan's chapter is the low point, as one continues to be mystified by the author's position that sexual perversions in women are NOT sexual.

23. **Kernberg OF:** Barriers to falling and remaining in love. *J Am Psychoanal Assoc* 22:486–511, 1974

24. **Kernberg OF:** Aggression and love in the relationship of the couple. *J Am Psychoanal Assoc* 39:45–70, 1991

These two articles represent a complex, brilliant, psychoanalytic conceptualization of sexual functioning and dysfunctioning in the context of the couple's relationship. The author's object relations approach to love and sex is extremely helpful for understanding some of the more complex cases of partner-specific sexual disorders.

25. *Kraft von Ebbing RF: *Psychopathia Sexualis* (1906). New York, Putnam, 1965

The author's classic, detailed, clinically valid descriptions of sexual perversions (which are currently termed *paraphilias*) stand up very well to the tests of time and culture.

26. **Money J:** *Gay, Straight and In-Between: The Sexology of Sexual Orientation.* Baltimore, MD, Oxford Press, 1988

27. **Money J, Ehrhardt AA:** *Man and Woman, Boy and Girl.* New York, Guilford, 1972

Money's books represent alternative and innovative views of sexual orientation, the paraphilias, and gender identity from a nonpsychoanalytic view, which stems from the author's long-term developmental studies of individuals with congenitally ambiguous genitalia or gender-incongruent hormone patterns. The books also introduce Money's interesting concept of "love maps," which is the author's term for the mental template of erotic desires that is the product of early pre- and postnatal biosocial factors.

Whether or not one agrees or entirely agrees with Money, he is an important voice in the fields of gender and perversions, and any serious student of sexuality should be familiar with his work.

28. **Person E:** Sexuality as the mainstay of identity: psychoanalytic perspectives. *Signs* 5:605–630, 1980

This is a creative and useful conceptualization of sex and identity from the perspective of modern psychoanalysis.

29. **Person E:** *Dreams of Love.* New York, WW Norton, 1988

This is a psychoanalytic study of the vicissitudes of romantic love. Topics discussed include the development of the capacity to love and the potentially positive, "transforming" effects of love, which can outlast the relationship, as well as an in-depth view of some psychic problems and obstacles to the achievement of rewarding love relationships.

30. **Rosen RC, Beck GJ:** Assessment and treatment of sexual deviation (paraphillias), in *Patterns of Sexual Arousal: Psychophysiological Processes and Clinical Applications.* Edited by Rosen R, Beck JG. New York, Guilford, 1988, pp. 120–343

This is a superb, comprehensive review of the behavioral concepts and treatments of sexual deviations and an excellent counterpoint to the psychodynamically oriented material cited in this section (Fogel and Myers 1991; Kernberg 1974, 1991; Person 1980, 1988; Stoller 1975, 1979).

31. **Sarrel LJ, Sarrel PN:** *Sexual Unfolding: Sexual Development and Sex Therapies in Late Adolescence.* Boston, MA, Little Brown, 1979

This is one of the few books, and the best, on adolescent sexuality. The authors direct the Human Sexuality Program at Yale University, and the material of this book is a product of their work with students at that institution.

32. **Stoller RJ:** *Perversion: The Erotic Form of Hatred.* New York, Pantheon, 1975

33. **Stoller RJ:** *Sexual Excitement.* New York, Pantheon, 1979

Stoller was a leading psychoanalytically oriented thinker on the subject of sexual perversion. Even if one does not agree with his position that sexual desire, fantasy, and perversions always have their roots in hatred toward the parents and wishes for vengeance, these books are modern classics in the field.

Sexual Orientation

Even though homosexuality is no longer classified as a sexual disorder, students of human sexuality should be aware of the excellent, variegated literature that is available on this topic. The following is only a small sample.

34. **Bell AP, Weinberg MS, Hammersmith SK:** *Sexual Preference: Its Development in Men and Women.* Bloomington, IN, Indiana University Press, 1981

    This presents a study of homosexual behaviors and comparisons to heterosexual behaviors by the Kinsey group. Because of the large and socially varied study population (1,500 persons were interviewed) and the detailed questions about significant parameters of sexual behaviors, relationships, and sexual practices, this book is considered a major reference work in the field.

35. **Green R:** *The Sissy Boy Syndrome and the Development of Homosexuality.* New Haven, CT, Yale University Press, 1986

    This is a fascinating, meticulously executed, long-term (15+ years follow-up) comparison of the psychosexual development of effeminate boys with a matched group of masculine boys, by one of the leading sex researchers. The text is enlivened by copious verbatim excerpts of recorded interviews with the boys and their families. The results confirm the widely held beliefs that effeminate behavior and the avoidance of "rough-and-tumble" play are fairly strong (but by no means perfect) predictors of adult homosexual orientation. The study underscores the importance of the father in the development of a masculine identity.

36. *Marmor J, Green R:** Homosexual behavior, in *Handbook of Sexology.* Edited by Money J, Mustoph J. New York, Elsevier, 1977, pp. 1051–1068

    This is an excellent, nonjudgmental review of contemporary concepts of male homosexuality.

37. **Masters WH, Johnson VE:** *Homosexuality in Perspective.* Boston, MA, Little Brown, 1979

    This is an interesting and apparently successful application of Masters and Johnson's brief sex therapy model to male homosexuals (more probably bisexuals) who suffer from performance-anxiety–related functional problems with women.

23

Eating Disorders

Joel Yager, M.D.

The eating disorders constitute a group of clinical syndromes in which the primary abnormalities concern perceptions, attitudes, emotions, and behaviors related to the ingestion of food, body weight, body image, and related issues. Although most people give some thought to their eating and to their weights, and many apply a degree of conscious control over what and how much they eat, for most these matters do not become all-preoccupying concerns. An eating disorder exists when the acts of eating, elimination, exercise, and related activities become the focus of unrelenting obsessional thoughts and compulsive behaviors; when those with these disorders feel that their eating is no longer under their own control; and when psychosocial adaptation and physiological health are impaired because of these self-damaging thoughts, emotions, and behaviors. DSM-IV lists the following types of eating disorders as "disorders of infancy, childhood, and adolescence": anorexia nervosa, bulimia nervosa, pica, rumination disorder of infancy, and eating disorder not otherwise specified. Simple obesity per se is not considered to be an eating disorder, because a great deal of obesity is accounted for by genetic and metabolic factors and the majority of obese patients appear not to differ from community control subjects with regard to psychopathology. Nevertheless, a large number of obese persons suffer self-image disparagement, and a sizable minority may have compulsive overeating.

Diagnostically, these primary eating disorders must be distinguished from abnormalities in thoughts and behaviors concerning the ingestion and handling of food that can occur in a variety of psychopathological conditions, including major depressions, schizophrenias, and obsessive-compulsive disorders, to name the most obvious. Clinically, these disorders appear to have increased in frequency over the past several decades, and they often occur concomitantly with other psychiatric diagnoses. Current views of both their pathogenesis and treatment argue strongly for a comprehensive biopsychosocial perspective, and the references selected for this chapter underscore this broad understanding. The articles were selected based on a recent review of the field in my capacity as Chair of the American Psychiatric Association's work group to develop recently completed practice guidelines for eating disorders and through my constant monitoring of the field as editor of *Eating Disorders Review*, a bimonthly professional newsletter.

General

1. **Agras WS:** *Eating Disorders: Management of Obesity, Bulimia and Anorexia Nervosa.* Oxford, England, Pergamon, 1987

   This is an excellent, brief monograph that provides a multifaceted account of these disorders and focuses primarily on behavioral and cognitive-behavioral treatments.

2. *American Psychiatric Association Practice Guidelines Work Group on Eating Disorders:** Practice guidelines for eating disorders. *Am J Psychiatry* 150:207–228, 1993

   The first American Psychiatric Association practice guideline to be published, this document contains a brief review of diagnostic and treatment issues followed by recommendations and options for the treatment of anorexia nervosa and bulimia nervosa. The guidelines were based on suggestions from the existing literature and from consensus derived through a process developed by the American Psychiatric Association that utilized the input of literally hundreds of psychiatrist and nonpsychiatrist expert consultants.

3. **Bruch H:** *Eating Disorders: Obesity, Anorexia Nervosa, and the Person Within.* New York, Basic Books, 1973

   This is a classic volume, sensitively written by a leading clinician who brought a psychodynamic and humanistic perspective to her study of scores of patients. Her work revealed their deficits in the sense of self and self-efficacy and in interoceptive awareness and has formed the basis of much psychodynamic, cognitive, and family work that has followed.

4. **Fallon P, Katzman MA, Wooley SC** (eds): *Feminist Perspectives on Eating Disorders*. New York, Guilford, 1994

This book provides an excellent, highly sensitive, and generally insightful collection of chapters concerning sociological, theoretical, and clinical aspects of eating disorders written by the foremost female and feminist authorities in the field.

5. **Garfinkel PE, Garner DM:** *Anorexia Nervosa: a Multidimensional Perspective.* New York, Brunner/Mazel, 1982

A volume written entirely by two leading authorities, a psychiatrist and psychologist who have contributed many original clinical and theoretical observations to the field, this is arguably the single most comprehensive text of the eating disorders thus far written.

6. *Hsu LKG:* *Eating Disorders.* New York, Guilford, 1990

This book is a highly readable, authoritative review of the clinical features and treatment of anorexia nervosa and bulimia nervosa by a leading clinical researcher.

7. **Johnson C, Connor ME:** *The Etiology and Treatment of Bulimia Nervosa.* New York, Basic Books, 1987

This is a thorough review of social, epidemiological, nutritional, and psychodynamic aspects of bulimia nervosa and its primarily psychological treatment, focusing on nutrition and cognitive and psychodynamic approaches. The book includes the authors' semistructured interview for eating disorders.

8. **Spitzer RL, Devlin M, Walsh BT, Hasin D, Wing R, Marcus M, Stunkard A, Wadden T, Yanovski W, Agras S, Mitchell J, Nonas C:** Binge eating disorder: a multisite field trial of the diagnostic criteria. *International Journal of Eating Disorders* 11:191–204, 1992

This study illustrates many contemporary issues in the delineation of a potential addition to the diagnostic nomenclature. Based on a study involving nearly 2,000 community residents and patients drawn from 11 different samples, a strong case is made for the fact that binge eating without purging is a clinically meaningful disorder, occurring in about 30% of people presenting to medically supervised weight loss programs and only about 2% of community residents.

Historical and Social Aspects

9. **Bell RM:** *Holy Anorexia.* Chicago, IL, University of Chicago Press, 1985

   This is a fascinating story about several hundred Italian women who were sainted by the church in the Middle Ages whose life patterns of self-starvation in the service of God sound remarkably similar to those of contemporary women with anorexia nervosa.

10. **Brumberg JJ:** *Fasting Girls: The Emergence of Anorexia Nervosa as a Modern Disease.* Cambridge, MA, Harvard University Press, 1988

    This is a well-written treatise that examines historical and sociological aspects of self-starvation and the transformation from spiritual to medical thinking about these phenomena that occurred in the late 18th and 19th centuries. The book follows anorexia nervosa, first described in modern form in the late 1870s, into the 20th century, discussing issues of gender role, changing societal expectations of women, and pressures on women in relation to their self-images and body images.

11. **Orbach S:** *Hunger Strike: The Anorectic's Struggle as a Metaphor for Our Age.* New York, WW Norton, 1986

    This provocative and influential feminist and self psychoanalytic perspective on the genesis of eating disorders suggests that early patterns of mothering that differ for boys and girls may have substantial subsequent effects on self-image.

Epidemiology

12. **Schotte D, Stunkard A:** Bulimia vs bulimic behaviors on a college campus. *JAMA* 258:1213–1215, 1981

    In this study of students at the University of Pennsylvania, Schotte and Stunkard suggest that the prevalence of frank eating disorders on campus is no more than 2%–3%.

13. **Szmukler GI:** The epidemiology of anorexia nervosa and bulimia. *J Psychiatr Res* 19:143–153, 1985

    In this review of the changing patterns in prevalence of eating disorders in America and Europe, the data support the view that increased rates in the past several decades are due not only to higher awareness but also to actual increases in prevalence.

Biological Aspects

14. **Brownell KD, Rodin J, Wilmore JH** (eds): *Eating, Body Weight and Performance in Athletes.* New York, Lea & Febiger, 1992

   This is an excellent collection of chapters examining basic issues concerning human weight, body composition, and nutrition; the etiology and prevalence of eating disorders among various groups of athletes; athletic amenorrhea; the influence of social and performance pressures; treatment; and other issues concerning eating disorders among an especially high-risk population.

15. **Fava M, Copeland P, Schweiger U, Herzog D:** Neurochemical Abnormalities of Anorexia Nervosa and Bulimia Nervosa. *Am J Psychiatry* 146:963–972, 1989

   This article reviews biological theories related to starvation and to available data and speculation regarding the roles of catecholamine, serotonin, and neuropeptides in the etiology and pathogenesis of eating disorders.

16. **Halmi KA:** Anorexia nervosa and bulimia. *Annu Rev Med* 38:373–380, 1987

   This article is an authoritative review of medical complications, virtually all secondary to starvation, malnutrition, and purging, found in patients with eating disorders. It provides a systematic system-by-system review.

17. **Mitchell JE, Seim HC, Colon E, Pomeroy C:** Medical complications and medical management of bulimia. *Ann Intern Med* 107:71–77, 1987

   Based on the study of several hundred patients seen at the University of Minnesota and on existing literature, this article reviews prominent medical findings with special focus on electrolyte, endocrine, cardiac, and renal findings.

18. **Rigotti NA, Neer RM, Skates SJ, Herzog DB, Nussbaum SR:** The clinical course of osteoporosis in anorexia nervosa: a longitudinal study of cortical bone mass. *JAMA* 265:1133–1138, 1991

   Following a cohort of anorexia nervosa patients for about 18 months, Rigotti et al. found roughly a seven times higher rate of pathological fractures than in control subjects and also found that vigorous attempts to replace calcium in bone were only marginally successful.

19. **Schneider LH, Cooper SJ, Halmi KA** (eds): *The Psychobiology of Human Eating Disorders: Preclinical and Clinical Perspectives,* Vol. 575. New York, New York Academy of Sciences, 1989

This book is the best available collection of papers concerning basic research, animal models, and clinical laboratory research in the neuroscience and physiology of hunger, satiety, feeding behavior, and eating disorders.

20. **Wadden TA, VanItallie TB** (eds): *Treatment of the Seriously Obese.* New York, Guilford, 1992

Chapters in this book review pathogenesis, negative health consequences, and medical and psychological concomitants of serious obesity (30% or more over recommended weight for height). Treatment studies focus on medical managements with very-low–calorie diets and exercise, but also cover psychological-behavioral, surgical, and pharmacological approaches.

Developmental Aspects

21. **Andersen AE:** A proposed mechanism underlying eating disorders and other disorders of motivated behavior, in *Males With Eating Disorders.* Edited by Andersen AE. New York, Brunner/Mazel, 1990, pp. 221–254

This scholarly, thoughtful, and satisfying theory of how eating disorders develop draws heavily on developmental and operational conditioning models in a biological context.

22. **Bemporad JR, Herzog DB** (eds): *Psychoanalysis and Eating Disorders.* New York, Guilford, 1989

This book provides essays by a group of psychoanalytically trained writers that vary widely in both theoretical perspectives and extent of field observations on which their views, informed opinions, and speculations are offered.

23. **Casper RC:** Personality features of women with good outcome from restricting anorexia nervosa. *Psychosom Med* 52:156–170, 1990

Based on a follow-up of women recovered from anorexia nervosa for about a decade compared with their own sisters, this study showed that those with a past history of the disorder tended to be generally more timid and avoidant than their sisters. The study suggests that such enduring personality traits may have been preexisting and may contribute to the vulnerability of some women to the initial development of eating disorders.

24. **Crisp A:** *Anorexia Nervosa: Let Me Be.* London, Academic Press, 1980

This book is the synthesis of a highly experienced and thoughtful British clinician and clinical researcher regarding the genesis of anorexia nervosa. He views anorexia nervosa primarily as avoidant behavior and the development of fat phobia in the face of adolescent challenges and sees the thinking and preoccupations of anorexia nervosa as progressively replacing the personality of the victim.

25. **Pope HG Jr, Hudson JI:** Is childhood sexual abuse a risk factor for bulimia nervosa? *Am J Psychiatry* 149:455–463, 1992

Clinicians frequently uncover histories of child sexual abuse in their eating disorders patients. Nevertheless, in a careful examination of existing epidemiological and clinical studies, Pope and Hudson found little evidence to support the view that child sexual abuse is more common among eating disorders than among either other psychiatric populations or, for that matter, among the female population at large. These highly controversial conclusions are likely to generate additional discussion and research. An alternative view, which thoughtfully evaluates the experience of sexual abuse in the lives of women with eating disorders, is presented by Wooley's chapter in Faloon et al. (1994) above.

26. **Schwartz HJ** (ed): *Bulimia: Psychoanalytic Treatment and Theory,* 2nd Edition. Madison, CT, International Universities Press, 1990

This is a collection of essays by psychoanalysts who have collectively treated several dozen patients regarding their insights into the genesis, transference aspects, and psychoanalytically oriented treatment of patients with bulimia nervosa. The views regarding psychoanalytic approaches to treatment offered here sometimes relegate physiological concerns to the background, in marked contrast to those proposed by more comprehensively schooled clinicians.

27. **Thompson JK:** *Body Image Disturbance: Assessment and Treatment.* New York, Pergamon, 1990

This is a theoretically and clinically rich book that considers body image, particularly but not exclusively in relation to eating disorders, from several developmental, perceptual, and attitudinal perspectives. Several therapeutic approaches to body image disturbances are described using psychodynamic and cognitive approaches, behavioral homework, and reduction of body image anxieties through the use of videotape sessions.

Family

28. **Minuchin S, Rosman BL, Baker L:** *Psychosomatic Families: Anorexia Nervosa in Context.* Cambridge, MA, Harvard University Press, 1978

    This is a classic book in which many seminal hypotheses about family functioning in anorexia nervosa were first presented, including the suggestion that enmeshment, rigidity, and conflict avoidance are more likely to be found in families of patients with anorexia nervosa (as well as families in which children have other major psychological overlay to so-called psychosomatic conditions such as asthma and juvenile-onset diabetes mellitus) than in other families.

29. **Russell GFM, Szmukler GI, Dare C, Eisler I:** An evaluation of family therapy in anorexia nervosa and bulimia nervosa. *Arch Gen Psychiatry* 44:1047–1056, 1987

    In an elegant, controlled study of more than 90 eating disorders patients and their families, these researchers showed that, for younger patients with anorexia nervosa, weekly family therapy for a year following discharge from a hospital was associated with better outcomes than weekly individual psychotherapy. For older-onset patients and for those with bulimia nervosa, outcomes for the two forms of psychotherapy were equivalent.

30. **Strober M, Lampert C, Morrell W, Burroughs J, Jacobs C:** A controlled family study of anorexia nervosa: evidence of familial aggregation and lack of shared transmission with affective disorders. *International Journal of Eating Disorders* 9:239–253, 1990

    This careful study of nearly 100 probands with anorexia nervosa, appropriate comparison group probands, and nearly 900 interviewed first-degree relatives demonstrated that anorexia nervosa was about eight times as common in their first-degree relatives as among those of the control probands and that affective disorder was higher among relatives of those anorexia nervosa patients who had concurrent mood disorder. Genetics and heritability of eating disorders are discussed in depth.

31. **Vandereyken W, Kog E, Vanderlinder J** (eds): *The Family Approach to Eating Disorders.* New York, PMA Publishing, 1989

    In this collection of excellent theoretical and practical clinically oriented chapters by a productive Belgian research and clinical group, chapters consider everything from systems to family group and family education programs.

Treatment

32. **Agras WS:** *Cognitive Behavior Therapy Treatment Manual for Bulimia Nervosa.* Stanford, CA, Department of Psychiatry and Behavioral Sciences, Stanford University School of Medicine, 1991

33. **Mitchell JE and Staff Members of the Eating Disorders Program:** *Bulimia Nervosa: Group Treatment Manual.* Minneapolis, MN, Department of Psychiatry, University of Minnesota Hospital and Clinic, 1989; **Mitchell JE and Staff Members of the Eating Disorders Program:** *Bulimia Nervosa: Individual Treatment Manual.* Minneapolis, MN, Department of Psychiatry, University of Minnesota Hospital and Clinic, 1989

These excellent treatment manuals are available for a modest fee (reproduction and mailing) from the authors. They provide a step-by-step guide for clinicians using structured forms of cognitive psychotherapy with patients suffering from bulimia nervosa.

34. **Agras WS, Rossiter EM, Arnow B, Schneider JA, Telch CF, Raeburn SD, Bruce B, Perl M, Koran LM:** Pharmacologic and cognitive-behavioral treatment for bulimia nervosa: a controlled comparison. *Am J Psychiatry* 149:82–87, 1992

This well-designed study showed advantages for treating patients with both types of therapy concurrently. Desipramine was the medication used in this study. For specifics of the cognitive therapy, see Piran and Kaplan (1990) below.

35. *American Psychiatric Association Task Force on Treatments of Psychiatric Disorders:* *Eating Disorders: Section 6: Treatment of Psychiatric Disorders: A Task Force Report of the American Psychiatric Association,* Vol. 1. Washington, DC, American Psychiatric Association, 1989, pp. 449–616

This is a series of chapters that detail the rationales, benefits, and limitations for each of the major medical, pharmacological, individual, group, and family psychotherapeutic approaches to the treatment of anorexia nervosa and bulimia nervosa.

36. *Andersen AE:* *Practical Comprehensive Treatment of Anorexia Nervosa and Bulimia.* Baltimore, MD, Johns Hopkins, 1985

Based on experience with several hundred eating disorders patients treated at Johns Hopkins' eating disorders program, this book offers a sensible almost cookbook approach, detailing the specific tasks for physicians, nurses, dietitians, and other staff members. It is an excellent guide for those planning inpatient treatment programs.

37. **Fairburn CG, Jones R, Peveler RC, Carr SJ, Solomon RA, O'Connor ME, Burton J, Hope RA:** Three psychological treatments for bulimia nervosa: a comparative trial. *Arch Gen Psychiatry* 48:463–469, 1991

Seventy-five patients randomly assigned to each of three treatment groups received 19 40- to 50-minute sessions over an 18-week period. Although all treatments were beneficial, on several dimensions of outcome cognitive-behavioral therapy was superior to interpersonal psychotherapy and to a simpler form of behavior therapy.

38. **Fluoxetine Bulimia Nervosa Collaborative Study Group:** Fluoxetine in the treatment of bulimia nervosa: a multicenter, placebo-controlled, double-blind trial. *Arch Gen Psychiatry* 49:139–147, 1992

Thirteen centers provided 387 patients for a study comparing 20 versus 60 mg/day of fluoxetine versus placebo for an 8-week trail. For this short period, higher-dose fluoxetine was superior to lower-dose fluoxetine, and both were superior to placebo in ameliorating the symptoms of bulimia nervosa.

39. ****Garner DM, Garfinkel PE** (eds): *Handbook of Psychotherapy for Anorexia Nervosa and Bulimia.* New York, Guilford, 1985

This is a superb, detailed, well-written, almost encyclopedic book containing chapters by internationally recognized experts in all aspects of psychodynamic, cognitive, behavioral, group, family, and educational psychotherapeutic approaches for eating disorders. The lengthy, authoritative chapters offer both scholarly theoretical as well as clinically focused reviews, making this a superb text on the preponderance of contemporary psychotherapies, useful far beyond its application to eating disorders alone.

40. **Johnson C** (ed): *Psychodynamic Treatment of Anorexia Nervosa and Bulimia.* New York, Guilford, 1991

This book provides excellent chapters on current psychodynamic themes relevant to eating disorders: self psychology, masochism, borderline and narcissistic personality formulations, feminist psychology, interpersonal approaches and integrative perspectives that combine object relations and family systems, disorders of self within an organismic-developmental perspective, and psychodynamic and behavioral approaches.

41. **McKenzie R** (ed): *Group Treatment for the Eating Disorders.* Washington, DC, American Psychiatric Press, 1992

From the extremely productive eating disorders research clinical and research programs at the University of Toronto, this book by large numbers of mental health professionals at that center covers all theoretical and practical aspects of group work with anorexia nervosa and bulimia nervosa patients in inpatient, partial hospitalization, and outpatient settings. Included are discussions of psychodynamic, cognitive, educational, nutritional, and family groups, and much more.

42. **Mitchell JE, Pyle RL, Eckert ED, Hatsukami D, Pomeroy C, Zimmerman R:** A comparison study of antidepressants and structured intensive group psychotherapy in the treatment of bulimia nervosa. *Arch Gen Psychiatry* 47:149–157, 1990

In a four-cell design study, outpatients were treated with intensive outpatient group psychotherapy (starting with several weeks of programming several hours per evening), imipramine, both, or neither. For this population, the intensive group program was very effective, so much so that adding medication appeared to offer little additional benefit. It must be emphasized that this is not your average outpatient group therapy program.

43. **Mitchell JE, Pyle RL, Eckert ED, Hatsukami D, Pomeroy C, Zimmerman R:** Response to alternative antidepressants in imipramine nonresponders with bulimia nervosa. *J Clin Psychopharmacol* 9:291–293, 1989

44. **Pope HG Jr, McElroy SL, Keck RE, Hudson J:** Long term pharmacotherapy of bulimia nervosa. *J Clin Psychopharmacol* 9:385–386, 1989

These two case series provide evidence to support the practice of treating bulimia nervosa patients who fail an initial antidepressant drug trial with a second and sometimes a third agent before knowing whether the patient may have a positive response to medication.

45. **Piran N, Kaplan AS** (eds): *A Day Hospital Group Treatment Program for Anorexia Nervosa and Bulimia Nervosa.* New York, Brunner/Mazel, 1990

This is an excellent description of program details and an early outcome evaluation of a complete day-hospital program from the University of Toronto's excellent eating disorders group. It is the best and most complete description of a day-hospital program currently available.

46. **Walsh BT, Stewart JW, Roose SP, Gladis M, Glassman AH:** Treatment of bulimia with phenelzine: a double-blind placebo controlled study. *Arch Gen Psychiatry* 41:1105–1119, 1984

This excellent study points out the difficulties in recruiting a large enough population of bulimic women to conduct a trial with monoamine oxidase inhibitors, the high rate of side effects in this population, and the superiority of phenelzine over placebo for those who stayed in the study.

Comorbidity and Other Conditions

47. Andersen AE (ed): *Males With Eating Disorders*. New York, Brunner/Mazel, 1990

Males constitute approximately 5% of patients with eating disorders, and this book offers the best available compilation of information regarding clinical, clinical research, and theoretical aspects of the development and treatment of eating disorders in males. A male clinical psychologist provides a compelling first-person account of his developing and struggling with anorexia nervosa. Andersen's (1990) chapter on the development of eating disorders, described above, by itself makes this book worth reading carefully.

48. Halmi KA, Eckert E, Marchi P, Sampugnaro V, Apple R, Cohen J: Comorbidity of psychiatric diagnoses in anorexia nervosa. *Arch Gen Psychiatry* 48:712–718, 1991

During a 10-year follow-up study, 62 women with anorexia nervosa were assessed for other lifetime psychiatric diagnoses. Much higher rates of current and lifetime affective (84%) and anxiety (65%) disorders were found among the anorexia nervosa population than among a nonclinical control group. The current and lifetime rate for obsessive-compulsive disorder in the anorexia nervosa group was 26%.

49. Yager J, Gwirtsman HE, Edelstein CK (eds): *Special Problems in Managing Eating Disorders*. Washington, DC, American Psychiatric Press, 1991

This is a collection of clinically focused chapters dealing with the assessment and management of eating disorders presenting concurrently with mood disorders, chemical dependency, personality disorders, pregnancy, diabetes mellitus, medical problems, and other concomitants.

50. Yates A: *Compulsive Exercise and the Eating Disorders: Toward an Integrated Theory of Activity*. New York, Brunner/Mazel, 1991

This is a thorough review of the relationship between activity and eating disorders by an authority whose provocative work on compulsive running as a potential male analogue of anorexia nervosa has stimulated considerable debate and discussion in medical and psychiatric circles.

Course and Outcome

51. Herzog D, Keller M, Lavori P: Outcome in anorexia nervosa and bulimia nervosa: a review of the literature. *J Nerv Ment Dis* 176:131–143, 1988

Herzog et al. are engaged in a long-term prospective naturalistic follow-up study of several hundred women with eating disorders initially assessed at the Massachusetts General Hospital. This review of the literature points out some of the difficulties in comparing studies that differ in definitions and outcome criteria. The prognosis for normal-weight bulimia nervosa patients is better than for anorexia nervosa patients. Controversy exists over the prognostic import of other clinical features.

52. **Ratnasuriya R, Eisler I, Szmukler GI, Russell GFM:** Anorexia nervosa: outcome and prognostic factors after 20 years. *Br J Psychiatry* 158:495–502, 1991

53. **Theander S:** Outcome and prognosis in anorexia nervosa and bulimia: some results of previous investigations, compared with those of a Swedish long-term study. *J Psychiatr Res* 19:493–508, 1985

These two studies report the long-term prognosis following initial hospitalization for anorexia nervosa. About 18%–20% of women were dead (word for index: death), due to malnutrition, cardiac arrest, and suicide. The remainder had mixed prognoses, with about one-third showing recovery.

Rumination Disorder

54. **Blinder BJ, Goodman SL, Goldstein R:** Rumination disorder: a critical review of diagnosis and treatment, in *The Eating Disorders: Medical and Psychological Basis of Diagnosis and Treatment.* Edited by Blinder BJ, Chaitin BJ, Goldstein R. New York, PMA Publishing, 1988, pp. 315–329

Rumination disorder occurs mostly in young children but may persist to adulthood. This chapter reviews what is known and speculated regarding its physiology, psychology, and treatment.

24

Substance-Related Disorders

Richard J. Frances, M.D.
Avram H. Mack, A.B.
William A. Frosch, M.D.

This has been an exciting decade of growth in addiction psychiatry. However, there is still a great need for a major expansion and emphasis of psychiatric education in the diagnosis and the treatment of addictive disorders. In the United States, not counting nicotine, approximately one-sixth of the population will develop a substance-related problem; for two-thirds of the individuals in this group, alcoholism is the major problem. In addition, in 1985 51.1 million American adults smoked cigarettes, and nicotine addictions account for approximately 300,000 deaths annually. Definitions of substance dependence have been developed by the World Health Organization in the ICD-10 and by the American Psychiatric Association both in DSM-III-R and in DSM-IV. Central to the concept of dependence is the development of the concepts of tolerance, withdrawal, and negative psychosocial consequences. Although the cocaine epidemic of the early 1980s has receded somewhat, drugs are as cheap and as available as ever in the nation's inner cities. The spread of acquired immunodeficiency syndrome (AIDS) and tuberculosis in the intravenous (IV)-drug–using population has contributed to a mounting death toll, and it poses an awesome challenge to providers of addiction treatment. The debate over decriminalization has been renewed in light of the frustration felt over both rising costs and rising numbers of drug-related prisoners, the lack of crime reduction, and the failure of interdiction to lessen the availability of drugs. Most addiction experts, however, remain solidly opposed to decriminalization.

In this chapter, we made selections among a burgeoning literature, with readings that are sometimes substance specific and that at other times cover substances generally and with many different levels of approach. Some of the writings were chosen for historical interest; others were picked to cover the most important developments in the field, especially those relevant to educating the general psychiatrist in clinical practice, with the inclusion of the most useful research. When equipped with skills and knowledge, the generalist is better able to assess the impact of substance-related disorders and their comorbidity in the patient and to match these patients with appropriate treatment in a way that increasingly will take into account cost effectiveness.

The writings are classified under the following sections: 1) assessment, diagnosis, definitions, and overview texts; 2) substance-specific readings; 3) epidemiology; 4) psychiatric and medical comorbidity; 5) models of addiction; 6) detoxification, treatment, and outcome; 7) familial, cultural, and socioeconomic aspects of substance abuse; 8) and special populations. Many high-quality addiction textbooks are available, and a growing number of addiction journals are backlogged for years with forthcoming articles. *The American Journal of Addictions* was founded in 1992, and it promises to be of special interest to clinicians. It is difficult to do justice to the literature in this short review, which attempts to pick classic influential articles, many of which are of recent vintage. The inclusion of textbooks that provide more comprehensive reviews is intended to help cover the breadth of the field. Traditionally underdiagnosed and undertreated, addicted patients are in need of well-informed professional care, as well as self-help.

Assessment, Diagnosis, Definitions, and Overview Texts

1. **Cala LA, Mastaglis FL:** Computerized tomography in chronic alcoholics. *Alcoholism: Clinical and Experimental Research* 5:283–294, 1981

   These striking and surprising findings of recovery from cortical thinning in chronic alcoholic persons provide some hope to organic patients who maintain long-term abstinence.

2. **Charness ME, De La Paz RL, Diamond I, Norman D:** MR imaging of atrophic mammillary bodies in chronic Wernicke disease. *Radiology Suppl* 157:344, 1985

   Magnetic resonance imaging allows noninvasive high-resolution anatomical data superior to computed tomography scans, including chemical and physiological information, and it led to findings of atrophy in mammillary bodies in live patients with chronic Wernicke's syndrome. In the past such anatomical diagnosis could be made only at autopsy.

3. **Frances RJ, Miller SI** (eds): *The Clinical Textbook of Addictive Disorders.* New York, Guilford, 1991

    This readable textbook contains well-written chapters by well-known clinical teachers. It begins with an overview that places addictions in an historical context, then goes on to describe the consequences of addiction to each drug, diagnostic issues, and problems with special populations. It also reviews the differential therapeutics of addiction treatment, providing descriptions of each modality.

4. **Johnson JL, Adinoff B, Bisserbe JC, Martin PR, Rio D, Rohrbaugh JW, Zubovic E, Eckardt MJ:** Assessment of alcoholism-related organic brain syndromes with positron emission tomography. *Alcoholism: Clinical and Experimental Research* 10:237–240, 1986

    Alcohol central nervous system deficits are correlated by this group in terms of functional alcohol-induced organic brain syndrome, computed tomography scans, electroencephalograms, cognitive measures, and pathophysiological data identified by positron-emission tomography (PET). The localized brain metabolism of substances such as glucose, a source of energy and localized brain receptors, can be measured by PET, providing data on biochemical processes in the live brain.

5. **Lowinson JH, Ruiz P, Millman RB, Langrod JG** (eds): *Substance Abuse: A Comprehensive Textbook,* 2nd Edition. Baltimore, MD, Williams & Wilkins, 1992

    This second edition includes authoritative reviews of the progress over the last decade in addictions and provides encyclopedic (80 chapters) coverage of subjects not as deeply handled in other textbooks, such as special populations, acquired immunodeficiency syndrome, psychiatric education, and public policy. It is useful for novices as a reference text and for selected readings.

6. **Schuckit MA:** The clinical implications of primary diagnostic groups among alcoholics. *Arch Gen Psychiatry* 42:1043–1049, 1985

    Issues of primary and secondary disorders and the implications of these interactions are discussed in this article. There has been increasing attention paid to the importance of psychiatric comorbidity and the full evaluation of mentally ill alcoholic patients.

7. **Schuckit MA:** *Drug and Alcohol Abuse: A Clinical Guide to Diagnosis and Treatment,* 2nd Edition. New York, Plenum Press, 1988

This is a useful, lucid, and practical textbook that is especially good for definitions, substance-specific descriptions, and the emergency management of intoxication and withdrawal. Because it is a single-author textbook, it is not repetitious, and it succinctly covers a great deal of material.

8. **Tarter R, Edwards K:** Brief and comprehensive neuropsychosocial assessment of alcoholism and drug abuse, in *Essentials of Neuropsychological Assessment.* Edited by Hartlage L, Ashen M, Hornsby L. New York, Springer, 1987, pp. 138–162

The screening, evaluation, and neuropsychological assessment of addicted patients is important since organicity is prevalent in substance-abusing persons. This chapter provides a good overview of instruments useful in this process.

Substance-Specific Readings

9. **Adams RD, Victor M:** *Principles of Neurology.* New York, McGraw-Hill, 1981

This volume contains the classic descriptions of the effects of alcohol intoxication and withdrawal, and these have yet to be described better.

10. **Department of Health and Human Services:** *Smoking and Health: A National Status Report: A Report to Congress.* Washington, DC, U.S. Department of Health and Human Services, 1987

This landmark report has had a wide impact on health care in relation to smoking. It covers nicotine addiction, the public health problem of smoking, and prevention and treatment.

11. **Dole VP, Nyswander ME:** A medical treatment of diacetylmorphine (heroin) addiction. *JAMA* 193:646–650, 1965

12. **Greenstein RA, Fiedala PJ, O'Brien CP:** Alternative psychotherapies for opiate addiction, in *Substance Abuse: A Comprehensive Textbook,* 2nd Edition. Edited by Lowinson JH, Ruiz P, Millman RB, Langrod JC. Baltimore, MD, Williams & Wilkins, 1992, pp. 562–571

13. **Lowinson JH, Marion IS, Joseph H, Dole VP:** Methadone maintenance, in *Substance Abuse: A Comprehensive Textbook,* 2nd Edition. Edited by Lowinson JH, Ruiz P, Millman RB, Langrod JC. Baltimore, MD, Williams & Wilkins, 1992, pp. 550–561

Dole and Nyswander pioneered methadone treatment and forged the model of drug substitution in the treatment of opioid-addicted persons. Methadone maintenance remains an effective means of reducing crime, and it has been valuable in helping prevent the spread of the human immunodeficiency virus. The method is updated in a chapter by Lowinson et al., and approaches to the psychotherapy of opioid addicts are well described in Greenstein et al.'s chapter in the same textbook.

14. **Frosch WA, Robbins ES, Stern M:** Untoward reactions to lysergic acid diethylamide (LSD) resulting in hospitalization. *N Engl J Med* 273:1235–1239, 1965

This article was one of the first scientific studies of "acid." Its findings are applicable to other drugs, such as marijuana and other hallucinogens as well.

15. **Jaffe JH:** Drug addiction and drug abuse, in *The Pharmacological Basis of Therapeutics*, 17th Edition. Edited by Gilman AF, Goodman LS, Rall TW, Murad F. New York, Macmillan, 1985, pp. 550–554

Along with the signs and symptoms of intoxication and withdrawal, this is the best place to learn the clinical pharmacology of addictive substances.

Epidemiology

16. **Johnston LD, O'Malley PM, Bachman JG:** *National Trends in Drug Use and Related Factors Among American High School Students and Young Adults 1975–1986.* Rockville, MD, National Institute on Drug Abuse, 1987

This important, large-population, databased research charts the rise and turnaround in drug use in young adults, with a decrease in cocaine seen shortly after the deaths of several famous athletes.

17. **Kandel D, Faust R:** Sequence and stages in patterns of adolescent drug use. *Arch Gen Psychiatry* 32:923–932, 1975

This classic article opened the door to the concept of "gateways" to substance abuse and confirmed what many had long suspected: that the use of tobacco, alcohol, and marijuana in adolescence predicts progression to other drug use and abuse.

18. **Nadelmann EA:** Drug prohibition in the United States: costs, consequences, and alternatives. *Science* 245:939–947, 1989

This thought-provoking article shows the many fronts of the drive to decriminalize drugs. It views the debate with respect to the history of past prohibitions, the nature of current drugs, the current efforts at interdiction, the ways in which people use both alcohol and other drugs, and the differences between the two. It suggests that such a move would aid in curtailing drug abuse.

Psychiatric and Medical Comorbidity

19. **Helzer JE, Pryzbeck FR:** The co-occurrence of alcoholism with other psychiatric disorders in the general population and its impact on treatment. *J Stud Alcohol* 49:219–224, 1988

Based on the Epidemiologic Catchment Area study data, this study spells out the high comorbidity of alcoholism and other psychiatric disorders. Antisocial personality disorder, manic depression disorder, and anxiety disorders are especially overrepresented here.

20. **Lieber CS** (ed): *Medical and Nutritional Complications of Alcoholism, Mechanisms and Management.* New York, Plenum, 1992

Given its multisystem involvement, to know alcoholism is to know all of medicine. The acute and chronic medical complications of alcoholism are well considered here in terms of pathogenesis, pathophysiology, and clinical management.

21. **Lieber CS, Leo MA:** Alcohol and the liver, in *Medical Disorders of Alcoholism: Pathogenesis and Treatment.* Edited by Lieber CS. Philadelphia, PA, WB Saunders, 1982, pp. 259–312

This is an authoritative review of alcohol's effect on the liver. It is important not only in terms of medical comorbidity, but also in the use of medications that are metabolized in the liver.

22. **McLellan AT, Woody GE, O'Brien CP:** Development of psychiatric illness in drug abusers: possible role of drug preference. *N Engl J Med* 301:1310–1314, 1979

This is a study of the "longitudinal relations between patterns of drug abuse and the development of psychiatric disorders" (p. 1310). There are clear, drug-specific changes. Some drugs are bad for mental health (psychostimulants and depressants); others (opiates) did not produce change over time.

23. **Meyer RE** (ed): *Psychopathology and Addictive Disorders.* New York, Guilford, 1986

The high level of depression, anxiety disorders, and other psychiatric disorders and the need to address these issues in treatment are the subjects of this pioneering textbook on comorbidity. This has led psychiatrists more frequently to diagnose and improve treatment of patients with comorbid psychiatric disorders.

Models of Addiction

24. **Bohman M, Sigvardsson S, Cloninger CR:** Maternal inheritance of alcohol abuse: cross-fostering analysis of adopted women. *Arch Gen Psychiatry* 38:965–969, 1981

25. **Cloninger CR, Bohman M, Sigvardsson S:** Inheritance of alcohol abuse: cross fostering analysis of adopted men. *Arch Gen Psychiatry* 38:861–868, 1981

These two studies of cross-fostering in men and women suggest heterogeneous etiology among alcoholic persons. This has led Cloninger et al. to develop a typology of familial alcoholism, separating those whose influences have tended to be genetic from those for whom the main force has been environmental.

26. **Khantzian EJ:** The self-medication hypothesis of addictive disorders. *Am J Psychiatry* 142:1259–1264, 1985

This is a modern exposition of the self-medication hypothesis by its current leading exponent. Khantzian discusses the use of medications to regulate affective experience, and he emphasizes the importance of self-care in treatment.

27. **Krystal H:** Alexithymia and the effectiveness of psychoanalytic treatment. *International Journal of Psychoanalytic Psychotherapy* 9:338–353, 1982

Krystal describes patients with substance-use disorders who have difficulty feeling, knowing, and regulating their affect. Psychodynamic psychotherapy may help these patients to label and cope with painful feeling states.

28. **Lorand S:** A summary of psychoanalytic literature on problems of alcoholism. *Yearbook of Psychoanalysis* 4:359–378, 1948

This is the best psychoanalytic review of the field up to 1948. Although psychodynamic theory has had lessened influence in recent years, it is important not to throw out the baby with the bathwater.

29. **Milkman H, Frosch WA:** On the preferential abuse of heroin and amphetamine. *J Nerv Ment Dis* 156:242–248, 1973

    This is one of the classic articles describing the matching of desired drug effects and a self-medication hypothesis.

30. **Skolnick P, Paul SM:** Benzodiazepine receptors in the central nervous system. *Int Rev Neurobiol* 23:103–140, 1982

    In this article, one of the striking findings are brain receptors for psychoactive substances such as endogenous benzodiazepine receptors.

31. **Vaillant GE:** *The Natural History of Alcoholism.* Cambridge, MA, Harvard University Press, 1983

    An instant classic, this book has excellent prospective data that argue against the self-medication hypothesis as the basis of most alcoholism and that help establish a rationale for alcoholism as usually being the primary illness in the patient.

Detoxification, Treatment, and Outcome

32. **Charney DS, Heninger GR, Kleber HD:** The combined use of clonidine and naltrexone as a rapid, safe, and effective treatment of abrupt withdrawal from methadone. *Am J Psychiatry* 143:831–837, 1986

    This article presents a fast and efficient way to detoxify heroin-addicted persons through the use of blockade of opiate effects and of withdrawal symptoms. It is an example of the use of sophisticated knowledge of pharmacological effects to improve treatment.

33. **Edwards G, Orford J, Egert S, Guthrie S, Hawker A, Hensman C, Mitcheson M, Oppenhiemer E, Taylor C:** Alcoholism: a controlled trial of "treatment" and "advice." *J Stud Alcohol* 38:1004–1031, 1977

    This classic and often-cited article set a standard for therapeutic nihilism and provides a challenge to those who seek proof that treatment works. It is very difficult, yet important, to do good controlled treatment-outcome studies that demonstrate the effectiveness of specific treatment formats.

34. **Emrick CD:** Alcoholics Anonymous: affiliation processes and effectiveness as treatment. *Alcoholism: Clinical and Experimental Research* 11:424–429, 1987

    This review finds support for the effectiveness of Alcoholics Anonymous (AA), but there is neither hard evidence nor controlled studies of AA.

The best evidence for 12-step self-help groups is patient acceptance and the fact that 1.5 million Americans vote with their feet in attending 80,000 AA groups each week.

35. **Gawin FH, Kleber HD:** Abstinence symptomatology and psychiatric diagnosis in cocaine abusers. *Arch Gen Psychiatry* 43:107–113, 1986

Treatment of prolonged abstinence from cocaine with desipramine followed from the findings of this article.

36. **Helzer JE, Robins LN, Taylor JR, Carey K, Miller RH, Combs-Orne T, Farmer A:** The extent of long-term moderate drinking among alcoholics discharged from medical and psychiatric treatment facilities. *N Engl J Med* 312:1678–1682, 1985

Most clinicians recommend an abstinence approach to addictions, and this article provides data to support this view. Although almost all patients wish and hope to learn controlled drinking, very few succeed, and no one can predict who they will be.

37. **Hester RK, Miller WR:** *Handbook of Alcoholism Treatment Approaches: Effective Alternatives.* New York, Pergamon, 1989

This excellent textbook of treatment approaches relies heavily on scientific study and is especially strong on cognitive-behavioral approaches. It leaves out discussion of psychodynamic psychotherapy.

38. **Marlatt GA, Gordon JR** (eds): *Relapse Prevention: Maintenance Strategies in the Treatment of Addictive Behaviors.* New York, Guilford, 1985

This is an instant classic that provides practical cognitive-behavioral tools in addiction treatment, which are rapidly being incorporated into most rehabilitation programs. This approach is also readily accepted by patients.

39. **Pettinati M, Sugarman A, Maurer HS:** Four year MMPI changes in abstinent and drinking alcoholics. *Alcoholism: Clinical and Experimental Research* 6:487–494, 1982

This article presents one of the better prospective treatment-outcome studies and shows the effects of long-term improvements. In those who remain abstinent, Minnesota Multiphasic Personality Inventory scale scores continue to improve over time.

40. **Woody GE, Luborsky L, McLellan AT, O'Brien CP, Beck AT, Blaine J, Herman I, Hole A:** Psychotherapy for opiate addicts: does it help? *Arch Gen Psychiatry* 40:639–645, 1983

This is one of the few controlled studies that demonstrates a benefit for dynamic psychotherapy for any population, and it is especially interesting in that it does so for opioid-addicted persons.

41. **Woody GE, McLellan AT, Luborsky L, O'Brien CP, Blaine J, Fox S, Herman I, Beck AT:** Severity of psychiatric symptoms as a predictor of benefits from psychotherapy: the Veterans Administration-Penn Study. *Am J Psychiatry* 141:1172–1177, 1984

This is one of the few good treatment outcome studies we have, and it provides useful predictions based on severity. It also uses the Addiction Severity Index, which is now widely applied to treatment outcome research. Addicted persons with additional problems do worse, but have greater improvement if these problems are treated.

Familial, Cultural, and Socioeconomic Aspects of Substance Abuse

42. **Cloninger RC, Sigvardsson S, Bohman M:** Childhood personality predicts alcohol abuse in young adults. *Alcoholism: Clinical and Experimental Research* 12:494–505, 1988

This group is trying to correlate personality traits to genetics and familial subtypes of alcoholism. Although it is not clear that any one personality type can encompass addictive behavior, temperament and certain personality disorders may correlate with addictive behavior.

43. **Goodwin DW:** Alcohol as Muse. *Am J Psychother* 46:422–433, 1992

This interesting article discusses the rise of alcoholism in western literary figures in the first half of the 20th century. Why do many writers drink alcoholically? Goodwin has a hypothesis regarding this problem, and he describes the ways in which the mind and product of the artist are affected by alcohol.

44. **Harwood HJ, Napolitano DM, Kristiansen PL:** *Economic Costs to Society of Alcohol and Drug Abuse and Mental Illness* (Publ. No. RTI/2734/00-001FR). Research Triangle Park, NC, Research Triangle Institute, 1980

This often-cited review estimates the broad range of costs of addictions to society. The cost effectiveness of treatment will face increasing scrutiny as tough choices are made in provision of health care to addicted patients.

45. **Helzer JE, Canino GJ, Hwu H, Bland RC, Neuman S, Jeh EK:** Alcoholism: a cross-national comparison of population surveys with the DIS, in

Alcoholism: Origins and Outcomes. Edited by Rose RT, Barnett J. New York, Raven, 1988, pp. 31–47

This is rapidly becoming a classic study. It indicates that each culture influences rates of alcohol disorders but that the signs and symptoms of alcohol disorders exist, and are similar, across cultures.

46. **Kaufman E, Kaufman P** (eds): *Family Therapy of Drug and Alcohol Abuse.* New York, Gardner Press, 1979

Family and systems approaches to addictive disorders have achieved increasing acceptance and importance, in part as a result of this now classic work.

47. **Lowry M:** *Lunar Caustic.* Edited by Birney E, Lowry M. London, Cape, 1968; **Styron W:** *Darkness Visible: A Memoir of Madness.* New York, Random House, 1990; **Waugh E:** *The Ordeal of Gilbert Pinfold.* Boston, MA, Little, Brown, 1979

These are three from-the-inside-out views of toxic drug experiences based on the novelists' personal experiences transmuted through art. An extraordinarily high percentage of American writers have had alcoholism; many have been suicidal and have written about their experiences with substances.

48. **Mensch BS, Kandel DB:** Do job conditions influence the use of drugs? *J Health Soc Behav* 29:169–184, 1988

Although many feel that the workplace environment is that which drives many to substance abuse, using a large national labor survey, this study suggests that this is not true. Instead, it argues that one's personal background is a better predictor of substance abuse than his or her occupational surroundings.

49. **Steinglass P, Bennett L, Wolin S, Reiss D:** *The Alcoholic Family.* New York, Basic Books, 1987

This is an excellent textbook for those who work with alcoholic families, written by authoritative research clinicians who have helped pioneer this area of family work, including data that suggest the contribution of family systems to sustaining an addiction.

50. **Westermeyer J:** Cultural patterns of drug and alcohol abuse: an analysis of host and agent in the cultural environment. *Bull Narc* 39:11–27, 1987

The biopsychosocial perspective is enriched by this in-depth look at the relationship between cultural patterns and the use of substances. Westermeyer, a brilliant psychiatrist and anthropologist, has done fascinating fieldwork that combines ethnographic and psychiatric expertise.

Special Populations

51. **Blume SB:** Women and alcohol. *JAMA* 256:1467–1470, 1986

Most studies of alcoholism have been done on men, and more needs to be learned about alcoholism in women. There are biological, psychological, and cultural differences between the ways in which men and women are affected by alcohol, all of which need to be taken into account by clinicians.

52. **Des Jarlais DC, Wish E, Friedman SR, Stoneburner R, Yaneovitz SR, Mildvan D, El-Sadr W, Brady E, Cuadrado M:** Intravenous drug use and the heterosexual transmission of the human immunodeficiency virus: current trends in New York City. *N Y State J Med* 87:283–286, 1987

The spread of human immunodeficiency virus (HIV) infection in the intravenous (IV) drug–using population is alarming, and it poses the greatest challenge as well as need for medical skills in those treating IV-addicted patients. IV-drug users pose a special threat to increasing heterosexual HIV risk.

53. **Finnegan LP, Kandall S:** Maternal and neonatal effects of alcohol and drugs, in *Substance Abuse: A Comprehensive Textbook*, 2nd Edition. Edited by Lowinson JH, Ruiz P, Millman RB, Langrod JG. Baltimore, MD, Williams & Wilkins, 1992, pp. 628–656

This chapter provides a thorough and recent update by one of the leading experts in the field and includes a wide range of fetal effects of a variety of drugs with means of approaching screening, evaluation, and treatment.

54. **Niven RG:** Adolescent drug abuse. *Hosp Community Psychiatry* 37:596–607, 1986

This article provides a good overview of issues in adolescent drug abuse. Adolescent drug abuse is a major risk factor for adolescent suicide.

55. **Rosett HL, Weiner L, Edelin KD:** Treatment experience with problem drinking pregnant women. *JAMA* 249:2029–2033, 1983

Now that fetal alcohol syndrome has been rediscovered (it had been recognized in London during the gin epidemic in the early 1700s), those at risk should be identified and treatment instituted. This article outlines an effective treatment approach and presents evidence that outcome is improved.

56. **Schilling RF, Schinke SP, Nichols SE, Zayas LH, Miller SO, Orlandi MA, Botvin GJ:** Developing strategies for AIDS prevention research with black and Hispanic drug users. *Public Health Rep* 104:1–12, 1989

This Columbia University group has pioneered acquired immunodeficiency syndrome prevention research in the black and Hispanic communities. It is important to take ethnographic considerations into effect in planning prevention programs.

57. **Stall R:** Prevention of HIV infection associated with drug and alcohol use during sexual activity. *Adv Alcohol Subst Abuse* 7:73–88, 1987

Based on large-scale statistical research of the San Francisco, California, population, the author links higher rates of substance abuse among homosexual persons with greater risks of human immunodeficiency virus transmission. Suggestions to alleviate the problem address social conditions, recognizing that education alone is no panacea.

25

Posttraumatic Stress Disorder

Robert S. Pynoos, M.D., M.P.H.
Alan M. Steinberg, Ph.D.

Trauma, disaster, and violence have been ever-present throughout the course of human history. Until recently, the psychiatric interest in posttraumatic stress reactions primarily waxed and waned with the occurrence of major military conflicts. However, long before the pioneering trauma studies arising out of World War I and World War II, Homer recounted the psychological horrors of war and the emotional odyssey of the returning veteran. Most recently, it has been the veterans of the Vietnam War who have brought renewed attention to the study of traumatic stress and who, through their perseverance, have contributed in the United States to a national commitment to a research and clinical agenda. The past two decades have seen a broadening of interest to include situations of interpersonal violence and natural and technological disasters as well as an investigation of trauma throughout the life cycle, including the interplay of child and adult traumatic experiences.

These new interests were also anteceded by many historical artistic and literary works. Painters have often attempted to communicate traumatic emotions through their transformation of traumatic imagery—for example, Rembrandt's depiction of Lucretia's condemning herself to suicide after rape; the plight of the unrescued disaster victims in Gericault's *Raft of the*

Medusa; and Picasso's communication of terror, the grotesqueness of a dismembered body and agonizing grief after the bombing of civilians in his depiction of *Guernica*. Writers have provided detailed personal accounts of their own traumatic experiences—for example, Samuel Pepys' description of his personal reactions to the Great London Fire of 1666, and Maxim Gorky's autobiographical remembrances of child abuse and witnessing of spousal abuse. Writers have also described in fictional accounts, trauma-related coping long before any terminology existed to categorize it. For example, in his 1929 novel, *A High Wind in Jamaica*, Richard Hughes described a "Stockholm syndrome" in children kidnapped by pirates.

The diagnosis of posttraumatic stress disorder (PTSD) remains controversial. In great measure, this is due to the special place PTSD occupies within psychiatric nosology where the diagnostic gateway is the occurrence of a specific personal experience. There has always been difficulty surrounding the characterization of traumatic reactions because of the problem of classifying these reactions within a traditional spectrum of normality and pathology. At the same time, there has been consistent recognition that there is something sui generis about the experience of and response to traumatic situations. Freud struggled with these questions and continued to deliberate about a special role for "traumatic helplessness and anxiety," leaving this determination uncompleted in his mature developmental model. Psychoanalysts, to this day, continue to debate whether these intrapsychic responses conform to a more general model of the human mind in conflict.

It has been more than a decade since the inclusion of PTSD in DSM-III, and 5 years since DSM-III-R made specific mention of the clinical presentation in children. Within a relatively short period of time, the field of traumatic stress has become increasingly complex, incorporating knowledge from a variety of biological, social science, psychological, and psychiatric disciplines. Advances in research methodology have included refined typologies of exposure and multidimensional psychometric instruments. Dose-of-exposure designs have permitted better identification of specific traumatic features associated with risk, premorbid factors that relate to outcome, and processes that affect recovery.

Diagnostic questions include what characterizes an event as traumatic, how well the diagnosis of PTSD accounts for trauma-related pathological states, and how cohesive is the symptomatology of PTSD across different types of traumatic stresses. There is also growing clinical consensus that the symptoms seen in victims of repeated or prolonged interpersonal brutality and abuse are not totally captured by the diagnostic criteria for PTSD. In addition, there is greater recognition that traumatic experiences are deeply embedded in a cultural context that influences the meaning and assimilation of traumatic stresses; expectations in regard to recovery; and family, community, and societal responsiveness.

One of the most active areas of current research is the neurobiology of traumatic stress. There is accumulating scientific evidence that extreme threat constitutes a major biological challenge that may result in acute and long-term alterations in neurobiological systems. These investigations have focused on the interrelatedness of neurohormonal responses, neurophysiological pathways, and neurocommunication processes both regional and global that may constitute a biological substrate of PTSD. The studies also suggest the self-preservative function of these neural mechanisms in enhancing memory, attention, and vigilance and their potential contribution to a mental set of traumatic expectations.

The field of traumatic stress studies has progressed to the point where there is a healthy trend toward rapprochement among those oriented to psychodynamic, cognitive-behavioral, and psychopharmacological approaches. The treatment articles were chosen to illustrate how the three modalities provide complimentary perspectives in addressing the attribution of meaning, the acquisition of new fears, reactivity to external and internal reminders, and disturbances in the stability of self-concepts and biological systems.

This selected annotated bibliography includes articles of historic importance as well as publications exemplifying the most recent research methodologies and findings. It reflects the wide spectrum of traumatic experiences and the complex interactions of trauma with development, personality, family, and social environment. Several of these articles were chosen because they communicate a sense of the subjective experience of traumatic situations and the posttrauma environment.

General Reviews

1. **Figley CR** (ed): *Trauma and Its Wake: The Study and Treatment of Posttraumatic Stress Disorder.* New York, Brunner/Mazel, 1985

   This book represents the first collection of important papers after the introduction of PTSD into the diagnostic classification nosology of DSM-III. The first section contains chapters summarizing the history of the concept of PTSD and theoretical perspectives on the shattering of assumptions and the need for a psychosocial framework. The section on research findings presaged the expanding range of traumatic stress studies. The section on treatment innovations includes important contributions on intergenerational issues among holocaust survivors and their children and the importance of ethnocultural identifications in the readjustment process.

2. *Horowitz MJ: Stress Response Syndromes,* 2nd Edition. Northvale, NJ, Jason Aronson, 1986

This revised text of the scholarly treatise on the interplay of traumatic stress responses and personality styles reviews the theory of phasic responses and their importance to strategies of treatment.

3. *Oldham JM, Riba MB, Tasman A (eds): *American Psychiatric Press Review of Psychiatry*, Vol. 12. Washington, DC, American Psychiatric Press, 1993

    This is a current overview of traumatic stress studies. Chapters address diagnostic issues; a developmental psychopathology model for children and adolescents; ethnocultural considerations in research, assessment, and treatment; the evidence for complimentary neurobiological models of physiological reactivity, neurohormonal responses, and memory processes; an integrated approach to treatment utilizing cognitive-behavioral, psychodynamic, and pharmacological approaches; and the assessment and treatment of rape victims.

4. *Wilson JP, Raphael B: *International Handbook of Traumatic Stress Syndromes*. New York, Plenum, 1993

    This is the most comprehensive volume of current perspectives on the traumatic stress syndromes. Section topics include theoretical and conceptual issues; assessment, methodology, and research strategies; war trauma and civilian violence; disasters of natural and human origins; impact of trauma on children and adolescents; torture, detention, and internment; recovery and treatment; and organizational and social policy issues. Taken together, the contributions in each section represent a multidimensional approach to the evolving issues in the field.

Selected Additional Theoretical and Diagnostic Issues

5. **Brett EA, Ostroff RO:** Imagery and posttraumatic stress disorder: an overview. *Am J Psychiatry* 142:417–424, 1985

    This article reviews the central role of traumatic imagery in clinical theories of PTSD and in shaping other symptomatic responses. It offers a two-dimensional conceptualization of PTSD based on 1) repetitions of trauma-related images, affects, somatic states, and actions; and 2) defensive functioning and argues that PTSD can best be understood and treated as an interplay between these two dimensions.

6. **Cooper AM:** Toward a limited definition of psychic trauma, in *The Reconstruction of Trauma*. Edited by Rothstein A. New York, International Universities Press, 1986, pp. 41–56

This chapter provides an overview of relevant, historical psychoanalytic concepts of psychic trauma, suggesting there is sufficient evidence to adopt a restricted definition of what constitutes traumatic stress. Cooper argues that the presentation of an isolated, uncharacteristic symptom may have a specific traumatic childhood etiology.

7. **Frederick C:** Effects of natural vs. human-induced violence upon victims, in *Evaluation and Change: Services for Survivors.* Edited by Kivens L. Minneapolis, MN, Minneapolis Medical Research Foundation, 1980, pp. 71–75

Based on clinical observations, this chapter proposes a model that emphasizes the importance of human agency in determining the nature of the individual or group experience and the course of traumatic reactions. Frederick addresses how issues of human accountability are central to the understanding and treatment of victims of violence.

8. **Freud S:** Inhibitions, symptoms and anxiety (1926), in *The Standard Edition of the Complete Psychological Works of Sigmund Freud,* Vol. 20. Translated and edited by Strachey J. London, Hogarth Press, 1959, pp. 87–156

This is a core essay in which Freud introduced anxiety as a response to a danger situation, identified the ego as the source of anxiety, and elaborated a developmental schema of internal dangers. The addendum provides an important discussion of traumatic helplessness and the relationship of internal and external dangers. Ways in which mental representations may be modified in subsequent reworking of a traumatic experience are described.

9. **Herman JL, Perry JC, van der Kolk BA:** Childhood trauma in borderline personality disorder. *Am J Psychiatry* 146:490–495, 1989

This article prompted research and clinical attention to the careful assessment of a developmental history of traumatic experiences in patients with this severe personality disorder. It raises questions about the traumatic contribution to the symptom profile, including self-destructive behaviors, the relative risk of exposures within the family environment, and the interaction over time of Axis I and II disorders.

10. **Hocking F:** Extreme environmental stress and its significance for psychopathology. *Am J Psychother* 24:4–26, 1970

Hocking introduced the principle that individual vulnerability factors will exert more influence on stress-related psychopathology up until a certain trauma threshold is reached, beyond which expectable traumatic reactions will be manifested in almost everyone. This article set the stage for the subsequent use of dose-of-exposure designs to study the relative contribution of degree of exposure and prior vulnerability.

11. ***Kardiner A:** Traumatic neuroses of war, in *American Handbook of Psychiatry.* Edited by Arieti S. New York, Basic Books, 1969, pp. 246–257

This chapter introduced the central notions of a "physio-neurosis" and "ego-contraction" secondary to traumatic war exposures. This work laid the conceptual groundwork for including arousal symptoms in PTSD (e.g., exaggerated startle as well as dysregulation of aggression as key symptoms).

12. ***Krystal H:** Trauma and affects. *Psychoanal Study Child* 33:81–116, 1978

This is a major psychoanalytic examination of the course of affective response to trauma, suggesting developmental vulnerabilities that can lead to, among other outcomes, the loss of affective discrimination and alexithymic conditions. It examines the significant effect of childhood trauma on symbolization, fantasy formation, and the capacity to verbalize emotion.

13. **Putnam FW, Guroff JJ, Silberman EK, Barban L, Post RM:** The clinical phenomenology of multiple personality disorder: review of 100 recent cases. *J Clin Psychiatry* 47:285–293, 1986

This article is a clinical descriptive report characterizing the symptom presentation of multiple personality disorder including depression, dissociation, self-destructive behavior, and sexual dysfunction. It provided the first substantive evidence of the prevalence and potential etiologic role of chronic sexual and physical abuse and other types of childhood traumas in this disorder.

14. **van der Kolk BA, van der Hart O:** Pierre Janet and the breakdown of adaption in psychological trauma. *Am J Psychiatry* 146:1530–1540, 1989

This article is a reexamination of the central tenets of Janet's theory of the traumatic influences on cognition and affect, including the origins of state responses that may relate to current concepts of dissociation.

Psychometric Assessment

15. **Blake DD, Weathers F, Nagy LM, Kaloupek DG, Klauminzer G, Charney DS, Keane TM:** A clinician rating scale for assessing current and lifetime PTSD: the CAPS-1. *The Behavior Therapist* 14:187–188, 1991

This article describes the psychometric properties of a widely used, structured, clinician-administered interview for PTSD. The instrument includes both frequency and intensity axes as well as ratings of social and occupational functioning.

16. **Horowitz M, Wilner N, Alvarez W:** Impact of Events Scale: a measure of subjective stress. *Psychosom Med* 41:209–218, 1979

    This presents the first, widely used self-report scale designed specifically to assess the severity of traumatic stress and bereavement reactions. The scale includes subscales of intrusion and avoidance.

17. **Keane TM, Wolfe J, Taylor KL:** Post-traumatic stress disorder: evidence for diagnostic validity and methods of psychological assessment. *J Clin Psychol* 43:32–43, 1987

    This article introduces the importance of a multiaxial approach for the assessment of PTSD, including the use of structured instruments, psychometrics, and psychophysiological procedures. It addresses the issue of comorbidity and of reliable discrimination of PTSD from other diagnoses.

18. **Keane TM, Caddell JM, Taylor KL:** Mississippi Scale for Combat-Related Posttraumatic Stress Disorder: three studies in reliability and validity. *J Consult Clin Psychol* 56:85–90, 1988

    This article presents a scale designed specifically to assess posttraumatic stress reactions after combat exposure and recently revised to include exposure to interpersonal violence. It illustrates the various issues in examining reliability and validity in the measurement of posttraumatic stress reactions.

Neurobiology

19. **Blanchard EB, Kolb LC, Gerardi RJ, Ryan P, Pallmeyer TP:** Cardiac response to relevant stimuli as an adjunctive tool for diagnosing PTSD in Vietnam veterans. *Behavior Therapy* 17:592–606, 1986

    This is a key report documenting potential cardiovascular changes apparent in Vietnam veterans with PTSD compared with control subjects. It introduced the concept that traumatic exposures may affect underlying physiological mechanisms that regulate basic cardiac responses (e.g., heart rate).

20. *Charney DS, Deutch AY, Krystal JH, Southwick SM, Davis M:** Psychobiologic mechanisms of posttraumatic stress disorder. *Arch Gen Psychiatry* 50:294–305, 1993

This current review focuses on the interrelated biological systems that govern fear-enhanced learning, the failure of extinction, neuromechanisms of behavioral sensitization and stress sensitivity, neurochemical effects that may underlie primary symptoms, and the relationship of the hippocampus and amygdala in traumatic remembrances. In each area, both the clinical implications and directions for future research are discussed.

21. **Ornitz EM, Pynoos RS:** Startle modulation in children with posttraumatic stress disorder. *Am J Psychiatry* 146:866–870, 1989

This is the first reported laboratory investigation of startle in PTSD, demonstrating disturbances in inhibitory startle modulation among a small group of children traumatized by extreme violence. It places consideration of the pathogenesis of PTSD within a neurodevelopmental perspective.

22. **Pitman RK, Orr SP, Forgue DF, de Jong JB, Clairborn JM:** Psychophysiologic assessment of posttraumatic stress disorder imagery in Vietnam combat veterans. *Arch Gen Psychiatry* 44:1970–1975, 1987

This is an important laboratory study demonstrating that physiological reactivity to trauma-related imagery can be used to distinguish veterans with and without PTSD, a technique that is being more widely employed in studying various trauma populations. It places physiological studies within a broader context, building on Lang's model of fear and arousal in anxiety disorders.

23. **Yehuda R, Southwick SM, Perry BD, Mason JW, Giller EL:** Interactions of the hypothalamic-pituitary-adrenal axis and the catecholaminergic systems in posttraumatic stress disorders, in *Biological Assessment and Treatment of Posttraumatic Stress Disorder.* Edited by Giller EL Jr. Washington, DC, American Psychiatric Press, 1990, pp. 115–134

This chapter provides a summary of evidence to suggest a specific hormonal profile for PTSD, distinct from depression and perhaps other anxiety disorders. It offers hypotheses regarding enhanced reactivity and feedback within the cortisol and adrenergic neurohormonal systems.

Massive Trauma

24. **Eitinger L:** Concentration camp survivors in the post war world. *Am J Orthopsychiatry* 32:367–375, 1962

This article summarizes a series of studies documenting the significant increased lifetime risk of physical morbidity and psychological impairment among survivors of World War II concentration camps.

25. *Lifton RJ: *Death in Life.* New York, Random House, 1976

This book contains explicit personal accounts of the overwhelming nature and sequelae of trauma experienced by survivors of Hiroshima. It includes the author's concept of the "death imprint" and "psychic numbing" following catastrophic life threat and loss and highlights the special nature of this exposure compared with other types of disasters.

26. **Randall GA, Lutz EL:** *Serving Survivors of Torture: a Practical Manual for Health Professionals and Other Service Providers.* Riverton, NJ, American Association for the Advancement of Science, 1991

This book provides an introduction to the nature and scope of state-sponsored violence, utilizing detailed clinical examples to characterize the physical and psychological abuse and their sequelae. It presents a model of intervention that focuses on the critical role of psychological care within a wider framework of rehabilitation and recovery. Particularly useful is the attention given to the training and support required of mental health professionals in light of the demanding occupational challenges of working with victims of torture.

Combat

27. **Fairbank JA, Hansen DJ, Fitterling JM:** Patterns of appraisal and coping across different stressor conditions among former prisoners of war with and without posttraumatic stress disorder. *J Consult Clin Psychol* 59:274–281, 1991

This study addresses the long-term psychological repercussions of repatriated prisoners of war from World War II. Among those who were found to suffer from PTSD, there was poorer general psychological functioning, less control over memories of World War II, and more frequent use of self-isolation and self-blame in their coping repertoire. The article addresses how the extreme nature of captivity-related events can restrict the range and flexibility of perceptual and behavior responses, promoting a highly practiced, rigid characteristic pattern of maladaptive coping to later stressful life events.

28. **Grinker RR, Spiegel JP:** Men Under Stress. Philadelphia, PA, Blakiston, 1945

This is a classic clinical study of wartime stress response during World War II that provided the first cogent evidence for the importance of frontline psychiatric interventions before maladaptive ego resolution becomes organized. This work highlighted specific types of exposures—for example, witnessing a combat buddy killed or maimed—that carried high risk for severe and chronic reactions and emphasized the importance of reintegration into the group, family, or community for successful adaptation.

29. *Kulka RA, Schlenger WE, Fairbank JA, Hough RL, Jordan BK, Marmar CR, Weiss DS: *Trauma and the Vietnam War Generation.* New York, Brunner/Mazel, 1990

This is the major comprehensive mental health epidemiological study describing the role of exposure, age, sex, gender, ethnicity, the recovery environment, utilization patterns for postwar medical and social services, and physical and psychological symptoms and disabilities. It provides refined measurements of combat exposures and documents significant rates of psychopathology in accordance with degree of exposure.

30. Solomon Z, Weisenberg M, Schwarzwald J, Mikulincer M: Posttraumatic stress disorder among frontline soldiers with combat stress reaction: the 1982 Israeli experience. *Am J Psychiatry* 144:448–454, 1987

This article describes the relationship of acute combat stress reactions among Israeli soldiers to subsequent development of PTSD and includes a discussion of factors that enhance recovery and the role of early intervention.

Disaster

31. *Erikson KT: Disaster at Buffalo Creek: loss of communality at Buffalo Creek. *Am J Psychiatry* 133:302–305, 1976

This article is a sociologist's perspective on the long-term ramifications of a major disaster in disrupting the fabric of community life. Erikson suggests that mental health intervention requires attention to public policy that promotes larger-scale community recovery to secure the recovery of individuals or families.

32. Shore JH, Tatum EL, Vollmer WM: Psychiatric reactions to disaster: the Mount St. Helens experience. *Am J Psychiatry* 143:590–595, 1986

Using a structured diagnostic instrument, Shore et al. found a significant prevalence of disaster-related psychiatric disorders, including depression, generalized anxiety, and posttraumatic stress reactions, with a dose-response pattern among the bereaved, property-loss victims, and those from a nearby, unaffected community.

33. **Ursano RJ, McCarrol JE:** The nature of the traumatic stressors: handling dead bodies. *J Nerv Ment Dis* 178:396–398, 1990

This article describes the mental health risks for rescue workers, pathologists, and other disaster workers after disasters involving multiple deaths and injuries. It indicates the importance of training, experience, and support in reducing the occupational risks.

34. **Weisueth L:** The stressors and the post-traumatic stress syndrome after an industrial disaster. *Acta Psychiatr Scand* 80 (suppl 355):25–37, 1989

This article reports the acute and subacute stress reactions of employees of a factory after an explosion and fire. It documents the high level of posttraumatic anxiety reactions associated with exposure to physical suffering, danger to one's own life, and witnessing death, which depended on the employees' location at the time of the explosion. Exaggerated startle reactions were found to be prominent and a significant early indicator of risk for chronicity. Posttrauma irritability and aggressiveness developed as a common complication and carried important psychosocial consequences.

Interpersonal Violence

35. **Breslau N, Davis GC, Andreski P, Peterson E:** Traumatic events and posttraumatic stress disorder in an urban population of young adults. *Arch Gen Psychiatry* 48:216–222, 1991

This article presents rates of exposure to a variety of traumatic events and the respective frequency of PTSD associated with each. This was the first population study of young urban adults to document the significant frequency of traumatic exposures. Of special note, these researchers found an extremely high rate of chronic PTSD among those reporting a history of rape.

36. *Burgess AW, Holmstrom LL:** Rape trauma syndrome. *Am J Psychiatry* 131:981–986, 1974

This study provided the first comprehensive description of acute postrape reactions and efforts at psychological reorganization. In doing so, it brought needed mental health attention to the incidence of rape and the high risk for severe and chronic posttraumatic stress reactions.

37. **Kilpatrick DG, Best CL, Veronen LJ, Amick AE, Villeponteaux LA, Ruff GA:** Mental health correlates of criminal victimization: a random community survey. *J Consult Clin Psychol* 53:866–873, 1985

This article illustrates the utility of community survey methodology to document the prevalence of exposure to civilian crime and the relationship of psychological reactions to the level of violent threat or injury.

38. **Rothbaum BO, Foa EB, Riggs DS, Murdock T, Walsh W:** A prospective examination of posttraumatic stress disorder in rape victims. *Journal of Traumatic Stress* 5:455–475, 1992

A major, current prospective study following victims of rape from soon after the assault, this initial report demonstrates extremely high rates of PTSD in the acute aftermath. Careful assessment within the first 2 weeks provided key indicators of risk for persistent PTSD, with important implications for the provision of psychological services.

39. **Rynearson EK:** Psychological adjustment to unnatural dying, in *Biopsychosocial Aspects of Bereavement.* Edited by Zisook S. Washington, DC, American Psychiatric Press, 1990, pp. 77–93

Rynearson emphasizes three important aspects of unnatural dying—violence (injury), violation (transgression), and volition (willful intention or negligence)—that affect the course of bereavement among family and peers. The article describes patterns of behavior (e.g., compulsive inquiry) in response to homicide, suicide, or accidental deaths.

Children and Adolescents

40. *****Eth S, Pynoos RS** (eds): *Posttraumatic Stress Disorder in Children.* Washington, DC, American Psychiatric Press, 1985

This book provides a clinical descriptive overview of children who witness the rape, suicide, or homicide of a parent; are exposed to war atrocities; suffer from physical or sexual abuse (including incest); survive natural or human-caused disasters; or recover from life-threatening illnesses and medical procedures.

41. **Hartman CR, Burgess AW:** Sexual abuse of children: causes and consequences, in *Child Maltreatment: Theory and Research on the Causes and Consequences of Child Abuse and Neglect.* Edited by Ciccheti D, Carlson V. New York, Cambridge University Press, 1989, pp. 95–128

This is one of the most comprehensive, selected reviews of child sexual abuse, providing a thoughtful discussion of typologies of traumatic exposures, symptom profile and course, psychodynamic and developmental impact, and treatment approaches.

42. **Kinzie JD, Sack WH, Angell RH, Manson S, Ben R:** The psychiatric effects of massive trauma on Cambodian children: the children. *J Am Acad Child Adolesc Psychiatry* 25:370–376, 1986

Using data from structured interviews by psychiatrists, Kinzie et al. report the psychiatric sequelae for 40 Cambodian high school students in the United States who suffered massive trauma under the Pol Pot regime. They point out the importance of residing with a family member in the recovery process, perhaps through maintaining or reestablishing a sense of family or historical continuity.

43. **Pynoos RS, Frederick C, Nader K, Arroyo W, Steinberg A, Eth S, Nunez F, Fairbanks L:** Life threat and posttraumatic stress in school age children. *Arch Gen Psychiatry* 44:1057–1063, 1987

This is a study of children exposed to a sniper attack at school, demonstrating a dose of exposure correlation between proximity to the violence and degree and type of posttraumatic stress reactions. This article established the utility and reliability of child self-report in the assessment of traumatized children.

44. *Terr LC:* Children of Chowchilla: a study of psychic trauma. *Psychoanal Study Child* 34:547–623, 1979

This is a pioneering, clinical, descriptive report of group findings among kidnapped children that emphasizes similarity of response across age groups and characterizes manifestations of posttraumatic reactions specific to childhood.

45. **Yule W, Williams R:** Posttraumatic stress reactions in children. *Journal of Traumatic Stress* 3:279–295, 1990

This is a report of children who survived a catastrophic ferry boat disaster, documenting the degree of posttraumatic stress and depression. It contains good descriptive material of the children's harrowing experiences and provides a clear discussion of issues of discordance among parent, child, and teacher reports of children's reactions. It also describes approaches to intervention, especially the utility of group therapy among adolescent survivors.

Selected Additional Treatment Issues

46. **Figley CR:** A five-phase treatment of post-traumatic stress disorder in families. *Journal of Traumatic Stress* 1:127–141, 1988

    This article presents a comprehensive approach to family intervention after trauma that incorporates recognition of the changing family dynamics over time. It addresses the implications of exposure of single or multiple members of the family for treatment strategies.

47. **Friedman MJ:** Biological approaches to the diagnosis and treatment of post-traumatic stress disorder. *Journal of Traumatic Stress* 4:67–91, 1991

    This article discusses the psychopharmacological treatment of PTSD in relation to various changes in neurobiological function and efficacy in ameliorating specific symptoms. It includes discussion of the relationship of pharmacotherapy to psychotherapy and alerts the clinician to the increased risk of alcohol, opiate, or other illicit drug use.

48. **Haley SA:** When the patient reports atrocities. *Arch Gen Psychiatry* 30:191–196, 1974

    This article addresses countertransference reactions of the clinician whose patient reports having committed atrocities during wartime. It suggests that proper attention to these reactions is necessary to ensure therapeutic engagement and strongly emphasizes that the clinician must be prepared to hear everything, however horrifying or sad.

49. **Kinzie JD, Fleck J:** Psychotherapy with severely traumatized refugees. *Am J Psychother* 41:82–94, 1987

    This article describes cross-cultural factors affecting psychotherapy, with careful attention to therapeutic issues and strategies that arise when Euro-American therapists treat non-Western refugees with PTSD. It includes illustrative case examples.

50. **Levine H** (ed): *Adult Analysis and Childhood Sexual Abuse*. Hillsdale, NJ, Analytic Press, 1990

    This collection of essays provides excellent discussions of clinical manifestations, impact on ego development, and transference and countertransference issues in the psychodynamic treatment of adults who were sexually abused as children. The detailed case studies clearly illuminate the conceptual discussions.

51. **Lindy JD:** The trauma membrane and other clinical concepts derived from psychotherapeutic work with survivors of natural disasters. *Psychiatric Annals* 15:153–160, 1985

This article describes the central notions of "the trauma membrane"; the recovery environment; primacy of the traumatic event; and its special, often complex, multilayered configuration. It is an excellent introduction to different concepts of guilt and employs these concepts as they pertain to transference and countertransference issues.

52. *Marmar CR, Foy D, Kagan B, Pynoos RS:** An integrated approach for treating posttraumatic stress, in *American Psychiatric Press Review of Psychiatry*, Vol. 12. Edited by Oldham JM, Riba MB, Tasman A. Washington, DC, American Psychiatric Press, 1993, pp. 239–272

This chapter provides a complimentary model of treatment incorporating psychodynamic, cognitive-behavioral, and psychopharmacologic approaches. It suggests guidelines for clinical decision making depending on the intensity of exposure, severity of psychopathology, chronicity of symptoms, frequency of traumatic reminders, and extent of posttrauma adversities.

53. **Pynoos R, Nader K:** Issues in the treatment of post-traumatic stress in children and adolescents, in *The International Handbook of Traumatic Stress Syndromes*. Edited by Wilson JP, Raphael B. New York, Plenum, 1993, pp. 535–549

This chapter proposes a model of types of intervention strategies for children, including psychological first aid; initial consultation; brief family, group, individual, and pharmacologic therapies; planned interventions over future development; and long-term treatment.

54. **Rose DS:** A model for psychodynamic psychotherapy with the Rape victim. *Psychotherapy* 28:85–95, 1991

This article presents a sophisticated model of extended psychodynamic psychotherapy with rape victims, emphasizing a detailed understanding of the traumatic experience and adjustments to the posttrauma environment. It addresses the importance of aggressive fantasies in response to the violence, as manifested in the patient's reenactments, inhibitions, and transference reactions.

55. **Somnier FE, Genefke IK:** Psychotherapy for victims of torture. *Br J Psychiatry* 149:323–329, 1986

This article summarizes the findings from an extensive sample of victims of torture from throughout the world, including in-depth clinical material from one of the major treatment centers, located in Copenhagen. It documents the psychological and physical methods of torture and the impact on victims and offers a conceptual framework for psychotherapy.

Bereavement and Grief

Kathleen Kim, M.D.
Selby Jacobs, M.D.

Normal grief is a process consisting of sadness, longing for the deceased person, somatic complaints, and subsequent recovery. Bereavement is a complex emotional response; it includes components of separation anxiety, mourning, despair, depression, and avoidance that evolve independently over time. On average, grief reaches peak intensity 4–5 months after a loss. However, for many people, grief is still moderately severe 1 year after a loss.

Although the majority of individuals do not suffer adverse consequences following bereavement, a significant minority experience increased morbidity and mortality. The health consequences of bereavement are multiple. These consequences include nonspecific psychological and psychophysiological symptoms; increased help-seeking from health care professionals; and increased morbidity and mortality from cardiovascular diseases, accidents, injuries, suicide, and perhaps other diseases of middle and later life.

The relationship between psychiatric disorders and bereavement is less well documented. According to DSM-IV, major depression can complicate bereavement if certain symptoms are present (i.e., preoccupation with worthlessness, significant functional impairment, and marked psychomotor retardation). Currently, there are no guidelines for diagnosing anxiety disorders in the context of bereavement. Finally, pathological grief does not appear in DSM-IV as the concept is not universally accepted. In addition, there is no current consensus on the criteria for pathological grief. However, most bereavement experts consider pathological grief a failure to resolve the separation distress following a loss. The most common psychiatric complications of bereavement are major depression, anxiety disorders, and pathological grief.

For unresolved grief and depressive syndromes that do not resolve spontaneously, psychotherapy is an effective intervention. For major depression and panic disorder that occur during acute bereavement, pharmacologic interventions are effective. To improve social adjustment, mutual support or self-help groups can be quite helpful.

Bereavement is a well-described response to a conspicuous and severe life stressor. It provides the opportunity to investigate several questions of psychiatric etiology and psychopathology. General theories of emotional distress, such as crisis theory, and brief treatment interventions, such as crisis intervention and brief psychodynamic therapy, are applicable to bereavement. It serves as a model for examining the relationship between stress and mental health and the nature of coping or defenses that may mediate between stress and mental health.

Bereavement can serve as a model for investigating depression, particularly in clarifying the difference between "normal" depressed mood and "clinical" depression. Among the elderly, bereavement may be an important precipitant of late life depression. Furthermore, in a developmental framework, childhood bereavement serves as a paradigm for elucidating the consequences of early life experiences for adult personality functioning and mental health. Finally, bereavement has served as a paradigm in psychiatry for thinking about prevention.

General

1. **Jacobs SC:** *Pathologic Grief: Maladaptation to Loss.* Washington, DC, American Psychiatric Press, 1993

   Jacobs discusses the psychiatric complications of bereavement: major depressions, anxiety disorders, and the concept of pathological grief. He describes the nature of these disorders, criteria for differential diagnosis, and an approach to treatment.

2. **Lewis CS:** *A Grief Observed.* New York, Bantam Books, 1976

3. **Mooney E:** *Alone: Surviving as a Widow.* New York, Putnam, 1981

   These autobiographical accounts of bereavement are useful in understanding the subjective experience of the acutely bereaved. Lewis' book is a modern classic that has a strong religious-philosophical tone rather than a psychological tone. Mooney's work provides the perspective of a widow.

4. *Parkes CM: *Bereavement: Studies of Grief in Adult Life.* New York, International Universities Press, 1972

Parkes is one of the most thorough and creative empirical investigators of grief. In this book, he summarizes the findings of his studies from the 1940s to the 1970s.

5. *Raphael B: *The Anatomy of Bereavement.* New York, Basic Books, 1983

This book is encyclopedic in scope and provides a comprehensive review of modern knowledge about bereavement. It incorporates a summary of Raphael's empirical investigations of the treatment of complicated bereavement, grief in children, and the relationship of trauma to loss.

6. Siggins LD: Mourning: a critical survey of the literature. *Int J Psychoanal* 47:14–25, 1966

This article is a good review of the psychoanalytical literature on bereavement. It incorporates Freud's ideas into the broader framework of subsequent psychoanalytic thought and clarifies that many of Freud's conclusions, such as the idea that ambivalence distinguishes melancholia from mourning, have not been proven over time.

Descriptive/Phenomenological

7. *Futterman EH, Hoffman I, Sabshin M: Parental anticipatory mourning, in *Psychosocial Aspects of Terminal Care.* Edited by Schoenberg B. New York, Columbia University Press, 1972, pp. 243–272

The chapter is the best of several reports on anticipatory grief. It reviews the literature on this concept and summarizes data from a large study done by Futterman et al. Anticipatory grief is no substitute for the actual separation distress that occurs following a loss.

8. *Horowitz MJ, Krupnick J, Kaltreider N, Wilner N, Leong A, Marmar C: Initial psychological response to parental death. *Arch Gen Psychiatry* 38:316–323, 1981

Horowitz et al. conducted the first systematic study of adults who experienced the death of a parent. Despite the lack of a control group, the article provides a useful discussion of the importance and consequences of parental bereavement.

9. *Lindeman E:** Symptomatology and management of acute grief. *Am J Psychiatry* 101:141–148, 1944

   Lindeman's observations on the survivors of the Coconut Grove fire are a classic description of the manifestations of grief. He notes the essential features of grief and describes several manifestations and syndromes associated with severe or unresolved grief. Lindeman provided the first descriptive characterization of pathological grief.

10. **Parkes CM:** The first year of bereavement. *Psychiatry* 33:444–467, 1970

    Parkes summarizes the findings of the first longitudinal study of 22 acutely bereaved widows. The article documents the evolving manifestations of grief over time and interprets them in light of attachment theory.

Epidemiologic

11. *Bornstein PE, Clayton PJ, Halikas JA, Maurice WL, Robins E:** The depression of widowhood after thirteen months. *Br J Psychiatry* 122:561–566, 1973

    Bornstein et al. document that a significant proportion of acutely bereaved persons experience a depressive syndrome during the early phases of grief. These syndromes met the criteria for major depressive disorder, but the majority of bereaved depressed persons did not seek help.

12. *Clayton PJ:** Mortality and morbidity in the first year of widowhood. *Arch Gen Psychiatry* 30:747–750, 1974

    Clayton document that bereaved persons experience significantly more psychological and physical symptoms. Although the bereaved may use general medical services, they do not utilize psychiatric services more often than others. Clayton concludes that mortality is not a risk associated with acute bereavement; this finding, however, is controversial.

Dynamic

13. **Bowlby J:** *Attachment and Loss,* Vols. I–III. New York, Basic Books, 1969

    An expanded account of Bowlby's attachment theory can be found in these three volumes. They are called "Attachment," "Separation," and "Loss," respectively.

14. *Bowlby J: The making and breaking of affectional bonds. *Br J Psychiatry* 130:201–210, 1977

This article is a brief summary of Bowlby's theory that attachment behavior is a type of behavior that is distinct from sexual and aggressive behaviors and is of at least equal significance in human life. Initially, Bowlby's theory was considered novel and controversial, and it is important to consider.

15. Bowlby J: The making and breaking of affectional bonds, II: some principles of psychotherapy. *Br J Psychiatry* 130:421–431, 1977

In a companion article, Bowlby discusses the implications of attachment theory for psychotherapy.

16. *Freud S: Mourning and melancholia (1917[1915]), in *Standard Edition of the Complete Psychological Works of Sigmund Freud,* Vol. 14. Translated and edited by Strachey J. London, Hogarth Press, 1957, pp. 237–258

This essay is a seminal work on grief and depression. In Freud's view, depression or melancholia is distinguished from mourning by ambivalence and, when a separation occurs, the internalization of interpersonal conflict between the two persons. In addition, Freud develops the psychoanalytical hypothesis that loss may cause depression in vulnerable persons through anger turned inward.

Childhood Loss

17. *Lloyd C: Life events and depressive disorder reviewed, I: events as predisposing factors. *Arch Gen Psychiatry,* 37:529–535, 1980

Lloyd reviews several studies of childhood loss of parents. He finds that the preponderance of data indicate that such losses increase the risk of depression in adulthood by two to three times. Parental loss in childhood also is associated with more severe depressive episodes and perhaps suicidal gestures. Trends in these studies suggest that the loss of a mother in early childhood and the loss of a father for girls in later childhood are particularly salient. Contrasting findings to this article are discussed by Tennant et al. (1980) below.

18. Silverman PR, Worden JW: Children's reactions in the early months after the death of a parent. *Am J Orthopsychiatry* 62:93–104, 1992

This article is one of the first to document the manifestations of bereavement in adolescents systematically. It complements Weller et al. (1991) below.

19. **Tennant C:** Parental loss in childhood. *Arch Gen Psychiatry* 45:1045–1050, 1988

In an editorial, Tennant emphasizes the protective importance of alternative nurturance for children who lose a parent.

20. **Tennant C, Bebbington P, Hurry J:** Parental death in childhood and risk of adult depressive disorders: a review. *Psychol Med* 10:289–299, 1980

Tennant et al. review the literature on the long-term risks of depressive disorder for children who suffer parental death. They carefully address methodological issues and the conceptual distinction between help-seeking behavior and illness occurrence. They conclude that long-term consequences are small.

21. **Weller RA, Weller EB, Fristad MA, Bowes JM:** Depression in recently bereaved prepubertal children. *Am J Psychiatry* 148:1536–1540, 1991

Weller et al. describe one of the first systematic studies of grief in children. The article documents that depressive symptoms and other manifestations of grief are common. Longitudinal follow-up of this sample will provide an idea of the risk of acute complications of bereavement in children.

Biological

22. **Bartrop RW, Luckhurst E, Lazarus L, Kiloh LG, Penny R:** Depressed lymphocyte function after bereavement. *Lancet* 1:834–836, 1977

This study is the first report of altered functioning of one component of the immune system—that is, the depressed response of T-lymphocytes to mitogens during acute bereavement. The depressed T-lymphocyte response is apparently not caused by hormonal changes. The immune system is now receiving considerable attention as a key mediator between stressful experiences and diseases that have an immunological basis.

23. *Hofer MA, Wolff CT, Friedman SB, Mason JW:** A psychoendocrine study of bereavement, parts I and II. *Psychosom Med* 4:481–491, 492–504, 1972

This two-part article reports on a study of 17-hydroxycorticosteroid excretion rates and the process of mourning of parents following the death of their children from leukemia. This study was conducted during the period of acute mourning. The style and effectiveness of ego defenses, which had been important in predicting levels of adrenocortical hormone excretion before the death of the child, did not prove to be determinants of adrenocortical function during bereavement.

24. **Irwin M, Weiner H:** Depressive symptoms and immune function during bereavement, in *Biopsychosocial Aspects of Bereavement.* Edited by Zisook S. Washington, DC, American Psychiatric Press, 1987, pp. 159–174

Irwin and Weiner review the relationship between depression and immune system functioning during bereavement. They summarize findings from animal research as well as studies of depressed patients. They postulate that immune system changes occur and account for an increase in infectious, neoplastic, or autoimmune diseases among bereaved individuals.

25. **Kim K, Jacobs S:** Neuroendocrine changes following bereavement, in *Handbook of Bereavement.* Edited by Stroebe MS, Stroebe W, Hansson RO. New York, Cambridge University Press, 1993, pp. 143–159

This chapter is a comprehensive review of the literature on neuroendocrine changes during bereavement. It briefly summarizes studies of the psychiatric complications of bereavement, the basic concepts of the neuroendocrine system and stress research, neuroendocrine findings in depression and anxiety disorders, and neuroendocrine studies of bereavement.

26. **Reite M, Field T** (eds): *The Psychobiology of Attachment and Separation.* New York, Academic Press, 1985

There has been increasing attention paid to the biological aspects of bereavement in the past 20 years, which may be a reflection that attachment behavior is a fundamental behavior in humans. This edited volume summarizes the literature in this area. The information from studies of primates and other social animals suggests that the prefrontal cortex, the amygdala, and the limbic system, as well as estrogen, oxytocin, and peptide transmitter systems, are involved in attachment and separation behavior.

27. **Reynolds CF, Hoch CC, Buysse DJ, Houck PR, Schlernitzauer M, Frank E, Mazumdar S, Kupfer DJ:** Electroencephalographic sleep in spousal bereavement and bereavement-related depression of late life. *Biol Psychiatry* 31:69–82, 1992

This study demonstrates that the changes in sleep physiology observed in major depression are also observed in bereaved, depressed persons but not those who are bereaved and have no depression. These changes include lower sleep efficiency, more early morning awakening, shorter rapid eye movement (REM) latency, greater percentage of REM sleep, and lower rates of delta wave generation in the first non-REM period. The changes were associated with depressive aspects of bereavement and not with separation distress in the absence of depression, suggesting that the underlying anatomical and physiological substrates of separation distress are independent from that of depression. This study is the first to study sleep physiology during bereavement, and future work of this kind promises to clarify the nature of the depressions of bereavement.

28. **Wolff CT, Friedman SB, Hofer MA, Mason JW:** Relationship between psychological defenses and mean urinary 17-hydroxycorticosteroid excretion rates, I: a predictive study of parents of fatally ill children. *Psychosom Med* 26:576–591, 1964

This was the first neuroendocrine study of parents of fatally ill children. The children were dying of leukemia. The authors measured the parents' urinary 17-hydroxycorticosteroid excretion rates, ego defenses, and the effectiveness of their ego defenses. The style and effectiveness of ego defenses were important predictors of the levels of adrenocortical hormone excretion.

Pathological Grief

29. **Bowlby J:** Pathological mourning and childhood mourning. *J Am Psychoanal Assoc* 11:500–541, 1963

Bowlby summarizes four variants of pathological grief in psychodynamic terms. He discusses these variants in relationship to childhood mourning and emphasizes the similarity between pathological and childhood mourning.

30. **Cavenar JO, Nash JL, Maltbie AA:** Anniversary reactions masquerading as manic-depressive illness. *Am J Psychiatry* 134:1273–1276, 1977

Cavenar et al. provide a brief, excellent review of the literature on anniversary phenomena; they describe several clinical examples of anniversary reactions that masquerade as affective disorders. Severe anniversary reactions are one manifestation of pathological grief.

31. *Horowitz M:** Stress response syndromes. *Arch Gen Psychiatry* 31:768–781, 1974

Horowitz characterizes the emotional response to loss and other traumatic experiences as a stress response syndrome and discusses variations related to personality style. He illustrates the application of this theory in the brief, focal, dynamic psychotherapy of persons undergoing a stressful experience. Horowitz emphasizes that many losses are traumatic and that bereavement includes traumatic distress.

32. Horowitz M: *Stress Response Syndromes.* New York, Jason Aronson, 1976

This book provides an expanded account of Horowitz's work on stress response syndromes, including an approach to diagnosis.

33. Horowitz M: *Personality Styles and Brief Psychotherapy.* New York, Basic Books, 1984

This book provides an expanded version of Horowitz's theory of personality style as well as his approach to brief dynamic psychotherapy.

34. Parkes CM: The psychosomatic effects of bereavement, in *Modern Trends in Psychosomatic Medicine.* Edited by Hill O. London, Butterworth, 1970, pp. 71–80

Many clinical studies have investigated the etiological role of loss in the occurrence of several "psychosomatic" disorders, and many claims have been made about the importance of loss in illnesses such as cancer, ulcerative colitis, and asthma. Parkes reviews the literature critically and raises skepticism about the claims of anecdotal clinical cases and uncontrolled reports.

Treatment

35. Pasternak RE, Reynolds CF, Schlernitzauer M, Hoch CC, Buysse DJ, Houck PR, Perel JM: Acute open-trial nortriptyline therapy of bereavement-related depression in late life. *J Clin Psychiatry* 52:307–310, 1991

Pasternak et al. report on an open trial of a tricyclic antidepressant in bereaved elderly persons with major depression. They found, similar to an earlier open trial, that the antidepressant affected the depressive symptoms but did not affect the manifestations of severe separation distress. This finding suggests that both psychotropic drugs and psychotherapy may be necessary for some bereaved patients.

36. Raphael B: Preventive intervention with the recently bereaved. *Arch Gen Psychiatry* 34:1950–1954, 1977

Raphael describes a well-designed prospective, controlled study of psychodynamically oriented crisis intervention for recently bereaved persons. She found a significant lowering of morbidity in the intervention group 13 months after the loss. The bibliography is a good introduction to the treatment literature.

Psychosomatic Medicine

M. Philip Luber, M.D.
Milton Viederman, M.D.

E very culture throughout history has held theories about the relationships between psyche and soma, between psychological experience and physical functioning. Many religious cultures have viewed this as the relationship of the transcendent spirit or soul to the material body. Modern scientific inquiry has struggled to go beyond the Cartesian separation of mind and body to study the complex interrelationships between conscious and unconscious mental processes, the structure of the brain and the peripheral nervous system, neuroendocrine and neuroimmune connections, and the functioning of the various organ systems of the body.

The field of modern psychosomatic medicine developed as a challenge to the narrow biomedical model of disease dominant in the late 19th century. Epitomized by infectious disease, that model conceived of illness as the result of exposure to a specific noxious pathogen. A more complex view began to emerge from the pioneering physiological work of Bernard and Cannon. These researchers emphasized the need of the organism to maintain an internal state of homeostasis and to adapt to threats, both external and internal, to it. Earlier in this century, Wolff, Dunbar, and Alexander attempted to characterize the impact of psychological phenomena on the individual's physiological homeostasis. Wolff established psychophysiological correlations emphasizing bodily changes specific to the nature of aroused affect. Dunbar attempted to correlate certain personality constellations with the propensity to develop certain illnesses. Alexander postulated that specific unconscious conflicts led to specific diseases, the so-called Chicago Seven: duodenal ulcer, ulcerative colitis, bronchial asthma, neurodermatitis, essential hypertension, rheumatoid arthritis, and thyrotoxicosis. Although Alexander acknowledged the role of (unspecified) genetic and physiological factors in illness, in many quarters the search for specificity led to a unicausal psychogenic model of illness as naive and limited as the biomedical model that preceded it.

Focusing on a different aspect of the maintenance of homeostasis, a number of prominent investigators, including Rose, Mason, Sachar, and Stein, elucidated neuroendocrine and neuroimmune underpinnings of the organism's response to stress. Other investigators have focused on the nature of the nonspecific and specific stressors (including "life-events" and physical illness), individual styles of psychological coping and adaptation to them, and their effects on physiological functioning and development of disease.

The leading paradigm in the field today, Engel's biopsychosocial model, attempts to account for the complex interplay of biological, psychological, and social factors in the development and course of all illness, not just a small group of so-called psychosomatic or psychophysiological ones. This conceptualization is one reason why the discrete group of psychophysiologic disorders of DSM-II did not appear in DSM-III or DSM-III-R. In DSM-IV, the category of "Psychological Factors Affecting Medical Condition" has been broadened to include factors that interfere with treatment and factors that constitute health risks to the individual. Subtypes are provided that allow specification of the particular type of psychological factor involved (i.e., mental disorder, psychological symptom, personality traits or coping style, maladaptive health behaviors, and stress-related physiological response. Recent work in the field tends to avoid oversimplified, linear, cause-and-effect models and investigates in detail particular components of the complex, multifactorial interaction of physical and psychosocial elements in the initiation, precipitation, and development of disease processes and illness behavior.

Examples of many of these approaches are incorporated in the following bibliography. Included are classic articles in the field, more general review articles that summarize the state of the literature, and the most recent findings about specific disease entities.

General References

1. *Engel GL:* The need for a new medical model: a challenge for biomedicine. *Science* 196:129–136, 1977

2. **Engel GL:** How much longer must medicine's science be bound by a seventeenth century world view? *Psychother Psychosom* 57:3–16, 1992

The first article is a classic presenting the biopsychosocial model; the second is a recent update by the author. Engel provides a convincing critique of the reductionistic, unicausal thinking of the traditional biomedical model. The recent paper emphasizes how unscientific it is to dismiss as unscientific the data of the human clinical encounter.

3. **Fava GA:** The concept of psychosomatic disorder. *Psychother Psychosom* 58:1–12, 1992

The clinical concepts related to the assessment of psychosocial factors in the medically ill are reviewed, with particular reference to DSM-III-R diagnostic categories.

4. **Kellner R:** *Psychosomatic Syndromes and Somatic Symptoms.* Washington, DC, American Psychiatric Press, 1991

This is a practical review of the literature and guide to management of medical complaints without definitive organic pathology, including fibromyalgia, chronic fatigue syndrome, nonulcer dyspepsia, irritable bowel syndrome, and various chronic pain syndromes.

5. **Kleinman A:** *The Illness Narratives: Suffering, Healing, and the Human Condition.* New York, Basic Books, 1988

This is a wide-ranging investigation showing the different ways patients, doctors, and cultures organize and construct meanings about common somatic complaints. It provides a fascinating account of how individuals and societies devise acceptable ways to categorize and express physical and emotional pain.

6. **Nemiah JC, Freyberger H, Sifneos PE:** Alexithymia: a view of the psychosomatic process, in *Modern Trends in Psychosomatic Medicine.* Edited by Hill OW. London, Butterworth, 1976, pp. 430–439

This chapter is a concise presentation of the controversial and now popular concept of alexithymia.

7. **Reiser MF:** *Mind, Brain, Body: Toward a Convergence of Psychoanalysis and Neurobiology.* New York, Basic Books, 1984

This book is one of the most sophisticated attempts to integrate psychological and biological data by one of the most thoughtful researchers in the field, known for his critique of both the "brainless" and the "mindless" theories in the field.

8. **Hammer JS, Strain JJ, Lewin C, Easton M, Mayou R, Smith GC, Huyse F, Lyons J, Malt U, Himelein C, Kurosawa H:** The continuing evolution and update of a literature database for consultation-liaison psychiatry: MICRO-CARES Literature Search System 1993. *Gen Hosp Psychiatry* 15 (suppl):1–73, 1993

   This is the most recent update of the extensive literature database on consultation-liaison psychiatry developed by Strain et al. It is also available in software form for personal computers. It is invaluable to any student in the field, whether searching for core articles or a larger bibliography.

9. **Weiner H:** *Psychobiology and Human Disease.* New York, Elsevier North-Holland, 1977

   This classic work reviews all of the available data pertinent to the "psychosomatic diseases" of Alexander, now including epidemiology, genetics, social factors, psychological factors, and early environmental factors. It focuses on the heterogeneity of all of these diseases, the multiple influences that go to create them, and the special problems of methodology in attempting to elucidate causes. A reference text, particularly useful in conjunction with the author's more recent articles, is provided.

Stress, Coping, and Adaptation

10. **Breznitz S:** The seven kinds of denial, in *The Denial of Stress.* Edited by Breznitz S. New York, International Universities Press, 1983, pp. 257–280

    This is a microscopic analysis that studies the various components of what is usually lumped together as the denial of illness.

11. **Cannon WB:** Stresses and strains of homeostasis. *Am J Med Sci* 189:1–14, 1935

    This is a classic and extremely well-written article describing bodily homeostasis as an adaptive process. Although focused entirely on physiology, it reveals a brilliant and imaginative mind attempting to understand bodily processes.

12. **Coelho G, Hamburg D, Adams J** (eds): *Coping and Adaptation.* New York, Basic Books, 1974

13. *****Monat A, Lazarus RS:** *Stress and Coping: An Anthology.* New York, Columbia University Press, 1977

These two excellent older anthologies of previously published articles cover a wide array of topics, including a discussion of the impact of psychological stress on the development of disease, the role of cognition and coping processes in emotion, and modes of adaptation and defense as they affect behavior. These are excellent source books for those interested in stress.

14. **Edwards JR, Cooper CL:** Research in stress, coping, and health: theoretical and methodological issues. *Psychol Med* 18:15–20, 1988

    This article is a concise summary of problems of definition and research strategies in the burgeoning field of stress, coping, and health.

15. **Elliott GR, Eisdorfer C** (eds): *Stress and Human Health: Analysis and Implications of Research.* New York, Springer, 1982

16. **Zales MR** (ed): *Stress in Health and Disease.* New York, Brunner/Mazel, 1985

    These are two excellent collections of essays on the relationship of stress to health and illness, with contributions by many of the top investigators in the field.

17. **Holmes TH:** Development and application of a quantitative measure of magnitude of life change. *Psychiatr Clin North Am* 2:289–306, 1979

    This article is an exposition by one of the founders (with Rahe) of the life-stress methodology. The Social Readjustment Rating Scale is described as are ancillary scales, such as Seriousness of Illness Rating Scale.

18. **Taylor SE, Lichtman RR, Wood JV:** Attributions, beliefs about control, and adjustment to breast cancer. *J Pers Soc Psychol* 46:489–502, 1984

    The authors' research leads them to contend that adjustment to cancer is not related to accurate knowledge of the disease and prognosis, but rather to a sense of control, even if based on "illusions."

19. **Vaillant GE, Vaillant CO:** Natural history of male psychologic health: effects of mental health on physical health. *N Engl J Med* 301:1249–1254, 1979

    A piece of the larger prospective study (published as *Adaptation to Life*) of college-age men followed for four decades, showing that good mental health as an independent variable protects against deterioration in physical health in adult life.

Animal Models of Disease

20. *Hofer MA:** Animal models in the understanding of human disease. *Psychiatr Clin North Am* 2:211–226, 1979

This is a thoughtful discussion of the application of animal models of disease to human beings.

21. **Weiner H:** From simplicity to complexity (1950–1990): the case of peptic ulceration, II: animal studies. *Psychosom Med* 53:491–516, 1991

This is a detailed review of studies on the formation of gastric erosions in rats, clarifying the role of gastric acid secretions; body temperature; secretion of thyrotropin-releasing hormone, corticotropin-releasing factor, and other peptides; and feedback mechanisms of the vagus nerve.

Developmental Models of Disease

22. **Dowling S:** Seven infants with esophageal atresia: a developmental study. *Psychoanal Study Child* 32:215–256, 1977

This is an elegant study of the critical aspects of early care on later ego development in children with esophageal atresia.

23. **Engel G, Schmale A:** Conservation withdrawal: a primary regulatory process for organismic homeostasis, in *Physiology, Emotion and Psychosomatic Illness.* Edited by Hill D. New York, Elsevier, 1972, pp. 57–75

This is a careful theoretical discussion of the concept of conservation withdrawal with description of the historical origin of the concept in the first observations of Engel's famous patient, Monica.

24. *Hofer MA:** Toward a developmental basis for disease predisposition: the effects of early maternal separation on brain, behavior, and cardio-vascular system, in *Brain, Behavior and Bodily Disease.* Edited by Weiner H, Hofer M, Stunkard A. New York, Raven, 1981, pp. 209–228

25. **Hofer MA:** Some thoughts on the "Transduction of Experience" from a developmental perspective. *Psychosom Med* 44:19–28, 1982

These two articles show the author's rigorous approach to problems in research methodology, including the intricate relationship between experimental design and theory formation.

Specificity

26. **Alexander F, French TM, Pollock GH:** *Psychosomatic Specificity.* Chicago, IL, University of Chicago Press, 1968

This book is a definitive statement of the early psychoanalytic viewpoint as expounded by Alexander that focuses on the role of specific unconscious conflicts in the genesis of specific "psychosomatic diseases."

27. *Engel GL, Schmale AH Jr:** Psychoanalytic theory of somatic disorder. *J Am Psychoanal Assoc* 15:344–365, 1967

In this thoughtful discussion of the relationship between conversion reactions and physiological changes, the authors discuss the issue of specificity and conceptualize somatopsychic-psychosomatic interaction, emphasizing a multiplicity of reciprocal interactions that include the predisposing biological factors present at birth. They discuss the significance of the disease onset situation and the "giving up—given up" complex as a nonspecific onset condition.

28. **Weiner H:** Specificity and specification: two continuing problems in psychosomatic research. *Psychosom Med* 54:567–587, 1992

This article is a detailed review of methodological problems in assessing the impact of specific and nonspecific psychosocial variables in different disease entities and subgroups.

Body Image

29. **Druss RG:** Changes in body image following breast augmentation. *International Journal of Psychoanalytic Psychotherapy* 2:248–256, 1973

This is an interesting article that runs counter to the view that low self-esteem related to dissatisfaction with body form is necessarily resistant to change with surgery.

30. **Kolb LC:** Disturbances of the body-image, in *American Handbook of Psychiatry*, 2nd Edition, Vol. 4. Edited by Arieti S. New York, Basic Books, 1975, pp. 810–837

This is a broad perspective on body image as it pertains to physical abnormalities and manifest changes in the body.

31. **Schilder P:** *The Image and Appearance of the Human Body.* New York, International Universities Press, 1950

Schilder provides a classic study of the mental representation of the body incorporating both neurological and psychodynamic perspectives.

Psychoimmunology and Psychoendocrinology

32. *Ader R, Felten D, Cohen N (eds): *Psychoneuroimmunology*, 2nd Edition. San Diego, CA, Academic Press, 1991

This book is an encyclopedic, up-to-date reference with detailed, technical discussions grouped under four headings: neurochemical links between the nervous and immune systems; neuroendocrine-immune system interactions; behavior-immune system interactions; and psychosocial factors, stress, disease, and immunity.

33. **Riley V:** Psychoendocrine influences on immunocompetence and neoplasia. *Science* 212:1100–1109, 1981

In this elegant study, Riley demonstrates that stress in animals leads to adrenocortical hyperplasia and thymic involution, making the animals more susceptible to takes of transplanted neoplastic tissue.

34. **Stein M, Miller AH, Trestman RL:** Depression, the immune system, and health and illness. *Arch Gen Psychiatry* 48:171–177, 1991

This article is a concise review of the literature on the relationship between depression, the immune system, and health, with a methodological critique that particularly highlights the limitations of "fishing-expedition" type research that is not focused on specific questions to be answered by specific research techniques.

35. **Tennes K:** The role of hormones in mother-infant transactions, in *The Development of Attachment and Affiliative Systems*. Edited by Emde RN, Harn RJ. New York, Plenum, 1982, pp. 75–80

This is an elegant study of the impact of 2 hours separation from their mothers on 1-year-old infants in terms of emotional arousal and cortisol excretion rates.

36. **Wolff CT, Friedman SB, Hofer MA, Mason JW:** Relationship between psychological defenses and mean urinary 17-hydroxycorticosteroid excretion rates, I: a predictive study of parents of fatally ill children. *Psychosom Med* 26:576–591, 1964

This is the classic study of the parents of leukemic children in which correlations are established between failing defenses and higher 17-hydroxycorticosteroid levels.

Specific Disease Entities

Asthma

37. **Knapp PH:** The asthmatic and his environment. *J Nerv Ment Dis* 149:133–151, 1969

This is an excellent review article on the data pertinent to psychosocial factors in asthma by one of the pioneering researchers in this area.

38. **Strunk RC, Mrazek DA, Wolfson Fuhrmann GSW, LaBrecque JF:** Physiologic and psychological characteristics associated with deaths due to asthma in childhood: a case controlled study. *JAMA* 254:1193–1198, 1985

This case-controlled study revealed eight characteristics, four of them psychological, associated with death in childhood asthmatics. Degree of psychological factors in the precipitation of acute events was not correlated with risk of death, but conflicts of the child's parents with hospital staff over medical management, self-care inappropriate to age, depressive symptoms, and disregard of asthmatic symptoms were.

Cardiovascular Disease

39. **Berkman LF, Leo-Summers L, Horwitz RI:** Emotional support and survival after myocardial infarction: a prospective, population-based study of the elderly. *Ann Intern Med* 117:1003–1009, 1992

Emotional support after myocardial infarction was independently related to risk of death in the subsequent 6 months. Patients who had no one on whom to rely for emotional support had twice the risk of death compared with those with two or more sources of support.

40. **Booth-Kewley S, Friedman H:** Psychological predictors of heart disease: a quantitative review. *Psychol Bull* 101:343–362, 1987

41. **Dembroski TM, MacDougall JM, Costa PT Jr, Grandits GA:** Components of hostility as predictors of sudden death and myocardial infarction in the Multiple Risk Factor Intervention Trial. *Psychosom Med* 51:514–522, 1989

These two studies are part of a growing body of evidence that the "Type A" paradigm is too diffuse and requires more specification of its core elements. Booth-Kewley and Friedman used meta-analysis to review three decades of research and found depression and hostility as well as

Type A behavior associated with coronary heart disease. Dembroski et al.'s analysis of the Multiple Risk Factor Intervention Trial data shows that an antagonistic interactional style rather than global Type A behavior is an independent risk factor for coronary heart disease.

42. **DiBona GF:** Stress and sodium intake in neural control of renal function in hypertension. *Hypertension* 17 (suppl III):2–6, 1991

In this good example of the demystification of the effect of psychological factors on physical illness, the author summarizes what is known about the effect of emotional stress on central nervous system opioid peptides that in turn modulate renal function alterations (antidiuresis, antinatriuresis, and renal vasoconstriction), which in turn contribute to the initiation, development, and maintenance of the hypertensive process.

43. **Friedman M, Thorenson CE, Gill JJ, Ulmer D, Powell LH, Price VA, Brown B, Thompson L, Rabin DO, Breall WS, Bourg E, Levy R, Dixon T:** Alteration of Type A behavior and its effect on cardiac recurrences in post-myocardial infarction patients: summary results of the Recurrent Coronary Prevention Project. *Am Heart J* 112:653–665, 1986

This study shows the important therapeutic implications of the Type A constellation, despite the conceptual limitations noted above. Of 1,013 postmyocardial-infarction patients studied for 4.5 years, those who received specific counseling to reduce Type A behavior had a significantly lower incidence of recurrence or death compared with those who did not receive such counseling.

44. **Hackett TP, Cassem NH, Wishnie HA:** The coronary care unit: an appraisal of its psychologic hazards. *N Engl J Med* 279:1365–1370, 1968

In this classic article, denial of anxiety is correlated with a decrease of morbidity and mortality of patients with acute myocardial infarction.

45. **Sloan RP, Bigger JT Jr:** Biobehavioral factors in Cardiac Arrhythmia Pilot Study (CAPS): review and examination. *Circulation* 83 (suppl II):52–57, 1991

This study found that Type B behavior, depression, and reduced heart rate reactivity were associated with increased clinical events. The authors hypothesize that this increase is mediated by diminished vagal tone.

Cerebrovascular Disorders

46. **Starkstein S, Robinson R:** Affective disorders and cerebral vascular disease. *Br J Psychiatry* 154:170–182, 1989

47. **Starkstein SE, Cohen BS, Fedoroff P, Parikh RM, Price TR, Robinson RG:** Relationship between anxiety disorders and depressive disorders in patients with cerebrovascular injury. *Arch Gen Psychiatry* 47:246–251, 1990

    These two articles provide a concise overview of findings about the incidence of depression and anxiety after a cerebrovascular accident and their correlation with the site of the lesion and preexisting brain dysfunction.

Diabetes Mellitus

48. **Clouse RE, Lustman R, Reidel W:** Correlation of esophageal motility abnormalities with neuropsychiatric status in diabetes. *Gastroenterology* 90:1146–1154, 1986

    The authors' careful study revealed that autonomic dysfunction resulting in motility abnormalities previously thought to be largely secondary to neuropathy were in fact more highly correlated with psychiatric disorder. Of diabetic patients with depressive or anxiety disorders, 87% had contraction abnormalities independent of neuropathy effects.

49. **Hinkle LE, Wolf SA:** Summary of experimental evidence relating life stress to diabetes mellitus. *Journal of Mt Sinai Hospital* 19:537–570, 1952

    This is an excellent older study with a thoughtful discussion of the issue of stress and carbohydrate metabolism across the life span of individuals with diabetes.

50. **Schwartz L, Coulson L, Toovy D, Lyons J, Flaherty JA:** Biopsychosocial treatment approach to the management of diabetes mellitus. *Gen Hosp Psychiatry* 13:19–26, 1991

    The authors demonstrate correlations between recent life stressful events and worsening of blood glucose control, between a decrease in social support and longer-term worsening of glucose control, and between an external locus of control and both short- and long-term control of blood glucose.

Gastrointestinal Disease

51. **Creed F, Gutrie E:** Psychological factors in the irritable bowel syndrome. *Gut* 28:1307–1318, 1987

    This study found an incidence of over 40% of psychiatric disorder in a series of patients with irritable bowel syndrome. The authors distinguish between patients who develop abdominal symptoms and psychiatric symptoms concurrently and those in which the primary psychiatric disorder leads to an increase in illness behavior with preoccupation with bowel symptoms.

52. **Drossman DA, Leserman J, Nachman G, Zhiming L, Gluck H, Toomey TC, Mitchell CM:** Sexual and physical abuse in women with functional or organic gastrointestinal disorders. *Ann Intern Med* 113:828–833, 1990

    This important clinical study demonstrates the high incidence of a history of sexual and/or physical abuse in women with "functional" gastrointestinal disorders as well as chronic abdominal and pelvic pain and multiple surgeries.

53. **Engel GL:** Psychological aspects of gastrointestinal disorders, in *American Handbook of Psychiatry*, 2nd Edition, Vol. 4. Edited by Arieti S. New York, Basic Books, 1975, pp. 653–692

    This is an excellent summary chapter on the wide array of gastrointestinal diseases. The physiological data are dated, but the discussion of psychosocial points of view remains unmatched.

54. **Helzer JE, Chammas S, Norland CC, Stillings WA, Alpers DH:** A study of the association between Crohn's and psychiatric illness. *Gastroenterology* 86:324–330, 1984

    Using a control group of patients with other chronic medical illness, the authors found a 50% incidence of frank psychiatric disorder in patients with Crohn's disease, including a 36% incidence of depression.

55. **Karush A, Daniels GE, Flood C, O'Connor JF:** *Psychotherapy in Chronic Ulcerative Colitis*. Philadelphia, PA, WB Saunders, 1977

    This book places ulcerative colitis patients in different categories based on psychopathology and psychodynamic constellations with different recommendations for psychotherapy.

56. **Mirsky IA:** Physiologic, psychologic and social determinants in the etiology of duodenal ulcer. *American Journal of Digestive Disorders* 3:285–314, 1958

57. *Weiner HM, Thaler M, Reiser MF, Mirsky IA: Etiology of duodenal ulcer, I: relation of specific psychological characteristics to rate of gastric secretion (serum pepsinogen). *Psychosom Med* 19:1–10, 1957

These are two articles from the classic study of army inductees correlating psychological traits and postulated unconscious conflicts with serum pepsinogen levels and duodenal ulcer disease.

58. North CS, Clouse RE, Spitznagel EL, Alpers DH: The relation of ulcerative colitis to psychiatric factors: a review of findings and methods. *Am J Psychiatry* 147:974–981, 1990

The authors reviewed 138 studies and found serious flaws in the research design of most of them (lack of control subjects, unspecified methods of data collection, absence of diagnostic criteria). Seven studies without such flaws revealed no association between ulcerative colitis and psychiatric factors.

59. Walker EA, Roy-Byrne PP, Katon WJ, Li L, Amos D, Jiranek G: Psychiatric illness and irritable bowel syndrome: a comparison with inflammatory bowel disease *Am J Psychiatry* 147:1656–1661, 1990

This study found a significantly higher incidence of psychiatric disorders (lifetime diagnoses of major depression, somatization disorder, generalized anxiety disorder, and panic and phobic disorders) and medically unexplained somatic symptoms in patients with irritable bowel syndrome compared with those with inflammatory bowel disease.

60. *Weiner H: From simplicity to complexity (1950–1990): the case of peptic ulceration, I: human studies. *Psychosom Med* 53:467–490, 1991

This is a comprehensive and critical review of 40 years of research on human subjects. The article emphasizes the movement from simplistic, linear cause-and-effect theories to more complex models taking into account heterogeneity, both physiological (e.g., seven genetically distinct forms of pepsinogen) and psychological (e.g., variable individual coping with "objective" external stressors).

28

Suicide

John T. Maltsberger, M.D.

"Know thyself, presume not God to scan," declared Alexander Pope; "The proper study of mankind is man." The study of suicide is the study of "mankind" at a concentrated moment uniquely human: the deliberate choice between life and death.

What you will find here is a selection of papers on suicide, mostly with specific clinical reference. They offer the necessary perspective for understanding the basic psychopathology and should help the reader plan treatment and management intelligently. A patient bent on suicide cannot be understood from the perspective of an hour's interview, however. One's arrival at that brink is more than the manifestation of some diagnosis of a mental illness. The capacity to contemplate the future, to form a judgment on its hopefulness or its horrors, and to decide whether to be, or not to be, belongs to our species alone. Suicidology lies as close to the humanities as it does to science; in science, it extends into psychology, psychiatry, psychoanalysis, medicine, anthropology, and biology, to name a few of the disciplines where its roots grow.

Clinicians have a specific clinical task to perform and perforce must approach despairing patients from a specific (necessarily constricted) perspective. These references were chosen to help those who assess, manage, treat, and plan for suicidal patients. They have been arranged in five sections: 1) general background, 2) suicide risk assessment, 3) understanding, 4) treatment, and 5) aftermath.

General Background

1. **Barraclough B, Bunch J, Nelson B, Sainsbury P:** A hundred cases of suicide: clinical aspects. *Br J Psychiatry* 125:355–373, 1974

   This paper makes the point that most of the people who commit suicide suffer from major mental illness. It discusses their personalities and their patterns of suicide communication and forms a trio with Dorpat and Ripley (1960) and Pfeffer et al. (1986), both below.

2. **Colt GH:** *The Enigma of Suicide.* New York, Summit Books, 1991

   This is the best suicide book for general readers in English. Encyclopedic in scope (it addresses history, range, prevention, "the right to die," and the survivor experience, among other subjects), it is not technical but highly absorbing and very well written. It is the best book for the broad overview.

3. **Dorpat TL, Ripley HS:** A study of suicide in the Seattle area. *Compr Psychiatry* 1:349–359, 1960

   This article should be read with Barraclough et al. (1974) above and Pfeffer et al. (1986) below as defining the population of patients who commit suicide.

4. *Fawcett J, Scheftner WA, Fogg L, Clark DC, Young MA, Hedker D, Gibbons R:** Time-related predictors of suicide in major affective disorder. *Am J Psychiatry* 147:1189–1194, 1990

   This standardized, prospective study of 954 patients with major affective disorders proved that nine clinical features point to suicide. Six of these (panic attacks, severe anxiety, diminished concentration, insomnia, moderate alcohol abuse, and loss of interest or pleasure) were associated with suicide within a year. Three (severe hopelessness, suicidal ideation, and a history of previous attempts) were associated with suicide within 6 months.

5. *Jacobs D, Brown HN** (eds): *Suicide: Understanding and Responding.* Madison, CT, International Universities Press, 1989

   There are 26 chapters in this book, one of the best of the many available suicidological portmanteaus. It has a good clinical handle. The editors include an interview with a suicidal woman to show some of the problems psychotherapists meet in treating these patients. Discussants review the problems as they appear in the interview.

6. **McIntosh JL:** Suicide among the elderly: levels and trends. *Am J Orthopsychiatry* 55:288–293, 1985

Although the high suicide rate among young people receives great attention in the general media, suicide among the elderly is more common. National levels and trends of suicide in the elderly are reviewed here, and the trends are discussed, with some attempts at explanation. The reader will find valuable information on the recognition of impeding suicide in the elderly.

7. **Murphy GE:** The physician's responsibility for suicide, II: errors of omission. *Ann Intern Med* 82:305–309, 1975

Impending suicide often goes unrecognized by medical generalists even though a very high fraction of patients visit their physicians before destroying themselves. Medical students in the United States are taught to ask systematically after the signs and symptoms of diseases rarer than depression, but receive little instruction in suicide prevention.

8. **Pfeffer CR, Plutchik R, Mizruchi MS, Lipkins R:** Suicidal behavior in child psychiatric inpatients and outpatients and in nonpatients. *Am J Psychiatry* 143:733–738, 1986

In this study, 100 child outpatients were compared with control groups of inpatients and nonpatients; recent general psychopathology, death preoccupation, and depression proved to be significantly associated with suicidal behavior in all three groups.

9. **Robins E, Murphy GE, Wilkinson RH, Gassner S, Kayes J:** Some clinical considerations in the prevention of suicide based on a study of 134 successful suicides. *Am J Public Health* 49:888–899, 1959

This article began the work that was followed by the efforts of Barraclough et al. (1974) above, Dorpat and Ripley (1960) above, and their colleagues. Taken together, these articles define the suicidal population as comprised almost entirely by mentally ill persons. Without affective disorder, schizophrenia, alcoholism, or a serious personality disorder, suicide hardly ever occurs.

10. *Roy A: *Suicide*. Baltimore, MD, Williams & Wilkins, 1986

This is an excellent collection of review articles dealing with many aspects of suicide: epidemiology, biology, management, and its clinical phenomena in various special groups (diagnostic, various ages). The best general reference source, unfortunately it is now out of print.

11. **Weissman MM, Klerman GL, Markowitz JS, Ovellette R:** Suicidal ideation and suicide attempts in panic disorder and attacks. *N Engl J Med* 321:1209–1214, 1989

This article, empirically demonstrating the importance of panic in suicide, underscores the clinical importance of agitation and terror as driving forces in many instances of suicidal anguish. It proves what Kraepelin believed about the importance of panic in manic-depressive disease.

Suicide Risk and Assessment

12. *Maltsberger JT: *Suicide Risk: The Formulation of Clinical Judgment.* New York, New York University Press, 1986

This book is a clinical guide to organizing the information of the patient's history and mental state examination in a way to arrive at a rational estimation of the likelihood of suicide in the near future.

13. *Maris RW, Berman AL, Maltsberger JT, Yufit RI: *Assessment and Prediction of Suicide.* New York, Guilford, 1992

This definitive compendium of 32 contributions exhaustively reviews every aspect of suicide from psychiatric, sociological, psychological, epidemiological, biological, and other perspectives. It summarizes all we know about the problem of risk assessment.

14. Pokorny AD: Prediction of suicide in psychiatric patients. *Arch Gen Psychiatry* 40:249–257, 1983

Why is it so difficult to predict confidently whether patients will commit suicide or not? This article shows how the low sensitivity and specificity of available procedures for the identification of suicidal patients coupled with the comparative rarity of suicide make prediction of suicide impossible and force clinicians to rely on less than satisfactory risk assessment measures. It is not clinical, but it gives perspective.

Understanding

15. Adler G, Buie DH: Aloneness and borderline psychopathology: the possible relevance of child development issues. *Int J Psychoanal* 60:83–96, 1979

Although this article discusses the subjective experience of suicidal borderline patients, aloneness is also a prominent characteristic of depressive anguish in others on the verge of self-destruction. The authors make it plain that aloneness is a very different matter from strong loneliness: it is the affect that accompanies impending self-disintegration and has strong links to separation panic.

16. **Allen TE:** Suicidal impulse in depression and paranoia. *Int J Psychoanal* 48:433–438, 1967

In recovering from a persecutory psychosis, many patients abruptly plunge into suicidal depressions, catch their caretakers off guard, and do away with themselves. Atypical hypomanic patients shifting from angry paranoid states into depression are notorious for these lethal switches. Allen discusses the psychodynamic relationship between paranoid states and melancholia. Those who read this article will forearm themselves against these startling and sometimes sudden transitions.

17. **Asberg M, Traskman L, Thoren P:** 5-HIAA in the cerebrospinal fluid. *Arch Gen Psychiatry* 33:1193–1197, 1976

This important article demonstrates that depressed patients with low levels of 5-hydroxyindoleacetic acid (5-HIAA) in the cerebrospinal fluid are more likely to commit suicide that those without; they are also more likely to do so by more violent means. Later publications have verified and expanded on this important finding. Asberg et al. have opened a door to deeper biological understanding of suicide and invite the development of biological tests for suicide risk.

18. *Friedlander K:** On the "longing to die." *Int J Psychoanal* 21:416–426, 1940

The Greek gods of sleep (Hypnos) and death (Thanatos) were brothers. Friedlander presents and discusses a case to illuminate suicidal patients' almost universal tendency to confuse death with peaceful dreamless sleep. Readers will recall that Hamlet, contemplating suicide, feared what he might dream, and checked himself. Many suicidal patients expect pleasant dreams in death, an ominous sign.

19. **Havens LL:** The anatomy of a suicide. *N Engl J Med* 272:402–406, 1965

Here is one of the most extraordinary case reports in the psychiatric literature. Haven describes the loss of a patient to suicide and how he came to understand it. Much of what is written here is generalizable.

20. *Hendin H:** Psychodynamics of suicide, with particular reference to the young. *Am J Psychiatry* 148:1150–1158, 1991

This broad, short overview of almost all important aspects of the psychodynamic understanding of suicide is necessarily telegraphic. (Editors at major journals commonly must spurn more discursive contributions.) It brings up to date a previous review of the subject the author published 30 years ago. The valuable bibliography of 86 references covers the territory in a highly satisfactory manner.

21. **Hendrick I:** Suicide as wish fulfillment. *Psychiatr Q* 14:30–42, 1940

The rich clinical detail of this case report shows how suicide expresses the unconscious fantasy that in death one may become another person. Incorporative identification with a dead person is an insufficiently appreciated but common suicidal aim. Read this together with Friedlander's (1940) article above if you want to see how good single case reports highlighting familiar phenomena help clinicians more than many nomothetic contributions filled with statistics.

22. **Jensen VW, Perry T:** The fantasy of being rescued in suicide. *Psychoanal Q* 27:327–339, 1958

Almost every suicide reflects ambivalence about living and dying; one side of the struggle is expressed in the almost universal bids for rescue discernible in attempts. Jensen and Perry discuss suicidal ambivalence in a clinically valuable way.

23. **Jones E:** On "dying together," with special reference to Heinrich von Kleist's suicide (1911), in *Essays in Applied Psychoanalysis,* Vol. 1. Edited by Jones E. London, England, Hogarth Press, 1951, pp. 9–15

Read this chapter if you want help in understanding the psychology of suicide pacts. It often goes unappreciated that suicide takes place in the context of a folie à deux.

24. **Litman RE, Swearingen C:** Bondage and suicide. *Arch Gen Psychiatry* 27:80–85, 1972

Occasionally suicides are reported in which the victims' bodies are found in bizarre circumstances suggesting complex masturbatory rituals. Litman and Swearingen present a rich array of clinical material gathered from patients drawn to hanging and other deadly behavior because death excites them erotically. Many suicidal patients who do not act out in the ways described here nevertheless find the suicide fantasy sexually stimulating, a fact often overlooked by clinicians unfamiliar with these phenomena.

25. **Menninger KA:** Psychoanalytic aspects of suicide. *Int J Psychoanal* 14:376–390, 1933

This famous article is included for those readers who want to learn first hand what Menninger meant when he asserted the three common unconscious wishes expressed in suicide were the wish to kill, the wish to be killed, and to die.

26. **Morse SJ:** The after-pleasure of suicide. *Br J Med Psychol* 46:227–238, 1973

The extended theoretical discussion that opens this article should not daunt the reader; those who persevere to the third section will find an excellent summary of 14 fantasies and interpersonal devices that suicidal patients hope to realize in death.

27. *Novick J: Attempted suicide in adolescence: the suicide sequence, in *Suicide in the Young*. Edited by Sudak HS. Boston, MA, John Wright/PSG, 1984, pp. 115–137

From a study of a number of suicidal adolescents in psychoanalytic treatment, the author infers a series of steps through which such patients move in fruitless efforts to extract themselves from emotional bondage to their mothers. Suicide is the last step. The psychology discussed here is not unique to adolescents; one meets it in other suicidal adults who cannot extricate themselves from intense ambivalent attachments to their parents or surrogates. This excellent book includes other worthwhile chapters.

28. Phillips DP: The influence of suggestion in suicide: substantive and theoretical implications of the Werther effect. *American Sociology Review* 39:340–354, 1974

This article, one of many by Phillips that establish suicide as a contagious disorder, shows how the suicide rate increases after a suicide is publicized in the newspapers. It illustrates the importance of suggestion.

29. *Richman J, Rosenbaum MA: A clinical study of role of hostility and death wishes by the family and society in suicidal attempts. *Israel Annals of Psychiatry and Related Disciplines* 8:213–231, 1970

The patients' relationships to their family and to others close to them are critically important in most cases and can trip the balance toward suicide or toward survival. These authors show how this is true; their work suggests valuable perspectives for successful treatment. Read this article with the works of Novick (1984) above, Rubenstein and Winston (1976) below, and Sabbath (1969) below. Taken together, these papers will impress the reader that suicide can be understood only in the context of relationships that work to preserve or destroy the patient.

30. Roy A: Suicide in chronic schizophrenia. *Br J Psychiatry* 141:171–177, 1982

The importance of depression as a factor in driving chronic schizophrenic patients over the brink is demonstrated and illustrated in this article.

31. **Roy A:** Family history of suicide. *Arch Gen Psychiatry* 40:971–974, 1983

    Studying a large number of patients with a variety of different diagnoses, the author found that a history of suicide in near relatives greatly increased the likelihood of suicide in the patients. These findings were replicated in a comparable study published a month later (**Tsuang M:** Risk of suicide in the relatives of schizophrenics, manics, depressives, and controls. *J Clin Psychiatry* 44:396–400, 1983).

32. **Rubenstein M, Winston A:** Suicide and the participation of others. *Diseases of the Nervous System* 37:534–536, 1976

    As in Sabbath's (1969) article below, the dyadic nature of suicide is emphasized here. Suicide usually requires at least the passive assent of others who have been alerted that death is near; often enough, there is active promotion of suicide from others who are emotionally important to the patient. The late Otto Will coined the aphorism, "In suicidal cases, ask who wants the patient dead."

Treatment

33. *Birtchnell J:** Psychotherapeutic considerations in the management of the suicidal patient. *Am J Psychother* 37:24–36, 1983

    The limitations of the therapist's responsibility for saving the patient's life are discussed here. The failure to appreciate these limitations can lead to countertherapeutic struggles for control and rescue.

34. **Gutheil EA:** Dream and suicide. *Am J Psychother* 2:283–294, 1948

    This important (often overlooked) article covers the dreams of seven patients, showing how the study of dreams is an ongoing aid in risk assessment and psychodynamic understanding in the progress of treatment.

35. *Hendin H:** Psychotherapy and suicide. *Am J Psychother* 35:469–480, 1981

    This is the best available discussion of coercive countertransference bondage, the mire in which so many therapists become lethally entangled with their patients. The author also addresses other essential treatment matters.

36. **Kullgren G:** Factors associated with completed suicide in borderline personality disorder. *J Nerv Ment Dis* 176:40–44, 1988

    The importance of countertransference acting out in provoking suicide in patients with borderline personality disorder is empirically demonstrated in this study. Borderline suicidal patients are exquisitely sensitive to abandonment and may act with deadly impulsivity when they perceive (or misperceive) rejection in their caretakers.

37. *Maltsberger JT, Buie DH: Countertransference hate in the treatment of suicidal patients. *Arch Gen Psychiatry* 30:625–633, 1974

This article discusses fully the problems of clinicians' aversion in working with suicidal patients. Rejection responses, direct and indirect, are often provoked by patients when painful impulses (especially cruel ones) are aroused in the people who care for them clinically.

38. *Sabbath JC: The suicidal adolescent: the expendable child. *Journal of the American Academy of Child Psychiatry* 8:272–289, 1969

This article demonstrates the importance of scapegoating within the family as a suicide-inviting phenomenon. What is described here as an adolescent phenomenon applies often to adult family or group members as well.

39. *Schwartz DA, Flinn DE, Slawson PF: Treatment of the suicidal character. *Am J Psychother* 28:194–207, 1974

Not every suicidal patient is driven to death by depression—there are those for whom life on the brink of suicide is an adaptational style; many suffer from borderline and other personality disorders. Their treatment requirements are described, compared with, and contrasted to those appropriate to acute depressive suicidal states.

Aftermath

40. Dunne EJ, McIntosh JL, Dunne-Maxim K (eds): *Suicide and Its Aftermath.* New York, WW Norton, 1987

Suicide has devastating effects on families, friends, and therapists. It has serious implications for schools, hospitals, and other communities. The chapters in this book discuss all these implications and suggest remedial action to help those left behind.

41. Sacks MH: When patients kill themselves, in *American Psychiatric Press Review of Psychiatry*, Vol. 8. Edited by Tasman A, Hales RE, Francis AJ. Washington, DC, American Psychiatric Association, 1989, pp. 563–579

This chapter reviews the literature on psychiatrists as survivors of their patients' suicides, demonstrating that the impact can be severe. Helps for therapist survivors are reviewed, and the attitudes of the professional community are discussed.

29

Violence

Kenneth Tardiff, M.D., M.P.H.

In this chapter I focus on violence defined as assaultive behavior or
physical aggression directed toward others. The focus is on the
pathological aspects of physical aggression by humans of interest
to the clinician, although some of the texts present research in animal
aggression and discuss instrumental forms of human aggression such as
organized crime, riots, and wars. The violent behaviors included in these
references represent a wide variety of different types of violence, including
assault and homicide directed toward family members such as children,
spouses, siblings, and parents as well as violence directed toward nonfamily
members and also rape. Epidemiological and multiple etiological perspectives are presented, as are approaches to the evaluation and treatment of
violent individuals, and the impact of violence on staff, patients, and society.

General

1. *American Psychiatric Association: Report of the Task Force on Clinician Safety.*
   Washington, DC, American Psychiatric Association, 1993

   This is a report by the task force on the frequency and nature of attacks
   on clinicians by patients. There is discussion of the issue of safety from
   how to approach a potentially violent patient to details on environment
   safety. The current state of knowledge on the proper evaluation of the

violent patient and means of controlling violence and using drugs and physical techniques are discussed. The need for education of residents and practitioners is emphasized.

2. **Benedek EP, Cowell DG:** *Juvenile Homicide.* Washington, DC, American Psychiatric Press, 1989

   This is a book that presents many aspects of an area not frequently covered in the literature. Juvenile murderers are described from a clinical perspective and from the vantage of the forensic examiner, courts, and other aspects of the legal system. There is a chapter on the psychiatric impact of adolescents' witnessing homicide. Data and references are included.

3. **Dickstein LJ, Nadelson CC:** *Family Violence: Emerging Issues of a National Crisis.* Washington, DC, American Psychiatric Press, 1989

   This book describes patterns of violence toward women and children in families. It also has a chapter on abuse of the elderly. Social programs and legal interventions are presented. There are good references on treatment and a list of agencies to contact for further information.

4. **Eichelman B:** Aggressive behavior: from laboratory to clinic. *Arch Gen Psychiatry* 49:488–492, 1992

   This article is a review of research on aggression using animal models to study temperament, sensory cues, neuroanatomy, biochemistry, and social conditions. Implications for the study of human aggression are examined. It contains many relevant references.

5. **Lion JR:** *Evaluation and Management of the Violent Patient: Guidelines in the Hospital and Institution.* Springfield, IL, Charles C Thomas, 1972

   This book outlines the emergency management of the violent patient as well as the evaluation process, including the anamnesis, mental status examination, and organic evaluation. Lion specifically describes techniques of treatment in a variety of settings.

6. **Lion JR, Reid W:** *Assaults Within Psychiatric Facilities.* New York, Grune & Stratton, 1983

   This is an extensive collection of papers written by clinicians who manage problems with violence in a variety of treatment settings, including emergency rooms and inpatient units of general hospitals, psychiatric hospitals, and state hospitals. It contains guidelines for clinical management as well as epidemiological information about violence within facilities.

7. **Mulvihill D, Tumin M:** *Crimes of Violence: A Staff Report to the National Commission on the Causes and Prevention of Violence,* Vol. 13. Washington, DC, U.S. Government Printing Office, 1969

This is a comprehensive collection of papers from scholars in a wide range of disciplines covering violence in terms of statistics, etiology, evaluation of individual's drug abuse, the correctional system, cross-cultural perspectives, and treatment. It has withstood the test of time in terms of providing this broad perspective.

8. **Reid W** (ed): *The Treatment of Antisocial Syndromes.* New York, Van Nostrand Reinhold, 1981

This series of papers reviews the literature on the treatment of antisocial syndromes, which are broadly defined and often are accompanied by violent behavior. These violent individuals range from the asocial child to criminal offenders. Treatment modalities range from psychotherapy to medication to community-based programs for offenders.

9. **Roth LH** (ed): *Clinical Treatment and Management of the Violent Person.* Rockville, MD, National Institute of Mental Health, 1985

This series of papers discusses broad topics in the management of violent individuals, including legal and ethical issues, evaluation of individuals, and treatment.

10. **Tardiff K:** *The Psychiatric Uses of Seclusion and Restraint.* Washington, DC, American Psychiatric Press, 1984

This book reflects years of deliberation by the American Psychiatric Association Task Force on the Psychiatric Uses of Seclusion and Restraint. This has served as a model for national standards on the use of seclusion and restraint to address violence and self-destructive behaviors. It presents the indications and contraindications as well as implementation of these techniques. Guidelines as they pertain to special populations (i.e., children, the elderly, and developmentally disabled patients) are presented. Legal aspects of seclusion and restraint are discussed.

11. *Tardiff K: *Assessment and Management of Violent Patients.* Washington, DC, American Psychiatric Press, 1989

This is a compact handbook that presents a comprehensive picture of causes of violence, dealing with the acutely violent patient with words, medication, seclusion and restraint, extended evaluation of the violent patient, long-term treatment using medication, psychotherapy and behavioral therapy, prediction of violence, and legal issues. It contains many references that are clinically relevant.

12. **Tardiff K:** The current state of psychiatry in the treatment of violent patients. *Arch Gen Psychiatry* 49:493–499, 1992

This is a review of progress over the last two decades in describing patterns of violence by psychiatric patients and the development of standards and guidelines for the evaluation and treatment of violent patients. The focus is on psychiatry as part of the medical profession being responsible and capable to treat violence by patients rather than general violence in society.

13. **Turner JT:** *Violence in the Medical Care Setting: A Survival Guide.* Rockville, MD, Aspen Systems Corporation, 1984

This book describes violence by patients in a number of hospital settings by a variety of types of patients. It describes security procedures to deal with violence, including hostage taking, by patients. A chapter describes the treatment of staff victims of violence.

Etiology

14. **Centerwall BS:** Television and violence: the scale of the problem and where to go from here. *JAMA* 267:3059–3063, 1992

This article is a review of studies that support a relationship between violence on television and the development of violence in children. Recommendations to decrease the amount of television children watch and the need for parents to monitor the programs children see are discussed.

15. **Crowell DH, Evans IM, O'Donnell CR:** *Childhood Aggression and Violence: Sources of Influence, Prevention and Control.* New York, Plenum, 1987

This is a report containing papers presented at a conference by experts in the United States. It describes the clinical phenomenology of childhood aggression as well as biological, social, and psychological causes. It is well referenced and cites research findings.

16. **Davis S:** Violence by psychiatric inpatients: a review. *Hosp Community Psychiatry* 42:585–590, 1991

A review of studies examining causes of violence by patients in psychiatric hospitals, this article examines the role of psychosis, other aspects of psychopathology, drug abuse, history of violence, and age in relation to situational factors such as overcrowding, provocation, and staff inexperience.

17. **Garza-Trevino ES:** Neurobiological factors in aggressive behavior. *Hosp Community Psychiatry* 45:690–699, 1994

    This is an excellent review of studies using neuroimaging, pathological techniques, and biochemical techniques focused on aggressive behavior, predominantly in humans, although some animal studies are cited when appropriate.

18. **Gaylin W:** *The Rage Within: Anger in Modern Life.* New York, Viking Penguin, 1989

    This book looks at anger and violence in terms of causes and ways of expression in modern life, particularly urban settings. The perspective is psychoanalytic but it is written without jargon for the lay reader.

19. **Goldstein PJ, Brownstein HH, Ryan PJ, Bellucci PA:** Crack and homicide in New York City, 1988: a conceptually based event analysis. *Contemporary Drug Problems* 6:651–687, 1990

    This is a study and discussion of how crack cocaine is related to violence in society. A distinction is made between the pharmacological effect of cocaine producing violence and two other indirect effects: violence used to steal money for the drug and violence used as part of the business of drug-dealing.

20. **Krakowski M, Volavka J, Brizer D:** Psychopathology and violence: a review of the literature. *Compr Psychiatry* 27:131–148, 1986

    This article is a comprehensive review of studies of diagnosis and psychopathology in relation to violence by patients. The studies are presented in the text and in tabular form. References are numerous and relevant.

21. **McNiel DE, Binder RL:** The relationship between acute psychiatric symptoms, diagnosis and short-term risk of violence. *Hosp Community Psychiatry* 45:133–137, 1994

    This is a large study of 330 inpatients using standardized rating instruments to measure psychopathology. Symptom patterns related to violence in the hospital are discussed, such as hostility, agitation, and thinking disturbances.

22. **Rabkin JG:** Criminal behavior of discharged mental patients: a critical appraisal of the research. *Psychol Bull* 86:1–27, 1979

    This article provides a complete, objective, and detailed review of the conflicting research literature on whether mentally ill patients are at greater risk of violence and other criminal behavior than are persons in the general population.

23. **Sharpe WD, Levey S** (eds): Homicide: the public health perspective. *Bull N Y Acad Med* 62:373–624, 1986

   This is a report containing papers presented by experts from throughout the United States at a symposium on homicide. It is very comprehensive and addresses the causes of homicide, including drugs, as well as the phenomenology of homicide from domestic violence to sensationalistic homicides. Strategies for prevention are presented.

24. **Taylor PJ:** The risk of violence in psychotics. *Integrative Psychiatry* 4:12–24, 1986

   This article is a review of the international literature on the risk of violence among psychotic patients and a study in England documenting an increase in violence by psychotic patients. Experts in the field comment on the article as a supplement.

25. **Widom CS:** The cycle of violence. *Science* 244:160–166, 1989

   This is a review of studies and presentation of some data exploring the relationship between being abused or neglected as a child and becoming a violent or criminal adult. Methodological problems in the study of this subject are discussed. A prospective study did find a relationship between child abuse and adult violence.

26. **Wolfgang ME, Ferracuti F:** *The Subculture of Violence: Towards an Integrated Theory in Criminology.* London, Tavistock, 1967

   This is a classic text on the theory synonymous with the name of the first author. It maintains that there are subcultures or systems of values and beliefs in certain populations, usually of the lower socioeconomic classes, that foster the use of violence as the major form of human interaction.

27. **Wolfgang ME, Weiner NA:** *Criminal Violence.* Beverly Hills, CA, Sage, 1982

   This is a book that describes the biological, psychological, and sociological determinants of criminal violence. It explores the role of firearms in violent crime. It preceded the rise of cocaine, particularly crack, and so it does not cover the impact of drugs on criminal violence.

Evaluation

28. **Beck JC:** *The Potentially Violent Patient and the Tarasoff Decision in Psychiatric Practice.* Washington, DC, American Psychiatric Press, 1985

This is a book that describes the legal cases courts throughout the United States have decided following the California Tarasoff decision that a psychotherapist of a potentially violent patient has a duty to protect the intended victims from the patient's threatened violence. It discusses the clinical implications of the cases.

29. **Brizer DA, Crowner M:** *Current Approaches to the Prediction of Violence.* Washington, DC, American Psychiatric Press, 1989

This book presents a number of studies of violence in variety of populations, such as psychiatric inpatients, criminals, and abused children who have grown up to be violent adults. Many chapters deal with clinical factors and the prediction of violence among patients.

30. **Dubin WR:** The role of fantasies, countertransference and psychological defenses in patient violence. *Hosp Community Psychiatry* 40:1280–1283, 1989

This article is a discussion of the dynamics of violence and how staff fantasies, countertransference, and defenses can trigger violence by patients. Interventions to address these problems are discussed, such as expression of feelings without the need to explore psychodynamics, education, and strong leaders to serve as role models for the treatment team.

31. **Petrie WM, Lawson EC, Hollender MH:** Violence in geriatric patients. *JAMA* 248:443–444, 1982

This article describes a number of geriatric patients who committed acts dangerous to others as well as the nature of the acts, which often involved guns or knives.

32. **Yudofsky SC, Silver JM, Jackson W, Endicott J, Williams D:** The overt aggression scale for the objective rating of verbal and physical aggression. *Am J Psychiatry* 143:35–39, 1986

This article provides a description of the development and use of a scale to measure verbal aggression, physical aggression against objects, physical aggression toward self, and physical aggression toward others. This is useful in measuring changes in aggression during drug trials aimed at treating violent patients.

Treatment

33. **Cornfield RB, Fielding SD:** Impact of the threatening patient on ward communications. *Am J Psychiatry* 137:616–619, 1980

Based on clinical observations, the authors describe ways that potentially violent patients provoke strained communication patterns among staff and patients on an inpatient unit. These patterns include apathy and emotional detachment, displaced affect, and mutual criticism. Staff intervention strategies are presented.

34. **Levy P, Hartocollis P:** Nursing aides and patient violence. *Am J Psychiatry* 133:429–431, 1976

This is a report of a study that decreased the incidence of violence in a psychiatric unit organized as a therapeutic community whose nursing staff was composed entirely of women. The use of nonconfrontational approaches on this special treatment unit is discussed.

35. ***Lion JR, Pasternak SA:** Countertransference reactions to violent patients. *Am J Psychiatry* 130:207–210, 1973

This is a short, practical article that presents clinical case examples of a number of reactions to violent patients that can interfere with treatment as well as threaten the safety of staff. These include anger, denial, identification with the aggressor, prejudice, and reinforcement of violence by staff.

36. ***Thackrey M:** *Therapeutics for Aggression: Psychological/Physical Crisis Intervention.* New York, Human Sciences Press, 1987

This book describes psychological and verbal techniques of responding to imminent or actual violence by patients as well as physical techniques to defend against attacks by patients. It is clearly written and well illustrated with photographs. References are plentiful.

Child and Adolescent Psychopathology

David A. Mrazek, M.D., F.R.C.Psych.
Penelope Krener, M.D.

The field of child and adolescent psychiatry has evolved in many ways to the status of a distinct discipline. In the same way that pediatrics gradually differentiated itself from internal medicine, child and adolescent psychiatry has become a new medical specialty with distinct diagnostic procedures, a unique set of psychiatric syndromes, and specialized therapeutic modalities and methodologies. The extent and rate of this process is reflected in the exponential increases in research and publication in this new specialty. This recent change is reflected in the selection process of core papers for this chapter. To underscore this point, choosing core papers was often difficult given the expansion of work in areas that range from obsessive-compulsive disorder to multiple personality.

This chapter focuses on the range of disturbances that define child and adolescent psychopathology. It is arranged primarily on the basis of syndromes; there is a section that focuses on the consideration of risk factors and new efforts that are targeted at the prevention of disturbance. Although much is included, it is not absolutely comprehensive; to achieve that goal would have been far beyond the scope of this book. However, a solid core of readings are represented. Chapter 51 (Krener and Mrazek, this volume), "Modalities in Child and Adolescent Psychiatry," is a companion chapter. It focuses primarily on the widening range of available treatment strategies used with children and adolescents and particularly highlights exciting developments in pediatric psychopharmacology. This current chapter focuses on papers that describe the etiology, course, and diagnostic criteria of the syndromes and diseases that affect children and adolescents. Chapter 51 addresses the practical issues of intervention and efficacy of treatments; a section critiquing the basic textbooks in child and adolescent psychiatry as they address these issues is included. The two chapters are designed to complement each other with the minimal amount of redundancy. In many ways, they should be considered two parts of a single whole.

Autism and the Pervasive Developmental Disorders

1. *Folstein S, Rutter M:** Infantile autism: a genetic study of 21 twin pairs. *J Child Psychol Psychiatry* 18:297–321, 1977

    This is a classic article that provided strong evidence for the role of genetic factors in the etiology of autism. A 36% pair-wise concordance rate for monozygotic pairs was found compared with a 0% rate for dizygotic pairs. The concordance of "cognitive abnormalities" was 82% in the monozygotic pairs and only 10% in the dizygotic pairs.

2. **Hobson RP:** Methodological issues for experiments on autistic individuals' perception and understanding of emotion. *J Child Psychol Psychiatry* 32:1135–1158, 1991

    The thesis that autistic children have an inability to discriminate or attend to the facial, vocal, or other bodily emotional expressions of others is examined in this article. The advantages and limitations of experimental approaches to addressing these questions are discussed.

3. *Kanner L:** Autistic disturbances of affective contact. *Nervous Child* 2:217–250, 1943

    This classic article describes the phenomena that are core features of autism: an inability to relate; an "anxiously obsessive desire for the maintenance of sameness" (p. 249); and peculiarities of language, including echolalia and pronoun reversal.

4. *Kanner L:** Follow-up study of eleven autistic children originally reported in 1943. *Journal of Autism and Childhood Schizophrenia* 1:119–145, 1971

    A highly illustrative report of the original 11 children who were described by Kanner, this article highlights the considerable variability in outcome as well as the relatively poor levels of ultimate adjustment.

It also highlights Kanner's original statement that these children "come into the world with an innate disability to form the usual, biologically provided contact with people" (p. 141).

5. **Lockyer L, Rutter M:** A five to fifteen year follow-up study of infantile psychosis, III: psychological aspects. *Br J Psychiatry* 115:865–882, 1969

   This is a careful follow-up study looking at differential outcome for autistic children with a discussion of risk factors and empirical evidence of outcome.

6. **Perner J, Frith U, Leslie AM, Leekam SR:** Exploration of the autistic child's theory of mind: knowledge, belief, and communication. *Child Dev* 60:689–700, 1989

   Autistic children have been hypothesized to have an inability to conceptualize easily a "theory of mind." This article provides empirical evidence to illustrate deficits in these thought processes.

7. **Sherman M, Shapiro T, Glassman M:** Play and language in developmentally disordered preschoolers: a new approach to classification. *J Am Acad Child Adolesc Psychiatry* 22:511–524, 1983

   Data are presented to support the strategy of using "functional status" rather than traditional diagnostic labels to assess and study severely developmentally delayed preschool children.

Schizophrenia and Childhood Psychosis

8. **Caplan R, Guthrie D, Foy JG:** Communication deficits and formal thought disorder in schizophrenic children. *J Am Acad Child Adolesc Psychiatry* 31:151–159, 1992

   The "discourse devices" of schizophrenic children are described and their relationship to measures of formal thought disorder are discussed. The effect of neuroleptic medication on loosening of associations is reported to be somewhat paradoxical in these patients.

9. **Fish B:** Antecedents of an acute schizophrenic break. *Journal of the American Academy of Child Psychiatry* 25:595–600, 1986

   This is an illustrative clinical description of the evolution of schizotypal symptoms prior to the onset of overt schizophrenia at age 19.

10. **Volkmar FR, Cohen DJ, Hoshino Y, Rende R, Paul R:** Phenomenology and classification of the childhood psychoses. *Psychol Med* 18:191–201, 1988

In examining a series of 228 children with a diagnosis of childhood psychosis, three subgroups were identified; 42 children were diagnosed as having "schizophreniform" features. Disorders of thought processes were used primarily to differentiate these children from autistic or atypical subjects. Recognition of disturbance was later for schizophreniform subjects, with the mean age of recognition being about 7.

11. **Werry JS, McClellan JM:** Predicting outcome in child and adolescent (early onset) schizophrenia and bipolar disorder. *J Am Acad Child Adolesc Psychiatry* 31:147–150, 1992

For schizophrenic patients, premorbid adjustment and degree of initial recovery after initial hospitalization were the two strongest predictors of outcomes. In contrast, for bipolar patients, IQ and premorbid adjustment were the best predictors. By far the best overall predictive risk factor was early premorbid function.

Mental Retardation

12. **Bregman JD:** Special article: current developments in the understanding of mental retardation, part II: psychopathology. *J Am Acad Child Adolesc Psychiatry* 30:861–872, 1991

The occurrence of psychopathology in mentally retarded children and adolescents has been reported to be as high as 66%. Specific risk factors include neurological disease and genetic etiology as well as psychosocial factors. Autism and pervasive developmental delays have been reported to occur in as many as one-third of the children with severe mental retardation.

13. **Freund LS, Reiss AL, Abrarns MT:** Psychiatric disorders associated with fragile X in the young female. *Pediatrics* 91:321–329, 1993

Females with fragile X show higher frequency of attention-deficit/ hyperactivity, withdrawal, and depression than control subjects. The size of the DNA insertion is associated with IQ, severity of attentional problems, and anxiety/withdrawal symptoms.

14. **Hobson RP, Ouston J, Lee A:** Recognition of emotion by mentally retarded adolescents and young adults. *Am J Ment Retard* 93:434–443, 1989

In this article, evidence for a selective inability to match emotional facial expression correctly with appropriate emotionally expressive recorded voices is demonstrated for mildly mentally retarded adolescents and young adults.

15. **Reiss AL, Freund L:** Fragile X syndrome, DSM-III-R, and autism. *J Am Acad Child Adolesc Psychiatry* 29:885–891, 1990

    The symptomatic behaviors of children with the fragile X syndrome are described. These include 1) deficits in social interaction, 2) abnormalities in verbal and nonverbal communication, 3) stereotypic motor behavior, and 4) unusual responses to sensory stimuli. Similarities to children with the diagnosis of autism are highlighted.

Attention-Deficit/Hyperactivity Disorder

16. **August GJ, Garfinkel BD:** The nosology of attention-deficit hyperactivity disorder. *J Am Acad Child Adolesc Psychiatry* 31:155–165, 1993

    Five central issues related to the classification of attention-deficit/ hyperactivity disorder are discussed. Very different samples of children were identified using different methodologies. Using pervasive criteria considerably lowered the incidence, suggesting that context of symptoms remains an important consideration. Using all of the methods considered, comorbidity was frequently reported.

17. **Biederman J, Munir K, Knee D, Armentano M, Autor S, Waternaux C, Tsuang MT:** High rate of affective disorders in probands with attention deficit disorder and in their relatives: a controlled family study. *Am J Psychiatry* 144:330–333, 1987

    This article reports on early results of an extensive ongoing study of comorbidity of affective disorders, with attention disorders reporting a 32% comorbidity in the probands.

18. **Douglas VI, Barr KG, Aman K, O'Neill ME, Britton BJ:** Dosage effects and individual responsivity to methylphenidate in attention deficit disorder. *J Child Psychol Psychiatry* 29:453–475, 1988

    This study carefully characterizes the response of children with attention-deficit/hyperactivity disorder to cognitive tasks measuring attention and impulsivity, and the changes in their responses with medication. For these children, their reaction time on a continuous performance task is longer and more variable. Their distractibility is greater when distracters are salient and when they are embedded in the task.

19. **Dykman RA, Ackerman PT:** Attention deficit disorder and specific reading disability: separate but often overlapping disorders. *Journal of Learning Disabilities* 24:96–108, 1991

The argument is put forward that it is of value to differentiate, rather than to lump together, children with externalizing behavioral symptoms and learning difficulties.

20. **Hinshaw SP:** On the distinction between attentional deficits/hyperactivity and conduct problems/aggression in child psychopathology. *Psychol Bull* 101:443–463, 1987

Impulsivity and aggression emerge independently on factor analysis of behaviors observed in group or playroom settings. This contributes to the differentiation between attention-deficit/hyperactivity disorder and conduct disorder.

21. **Lahey BB, Pelham WE, Schaughency EA, Atkins MS, Murphy HA, Hynd G, Russo M, Hartdagen S, Lorys-Vernon A:** Dimensions and types of attention deficit disorder. *J Am Acad Child Adolesc Psychiatry* 27:330–335, 1988

Factor analysis of a teacher rating instrument yields three clinical clusters: children without attention deficit disorder, children with inattention and hyperactivity, and children with inattention but who are sluggish in their movement rather than hyperactive.

22. **Lambert NM, Hartsough CS, Sassone D, Sandoval J:** Persistence of hyperactivity symptoms from childhood to adolescence and associated outcomes. *Am J Orthopsychiatry* 57:22–32, 1987

This study followed 59 hyperactive boys and matched control subjects for at least 3 years to age 12 using comparison on parent and teacher reports and assessments of attention, achievement, and intellectual function. Attention-deficit/hyperactivity disorder children had significant differences from control subjects in IQ and achievement; both spatial perspectives and formal reasoning cognitive tasks were lower. Hyperactive subjects were also more field dependent, had been suspended from school more, had had trouble with law enforcement, and had more psychological disorders.

23. **Loney J, Milich R:** Hyperactivity, inattention and aggression in clinical practice, in *Advances in Developmental and Behavioral Pediatrics.* Edited by Routh D, Wolraich M. Greenwich, CT, JAI Press, 1982, pp. 113–147

Following an empirical/statistical approach to developing research diagnostic criteria, a short list of symptoms of hyperactivity can be empirically separated from a short list of aggression symptoms, creating two semi-independent constructs.

24. **Lou HC, Henriksen L, Bruhn P, Borner H, Nielsen JB:** Striatal dysfunction in attention deficit and hyperkinetic disorder. *Arch Neurol* 46:48–52, 1989

These studies on cerebral blood flow on children with attention-deficit/ hyperactivity disorder reveal patterns of underactivity in the prefrontal areas of the central nervous system and their rich connections to the limbic system via the striatum. This would endorse the motivational model of attention-deficit/hyperactivity disorder with neuroanatomical studies suggesting decreased activation of brain reward centers and their cortical-limbic regulating circuits.

25. **Satterfield JH, Schell AM, Backs RW:** Topographic study of auditory event related potentials in normal boys and in boys with attention deficit disorder with hyperactivity. *Psychophysiology* 25:591–606, 1988

Comparisons are presented of the responses of 6-year-old nondisabled children and children with attention-deficit/hyperactivity disorder in a task requiring selective attending to tones while ignoring flashes. Differences in auditory event-related potentials between the two groups are identified.

26. **Swanson JM, Posner M, Potkin S, Bonforte S, Youpa D, Fiore C, Cantwell D, Crinella F:** Activating tasks for the study of visual-spatial attention in ADHD children: a cognitive anatomic approach. *J Child Neurol* 6:S119–S127, 1991

This is an important study of the application of specific cognitive tasks, such as the Posner covert-orienting paradigm, to the study of children with attention-deficit/hyperactivity disorder.

27. **Zametkin J, Rapoport JL:** Neurobiology of attention deficit disorder with hyperactivity: where have we come in 50 years? *J Am Acad Child Adolesc Psychiatry* 26:676–686, 1987

The role of catecholamine modulation in the pathogenesis of attention- deficit/hyperactivity disorder is reviewed. A comprehensive model of the pathophysiology of this disorder and drug action should postulate the inhibitory influences of frontal cortical activity, predominantly noradrenergic acting on lower (striatal) structures that are driven by both direct dopamine agonists and controlled or modulated by higher inhibitory structures sensitive to adrenergic agents.

Conduct Disorder

28. **Boyle MH, Offord DR:** Primary prevention of conduct disorder: issues and prospects. *J Am Acad Child Adolesc Psychiatry* 29:227–233, 1990

The issues of the prevention of conduct disorder are discussed within the context of a longitudinal study of an epidemiological sample of children. The review concludes that 1) design characteristics can dramatically affect the relative risk rating of risk factors, 2) targeting multiple risk factors is sensible, and 3) identifying children at greatest risk for disorder is cost effective.

29. **Dishion TJ, Patterson GR, Stoolmiller M, Skinner ML:** Family, school, and behavioral antecedents to early adolescent involvement with antisocial peers. *Developmental Psychology* 27:172–180, 1991

This is a comprehensive assessment of 206 boys and their families at age 10, using structured individual and family interview, school and home observation, and follow-up at age 12. School failure and peer rejection were most strongly associated with these children's later deviant relationships.

30. **Dodge KA:** Nature versus nurture in childhood conduct disorder: it is time to ask a difficult question. *Developmental Psychopathology* 26:698–701, 1990

This critical review highlights the role that child factors play in the development of conduct disorder. Noting the heterogeneity of the construct of conduct disorder and methodological limitations or confounds in the study of biological factors, this review focuses on mechanisms that operate during the transactional development of the child within his or her environment.

31. **Elliott DS, Huizinga D:** *The Relationship Between Delinquency, Alcohol, Drug, and Mental Health Problems.* Boulder, CO, Behavior Research Institute, 1984

Three theories of the cause of delinquency are reviewed: 1) strain theory, which emphasizes the discrepancy between aspirations and expectations of school and work; 2) social control theory, which emphasizes inadequate socialization; and 3) social learning theory, which emphasizes socialization to the attitudes and behaviors of delinquent peers. Antisocial behavior, the use of alcohol and street drugs, and a high incidence of psychiatric symptomatology are shown to be frequently comorbid during adolescence.

32. **Hughes JR, Zagar R, Sylvies RB, Arbit J, Busch KG, Bowers ND:** Medical, family, and scholastic conditions in urban delinquents. *J Clin Psychol* 47:448–464, 1991

Medical, family, and school conditions of 1,962 children and adolescents ages 6–17 who had been referred to a juvenile court evaluation team were documented. Children in this study were found to have central nervous system and birth conditions leading to cognitive, communicative, and perceptual deficits that influenced academic and behavioral functioning.

33. **Inamdar SC, Lewis DO, Simopoulos G, Shanock SS, Lamels M:** Violent and suicidal behavior in psychotic adolescents. *Am J Psychiatry* 139:932–935, 1982

Histories of assaultive violence were noted in 83.3% of boys and 42.9% of girls who were hospitalized for psychotic and other serious psychiatric symptomatology.

34. **Kolko DJ, Kazdin AE, Meyer EC:** Aggression and psychopathology in childhood firesetters: parent and child reports. *J Consult Clin Psychol* 53:377–385, 1985

When compared with children with conduct disorders but who did not set fires, firesetters were found to have more delinquent and antisocial behaviors. It is suggested that firesetting represents a marker for the most extreme form of conduct disorder.

35. **Lewis DO, Lovely R, Yeager C, Della Femina D:** Toward a theory of the genesis of violence: a follow-up study of delinquents. *J Am Acad Child Adolesc Psychiatry* 28:431–436, 1989

This is an evaluation and follow-up of securely incarcerated juveniles, including those who had committed violent crimes and been sentenced to death. Unrecognized psychotic symptomatology, especially paranoid ideation, was immediately related to their violent acts. Abusive homes during childhood and intrinsic neuropsychiatric vulnerabilities were predictive of violent crimes in adulthood.

36. **Loeber R:** The stability of antisocial and delinquent behavior: a review. *Child Dev* 53:1431–1446, 1982

Extreme antisocial behavior is more stable through childhood and adolescence. Most vulnerable to chronic delinquency are children with early high rates of a range of antisocial behaviors that occur in more than one setting. Children who had families with persistent disruption and rejection were also at risk.

37. **Lytton H:** Child and parent effects in boys' conduct disorder: a reinterpretation. *Developmental Psychology* 26:683–697, 1990

This literature review evaluates theories explaining origins of conduct disorder in terms of family environment, factors residing in the child, or reciprocal effects arising from the interaction between family and child factors. The author argues for primacy of child factors.

38. **Mitchell J, Varley C:** Isolation and restraint in juvenile correctional facilities. *J Am Acad Child Adolesc Psychiatry* 29:251–255, 1990

   Incidents are documented that lead to the isolation of 30 randomly selected residents in a maximum security isolation unit in a large training school. Psychiatrically hospitalized juveniles and those incarcerated for legal infractions are both isolated. It is suggested that programs that rely on excessive isolation actually experience higher rates of aversive behavior. A discussion of physical restraint is also included.

39. **Nagin DS, Farrington DP:** The stability of criminal potential from childhood to adulthood. *Criminology* 30:235–260, 1992

   Two interpretations of the positive association between past and future criminal behavior are discussed. One states that prior antisocial involvement itself has a behavioral impact on future behavior. The second is based on the observation of persistent population heterogeneity and posits that criminal behavior is a manifestation of a persisting underlying criminal potential, which is a population variant. A panel analysis of 403 youths with conviction histories modeled measures of personal and familial characteristics. Early criminal history, IQ, and behaviors characterized as "daring" were stable constructs associated with ongoing criminal behavior. Poor parenting was not.

40. **Rowe DC, Rodgers JL, Meseck-Bushey S:** Sibling delinquency and the family environment: shared and unshared influence. *Child Dev* 63:59–67, 1992

   Data from 5,863 respondents with siblings in the National Longitudinal Survey of Youth were analyzed to evaluate shared and unshared family environmental influences. The data analyses revealed substantial shared environmental and genetic influences for siblings, suggesting that family-based interventions addressing the delinquent behavior of older siblings may be preventive for their younger siblings.

Eating Disorders

41. **Chatoor I, Egan J, Getson P, Menvielle E, O'Donnell R:** Mother-infant interactions in infantile anorexia nervosa. *J Am Acad Child Adolesc Psychiatry* 27:535–540, 1988

   Children with a feeding disorder described as infantile anorexia nervosa were found to have atypical interactions with their mothers. Feeding was characterized by 1) less dyadic reciprocity, 2) less maternal contingency, 3) more dyadic conflict, and 4) a struggle for control. Similar patterns of interaction were also noted during play between the mother and child.

42. **Gold PW, Gwirtsman H, Avgerinos PC, Nieman LK, Gallucci WT, Kaye W, Jimerson D, Ebert M, Rittmaster R, Loriaux L, Chrousos GP:** Abnormal hypothalamic pituitary adrenal function in anorexia nervosa. *N Engl J Med* 314:1335–1342, 1986

Underweight anorexic girls were shown to have marked hypercorticism but normal basal plasma adrenocorticotropin hormone (ACTH). The plasma ACTH response to corticotropin-releasing hormone was markedly reduced during their period of hypercorticism. However, 6 months after successful weight gain, their ACTH responses had returned to normal.

43. *Herzog DB, Keller MB, Lavori PW:** Outcome in anorexia nervosa and bulimia nervosa. *J Nerv Ment Dis* 176:131–143, 1988

This review of 40 empirical studies highlights the mortality rate and morbidity of anorexia nervosa; 88 deaths associated with anorexia are reported. The illness was noted to be chronic in about one-third of those studied.

44. **Marchi M, Cohen P:** Early childhood eating behaviors and adolescent eating disorders. *J Am Acad Child Adolesc Psychiatry* 29:112–117, 1990

Early predictors of anorexia nervosa included very "picky eating" throughout childhood; bulimia nervosa was preceded by pica in early childhood.

45. **Swift WJ, Ritholz M, Kalin NH, Kaslow N:** A follow-up study of thirty hospitalized bulimics. *Psychosom Med* 49:45–55, 1987

A 2- to 5-year follow-up study of bulimic girls revealed a highly variable outcome. Some girls recovered completely, whereas others remained severely effected.

46. **Yates A:** Current perspectives in the eating disorders, I: history, psychological and biological aspects. *J Am Acad Child Adolesc Psychiatry* 28:813–828, 1989

This article provides a comprehensive review of the history of eating disorders, including recent developments in classification, criteria, epidemiology, and a range of etiological theories.

Epidemiology

47. **Brandenburg NA, Friedman RM, Silver SE:** The epidemiology of child-hood psychiatric disorders: prevalence findings from recent studies. *J Am Acad Child Adolesc Psychiatry* 29:76–83, 1990

    Based on eight recent studies, the prevalence of psychiatric disorder is estimated to be between 14% and 20%. The prevalence of severe disorder is roughly 7%. Methodological issues responsible for variability in these estimates are reviewed.

48. **Jensen PS, Bloedau L, Degroot J, Ussery T, Davis H:** Children at risk, I: risk factors and child symptomatology. *J Am Acad Child Adolesc Psychiatry* 29:51–59, 1990

    Parental psychopathology, marital difficulties, and life stressors were consistently shown to be strong risk factors for the development of childhood symptomatology.

49. *Rutter M: Isle of Wight revisited: twenty-five years of child psychiatric epidemiology. *J Am Acad Child Adolesc Psychiatry* 28:633–653, 1989

    The father of child psychiatric epidemiology places the field in perspective and looks toward future objectives.

Enuresis and Encopresis

50. **Foxman B, Valdez RB, Brook RH:** Childhood enuresis: prevalence, perceived impact, and prescribed treatments. *Pediatrics* 77:482–487, 1986

    Of a larger pediatric sample, 14% between ages 5–13 years had wet their bed at least once during the previous 3 months, whereas 7% wet their bed every week. Despite most children reporting that they were distressed by their enuresis, only 38% of the sample had seen a physician concerning the problem.

51. **Levine M:** Encopresis: its potentiation, evaluation, and alleviation. *Pediatr Clin North Am* 29:315–330, 1982

    This article is a practical guide to the evaluation and treatment of encopresis.

52. **Moffatt ME, Kato C, Pless IB:** Improvements in self concept after treatment of nocturnal enuresis: randomized controlled trial. *J Pediatr* 110:647–652, 1987

In children between the ages of 8 and 14 who were successfully treated for enuresis, higher levels of self-esteem were documented.

53. *Rapoport JL, Mikkelsen EJ, Zavadil A, Nee L, Gruenau C, Mendelson W, Gillin JC: Childhood enuresis, II: psychopathology, tricyclic concentration in plasma, and antienuretic effect. *Arch Gen Psychiatry* 37:1146–1152, 1980

The efficacy of tricyclic antidepressants in the treatment of enuresis is demonstrated in 7- to 12-year-old boys. Of these boys, 58% were classified as good responders; only 10% were totally dry.

54. Steinhausen HC, Gobel D: Enuresis in child psychiatric clinic patients. *J Am Acad Child Adolesc Psychiatry* 28:279–281, 1989

This study considers psychiatric outpatients between ages 6 and 8 years who were noted to be enuretic. Although these children had delayed developmental milestones and lower socioeconomic status, no specific profiles of psychopathology were noted.

Gender Identity Disorders

55. *Green R, Roberts CW, Williams K, Goodman M, Mixon A: Specific cross-gender behaviours in boyhood and later homosexual orientation. *Br J Psychiatry* 151:84–88, 1987

This study considered a cohort of boys who frequently played with dolls, role-played as females, dressed in girls' clothes, had girls as friends, and said that they wanted to be girls. Of those boys who had become sexually active, 47% were primarily homosexual and 33% were clearly bisexual. Homosexual orientation was most associated with dressing as a girl, playing with dolls, and having a female peer group.

56. Pleak RR, Meyer-Bahlburg HFL, O'Brien JD, Bowen HA, Morganstein A: Cross-gender behaviour and psychopathology in boy psychiatric outpatients. *J Am Acad Child Adolesc Psychiatry* 28:385–393, 1989

Between 30% to 50% of a sample of boys between ages 5 and 12 years who came for outpatient psychiatric evaluation were noted to have cross-gender behavior. These behaviors were not identified by the Child Behavior Checklist and require explicit assessment to determine their presence.

57. Roberts CW, Green R, Williams K, Goodman M: Boyhood gender identity development: a statistical contrast of two family groups. *Developmental Psychology* 23:544–557, 1987

This thoughtful discussion of the formation of gender identity in boys supports the commonsense view that boys who grow up in a home without a father are more likely to be feminine.

Tourette's Syndrome and Other Tic Disorders

58. *Gilles de la Tourette G:** Etudes sur une affection nerveuse caracterise ar de l'incoordination motrice accompagnee d'echolalie et de copralalie. *Arch Neurol* 9:19–42, 158–200, 1885

This article is the original description of Tourette's syndrome.

59. **Pauls DL, Leckman JF:** The inheritance of Gilles de la Tourette syndrome and associated behaviors: evidence for autosomal dominant transmission. *N Engl J Med* 315:993–997, 1986

Analyses support the conclusion that obsessive-compulsive disorder is etiologically related to Tourette's syndrome, and that Tourette's syndrome is inherited as a highly penetrant, sex-influenced, autosomal-dominant trait.

Mood Disorders

60. *Beardslee WR, Bemporad J, Keller M, Klerman GL:** Children of parents with major affective disorder: a review. *Am J Psychiatry* 140:825–883, 1983

Approximately 40% of the children of parents with major affective disorder were reported to have psychiatric diagnoses based on a review of major studies. Depressive symptoms were frequently reported. However, a wide range of other psychiatric symptoms were also noted.

61. *Kovacs M, Feinberg TL, Crouse-Novak M, Parkansas SL, Pollock M, Finkelstein R:** Depressive disorders in childhood, II: a longitudinal study of the risk for a subsequent major depression. *Arch Gen Psychiatry* 41:643–649, 1984

Of a longitudinal cohort of depressed children with major depressive disorder and dysthymic disorder, 40% were shown to relapse within 2 years. Children who had been diagnosed as having adjustment disorder with depressed mood had a minimal risk for subsequent major depression.

62. **McCracken JT:** The epidemiology of child and adolescent mood disorders. *Child and Adolescent Psychiatric Clinics of North America* 1:53–72, 1992

Considerable variability in estimates of the prevalence of childhood depression is reviewed. Depression in prepubertal children is relatively uncommon (1%–3%), whereas the rate at least doubles after puberty. Some reports suggest that the incidence of depression peaks in late adolescence.

63. *Puig-Antich J, Perel JM, Luptakin W, Chambers WJ, Tabrizi MA, King J, Goetz R, Davies M, Stiller RL: Imipramine in prepubertal major depression. *Arch Gen Psychiatry* 44:81–89, 1987

No therapeutic effect of imipramine in depressed prepubertal children is reported in this well-controlled study. Discussion of this negative finding includes consideration of the dosage being too low.

64. Radke-Yarrow M, Nottelman E, Martinez P, Fox MB, Belmont B: Young children of affectively ill parents: a longitudinal study of psychosocial development. *J Am Acad Child Adolesc Psychiatry* 31:68–77, 1992

Children of unipolar depressed mothers were reported to have more disruptive behavior and to be more depressed by the time they are 5 years old when compared with control children and the children of bipolar depressed mothers. By ages 8–11, children of both bipolar (61%) and unipolar (68%) mothers developed problems, but the onset of the disturbance was earlier in the children with bipolar mothers.

65. Ryan ND, Puig-Antich J, Ambrosini P, Rabinovich H, Robinson D, Nelson B, Iyengar S, Twomey J: The clinical picture of major depression in children and adolescents. *Arch Gen Psychiatry* 44:854–861, 1984

This empirical report stresses the similarity in symptom picture between children and adolescents. Adolescents were noted to show greater anhedonia, hopelessness, hypersomnia, weight gain, use of alcohol and illicit drugs, and lethality of suicide.

66. Strober M, Morrell W, Lampert C, Burroughs J: Relapse following discontinuation of lithium maintenance therapy in adolescents with bipolar I illness: a naturalistic study. *Am J Psychiatry* 147:457–461, 1990

Adolescents with bipolar I illness were three times more likely to relapse after initial remission if lithium maintenance treatment was discontinued.

Suicide and Attempted Suicide

67. Brent DA, Perper JA, Goldstein CE, Kolko DJ, Allan MJ, Allman CJ, Zelenak JP: Risk factors for adolescent suicide. *Arch Gen Psychiatry* 45:581–588, 1987

Four putative risk factors for successful adolescent suicide are documented. These include diagnosis of bipolar disorder, affective disorder
with comorbidity, the absence of mental health treatment, and availability of firearms.

68. **Brent DA, Johnson B, Bartle S, Bridge J, Rather C, Matta J, Connolly J,
Constantine D:** Personality disorder tendency to impulsive violence and
suicidal behavior in adolescents. *J Am Acad Child Adolesc Psychiatry* 32:69–
75, 1993

    Hospitalized adolescent suicide attempters were found to have more
    borderline symptoms than nonsuicidal adolescent control subjects.
    Those adolescents with personality disturbance were also more likely to
    have made previous suicidal attempts.

69. **Kovacs M, Goldston D, Gatsonis C:** Suicidal behaviors and childhood-
onset depressive disorders: a longitudinal investigation. *J Am Acad Child
Adolesc Psychiatry* 32:8–20, 1993

    Two-thirds of a cohort of depressed children reported suicidal ideation,
    and 9% had made a suicide attempt over the course of the study.
    Despite variable durations of follow-up, the mean number of at-risk
    years was 6.6. The rate of attempted suicide was highest when the
    children reached age 17, at which point it was 24%.

70. *Pfeffer CR, Newcorn JH, Kaplan G, Mizruchi MS, Plutchik R:** Suicidal
behavior in adolescent psychiatric inpatients. *J Am Acad Child Adolesc
Psychiatry* 27:357–362, 1988

    Significant predictors of suicide attempts in hospitalized adolescent
    psychiatric inpatients included alcohol abuse, depression, aggressive
    behavior, and past suicidal behavior.

71. **Pfeffer CR, Klerman GL, Hurt SW, Kakuma T, Peskin JR, Siefker CA:**
Suicidal children grow up: rates and psychosocial risk factors for suicide
attempts during follow-up. *J Am Acad Child Adolesc Psychiatry* 32:106–113,
1993

    Children who had attempted suicide were six times more likely than
    nonpatients to attempt suicide during a 6- to 8-year follow-up. Poor
    social adjustment and recent mood disorder are the two strongest
    predictors of reoccurrence.

72. **Shaffer D, Garland A, Gould M, Fissher P, Trautman P:** Preventing
teenage suicide: a critical review. *J Am Acad Child Adolesc Psychiatry*
27:675–687, 1988

Concern regarding the efficacy of many suicide-prevention strategies was raised by this review. The point is made that most children who commit suicide have a psychiatric disorder and that addressing risk factors for these illnesses may be a promising strategy.

Anxiety Disorders

73. **Bernstein GA, Borchardt CM:** Special article: anxiety disorders of childhood and adolescence: a critical review. *J Am Acad Child Adolesc Psychiatry* 30:519–532, 1991

This article is a comprehensive recent review of anxiety disorders. Epidemiological studies highlight the widespread occurrence of these problems. Rates up to 8.9% have been reported in children when impairment is considered; rates as high as 8.7% were reported for adolescents. Comorbidity with depression is reviewed.

74. **Keller MB, Lavori PW, Wunder J, Beardslee WR, Schwartz CE, Roth J:** Chronic course of anxiety disorders in children and adolescents. *J Am Acad Child Adolesc Psychiatry* 31:595–599, 1992

A persistent course of anxiety disorder is reported as 46% of the longitudinal cohort remained symptomatic after 8 years. Median age at onset of separation disorders was 8 years of age; median age at onset for overanxious disorder was 10 years.

75. **Mattison R, Bagnato S:** Empirical measurement of overanxious disorder in boys 8 to 12 years old. *J Am Acad Child Adolesc Psychiatry* 26:536–540, 1987

Using consensual clinician diagnostic rating as the criterion standard, the combination of a parental behavioral rating score and a self-rating of manifest anxiety by the child was sufficient to identify 70% of the cases of overanxious disorder.

Obsessive-Compulsive Disorder

76. **Berg CZ, Rapoport JL, Whitacker A, Davies M, Leonard HL, Swedo SE, Braiman S, Lenane MC:** Childhood obsessive-compulsive disorder: two year prospective follow-up of a community sample. *J Am Acad Child Adolesc Psychiatry* 28:528–533, 1989

This article is the landmark natural history study of obsessive-compulsive disorder in adolescence. Analysis of the course and symptoms in students in a public high school cohort supports the idea that obsessive-compulsive disorder is a heterogenous disorder. Symptom severity waxes and wanes over time.

77. **Leonard HL, Goldberger EL, Rapoport JL, Cheslow DL, Swedo SE:** Childhood rituals: normal development of obsessive compulsive symptoms? *J Am Acad Child Adolesc Psychiatry* 29:17–23, 1990

Parents of 38 children with severe primary obsessive-compulsive disorder were interviewed regarding the early development of rituals and superstitions. A history of "marked patterns of early ritualistic behaviors" was elicited for 70% of the index children. However, when behaviors resembling obsessions are eliminated from the analysis, no difference between the index and control groups is evident. The possibility exists that these early rituals are the first symptoms of the disorder and could be considered a marker for the disease.

78. **Luxenberg JS, Swedo SE, Flament MF, Friedland RP, Rapoport J, Rapoport SI:** Neuroanatomical abnormalities in obsessive-compulsive disorder detected with quantitative X-ray computed tomography. *Am J Psychiatry* 145:1089–1093, 1988

The caudate nucleus volume in children with primary severe obsessive-compulsive disorder is demonstrated to be smaller than caudate nucleus volume in control children.

79. **Rettew DC, Swedo SE, Leonard HL, Lenane MC, Rapoport JL:** Obsessions and compulsions across time in 79 children and adolescents with obsessive-compulsive disorder. *J Am Acad Child Adolesc Psychiatry* 31:1050–1056, 1992

The presence of obsessive-compulsive symptoms is shown to be persistent but the precise form of the symptoms change over time. Interestingly, 47% of the patients demonstrated both washing and checking compulsions at some time in their illness.

80. **Riddle MA, Scahill L, King R, Hardin MT, Towbin KE, Ort SI, Leckman JF, Cohen DJ:** Obsessive compulsive disorder in children and adolescents: phenomenology and family history. *J Am Acad Child Adolesc Psychiatry* 29:766–772, 1990

Comorbid psychopathology was noted in 62% of the children. A positive parental family history, defined as having a parent with either obsessive-compulsive disorder or obsessive-compulsive symptoms, was noted for 71% of the children.

81. **Swedo SE, Schapiro MB, Grady CL, Cheslow DL, Leonard HL, Kumar A, Friedland R, Rapoport SI, Rapoport JL:** Cerebral glucose metabolism in childhood onset obsessive compulsive disorder. *Arch Gen Psychiatry* 46:518–527, 1989

Cerebral glucose metabolism was increased in the 1) left orbital frontal, 2) right sensorimotor, and 3) bilateral prefrontal and anterior cingulate regions. Right anterior cingulate and right orbital frontal regions had a higher rate of metabolism in those children with obsessive-compulsive disorder who were clomipramine nonresponders.

Sleep Disorders

82. **Benoit D, Zeanah CH, Boucher C, Minde KK:** Sleep disorders in early childhood: association with insecure maternal attachment. *J Am Acad Child Adolesc Psychiatry* 31:86–93, 1991

Mothers with toddlers with sleep disorders were uniformly classified as having had an insecure attachment. In contrast, they did not have a disproportionate frequency of marital difficulties or absence of social support. These findings are used to emphasize the importance of maternal relationship history for establishing normal sleep patterns.

83. **Emslie GJ, Roffwarg HP, Rush AJ, Weinberg WA, Parkin-Feigenbaum L:** Sleep EEG findings in depressed children and adolescents. *Am J Psychiatry* 144:668–670, 1987

The sleep architecture of depressed pubertal adolescents were documented to be similar to depressed adults. This included a shorter rapid eye movement (REM) latency, fewer arousals, and more REM activity and REM periods.

84. **Richman N:** Sleep problems in young children. *Arch Gen Psychiatry* 56:491–493, 1981

About 20% of children between ages 1 and 2 years have persistent sleep problems. By age 3, this rate decreased to 13%.

85. **Schmitt BD:** The prevention of sleep problems. *Clin Perinatol* 12:453–457, 1985

This short article provides a practical guide to the management of sleeping in young children. The prevention of more serious sleeping problems is achieved by providing proactive advice about the sleeping needs and patterns of infants.

86. **Simonds JF, Parraga H:** Prevalence of sleep disorders and sleep behaviors in children and adolescents. *Journal of the American Academy of Child Psychiatry* 21:383–388, 1982

Maternal reports of sleep problems in school-age children and adolescents are documented. Most children (93.5%) had no problems although a wide range of isolated difficulties existed. Almost 17% of the sample had experienced a nightmare, and nearly 3% reported an episode of night terrors in the previous 6 months.

Posttraumatic Stress Disorders

87. **Galante R, Foa D:** An epidemiological study of psychic trauma and treatment effectiveness for children after a natural disaster. *Journal of the American Academy of Child Psychiatry* 25:357–363, 1986

    An Italian study of 300 children found that community response and family response after a devastating earthquake were more closely related to subsequent adaptation than the amount of destruction in the village. A large-scale intervention program is described.

88. **Kinzie JD, Sack WH, Angell RH, Manson S, Ben R:** The psychiatric effects of massive trauma on Cambodian children: the children. *Journal of the American Academy of Child Psychiatry* 25:370–376, 1986

    Half the children assessed after experiencing severe abuse and living for 2 years in Cambodian refugee camps developed posttraumatic stress disorder. Symptoms were more severe if the children had been separated from all of their family.

89. **Kinzie JD, Sack WH, Angell RH, Clarke G, Ben R:** A three year follow-up of Cambodian young people traumatized as children. *J Am Acad Child Adolesc Psychiatry* 28:501–504, 1989

    Posttraumatic stress disorder persisted for 3 years in children in the Cambodian study. Of the children, 30% had persistent symptoms, whereas at least a quarter of the original cohort never developed the disorder.

90. **Pynoos RS, Eth S:** Witness to violence: the child interview. *J Am Acad Child Adolesc Psychiatry* 25:306–319, 1986

    This article is a practical guide to conducting an interview with a child who has recently been traumatized. Therapeutic aspects are highlighted.

91. **Pynoos RS, Frederick C, Nader K, Arroyo W, Steinberg A, Eth S, Nunez F, Fairbanks L:** Life threat and posttraumatic stress in school-age children. *Arch Gen Psychiatry* 44:1057–1063, 1987

    This is an empirical report of the symptoms of children exposed to the random killing of a child on the playground by a sniper. Thirteen other children were injured. The degree of disturbance of survivors was related to proximity rather than sex, ethnicity, or age.

92. [*]**Terr LC:** "Forbidden games": post-traumatic child's play. *Journal of the American Academy of Child Psychiatry* 20:741–760, 1981

This is a classic article that skillfully describes 11 characteristics of posttraumatic play. Compulsive repetitiveness and the failure of the play initially to relieve anxiety are key features.

93. **Yule W, Udwin O, Murdoch K:** The "Jupiter" sinking: effects on children's fears, depression and anxiety. *J Child Psychol Psychiatry* 31:1051–1061, 1990

Survivors of a major disaster were shown to develop quite persistent fears related to the traumatic event rather than a more generalized increase in level of fearfulness.

Multiple Personality

94. **Bowman E, Blix S, Coons PM:** Multiple personality disorder in adolescence: relating to incestual experiences. *J Am Acad Child Adolesc Psychiatry* 24:109–114, 1985

This is a discussion of the case of a 14-year-old girl who had an incestuous relationship with her father for 3 years that began when she was 5. During this time, she developed a multiple personality disorder with three personalities. Problems with making the diagnosis in young children are discussed.

95. **Fagan J, McMahon PP:** Incipient multiple personality in children: four cases. *J Nerv Ment Dis* 172:26–36, 1984

A set of 20 behavioral signs thought to be characteristic of children with multiple personality disorder is described. The advantages of early intervention for incipient cases are discussed.

96. **Putnam FW, Guroff JJ, Silberman EK, Barban L, Post RM:** The clinical phenomenology of multiple personality disorder: 100 recent cases. *J Clin Psychiatry* 47:285–293, 1986

This empirical review supports the position that the onset of multiple personality disorder occurs in childhood. The mean age at onset was 6 years; in nearly 90% of the cases, the onset was before 12 years. Sexual abuse occurred in 83% of the cases and was often incestuous.

Adjustment Disorder

97. **Newcorn JH, Strain J:** Adjustment disorder in children and adolescents. *J Am Acad Child Adolesc Psychiatry* 31:318–326, 1992

    This review of adjustment disorder suggests that it has a high prevalence of between 4.2% and 7.6% as well as considerable morbidity. Problems with making this diagnosis include a relatively low level of interrater reliability using current diagnostic methods, the predominance of a mixed symptom pattern rather than discrete symptoms, and the reality that these symptoms often persist for more than 6 months.

98. **Woolston JL:** Theoretical considerations of the adjustment disorders. *J Am Acad Child Adolesc Psychiatry* 27:280–287, 1988

    A theoretical framework for assessing adjustment disorders using a developmentally sequential model is put forward. Key features of the model and its clinical implications are discussed.

Borderline Disorders

99. **Greenman DA, Gunderson JG, Cane M, Saltzman PR:** An examination of the borderline diagnosis in children. *Am J Psychiatry* 143:998–1003, 1986

    Using a modification of the Diagnostic Interview for Borderlines, 27 children were identified as borderline and compared with other psychiatrically hospitalized children who did not meet these criteria. Relatively few differences were noted between the two groups, although those children who were designated as borderline were more likely to be psychotic, be characterized by angry actions, and have hostile interpersonal relationships. The validity of the diagnosis is discussed.

100. **Herman JL, Perry JC, van der Kolk BA:** Childhood trauma in borderline personality disorder. *Am J Psychiatry* 146:490–495, 1989

    When interviewed about childhood trauma, 81% of a sample of adult borderline patients gave a history of childhood abuse. Both physical abuse (71%) and sexual abuse (62%) were reported.

101. **Petti TA, Vela RM:** Special article: Borderline disorders of childhood: an overview. *J Am Acad Child Adolesc Psychiatry* 29:327–337, 1990

    The need for a better definition of borderline personality disorder is highlighted. Two possible subcategories are put forward. The first is characterized as "borderline spectrum"; the second is referred to as the "schizotypal spectrum."

Alcohol and Drug Abuse in Adolescents

102. **Estroff TW, Schwartz RH, Hoffmann NG:** Adolescent cocaine abuse: addictive potential, behavioral and psychiatric effects. *Clin Pediatr (Phila)* 28:550–555, 1989

The powerful addictive properties of cocaine in adolescents are documented. A wide range of psychiatric symptoms were evident in a majority of the moderate to heavy users, including nervousness, suspiciousness, aggressiveness, fatigue, insomnia, anorexia, and depression.

103. **Kandel DB:** Epidemiological and psychosocial perspectives on adolescent drug use. *Journal of the American Academy of Child Psychiatry* 21:328–347, 1982

This article supports the position that alcohol use precedes the use of illicit drugs in most adolescents. It highlights the similarities in risk factors for both substance abuse and other forms of psychopathology. A "pattern of disaffection from major institutions" (p. 336) was typical of users of marijuana in both 1967 and 1980.

Somatoform Disorders

104. **Livingston R, Martin-Cannici C:** Multiple somatic complaints and possible somatization disorder in prepubertal children. *Journal of the American Academy of Child Psychiatry* 24:603–607, 1985

The range and types of somatic symptoms in prepubertal children that would qualify for the diagnosis of somatization disorder are reviewed. A cluster of seven symptoms were present in each of the five cases discussed.

105. *Maloney MJ:** Diagnosing hysterical conversion reactions in children. *J Pediatr* 97:1016–1020, 1980

A chart audit of pediatric inpatients with the diagnosis of conversion reaction were compared with a control group of pediatric patients who had been evaluated psychiatrically and found to have no organic brain disease, psychotic illness, or conversion reactions. Of the 105 children with conversion reactions that were identified, there was a greater frequency of life stress, family communication problems, and grief reactions than there was with the control subjects.

106. **Steinhausen HC, von Aster M, Pfeiffer E, Gobel D:** Comparative studies of conversion disorders in childhood and adolescence. *J Child Psychol Psychiatry* 30:615–621, 1989

Twenty-six children and adolescents with the diagnosis of conversion disorder were compared with other clinical groups. Of the patients with conversion disorder, 85% were older than 11 years and 65% were female. They were more likely to be migrants and of a lower social class. Of these children, 71% of their fathers and 31% of their mothers had a physical problem.

107. **Volkmar FR, Poll J, Lewis M:** Conversion reactions in childhood and adolescence. *Journal of the American Academy of Child Psychiatry* 23:424–430, 1984

Thirty children with conversion disorder were compared with children with adjustment disorders. The four features that differentiated the children with conversion disorders were referral by physician, complaints of neurological symptoms, previous hospitalization, and presence of sexually stressful life events. Sexually stressful life events had occurred in 70% of the children with conversion disorder.

Pediatric Psychiatry

108. **Fritz GK:** Consultation-liaison in child psychiatry and the evolution of pediatric psychiatry. *Psychosomatics* 31:85–90, 1990

A plan for the provision of psychiatric care for pediatric patients is put forward. Successful models at major pediatric centers serve as the focus of this discussion.

109. **Fritz GK, Williams JR:** Issues of adolescent development for survivors of childhood cancer. *J Am Acad Child Adolesc Psychiatry* 27:712–715, 1988

Only 17% of adolescent survivors were having serious adjustment problems when assessed 2–8 years after their treatment. Only 7% of the sample had clearly documented depression. A quarter of the children were preoccupied with physical symptoms.

110. **Kovacs M, Feinberg TL, Paulauskas S, Finkelstein TL, Pollock M, Crouse-Novak M:** Initial coping responses and psychosocial characteristics of children with insulin-dependent diabetes mellitus. *J Pediatr* 106:827–834, 1985

Two modes of coping are described in a cohort of children with recent onset of insulin-dependent diabetes mellitus. Two-thirds show a subdued reaction accompanied by withdrawal; one-third met criteria for a psychiatric diagnosis. Within 7–9 months. 93% of these children recovered.

111. **Mrazek DA, Klinnert MD, Mrazek P, Macey T:** Early onset asthma: consideration of parenting issues. *J Am Acad Child Adolesc Psychiatry* 3:277–282, 1991

Parenting difficulties were assessed shortly after the birth of infants at genetic risk for the development of asthma. The children of parents who were exhibiting problems with parenting were more likely to have developed asthma based on the longitudinal maternal report of wheezing and illness episodes.

112. *Ravenscroft K:** Psychiatric consultation to the child with acute physical trauma. *Am J Orthopsychiatry* 52:298–307, 1982

This article is a practical guide to dealing with a traumatized child within the context of a pediatric hospital.

113. **Steinhausen H, Schindler H, Stephan H:** Correlates of psychopathology in sick children: an empirical model. *Journal of the American Academy of Child Psychiatry* 22:559–564, 1983

In asthmatic children, the presence of psychopathology was associated with family problems, disturbed parental behavior, marital problems, and the occurrence of undesirable life events, but not severity of illness. For children with cystic fibrosis, the reverse was true, with severity as measured by vital capacity being the strongest predictor of psychiatric disturbance.

114. **Strunk RC, Mrazek DA,Wolfson Fuhrmann GS, LaBrecque JF:** Physiologic and psychological characteristics associated with deaths due to asthma in childhood. *JAMA* 254:1193–1198, 1985

A set of seven risk factors are presented that could be used to identify children who had died from a fatal asthmatic attack. Chronic conflicted relationship between the family and caregivers and a history of recent depression in the child were among the strongest predictors.

HIV

115. **Belfer ML, Krener PK, Miller FB:** AIDS in children and adolescents. *J Am Acad Child Adolesc Psychiatry* 27:147–151, 1988

The danger of widespread dissemination of the human immunodeficiency virus as a consequence of the sexual behavior of asymptomatic infected adolescents is highlighted. Clinical efforts both at the level of individual children and families as well as involving the provision of liaison support to pediatric professionals is projected to increase dramatically. The special problems of helping patients cope with terminal disease are reviewed.

116. **Brown LK, Fritz GK:** Children's knowledge and attitudes about AIDS. *J Am Acad Child Adolesc Psychiatry* 27:504–508, 1988

This study of youths' knowledge about acquired immunodeficiency syndrome (AIDS) extended the inquiry about teaching youth about AIDS beyond factual education itself (as measured by correct responses to a questionnaire) to include attitudes, coping styles, and behaviors. Translation of knowledge into behavior was related to attitude and coping style, indicating that affective issues must be engaged for effective education.

117. **Krener PK, Miller FB:** Psychiatric response to HIV spectrum disease in children and adolescents. *J Am Acad Child Adolesc Psychiatry* 28:596–605, 1989

Through a series of vignettes, the biological, psychosocial, and treatment aspects of the clinical spectrum of human immunodeficiency virus (HIV) infection in children and adolescents is presented. Perinatal infection, transfusion-acquired HIV in a hemophiliac, and high-risk adolescent sexual behavior in heterosexual and homosexual youth are discussed.

Assessment

31

Psychiatric Interviewing

Shawn Christopher Shea, M.D.

R apid advancements in the field of mental health have necessitated an evolution in the craft of assessment interviewing.
In the past 40 years an impressive array of new therapeutic
interventions has emerged. These revolutionary advances include modalities such as tricyclic antidepressants, antipsychotic medications, behavior
modification, family therapy, group therapy, and more sophisticated forms
of dynamic, cognitive, and hypnotic psychotherapies, to name only a few.

The development of so many new tools has presented a startling
challenge to the initial interviewer, especially when the interviewer is functioning as a triage agent or consultant who may never see the patient again.
More specifically, to determine an effective treatment plan and disposition,
the interviewer must gather an amount of information in 50 minutes that
might have staggered an interviewer of 40 years ago. At that time, one did
not need to elicit the neurovegetative symptoms of depression, because
tricyclic antidepressants and serotonin-selective reuptake inhibitors did not
exist. One did not have to delineate the diagnosis of agoraphobia, because
behavioral tools such as flooding were unavailable. It did not matter
whether the interviewee had symptoms suggestive of mania, because lithium was a dream waiting to crystallize in John Cade's mind. In short, the
therapeutic explosion has created a substantially increased need for more
precise and more thorough data gathering in the initial encounter.

The challenge of the interview revolves around the manner in which the initial interviewer collects critical data, while constantly attending to rapport. With each unique pairing of interviewer and interviewee, this tension must be creatively resolved. A skilled interviewer is remarkably flexible. As has always been the case, the validity of the data depends directly on the strength of the therapeutic engagement. In fact, if anything, the importance of the therapeutic alliance has increased over the years. In the long run, reliable diagnosis, effective treatment planning, treatment compliance, and family support of therapeutic intervention are all limited by a common factor: the therapist's ability to engage the patient. Consequently, the initial interview remains the foundation of all mental health interventions.

Critical reading is one of the first steps that a trainee takes when embarking on the great challenge of mastering this most crucial of practical arts. When the resident asks where to start, the answer is not immediately obvious, for the resident is frequently confused by the overwhelming wealth of possibilities available. In the past 7 years alone, seven major textbooks on interviewing have appeared. Consequently, I have been faced with the unenviable task of being highly selective with asterisks (essential reading); my own personal preference would be to use an asterisk with most of the following selections because I have included only works of very high quality. But, it seems to me, that such an "asterisk-heavy" approach risks leaving the time-burdened trainee (or faculty) only more confused, compounded by a growing guilt that one has "not even read what is essential." Instead, with the selective use of the asterisk and in the annotations themselves, I have attempted to point out the strengths and weaknesses of the works listed, in an effort to help the reader piece together a realistic reading program that thoroughly meets the trainee's core educational needs, while providing direction for individualized interests, whether psychodynamic, diagnostic, or phenomenological.

For an introductory psychiatric curriculum to interviewing, I suggest beginning by reading a broad-based core textbook, such as the one I attempted to produce (Shea 1988). This text introduces the reader to the rich insights that can be gleamed from the classic interviewing literature of all mental health disciplines and immediately addresses the beginning resident's urgent need to integrate DSM-III-R diagnosis with other critical tasks such as suicide assessment, handling resistance, and assessing for psychotherapy. (Please note that, at the time of this writing, many of the standard texts, such as my own, are being updated with new editions to include DSM-IV.)

I suggest following this hopefully very stimulating initial incursion by picking one of the outstanding texts that are more focused on specific topics—for example, MacKinnon and Michels (1971) for an in-depth look at psychodynamics, Othmer and Othmer (1994) for more polish on DSM-III-R differential diagnosis, or Harry Stack Sullivan (1970) for further development of the interpersonal perspective. From there interested readers can use this annotated bibliography to find the clinical gems that match their individualized interests. If the novice resident follows this simplifying approach to the vast wealth of interviewing literature currently available, he or she is guaranteed not only a sound theoretical foundation in one of the cornerstone skills of our profession, but also many hours of provocative and fun reading.

Textbooks

1. **Bandler R, Grinder J:** *The Structure of Magic I.* Palo Alto, CA, Science & Behavior Books, 1975

   In an innovative fashion, Bandler and Grinder give specific techniques for uncovering the real meaning (deep structure) masked by patient's superficial statements (surface structure). The book is well written and stimulating; it utilizes aspects of a programmed text, forcing the reader immediately to apply the techniques as they are described. This book does not address diagnosis at all and is not a general text, but it is a nice complement to other texts described in this section.

2. **Benjamin A:** *The Helping Interview With Case Illustrations.* Boston, MA, Houghton Mifflin, 1987

   In this well-written and warm book, Benjamin further improves his brief classic, which first appeared in 1969. Benjamin presents down-to-earth advice, and one senses his mastery of what he speaks. If a psychiatric resident wants to read one text that gives a good feel for the approach of the counseling field to the initial encounter, this is it. Unfortunately, it is limited as a general text because it is weak on clinical tasks such as suicide assessment and does not consider differential diagnosis or the DSM.

3. **Cormier WH, Cormier LS:** *Interviewing Strategies for Helpers,* 2nd Edition. Monterey, CA, Brooks/Cole, 1985

   This text covers much more than interviewing skills, examining strategies for four counseling stages (assessment, goal setting, strategy selection, and evaluation-termination). The book is filled with good examples, and role-playing exercises are provided. Although this text does not consider the DSM or specific critical clinical tasks such as suicide assessment, it is a very nice introduction to counseling approaches and can serve as a complement to a more "psychiatric-specific" general text.

4. **Craig RJ** (ed): *Clinical and Diagnostic Interviewing.* Northvale, NJ, Jason Aronson, 1989

This edited book has four sections: 1) basic elements in the clinical interview, 2) approaches to interviewing (psychoanalytic, existential/humanist, behavioral, and family), 3) interviewing patients with specific psychopathologies, and 4) focused interviews (such as the mental status and suicide potential). It has an excellent breadth of coverage; the chapters on psychoanalytic and existential/humanist perspectives are particularly thought provoking. The editor made a significant error, however, in not directing the contributors to illustrate their interviewing techniques through the use of specific sample questions and interview vignettes. The book consequently seems to talk more about interviewing than demonstrating for the reader practical advice on how to interview. There is little satisfying advice on how to structure interviews sensitively while arriving at a DSM-III-R formulation. Little effort is given to synthesizing the differing interview perspectives presented in the second and third sections. As one would expect from an edited book, some of the writing is a bit dry. This is an excellent sourcebook but not a particularly good core textbook.

5. Egan G: *The Skilled Helper: A Model for Systematic Helping and Interpersonal Relating,* 3rd Edition. Monterey, CA, Brooks/Cole, 1986

Integrating many of the best strategies from the counseling perspective, Egan has produced a concise and clear guide to interviewing techniques and early treatment principles. The book is ripe with explicit examples; and an accompanying workbook is available. The lack of DSM-III-R differential diagnosis and any guide for suicide assessment or mental status limits the book as a general text.

6. Greenspan SI, in collaboration with Greenspan NT: *The Clinical Interview of the Child,* 2nd Edition. Washington, DC, American Psychiatric Association Press, 1991

This is a well-written and enjoyable text. The clinical vignettes are rich with realism and sensitivity. Greenspan thoughtfully describes the role of development and its interplay with normal and abnormal behavior. There is a practical chapter on interviewing parents at the end. There is not much on adolescence here. The book is heavy on the psychodynamic-developmental approach and light on DSM-III-R, with which the author does not sound particularly enthused.

7. Halleck SL: *Evaluation of the Psychiatric Patient: A Primer.* New York, Plenum Medical, 1991

When reading Halleck's book, one is reminded of the provocative and charming writing of Harry Stack Sullivan. Halleck has the same knack for providing practical advice on how to understand the person beneath the diagnosis. The book is particularly strong when pointing out the interviewer's potential impact on the patient's responses, feelings, and symptom picture. The chapter on developmental history is quite strong as is the mental status material. Because of its more contemporary feel, some residents may even prefer it to Sullivan's classic text as a foray into the complexities of the interpersonal perspective of interviewing. Compared with several other recent texts, the book is relatively weak on DSM-III-R differential diagnosis and does not adequately show effective ways for sensitively structuring interviews or handling time management well, topics of marked importance for contemporary residents. Suicide assessment is not covered in depth. Another problem is the lack of reference to practical findings from previous writers on interviewing, making the book unnecessarily idiosyncratic.

8. **Hersen M, Turner SM:** *Diagnostic Interviewing.* New York, Plenum, 1985

This book begins with some useful but brief material concerning basic interviewing process and the mental status, and it quickly turns to a series of chapters addressing specific DSM-III-R diagnostic clusters. It ends with some chapters concerning special populations such as families, children, and the elderly, with the latter chapter, in particular, providing some nice insights. The authors were pioneering in recognizing the marked evolution of interviewing necessitated by the advent of DSM-III-R and the subsequent need to teach new interviewing skills related to sensitive structuring and differential diagnosis. The book demonstrates the problems so common to edited works, however, such as uneven quality of chapters and not enough focus on unifying principles. The book is also light on interview vignettes and sample questions. Many key interviewing authors and their innovations are simply not mentioned, limiting the book as a general text.

9. **Hughes JN, Baker D:** *The Clinical Child Interview.* New York, Guilford, 1990

The text here is nicely written, and the authors provide a fine introduction to three broad theoretical perspectives: structured interviews, psychodynamic interviews, and behavioral interviews. They provide a very practical chapter on altering interview style to meet the developmental needs of the child. Overall, this is an excellent book that is somewhat hampered by not enough advice on arriving at a DSM-III-R diagnosis, although DSM-III-R is favorably addressed.

10. **Leon RL:** *Psychiatric Interviewing: A Primer.* New York, Elsevier, 1982

This book is a short and reasonable introduction to psychiatric interviewing for medical students. Psychiatric residents will find it unfulfilling, but it was not intended for them. It has some nice sections on nonverbal communication and cross-cultural issues, which are often not given enough attention even in major textbooks. Leon also conveys a deep sense of compassion and the importance of empathy and openness. The book has problems, however, wedding nondirective and directive techniques. The author overemphasizes the former and misses the value of the latter in arriving at a sound diagnosis. Suicide assessment is barely mentioned and, having been written before both DSM-III-R and DSM-IV, good strategies for DSM differential diagnosis are not well presented, two major omissions that significantly limit this text even for medical students.

11. *MacKinnon RA, Michels R: *The Psychiatric Interview in Clinical Practice.* Philadelphia, PA, WB Saunders, 1971

Here is a gem of a book. I believe it to be the best book concerning the psychodynamics of interviewing ever written. The writing style is pleasingly easy to read, and one feels that one is being guided by master clinicians, which is exactly the case. Commonly encountered, yet potentially problematic situations, such as chance meetings with patients outside of the office and unexpected telephone calls, are insightfully discussed. Useful interviewing techniques are reviewed by syndrome, such as obsessive patients or phobic patients. The book is packed with wisdom and psychodynamic tips. Unfortunately, as a general textbook, the book has shown its age. There is no guidance for the use of the DSM-III-R or DSM-IV; minimal help is provided on how to structure interviews efficiently in the age of managed care; and the advice on suicide assessment is inadequate. With these problems in mind, the contemporary resident must look elsewhere for a general text, but MacKinnon and Michels' remains "the book to read" on psychodynamic interviewing, a true classic in this respect and a delight to explore.

12. *MacKinnon RA, Yudofsky SC: *Principles of the Psychiatric Evaluation,* Revised Edition. Philadelphia, PA, JB Lippincott, 1991

This brilliantly conceived and executed book covers the following areas: the psychiatric interview, the clinical examination of the patient, biological testing in psychiatry, evaluation of regional cortical functioning, psychological testing and psychiatric rating scales, and DSM-III-R diagnosis and the psychodynamic formulation. The two brief sections on interviewing are nicely done but introductory in nature. The resident must go elsewhere for a satisfying exploration of the complexities of interviewing, and even some basics such as suicide assessment are barely discussed. Nor will the resident find any mention of the enormous wealth of interviewing knowledge provided by psychology and counseling here. However, this is not really a book focusing primarily on interviewing and should not be judged as such. Instead, it is an ambitious and highly successful introduction to the overall psychiatric assessment process from intake interview to computed tomography scan and psychological testing. The remaining chapters are outstanding, with a great section on structured interviews and a "must-read" chapter on psychodynamic formulation hiding at the end of the book. Excellent examples of assessment write-ups are given. The information on biological tests and psychiatric rating scales is top-notch and very practical. All information is presented in a concise and clear fashion, and I recommend the book to all residents.

13. **Morrison J:** *The First Interview: A Guide for Clinicians.* New York, Guilford, 1993

This book has a pleasant writing style, and the author has a good instinct for some of the common errors of beginning students. There is an ample supply of excellent model questions and some good tips on resistance and interviewing informants. Unfortunately, these good points are marred by some significant flaws. Differential diagnosis by DSM-III-R criteria is given relatively little attention. Moreover, time management, while integrating differential diagnosis, is also handled relatively weakly and in a somewhat misleading fashion. For instance, the author suggests that only 30% of interview time (just 18 minutes of a full hour) is needed to explore the combined tasks of Axis I differential diagnosis, suicide assessment, history of violence, and history of drug abuse (a daunting task for even the most experienced of clinicians). Another problem for the beginning student is the author's choice to ignore the numerous innovations to be found in the wealth of recent textbooks, an omission that results in a curiously dated work. Despite some very nice points, for a general introduction for medical students or residents, it is probably best to look elsewhere.

14. *Othmer E, Othmer SC:* *The Clinical Interview Using DSM-IV, Vol. 1: Fundamentals.* Washington, DC, American Psychiatric Press, 1994

This text provides an outstanding introduction to the use of the DSM-IV system. There are some excellent tips on differential diagnosis and methods of structuring the interview. The authors do a fine job of operationally defining interview techniques and strategies, and they reinforce this material with well-chosen illustrative examples of dialogue. The mental status is nicely covered with a well-conceived chapter on testing. There are also some insightfully annotated interviews. Unfortunately, for a general text, the book is somewhat limited by the focus on DSM-IV and a relative lack of reference to the wealth of practical tips to be found in the previous literature on interviewing.

Areas critical to all initial interviews, such as suicide-homicide assessment, social and family history, nonverbal communication, and assessment for psychotherapy are given less attention than one would hope to see in an introductory text. The result is a somewhat dry and idiosyncratic book, with many strengths, that provides an array of important insights into the practical use of DSM-IV.

15. **Pascal GR:** *The Practical Art of Diagnostic Interviewing.* Homewood, IL, Dow Jones-Irwin, 1983

Far too brief in nature (about 100 pages) and too minimally focused on DSM-III-R diagnosis to be of value as a core textbook, this small text is a curious delight. Pascal jumps directly into the complex nature of how interviewer style can distort and change the validity and reliability of data. The book is filled with insights and practical suggestions, woven together by an informal and sensitive writing style. Pascal also describes a specific technique, known as the "behavioral incident," which is one of the most powerful interviewing tips I have ever encountered. For the resident particularly interested in the complexities of interviewing, this book is a real find.

16. *Shea SC: *Psychiatric Interviewing: The Art of Understanding.* Philadelphia, PA, WB Saunders, 1988

In this book I attempted to provide a stimulating introduction to both basic and advanced principles of psychiatric interviewing, while distilling the "clinical pearls" of experts from many schools of thought from psychoanalysis to counseling. I felt it was critical to provide both the resident and medical student a concrete set of strategies for rapidly arriving at a sound DSM-III-R diagnosis, while sensitively engaging the patient and efficiently structuring the flow of the interview in this "age of managed care." Always trying to illustrate practical advice with actual interview excerpts, I devoted separate chapters to key areas such as engagement techniques, suicide and homicide assessment, nonverbal communication, and handling common resistances such as the shut-down, wandering, or hostile patient. Concerning the mental status, specific examples of a well-written mental status are contrasted with examples that highlight common beginner errors. I feel that the assessment for psychodynamic therapy was nicely explored, but note that no specific examples of a psychodynamic formulation are given. The text lacks, due to space limitations, a chapter on anxiety disorders, and perhaps it would have benefited from more time spent exploring substance abuse assessment. Nevertheless, it was my hope, that by using a fast-paced and informal writing style to illustrate practical techniques from many perspectives, that a powerful introductory textbook would result, a text that would resonate with the warmth and compassion so central to our art. (A new edition, updated to consider DSM-IV, will also include an annotated initial interview and sample write-up with tips on preparing the written document.)

17. **Simmons JE:** *Psychiatric Examination of Children,* 4th Edition. Philadelphia, PA, Lea & Febiger, 1987

This book is straightforward and well written. It has nice chapters on interviewing the family as a group, the individual child, and the parents alone. DSM-III is discussed, but not much specific advice is given on how to arrive at DSM-III diagnosis. The book is filled with realistic clinical descriptions and sound advice. It has had good longevity, being originally published in 1969.

18. *Sullivan HS: *The Psychiatric Interview.* New York, WW Norton, 1970

For many years following its initial appearance in 1954, this book was "the book" when it came to interviewing. Several generations of psychiatrists grew up on it, and it is still filled with wisdom, compassion, and practical information. Sullivan was a gifted writer, and he possessed an almost uncanny way of "getting into the patient's world." This is an ideal introduction to Sullivan's interpersonal framework for understanding interviewing process and psychopathology in general. It is also a fun read. Because of its age (no reference to DSM-III-R or DSM-IV, no reference to the practical writings and techniques of subsequent interviewing educators), the book can no longer be recommended as a general text. In this regard, the reader should be forewarned that Sullivan's "initial interview" sometimes spanned seven or nine sessions, a timeframe simply not practical in the age of managed care and time-limited therapies. Nevertheless, *The Psychiatric Interview* is still packed with practical insights and will stand forever as a psychiatric classic.

19. **Trzepacz PT, Baker RW:** *The Psychiatric Mental Status.* New York, Oxford University Press, 1993

The authors have put together an excellent resource book. It is the single-best reference book on the mental status currently available, filled with concise definitions and clinical applications. There are some nice illustrations of model mental status write-ups at the end of the book that are directly drawn from clinical vignettes. The book is too encyclopedic and dry, however, for required use with medical students, and even many busy psychiatric residents would probably not read the whole text. For the medical student and beginning resident, the practical use of the mental status is more manageably covered in most of the recent interviewing texts cited above (Halleck 1991; MacKinnon and

Yudovsky 1991; Morrison 1993; Othmer and Othmer 1989; Shea 1988). It also lacks some of the sense of warmth and sensitivity seen in the classic book by Strub and Black (1977) below. The authors are explicit that theirs is not a general text on interviewing but meant to be an in-depth foray into the intricacies of the mental status itself. In this regard, they have produced an admirable work.

20. *Whitehorn JC:* Guide to interviewing and clinical personality study. *Archives of Neurology and Psychiatry* 52:197–216, 1944

More than 50 years after its publication, this educational gem still shines. Whitehorn brings to life the "interpersonal" framework for which Harry Stack Sullivan would become famous. Indeed, if the resident does not have time to tackle Sullivan's masterpiece, Whitehorn's article can substitute in a remarkably effective manner for its size. Whitehorn's work reminds the interviewer constantly to attempt to understand the patient's attitudes toward key circumstances such as their own symptoms and their self-image and even toward the interviewer. Some of the subtitles of this article give a flavor of the stimulating and provocative nature of its contents: "Irrelevant Talk and Its Relevance for Personality" and "The Interview as a Constructive Experience for the Patient." The reader can be assured that time spent with this article will, likewise, be a highly constructive experience.

Empathy and Engagement

21. **Barrett-Leonard GT:** The empathy cycle: refinement of a nuclear concept. *Journal of Counseling Psychology* 28:91–100, 1981

The author presents a practical and aesthetically pleasing theoretical framework for understanding clinical empathy. He describes five states to the development of empathy, involving a slowly evolving empathic resonance between the clinician and patient.

22. *Havens L:* Experience in the uses of language in psychotherapy: counterprojective statements. *Contemporary Psychoanalysis* 16:53–67, 1980

Havens engagingly presents his concept of counterprojection and clarifies it with some nice examples. Counterprojection may well represent the single most effective technique for decreasing paranoia. This is a highly recommended article for all psychiatric residents.

23. **Havens L:** *Making Contact.* Cambridge, MA, Harvard University Press, 1986

This well-written and short book nicely summarizes much of Haven's pivotal work on engagement. Key concepts such as simple empathy, complex empathy, and counterprojection are summarized in the stimulating style so typical of Havens.

24. *Margulies A:** Toward empathy: the uses of wonder. *Am J Psychiatry* 141:1025–1033, 1984

This stimulating article pushes the clinician to understand two subtly different empathic listening perspectives. The discussion regarding the clinician's need to project imaginatively into the patient's world is particularly thought provoking.

25. *Margulies A:** *The Empathic Imagination.* New York, WW Norton, 1989

This book is more focused on ongoing therapy than the initial interview, but remains highly pertinent to the initial encounter as well. It is a marvelous book, written with elegance, humor, and warmth. It is a great book to read as one begins the transition from interviewing training into the enigmatic world of psychotherapy proper.

26. *Margulies A, Havens L:** The initial encounter: what to do first. *Am J Psychiatry* 138:421–428, 1981

This is a nicely written article that reminds the reader of the constant need to empathize with patients throughout the initial interview and provides tips on how to do just that.

27. **Rogers CR, Truax CB:** The therapeutic conditions antecedent to change: a theoretical view, in *The Therapeutic Relationship and Its Impact.* Edited by Rogers C. Madison, WI, University of Wisconsin Press, 1967, pp. 97–108

One cannot leave the topic of empathy without mentioning Carl Rogers, the master himself. Sometimes overlooked by psychiatric educators, Rogers was innovative and charismatic. His theories are almost universally known by counselors and psychologists and, consequently, should be part of any psychiatric trainee's knowledge base.

Special Situations and Research

28. **Ekman P:** *Telling Lies: Clues to Deceit in the Marketplace, Politics, and Marriage.* New York, WW Norton, 1985

Ekman has spent years studying deceit. This is a fun book that provides state-of-the-art information of use in detecting malingering, sociopathy, and family secrets.

29. **Gorden RL:** *Interviewing: Strategy, Techniques, and Tactics,* 4th Edition. Chicago, IL, Dorsey Press, 1987

   This is not a book primarily about psychiatric interviewing. It discusses all types of interviews from initial counseling sessions to police interrogations, with a special emphasis on the role of interviewing in social research. The text stands as a remarkable accomplishment, carefully detailing almost any aspect of interviewing one could imagine, from nonverbal communication to strategies for handling resistance. Encyclopedic in nature, it is not for the novice nor will the typical trainee have time for it. If one has any interest in doing research on interviewing, however, it can quickly become "the bible."

30. **Harper RG, Wiens AN, Matarazzo JD:** *Nonverbal Communication: the State of the Art.* New York, Wiley, 1978

   Although somewhat dated, this book provides an excellent background on nonverbal communication and research. If you want to do research in this area, it is a great place to start.

31. *****Kernberg OF:** Structural interviewing, in *The Psychiatric Clinics of North America: Borderline Disorders,* Vol. 4. Edited by Stone M. Philadelphia, PA, WB Saunders, 1981, pp. 169–195

   Otto Kernberg somehow always manages to shed new light on work with difficult patients. This brief chapter is yet another example of Kernberg magic at work. He presents a systematic method of questioning patients that helps the interviewer determine the degree of damage to the underlying personality structure (hence the name *structural interviewing*) of the patient. This line of questioning nicely complements the approach of DSM-III-R. The chapter is a "good read" and a nice introduction to Kernberg.

32. **Morris D:** *Manwatching: A Field Guide to Human Behavior.* New York, Harry N Abrahams, 1977

   Morris is writing for the general public, but this fascinating book, which is packed with excellent photographs, is both fun and useful for any mental health professional. Nonverbal cues for impending violence, deceit, and fear are covered in detail.

33. *****Perry S, Cooper AM, Michels R:** The psychodynamic formulation: its purpose, structure, and clinical application. *Am J Psychiatry* 144):543–550, 1987

   This is a splendid article that provides, in a surprisingly brief amount of space, a sound foundation for understanding the important role of psychodynamic formulation from the combined perspectives of ego psychology, object relations, and the psychology of the self.

34. *Platt FW, McMath JC:** Clinical hypocompetence: the interview. *Ann Intern Med* 91:898–902, 1979

Here is another splendid article, focusing on five common, problematic approaches taken by physicians during the standard medical history and physical. These common errors are nicely defined and then illustrated with well-chosen examples. These same errors are, unfortunately, all too common with psychiatric residents as well. A "must read" for any medical student interviewing course.

35. **Pomeroy WB, Flax CC, Wheeler CC:** *Taking a Sex History.* New York, Free Press, 1982

Building on extensive clinical and research experience, the authors have produced a well-written and highly practical text filled with specific tips and examples.

36. **Rogers R** (ed): *Clinical Assessment of Malingering and Deception.* New York, Guilford, 1988

Everything a resident could want to know about the assessment of malingering is in here, including nice chapters on malingered psychosis and malingered posttraumatic stress disorder. The book also includes many chapters on testing instruments and even the polygraph. On a practical level, most time-conscious residents will probably be drawn to earlier (more clinical) works; those interested in research on malingering will find this comprehensive book almost too good to be true.

37. **Shea SC:** Contemporary psychiatric interviewing: integration of DSM-III-R, psychodynamic concerns, and mental status, in *Handbook of Psychological Assessment,* 2nd Edition. Edited by Goldstein G, Hersen M. New York, Pergamon, 1990, pp. 283–307

This chapter contains a succinct history of the technical developments and books related to psychiatric interviewing, followed by a review of interviewing research in the following areas: clinician response modes, nonverbal behavior, clinician characteristics, reliability and validity concerns, and educational techniques.

38. **Shea SC, Rancurello M:** Faculty and resident response to an innovative Mock Board. *Academic Psychiatry* 13:137–144, 1989

The authors describe a format for mock oral boards that was enthusiastically received both by residents and faculty. The format does not use grades and focuses solely on constructive feedback.

39. *Strub RL, Black FW: *The Mental Status Examination in Neurology.* Philadelphia, PA, FA Davis, 1977

This book is written in an informal and fluid style. It is a great introduction to the cognitive aspects of the mental status and painlessly helps the resident understand complex concepts such as the localization of brain lesions. The authors convey a deep sense of compassion that makes this book something special. All residents should read this brief classic.

40. **Wiens AN:** The assessment interview, in *Clinical Methods in Psychology,* 2nd Edition. Edited by Weiner IB. New York, Wiley, 1983, pp. 3–57

Wiens reviews the research on interviews in a concise and well-organized fashion. Topics include validity, speech characteristics, nonverbal considerations, and interviewer role. This is a good introduction to research concerns with a nice bibliography.

41. **Wiens AN:** Structured Clinical Interviews for Adults, in *Handbook of Psychological Assessment,* 2nd Edition. Edited by Goldstein G, Hersen M. New York, Pergamon, 1990, pp. 324–341

Wiens provides a concise introduction to structured interviews such as the Diagnostic Interview Schedule and the Comprehensive Drinker Profile. The chapter is good at discussing the benefits and potential problems encountered with structured formats.

Research on Interview Training

42. **Benedek EP, Bieniek CM:** Interpersonal process recall: an innovative technique. *Journal of Medical Education* 52:939–941, 1977

This article considers videotape supervision at its best. The authors describe a technique in which the supervisor helps the trainee to reexperience the trainee's emotional response and cognitive processes during specific sections of interview played back on videotape. This is a slick technique that can be utilized in conjunction with more traditional videotape work.

43. *Dobbs HI, Carek DJ: The conceptualization and teaching of medical interviewing. *Journal of Medical Education* 47:272–276, 1972

I have included this citation for two reasons. First, it is a beautiful description of the many processes occurring during interviewing training and is equally applicable to psychiatric interviewing as it is to medical interviewing. Second, psychiatrists and psychiatric residents are often asked to coordinate medical student interviewing programs, and this article can serve as a wonderful guide even though it is somewhat dated.

44. **Gibbon M, McDonald-Scott P, Endicott J:** Mastering the art of research interviewing: a model training procedure for diagnostic evaluation. *Arch Gen Psychiatry* 38:1259–1262, 1981

This article focuses on a four-phase training program for research interviewers interested in using the Schedule for Affective Disorders and Schizophrenia and Research Diagnostic Criteria. The four phases (case vignettes, observation of videotapes, live interviews, and continued monitoring of raters) represent a sound approach to interviewing training in general. It also highlights the frequently underplayed fact that the mere use of semistructured interviews in no way guarantees high validity or reliability, unless the interviewers are meticulously trained and on-site interrater reliability is tested.

45. **Ivey AE:** *Microcounseling: Innovations in Interviewing Training,* 2nd Edition. Springfield, IL, Charles C Thomas, 1978

This large volume does justice to the innovative work of Ivey, who has developed one of the best methods of teaching interviewing skills. The strategy involves focusing on a specific, single interviewing technique (hence the name "microtraining"). Role-playing, readings, direct feedback, and videotape work are used until the trainee literally has perfected the identified skill. I believe microtraining to be the single biggest advance in interviewing training to date.

46. **Junek W, Burra P, Leichner P:** Teaching interviewing skills by encountering patients. *Journal of Medical Education* 54:402–407, 1979

This article describes an interviewing course for first-year psychiatric residents utilizing a group setting with live patients. Residents improved in areas of empathy, congruence, and level of regard as evidenced by self-report and videotape rating. This course was partially based on the work by Ward and Stein (1975) described below and once again demonstrated the efficacy of interviews performed directly in front of the trainees.

47. *Shea SC, Mezzich JE:** Contemporary psychiatric interviewing: new directions for training. *Psychiatry: Interpersonal and Biological Processes* 51:385–397, 1988

This article introduced the interviewing-educational technology known as facilic analysis. Facilic analysis is the study of the structuring strategies and transitions used during an interview. Schematics have been developed that allow the supervisor quickly to "map-out" the interviewer's structuring movements as they unfold. This visual map is then used immediately in supervision and as a springboard for discussion in group formats. It also provides a permanent record of the resident's progress.

48. *Shea SC, Mezzich JE, Bohon S, Zeiders A:* A comprehensive and individualized psychiatric interviewing training program. *Academic Psychiatry* 13:61–72, 1989

This article is a description of a state-of-the-art interviewing training program that emphasized individualized training goals, videotape work, direct supervision, role-playing, and directed reading—all integrated around a 17-session course in which patients were interviewed in front of a group of trainees (see Junek et al. 1979 above and Ward and Stein 1975 below). This is an excellent article for residents to use as a "measuring stick" of their own interviewing training programs and when developing interviewing courses for medical students. The appendix contains a detailed outline of the individual classes.

49. *Ward NG, Stein L:* Reducing emotional distance: a new method to teach interviewing skills. *Journal of Medical Education* 50:605–614, 1975

This article was one of the first descriptions of an interviewing training program in which direct supervision of the psychiatric resident was emphasized. In addition, it placed the fellow seminar participants in the same room as the interviewer and interviewee, proving that many patients were comfortable with this format and that participants found it more energizing and discussion-provoking than one-way mirrors.

32

Diagnostic Psychological Testing

Donald M. Quinlan, Ph.D.

D iagnostic psychological testing is employed to derive and elaborate information regarding a patient's psychopathology, personality and character structure, and cognitive functioning. A broad definition of a test is a sample of behavior used to predict other behavior (Anastasi 1988). Tests used in clinical work are selected from the thousands of tests developed for a broad spectrum of uses within and outside of the clinical setting. As distinguished from interview and other assessment procedures, tests employ standard stimuli (questions, visual materials, or other apparatus), the answers to which are compared with norms from relevant samples, and the results measure a specific characteristic with a demonstrated degree of reliability and validity. Tests may measure behavior observable by a clinician or may measure behavior that can be observed only under specific conditions with stimuli not generally available.

The characteristics of the range of test responses are evaluated across broad samples to represent general and specific populations (e.g., patients with particular psychiatric diagnoses, patients with specific neurological dysfunction or abnormalities, and individuals from different ethnic and cultural backgrounds). Items (questions or stimuli) are selected to sample from domains of relevant characteristics (e.g., intelligence, level of pathology). Tests or scales on tests summarize items to represent an ordering of the individuals according to the specific characteristic. For example, digit span, or the presentation of series of digits with the subject being required to repeat the series forward and backward, is part of the mental status exam. Knowing a patient completed up to 6 digits forward and 5 digits backward means relatively little unless one knows what is the general performance for individuals of the same age—the digit span subtest of the Wechsler scales would give a scale score that places the subject along a known distribution of performance on this test, or norms, with additional norms taking into account the age of the subject.

The degree to which scores or scales can give the information consistently is the reliability of the test or scale. Up to a point, the more reliable a test, the more useful it is. The validity of a test or scale is the degree to which it measures the characteristic it is designed to measure. Establishing reliability and validity are prerequisites for development of a test or scale. Reliability and validity are established over a series of studies over a broad range of target populations, and the reliability and validity of a test for a specific purpose are affected by the range of individuals within the target population.

Tests used in clinical practice derive from at least four different sources representing distinct differences in approach and focus: ability testing (e.g., intelligence), projective techniques, "objective" testing of personality and psychopathology, and neuropsychological assessment. Other procedures that share some of the characteristics of diagnostic testing (e.g., structured clinical interviews) are not covered in this chapter.

General Background in Testing

The field of psychometrics represents a broad field of research going well beyond the clinical testing field. Statistics for assessing item characteristics are extensive. Books in this area can be useful for background in developing scales for research work. Some general reference texts for the field follow.

1. **Anastasi A:** *Psychological Testing,* 6th Edition. New York, Macmillan, 1988

   This is a general text for courses in psychological testing. General issues of reliability and validity are covered, and tests from major areas of testing are reviewed, including ability and achievement, personality, and personnel selection.

2. **Maloney MP, Ward MP:** *Psychological Assessment: A Conceptual Approach.* New York, Oxford University Press, 1976

   This work provides an overview of psychological assessment in a clinical setting. Written by two authors in a department of psychiatry, the book discusses integration of data collection approaches with psychological testing. Sections cover the assessment process, report writing, diagnosis, personality testing, intelligence testing, low intelligence, projective testing, objective testing, and assessment of brain damage.

Ability and Intelligence Assessment

The use of ability tests such as intelligence scales in clinical work is aimed at a different goal than the usual uses of ability testing—measuring an individual's potential for intellectual tasks and academic achievement. Clinical testing is more focused on impairment, often due to psychopathology. Nonetheless, ability testing forms one of the core areas of clinical testing. The following works provide coverage of specific aspects of ability testing.

3. **Lezak MG:** *Neuropsychological Assessment,* 2nd Edition. New York, Oxford University Press, 1983

   The chapter on assessment of intelligence reviews the use of the intelligence test as a measurement of basic intellectual functions and their general psychological import, as well as the basis for neuropsychological assessment.

4. **Matarazzo JG:** *Wechsler's Measurement and Appraisal of Adult Intelligence,* 5th and Enlarged Edition. New York, Williams & Wilkins, 1972

   Matarazzo revised and expanded the book by Wechsler on the principal scale for assessment of adult intelligence. A detailed discussion of intelligence and the Wechsler scales in particular (Wechsler Bellevue I and II, Wechsler Adult Intelligence Scale, Wechsler Adult Intelligence Scale—Revised) is expanded with numerous chapters on the research and clinical applications of the scales.

5. **Rapaport MM, Gill MM, Schafer R:** *Diagnostic Psychological Testing,* Revised Edition. Edited by Holt RR. New York, International Universities Press, 1968

   A discussion of the clinical interpretation of the Wechsler scales. It remains a notable statement of the ego-psychological approach to use of diagnostic testing.

Projective Techniques

These techniques, represented by the Rorschach and the Thematic Apperception Test, grew out of a clinical and interpretive tradition of European psychology. Modern adaptations have extended the principles for interpretation and added scoring approaches with a body of research.

6. **Allison J, Blatt SJ, Zimet C:** *The Interpretation of Psychological Tests.* New York, Harper & Row, 1968

    This text is intended as an introduction for clinical psychologists to the interpretation of psychological testing from the ego psychoanalytic point of view. Tests are introduced, techniques for administration and interpretation are discussed, and a case history of a patient is introduced as an example of the techniques.

7. **Exner J:** *The Rorschach: A Comprehensive System,* 2nd Edition. New York, Wiley, 1986

    This comprehensive system, originally defined by John Exner, and extended in collaboration with his colleague, Irving Weiner, provides the basis for a comprehensive scoring system for the Rorschach, along with a presentation of extensive research on multiple aspects of the Rorschach.

8. **Rapaport D, Gill MM, Schafer R:** *Diagnostic Psychological Testing,* Revised Edition. Edited by Holt RR. New York, International Universities Press, 1968

    This work, described above for the interpretation of intellectual assessment, provides a detailed discussion of the scoring and interpretation of the Rorschach, along with use of the Thematic Apperception Test and the Babcock Story Recall. Although the original work is dated, it remains, especially with Robert R. Holt's revisions, a classic text and a statement of an influential viewpoint within the field.

"Objective" Testing

This approach measures psychological states by questionnaire methods. Eschewing the clinical approach of projective techniques, psychologists have developed a large group of tests based on empirical derivation of scales. The most widely used clinical instrument is the Minnesota Multiphasic Personality Inventory (MMPI), with the new, revised, and renormed version MMPI-2 and a separate version for adolescents, MMPI-A.

9. **Butcher JN:** *MMPI-2 in Psychological Treatment.* New York, Oxford University Press, 1990

    This is a description of the new version, MMPI-2, with clinical case studies illustrating the use of the instrument in clinical diagnosis. It is a useful introduction for the reader working with this version.

10. **Dahlstrom WG, Welsh GS, Dahlstrom LE:** *An MMPI Handbook,* Vols. 1 & 2. Minneapolis, MN, University of Minnesota Press, 1972/1975

Published as two volumes, this is a classic work, describing the derivation of the MMPI scales, describing their clinical applications, and summarizing research developing and validating the scales. Volume 1 is a handy reference work for anyone using the scales. Volume 2 reviews the research on the principal scales and some research scales.

11. **Graham JR:** *The MMPI: A Practical Guide.* New York, Oxford University Press, 1977

This work provides a clinical approach to the use of the MMPI in diagnosis. The author takes the reader through the steps of reading and interpreting an MMPI profile. Although somewhat dated by advances in diagnostic terminology, the text remains useful as an introduction to the clinical use of the MMPI.

Neuropsychological Assessment

One of the most rapidly growing fields of psychology, neuropsychology has exploited advanced imaging techniques to describe relationships between brain pathology and behavioral consequences.

12. **Benton AL:** *Studies in Neuropsychology: Selected Papers of Arthur Benton.* Edited by Costa L, Spreen O. New York, Oxford University Press, 1985

A collection of papers by Arthur Benton, this book represents the reasoning processes used in neuropsychological assessment and presents the research basis for the instruments.

13. **Benton AL, Hamsher K, Varney N, Spreen O:** *Contributions to Neuropsychological Assessment: A Clinical Manual.* New York, Oxford University Press, 1983

This is a description of the principal neuropsychological tests by one of the leading contributors to the field. Psychological tests are reviewed, with an interpretation of their relationship to psychophysiology and neuropsychology. Although neuropsychologically oriented, this text is accessible to the serious reader.

14. **Goodglass H, Kaplan E:** *The Assessment of Aphasia and Related Disorders,* 2nd Edition. Philadelphia, PA, Lea & Febiger, 1983

A description of assessment of a major class of neuropsychological disorders by two of the major figures, this book is useful for demonstrating the process approach to the understanding of neuropsychology.

See also Lezak (1983) above.

The Clinical Neuropsychological Examination

William J. Waked, Ph.D.
Steven Mattis, Ph.D.

D ue to great strides in the neurosciences, the closing years of the 20th century are being called the "Decade of the Brain." Clinical neuropsychology, having firmly established its place within the neurosciences, is forging a partnership with psychiatry, behavioral neurology, and medicine. Whereas psychiatry has become more medicalized, neurology has renewed its interest in the study of mind and brain-behavior relationships. This trend is partly in response to the rapid development during the 1980s of brain imaging technologies such as magnetic resonance imaging and positron-emission tomography. Growing interdisciplinary partnership has stimulated theory building and revisionist ideas concerning brain-behavior relationships and the underlying mechanisms of neuropsychological syndromes and psychopathology.

Over the past two decades, major changes within neuropsychology have taken place. The traditional antithesis between theories of equipotentiality and localization of brain function that dominated the late 19th and early to middle 20th centuries has been replaced by dynamic models of higher cortical function. Contemporary paradigms hold that information processing and hierarchically organized cortical systems with intra- and interhemispheric communication and feedback loops are hypothesized to account for all cognitive, emotional, and behavioral output. Continuing developments in brain imaging technology, psychophysiology, neurochemistry, and neuropsychological test construction are now making it possible to study simultaneously and in vivo normal and brain-damaged individuals. These newer developments promise to elucidate further the underlying neural processes and mediating structures of neuropsychological functions in humans. Clinical neuropsychology has also shifted its primary focus away from diagnosis and lesion localization. Research and practice have broadened to include conducting differential diagnosis (e.g., psychogenic-versus neurogenic-based etiology), documenting the effects of medical and neurologic disease on neuropsychological and psychosocial functioning, assessing the response to pharmacotherapy and rehabilitation, and conducting forensic evaluation. The expanded clinical practice and extensive database of knowledge collected in the 1980s and early 1990s has led to the development of more than one dozen neuropsychology and neuropsychiatric journals and many new chapters and books covering diverse topics bearing direct relevance to the understanding of the neuropsychology of psychiatric, neurologic, and medical disorders. Growing interest in evaluating neuropsychological status in diverse patient populations is testimony to the value of neuropsychology both in research and in treatment of the whole person who comes to the attention of a medical specialist.

The bibliography presented below highlights major conceptual issues in clinical neuropsychology and its interface with psychiatry, behavioral neurology, and medicine.

Brain-Behavior Relationships and Related Neuropsychological Syndromes Following Brain Damage

1. **Filskov SB, Grimm BH, Lewis JA:** Brain-behavior relationships, in *Handbook of Clinical Neuropsychology.* Edited by Filskov SB, Boll TJ. New York, Wiley, 1981, pp. 39–73

   In this excellent introduction to clinical neuropsychology and the study of brain-behavior relationships, the authors summarize conceptual models of cerebral organization and highlight cognitive and personality changes associated with prefrontal and frontal, parietal, temporal, occipital, and subcortical brain-stem damage. Descriptions of neuropsychological assessment methods and neuropsychological syndromes are successfully woven into the discussion.

2. **Heilman KM, Valenstein E:** *Clinical Neuropsychology*, 3rd Edition. New York, Oxford University Press, 1993

    This is a basic text for the student and clinician of psychiatry, psychology. and neurology interested in brain-behavior relationships, mechanisms of brain dysfunction, and major neuropsychological syndromes. Chapters are written by noted authorities and provide a thorough review of relevant theory and research findings.

3. **Kolb B, Whishaw IQ:** *Fundamentals of Human Neuropsychology*, 3rd Edition. New York, WH Freeman, 1990

    This basic text for the study of human neuropsychology as an applied science contains a review of general principles of brain function; human neuropsychology; recovery of function; and assessment of neurologic, neuropsychiatric, and medical conditions. The authors successfully integrate historical background with current conceptualizations and research findings.

4. **Luria AR:** *The Working Brain: An Introduction to Neuropsychology.* New York, Basic Books, 1973

    This classic work is one of Luria's seminal contributions to the history and development of clinical neuropsychology. The Lurian legacy can be traced to many of the ideas and clinical findings that are elucidated in this highly readable text for the student and advanced clinician.

The Mental Status Examination

5. **Gallo JJ, Reichel W, Andersen L:** Mental status testing, in *Handbook of Geriatric Assessment.* Edited by Gallo JJ, Reichel W, Anderson L. Rockville, MD, Aspen Publishers, 1988, pp. 11–64

    This chapter presents an overview of systems and description of the mental status exam in medical and psychiatric patients. Some commonly used mental status exams, dementia rating scales, and symptom inventories are provided, with emphasis on their clinical utility for an aged population.

6. **Keller MB, Manschreck TC:** The mental status examination, II: higher intellectual functioning, in *Outpatient Psychiatry: Diagnosis and Treatment*, 2nd Edition. Edited by Lazare A. Baltimore, MD, Williams & Wilkins, 1989, pp. 188–199

    This chapter focuses on the clinical assessment of higher intellectual functioning in elderly individuals in medical and psychiatric settings.

A review of reliability and validity of a variety of mental status screening exams is provided.

7. **Schmitt FA, Ranaseen JD, DeKosky ST:** Cognitive mental status examinations. *Clin Geriatr Med* 5:545–564, 1989

   A variety of mental status exams for use in a medical, neurologic, and psychiatric setting are reviewed. Discussions of test validity and reliability and clinical and research utility in studying geriatric populations and progression of disease are included.

8. **Strube RS, Black FW:** *The Mental Status Examination in Neurology*, 3rd Edition. Philadelphia, PA, FA Davis, 1993

   An excellent introduction to the mental status exam for the student of psychiatry, neurology, and medicine, this little book provides many practical tips, useful illustrations, and concrete guidelines for conducting a comprehensive neuropsychiatric screening examination.

Neuropsychological Tests and Measurement

9. **Frazen MD, Robbins DE, Sawicki RF:** *Reliability and Validity in Neuropsychological Assessment.* New York, Plenum, 1989

   This book addresses validity and reliability in neuropsychological and intelligence test construction and assessment. The authors emphasize test construction as an active process that is ongoing and requires the scrutiny of test users to decide under what conditions and with which populations such tests are best suited.

10. **Kane RL:** Standardized and flexible batteries in neuropsychology: an assessment update. *Neuropsychology Review* 2:281–339, 1991

    This is an excellent review of the theoretical underpinnings of the standardized and flexible neuropsychological test battery, recognizing the need for continued research and refinement of neuropsychological tests and the abilities they purport to measure.

11. **Lezak M:** *Neuropsychological Assessment*, 3rd Edition. New York, Oxford University Press, 1995

    This is the definitive handbook of neuropsychological assessment with a focus on test procedures and their application to brain-behavior relationships. Descriptions of standardized tests and use with specific populations and clinical norms are provided. Chapters were updated to include discussions of aging, cerebral lateralization, handedness, motor functions, and executive functions.

12. **Reitan R:** Theoretical and methodological bases of the Halstead-Reitan Neuropsychological Test Battery, in *Neuropsychological Assessment of Neuropsychiatric Disorders.* Edited by Grant I, Adams KM. New York, Oxford University Press, 1986, pp. 3–30

    Reitan describes the historical and theoretical development of the Halstead-Reitan Neuropsychological Test and its emphasis on the central processing functions of problem solving and brain-behavior relationships.

13. **Spreen O, Strauss E:** *A Compendium of Neuropsychological Tests, Administration, Norms, and Commentary.* New York, Oxford University Press, 1991

    This compendium of neuropsychological and intellectual tests is a valuable resource to the psychiatrist and neurocognitive scientist. Tests with demonstrated brain-behavior relationships are described in their composition, purpose, administration, scoring, and norms. Many tests are corrected for age, sex, education level, and IQ.

Intellectual Measurement and Brain Damage

14. **Kaufman AS:** *Assessing Adolescent and Adult Intelligence.* Needham Heights, MA, Allyn & Bacon, 1990

    This is a comprehensive text devoted to the assessment of intelligence in adolescents and adults. Detailed review of the Wechsler Adult Intelligence Scale—Revised is provided, including a description of other newly developed tests of intelligence and supplementary cognitive tests for use as part of a neuropsychological evaluation.

15. **Matarazzo JD:** *Wechsler's Measurement and Appraisal of Adult Intelligence,* 5th Edition. New York, Oxford University Press, 1972

    This text outlines the history of measured intelligence, IQ, and development of the Wechsler-Bellevue and Wechsler Adult Intelligence Scale subscales. Brain-behavior relationships reflected in the verbal-performance scales and the effects of age, sex, education, socioeconomic status, and brain damage on measured IQ using the Wechsler scales are also discussed.

Disorders of Memory

16. **Baddeley A, Harris J, Sunderland A, Watts KP, Wilson BA:** Closed head injury and memory, in *Neurobehavioral Recovery From Head Injury.* Edited

by Levin HS, Grafman J, Eisenberg HM. New York, Oxford University Press, 1987, pp. 295–317

This is a review of clinical neuropsychological assessment and research findings of functional memory disorders following closed head injury, using research-generated paradigms of normal memory processes.

17. **Bauer RM, Tobias B, Valenstein E:** Amnesic disorders, in *Clinical Neuropsychology*, 3rd Edition. Edited by Heilman KM, Valenstein E. New York, Oxford University Press, 1993, pp. 523–602

This is an excellent review of the amnesic disorders and their clinical presentation. The neuropsychological features of various amnesic states with differing brain localization and etiologies are identified and compared. The work of many influential memory investigators is well integrated into the discussion.

18. **Heindel WC, Salmon DP, Butters N:** Neuropsychological differentiation of memory impairments in dementia, in *Memory, Aging, and Dementia: Theory, Assessment, and Treatment*. Edited by Gilmore GC, Whitehouse PJ, Wykle ML. New York, Springer, 1989, pp. 112–139

This chapter summarizes contemporary memory research and neuropsychological practice regarding specific cognitive processes that are believed to underlie anterograde and retrograde memory deficits associated with forms of amnesia and dementia in conditions such as Alzheimer's, Huntington's, and alcoholic Korsakoff disease.

19. **Kaszniak A:** The neuropsychology of dementia, in *Neuropsychological Assessment of Neuropsychiatric Disorders*. Edited by Grant I, Adams KM. New York, Oxford University Press, 1986, pp. 172–220

This is an overview of dementia from the diagnostic, anatomic and biochemical, epidemiological, and neuropsychological assessment perspectives. Issues concerning the mental status exam, dementia rating scales, assessment of premorbid intelligence, memory, and major research findings on memory and other deficits in dementia are reviewed.

20. **Knight RG, Longmore BE:** What is an amnesic?, in *Memory Mechanisms: A Tribute to GV Goddard*. Edited by Abraham WC, Corballis M, White KG. Hillsdale, NJ, Lawrence Erlbaum, 1991, pp. 149–174

This chapter provides an excellent review of conceptual and methodological problems inherent in the definition, assessment, and study of amnesia. The clinical and research findings on the amnesias and the adequacy of some common procedures for assessing amnesia syndromes are considered.

21. **Ogden JA, Corkin S:** Memories of H M, in *Memory Mechanisms: A Tribute to GV Goddard.* Edited by Abraham WC, Corballis M, White KG. Hillsdale, NJ, Lawrence Erlbaum Associates, 1991, pp. 195–215

This is an update on the celebrated case of H M, who was left with a dense amnesia following a bilateral medial temporal-lobe resection for the relief of intractable temporal lobe epilepsy. Ogden and Corkin discuss their interview with H M at age 62 in light of contemporary theories of amnesia. Verbatim record of their warm and lively interview with H M is presented.

22. **Shimamura A:** Aging and memory disorders: a neuropsychological analysis, in *Cognitive and Behavioral Performance Factors in Atypical Aging.* Edited by Howe ML, Stones MJ, Brainerd CJ. New York, Springer-Verlag, 1990, pp. 37–55

Clinical and research findings relevant to declarative, implicit, and prospective memory systems in "normal" and pathological aging and the development of amnestic states and the dementias are reviewed and offer new directions for clinical study.

23. **Squire LR:** *Memory and Brain.* New York, Oxford University Press, 1987

This is a historic and contemporary overview of the state of knowledge regarding human memory and its disorders. Using rich clinical descriptions and research findings, Squire discusses memory organization at the level of the neuron on up to complex memory systems and forges a synthesis of knowledge that will help inform the direction of future research in memory.

Neuropsychology of Language and Related Disorders

24. **Benson FD:** Aphasia, in *Clinical Neuropsychology*, 3rd Edition. Edited by Heilman KM, Valenstein E. New York, Oxford University Press, 1993, pp. 18–32

This chapter provides an overview of the historical background of brain-behavior relationships associated with language, clinical descriptions of aphasia syndromes and related disorders, and clinical assessment of aphasia and treatment strategies.

25. **Chaika EO:** *Understanding Psychotic Speech: Beyond Freud and Chomsky.* Springfield, IL, Charles C Thomas, 1990

This book provides a linguistic analysis of schizophrenic and psychotic speech. Recognizing that schizophrenic speech can occur in mania and other patients, the author, a linguist, argues that schizophrenic speech is different in degree but not in kind from other forms of psychotic speech. Issues concerning thought disorder versus ungrammatical speech, grammatical structures, metaphor, cohesion and coherence, intentionality, and meaning are closely examined and discussed.

26. **Damasio AR, Damasio H:** Brain and language. *Sci Am* 267:89–95, 1992

This article is a thought-provoking review of historical considerations, current research, and conceptual models of normal language and aphasia syndromes based on years of neuropsychological and neuroimaging studies of healthy and brain-damaged individuals.

27. **Goodglass H:** The assessment of language after brain damage, in *Handbook of Clinical Neuropsychology*, Vol. 2. Edited by Filskov SB, Boll TJ. New York, Wiley, 1986, pp. 172–197

This is an excellent overview of brain-behavior relationships, neuropsychological assessment, and treatment of aphasia and related phenomena of dysarthria, mild word finding problems, and tangentiality of thought that are not technically aphasic in origin.

28. **Grant I, Adams KM:** *Neuropsychological Assessment of Neuropsychiatric Disorders.* New York, Oxford University Press, 1986

This book is an excellent reference for in-depth description of comprehensive neuropsychological assessment and review of major studies and test findings pertinent to neuropsychiatric syndromes such as schizophrenia, depression and pseudodementia, dementia, epilepsy, closed head injury, and long-term alcoholism and substance abuse.

Neuropsychology and the Interface With Psychiatry

29. **Cassens G, Wolfe L, Zola M:** The neuropsychology of depressions. *Journal of Neuropsychiatry and Clinical Neuroscience* 2:202–213, 1990

Clinical neuropsychological studies of depression and pseudodepression are summarized, as are the findings on measures of attention, vigilance, abstraction, memory, visuospatial, and executive/motor skills. The need to identify reversible cognitive deficits as a means to generate new hypotheses about subtypes and associated brain-behavior relationships in depression is emphasized.

30. **Gold J, Goldberg TE, Kleinman JE, Weinberger DR:** The impact of symptomatic state and pharmacological treatment on cognitive functioning of patients with schizophrenia and mood disorders, in *Handbook of Clinical Trials: The Neurobehavioral Approach.* Edited by Mohr E, Brouwers P. Amsterdam, Netherlands, Swets & Zeitlinger, 1991, pp. 185–214

This chapter provides a comprehensive review of the effects of symptomatic state and pharmacological side effects on intellectual and neuropsychological assessment in schizophrenia and major affective disorders.

31. **Joseph R:** *Neuropsychology, Neuropsychiatry, and Behavioral Neurology.* New York, Plenum, 1990

This is an excellent basic text for those interested in the interface between clinical neuropsychology, psychiatry, and behavioral neurology. Chapters elucidate the structure and function of major brain regions, associated neuropsychological deficits, and resulting clinical syndromes. This book has appeal to both the novice and experienced clinician and researcher.

32. **Kaplan E:** The process approach to neuropsychological assessment of psychiatric patients. *Journal of Neuropsychiatry and Clinical Neuroscience* 2:72–87, 1990

This article highlights Kaplan's "process approach," which emphasizes both the qualitative (process) and quantitative (achievement) aspects of problem solving and its relevance to assessment of cognitive impairment in psychiatric disorders. By use of rich clinical examples and diagrams, she demonstrates the power of this method in generating hypotheses about brain-behavior relationships and rehabilitation treatment strategies.

33. **Seidman LJ:** The neuropsychology of schizophrenia: a neurodevelopmental and case study approach. *Journal of Neuropsychiatry and Clinical Neuroscience* 2:301–312, 1990

This article is a selected review of the neurobiology of schizophrenia and three clinical records illustrating the case study approach to neuropsychological assessment. The clinical utility of assessment in helping to evaluate response to treatment, stability of cognitive impairments over time, and treatment planning and outcome are shown.

Neuropsychology and the Interface
With Behavioral Neurology and Medicine

34. **Bornstein RA, Kelly MP:** Risk factors for stroke and neuropsychological performance, in *Neurobehavioral Aspects of Cerebrovascular Disease.* Edited by Bornstein RA, Brown G. New York, Oxford University Press, 1991, pp. 182–201

   This is a contemporary review of the effects of stroke risk factors such as hypertension, diabetes mellitus, cholesterol, tobacco use, and cardiac disease on neuropsychological status, with implications for treatment and future study.

35. **DeLuca J:** Cognitive dysfunction after aneurysm of the anterior communicating artery. *J Clin Exp Neuropsychol* 14:924–934, 1992

   This article describes the neuropsychology of the "ACoA syndrome" as a type of amnesia occurring in combination with personality changes and/or confabulation, as distinct from other amnestic states following focal brain damage or stroke.

36. **Ingraham LJ, Bridge TP, Janssen R, Stover E, Mirsky AF:** Neuropsychological effects of early HIV-1 infection: assessment and methodology. *Journal of Neuropsychiatry and Clinical Neuroscience* 2:174–182, 1990

   This review of research and clinical findings on the effects of early human immunodeficiency virus (HIV)-1 infection on neuropsychological processes highlights the variability of research findings regarding the presence and severity of cognitive deficits in infected individuals. A variety of methodological problems are identified and discussed.

37. **Tarter RE, Van Thiel DH, Edwards KL:** *Medical Neuropsychology: The Impact of Disease on Behavior.* New York, Plenum, 1988

   This compendium reviews some common medical conditions with neuropsychological and psychiatric sequelae. The breadth of subject matter includes diseases of the pulmonary, vascular, liver, renal, pancreas, pituitary, and thyroid systems and the effects of neurotoxins, cancer, and malnutrition on cognitive functioning.

38. **White RF:** Emotional and cognitive correlates of multiple sclerosis. *Journal of Neuropsychiatry and Clinical Neuroscience* 2:422–428, 1990

   This review article summarizes the neuropsychology of multiple sclerosis, with particular emphasis on the interface between neuropsychological test findings, emotional changes, and progression of illness.

Special Topics

39. **Damasio H, Damasio AR:** *Lesion Analysis in Neuropsychology.* New York, Oxford University Press, 1989

Written by two internationally known figures in behavioral neurology, Damasio and Damasio describe the lesion method as applied to healthy and brain-damaged individuals. Using many computed tomographic and magnetic resonance images, it illustrates how modern neuroimaging is modifying theories of neuropsychological function and elucidating the underlying neural substrates of language, perception, memory, and complex problem solving.

40. **Meier M, Benton A, Diller L:** *Neuropsychological Rehabilitation.* New York, Guilford, 1987

This book illustrates the expanding role of neuropsychology in the field of clinical practice, assessment, and individualized treatment of disabled persons with cognitive deficits. An impressive list of contributors makes this book well worth reading.

41. **Mitrushina M, Satz P:** Changes in cognitive functioning associated with normal aging. *Archives of Clinical Psychology* 6:49–60, 1991

The study of normal aging is emphasized in this 3-year prospective study of intellectual and cognitive functioning in four groups of older subjects ranging in age from 57 to 85. Discussion of results reflects current views on aging and methodological problems.

42. **Parsons OA, Farr SP:** The neuropsychology of alcohol and drug use, in *The Handbook of Clinical Neuropsychology.* Edited by Filskov SB, Boll TJ. New York, Wiley, 1981, pp. 320–365

This comprehensive review focuses on the long-term effects of alcohol and drugs on neuropsychological functioning. Clinical methods and research findings are largely derived from studies using the Halstead-Reitan Neuropsychological Battery.

43. **Prigatano GP, Schacter DL:** *Awareness of Deficit After Brain Injury: Clinical and Theoretical Issues.* New York, Oxford University Press, 1991

This excellent book offers a multidisciplinary perspective regarding awareness of deficits in patients with traumatic brain injury, dementia, and neuropsychiatric disorders. Historical and contemporary references to the problem of denial and altered awareness, evaluation, etiology, and implications for treatment are discussed.

34

Neurology for Psychiatrists

David A. Silbersweig, M.D.

I t is now extremely important for psychiatrists to have a working knowledge of the nervous system. The brain is the organ of the mind. Neural mechanisms underlie normal and abnormal perception, cognition, emotion, and behavior. Even consciousness is instantiated in neural networks. As such, the distinction between "psychiatric" and "neurologic" is dissolving. Neurologic disorders may have a psychiatric presentation, and effective pharmacologic treatments for psychiatric disorders affect specific brain systems. Ongoing technical and methodological developments are providing researchers and clinicians with a greater understanding of the specific neuroanatomical and neurochemical systems implicated in the pathophysiology of neuropsychiatric symptoms and syndromes. These advances have implications for the diagnosis, classification, and treatment of psychiatric diseases.

The core readings in this chapter have been selected to reflect the classic neurologic approach to patients and the exciting new insights that are fueling the field of neuropsychiatry and are of great relevance to all psychiatrists today. The selections are grouped into categories that cover 1) clinical neurology, 2) neurologic differential diagnosis and examinations, 3) common neurologic problems encountered by psychiatrists, 4) neurologic treatment, 5) neuroscience and neuroanatomy, 6) neurochemistry and neuropharmacology, 7) behavioral neurology and behavioral neuroanatomy, 8) neuropsychiatry and psychiatric presentations/ complications of neurologic illness, 9) dementia, 10) neuropsychology and cognitive neuroscience, 11) brain imaging and electrophysiology, 12) neurobiological models of psychiatric disease, and 13) biological theories of mind. The subject index may be helpful for locating references on particular topics or clinical conditions. The works chosen are almost exclusively new because of the rapidly advancing state of knowledge in the field of behavioral neuroscience. A number of current editions of classic textbooks are included because of their great reference value. The articles are meant to serve as excellent reviews or important examples of current work in this exciting field.

Clinical Neurology

1. *Adams RD, Victor M:** *Principles of Neurology,* 4th Edition. New York, McGraw-Hill, 1989

   This classic textbook of neurology has clear, substantive discussions of the cardinal signs and symptoms and the major categories of neurologic disease. It also contains sections on normal and disordered development and aging of the nervous system. The dual authorship provides a continuity of style not usually seen in major textbooks.

2. **Rowland LP** (ed): *Merritt's Textbook of Neurology,* 8th Edition. Philadelphia, PA, Lea & Febiger, 1989

   This superb textbook is encyclopedic in form, with discrete sections on specific diseases or syndromes written by experts in each field.

3. **Weiner HL, Levitt LP:** *Neurology for the House Officer,* 4th Edition. Baltimore, MD, Williams & Wilkins, 1989

   In this invaluable little book, chapters outline the approach to diagnosis and treatment of the most common neurologic presentations.

4. **Weiner HL, Urion DK, Levitt LP:** *Pediatric Neurology for the House Officer.* Baltimore, MD, Williams & Wilkins, 1988

   This gem does for pediatric neurology what Weiner and Levitt's (1989) *Neurology for the House Officer* above does for adult neurology. Its explanations of developmental milestones and the workup of a child who fails to achieve or loses milestones is particularly helpful.

Neurologic Differential Diagnosis and Examinations

5. *Mayo Clinic and Mayo Foundation for Medical Education and Research:** *Clinical Examinations in Neurology,* 6th Edition. St. Louis, MO, CV Mosby Year Book, 1991

This is a single book with "everything you need to know" about taking a neurologic history, doing a child and adult neurologic examination (including an excellent mental status–higher cognitive function exam), and performing an appropriate workup. It has chapters with clear descriptions of relevant neuroradiologic, electrophysiologic, cerebrospinal fluid, and laboratory examinations.

6. *Patten JP: *Neurological Differential Diagnosis: An Illustrated Approach.* London, Springer-Verlag, 1987 (reprint of 1977 edition)

This is perhaps the best exposition of traditional neurologic differential diagnosis because of its concise presentation of clinical "pearls" and its superlative three-dimensional drawings that clarify the effect of lesions at various neuroanatomical sites.

Also see general neurology texts above, imaging references below, and mental status exam chapters in Mesulam (1985) and Cummings (1985), both below.

Common Neurologic Problems Encountered by Psychiatrists

7. **Devinsky O, Feldmann E, Bromfield E, Emoto S, Raubertas R:** Structured interview for partial seizures: clinical phenomenology and diagnosis. *Journal of Epilepsy* 4:107–116, 1991

"Does that symptom represent a seizure?" This article, based on recent neuropsychiatric findings in seizure patients with intracranial electrophysiological monitoring, describes an empirically validated approach to this common clinical question.

8. **Diamond S** (guest ed): Headache. *Med Clin North Am,* Vol. 75, No. 3, 1991

This volume covers the evaluation and treatment of headaches of many etiologies. There are good reviews of differential diagnosis, migraine, cluster headache, tension headache, headaches secondary to other neurologic disease, psychiatric aspects of headache, and emergency management. For a discussion of a new pharmacologic agent for migraine, see Fullerton and Gengo (1992) below.

9. **Ojala M, Palo J:** The aetiology of dizziness and how to examine a dizzy patient. *Ann Med* 23:225–230, 1991

This article is a nice approach to a very common complaint that can be difficult to evaluate.

10. **Plum F, Posner JB:** Approach to the unconscious patient, in *The Diagnosis of Stupor and Coma,* 3rd Edition. Edited by Plum F, Posner JB. Philadelphia, PA, FA Davis, 1980, pp. 345–364

This chapter of this classic book provides a clinical regimen for the differential diagnosis, examination, and emergency management of patients with unresponsiveness of structural, toxic (including overdose), metabolic, or psychiatric etiology.

11. **Rubino FA:** Neurologic complications of alcoholism. *Psychiatr Clin North Am* 15:359–372, 1992

This material is valuable for psychiatrists given the prevalence and psychiatric aspects of alcohol abuse.

Also see neuropsychiatry references below.

Neurologic Treatment

12. **Fullerton T, Gengo FM:** Sumatripton: a selective 5-hydroxytryptamine receptor agonist for the acute treatment of migraine. *Annals of Pharmacotherapy* 26:800–808, 1992

This article provides an assessment of the pharmacology, efficacy, and adverse effects of this promising new treatment for migraine attacks.

13. **Johnson RT** (ed): *Current Therapy in Neurologic Diseases,* No. 3. Philadelphia, PA, CV Mosby, 1990

The value of this book lies in its flow diagram synopses of the evaluation and treatment of the major neurologic complaints and presentations.

14. *Samuels M** (ed): *Manual of Neurologic Therapeutics,* 3rd Edition. Boston, MA, Little, Brown, 1986

In the best tradition of the "spiral" manuals, this volume serves as an easy-to-read bible of essential diagnostic points and therapeutic interventions for the whole range of neurologic symptoms and diseases. The sections on headache and alterations in consciousness may be especially relevant for psychiatrists. See also the general neurology texts above.

Neuroscience and Neuroanatomy

15. **Gilman S, Winans SS:** *Manter and Gatz's Essentials of Clinical Neuroanatomy and Neurophysiology,* 8th Edition. Philadelphia, PA, FA Davis, 1992

This is an excellent review of the anatomy and function of the major neural tracts and systems. Familiarity with this material is a prerequisite for neurologic diagnosis. The numerous multitoned drawings highlight the important connections and relations among key structures.

16. **Kandel ER, Schwartz JH** (eds): *Principles of Neural Science*, 3rd Edition. New York, Elsevier, 1991

This definitive neuroscience textbook presents the latest information about everything from genes to behavior in a lucid, readable fashion. The sections on neuronal physiology and synaptic transmission may be particularly useful.

Neurochemistry and Neuropharmacology

17. **Arana GW, Hyman SE:** Psychiatric uses of anticonvulsants, in *Handbook of Psychiatric Drug Therapy*, 2nd Edition. Edited by Arana GW, Hyman SE. Boston, MA, Little, Brown, 1991, pp. 108–127

Anticonvulsants are now part of the psychopharmacologic armamentarium. Psychiatrists may not have as much experience administering these medications as neurologists do. This phenomenal chapter provides an up-to-date report on the pharmacology, mechanisms of action, indications, therapeutic use, side effects, and drug interactions of carbamazepine, valproic acid, and clonazepam. The rest of this psychopharmacology handbook is also outstanding.

18. **Cooper JR, Bloom FE, Roth RH:** *The Biochemical Basis of Neuropharmacology*, 6th Edition. New York, Oxford University Press, 1991

This is a detailed presentation of the current understanding of the mechanisms underlying neurotransmitter and neuropeptide function. A greater familiarity with this material will help one to keep up with new developments in the ever-changing pharmacopoeia.

19. **Javitt DC, Zukin SR:** The role of excitatory amino acids in neuropsychiatric illness. *Journal of Neuropsychiatry and Clinical Neuroscience* 2:44–52, 1990

This article provides a review of the neurotransmitter functions and neurotoxicity of excitatory amino acids and of their implication in the pathophysiology of psychiatric and neuropsychiatric disorders.

20. **Risby ED:** G proteins in neuropsychiatric disorders. *Current Opinion in Psychiatry* 5:74–78, 1992

This is a review of the new literature concerning G protein abnormalities found in several neuropsychiatric disorders. The family of guanosine 5'-triphosphate (GTP)-binding proteins plays a key role in trans-membrane signal transduction and may be involved in pathogenesis and response to psychopharmacologic treatment.

Behavioral Neurology and Behavioral Neuroanatomy

21. **Culebras A:** Neuroanatomic and neurologic correlates of sleep distur-bances. *Neurology* 42 (suppl 6):19–27, 1992

This article provides a clear discussion of the neurobiology of sleep and wakefulness and of the sleep changes seen with various neurologic conditions.

22. **Fuster JM:** *The Prefrontal Cortex,* 2nd Edition. New York, Raven, 1989

This is an important work on the anatomy, physiology, and neuro-psychology of the lobe, which is the substrate for much of our higher mental abilities.

23. **Joseph R:** *Neuropsychology, Neuropsychiatry, and Behavioral Neurology.* New York, Plenum, 1990

This book is organized neuroanatomically. It is therefore an ideal source for quick information about the behavioral function of any particular brain area of interest. Hemispheric laterality of function is reviewed. In addition, there are sections on the neuropsychological sequelae of brain trauma, cerebrovascular diseases, and neoplasms. A similar, and perhaps more readily available, source for this type of information is M.-M. Mesulam's chapter, "Neural Substrates of Behav-ior: The Effects of Brain Lesions Upon Mental State," in *The New Harvard Guide to Modern Psychiatry* (Cambridge, MA, Belknap Press, 1988, pp. 91–128).

24. *Mesulam M-M (ed): *Principles of Behavioral Neurology.* Philadelphia, PA, FA Davis, 1985

This is the preeminent textbook in this field. The chapter on behavioral neuroanatomy provides a clear approach to structure-function relation-ships within and among different areas of the brain. The chapter on mental state assessment provides a superb battery of neuropsychologi-cal tests of abilities associated with specific language, cognitive, and perceptual functions and with the different lobes and hemispheres of the brain. Chapters on the various deficit syndromes, right hemisphere modulation of affect and nonverbal communication, electrophysio-logic tests, and imaging modalities complete this outstanding volume.

25. *Mesulam M-M:* Large scale neurocognitive networks and distributed processing for attention, language and memory. *Ann Neurol* 28:597–613, 1990

This article is a fine example of current thinking about how parallel distributed processing in regionally distributed brain networks gives rise to our most important cognitive functions.

26. *Mind and brain. *Sci Am,* Vol. 267, No. 3, 1992

This special issue brings together world experts, each of whom has written a review article on the latest findings concerning the brain mechanisms underlying vision, memory, learning, language, consciousness, and mental disorders. Brain development, aging, and sexual differences are covered as well.

27. **Silberman EK, Weingartner H:** Hemispheric lateralization of functions related to emotion. *Brain Cogn* 5:322–353, 1986

This is a review of hemispheric differences in the recognition, expression, and experience of positive and negative emotions.

Neuropsychiatry and Psychiatric Presentations/ Complications of Neurologic Illness

28. **Bear D, Herman B, Fagel B:** Interictal behavior syndrome in temporal lobe epilepsy: the views of three experts. *Journal of Neuropsychiatry and Clinical Neuroscience* 1:308–318, 1989

This article provides three vantage points on the clinically important, fascinating, and controversial topic of personality and behavior changes in patients with chronic temporal lobe epilepsy.

29. **Cohen DJ, Riddle MA, Leckman JF:** Pharmacotherapy of Tourette's syndrome and associated disorders. *Psychiatr Clin North Am* 15:109–129, 1992

This is a fine review of Tourette's syndrome, stressing developmental context, associated disorders (obsessive-compulsive disorder, attention-deficit/hyperactivity disorder), and current pharmacotherapy.

30. *Cummings, JL:* *Clinical Neuropsychiatry.* Orlando, FL, Grune & Stratton, 1985

This book is a tremendous wealth of useful information. With a discerning clinical perspective, Cummings provides an introduction to neuropsychiatry, a sophisticated neuropsychiatric interview and mental status exam, and a complete review of the neurologic and psychiatric etiologies (and differential diagnosis) of classic symptoms and syndromes. There are particularly enlightening chapters on acute confusional states; dissociative states; violence and aggression; and disturbances of sleep, appetite, and sexual behavior.

31. **Devinsky O, Bear DM:** Varieties of depression in epilepsy. *Neuropsychiatry, Neuropsychology, and Behavioral Neurology* 4:49–61, 1991

   This article by two authorities on the neuropsychiatry of epilepsy makes the extremely important clinical distinctions between pre-ictal, ictal, post-ictal, and inter-ictal psychiatric symptoms in patients with seizure disorders.

32. *Hyde TM, Hotson JR, Kleinman JE:** Differential diagnosis of choreiform tardive dyskinesia. *Journal of Neuropsychiatry and Clinical Neuroscience* 3:255–268, 1991

   This is an excellent guide to the differential diagnosis and the clinical and laboratory evaluation of orofacial and appendicular choreiform involuntary movements.

33. **Lipowski ZJ:** Update on delirium. *Psychiatr Clin North Am* 15:335–346, 1992

   This article is a welcome update by a recognized authority on the differential diagnosis and management of confusional states.

34. **Marin RS:** Apathy: a neuropsychiatric syndrome. *Journal of Neuropsychiatry and Clinical Neuroscience* 3:243–254, 1991

   This article demonstrates the impact that a neurobiologically informed approach can have on the classification of disorders. Based on the neurology of intentional behavior, Marin makes the distinction between the primary syndrome and the secondary symptom of motivational loss. It is also a fine literature review on the topic.

35. *Psychiatric syndromes associated with neurologic disease. *Semin Neurol* 10:221–317, 1990

   This journal edition contains reviews of great relevance to the psychiatrist. The topics covered are conversion symptoms, organic delusional syndrome, depressive syndromes associated with central nervous system disease, depression following cerebrovascular lesions, psychiatric and cognitive aspects of multiple sclerosis, psychiatric consequences of basal ganglia disease, the neuropsychiatry of human immunodeficiency virus, the brain in schizophrenia, psychopathology of frontal lobe syndromes, neurologic side effects of psychiatric treatments, and the neurology of aggression and episodic dyscontrol.

36. **Rogers D:** Catatonia: a contemporary approach. *Journal of Neuropsychiatry and Clinical Neuroscience* 3:334–340, 1991

Rogers provides a history of the conceptualization of patients who present with severe abnormal movement accompanying psychiatric illness and an up-to-date clinical approach to such patients.

37. **Trimble MR:** The schizophrenia-like psychosis of epilepsy. *Neuropsychiatry, Neuropsychology, and Behavioral Neurology* 5:103–107, 1992

A leading figure in this field discusses specific psychotic symptoms seen in some patients with seizure disorders, the similarities with and differences from schizophrenic psychosis, relevant positron-emission tomography studies, and a resultant model for the pathophysiology of psychosis.

38. **Yudofsky SC, Silver J, Hales RE:** Neuropsychiatry of brain injury. *Current Opinion in Psychiatry* 5:103–108, 1992

This is a review of the cognitive, affective, and psychosocial changes that occur after brain injury, written by leaders in this field.

Dementia

39. **Cummings JL:** Dementia and depression: an evolving enigma. *Journal of Neuropsychiatry and Clinical Neuroscience* 1:236–242, 1989

An overview of the various interrelated clinical presentations of dementia and depression, this review provides an insight into the causal relationships, differential diagnosis, and treatment of these conditions.

40. **Cummings JL, Victoroff JI:** Noncognitive neuropsychiatric syndromes in Alzheimer's disease. *Neuropsychiatry Neuropsychology and Behavioral Neurology* 3:140–158, 1990

This article is a guide to the delusions, hallucinations, mood changes, appetite changes, sleep changes, sexual changes, and psychomotor disorders that the psychiatrist is likely to encounter in patients with the most common form of dementing illness.

41. *Cummings JL, Benson DF, Dementia A: *Clinical Approach,* 2nd Edition. Boston, MA, Butterworth-Heineman, 1992

This is a definitive, up-to-date text about all clinical aspects of dementia by two experts in the field. There are excellent discussions of the definition, epidemiology, ethics, workup, treatment, and management (including working with the caregivers) of the syndromes. There are chapters on the cortical dementias (e.g., Alzheimer's disease and Pick's disease) and the subcortical dementias that can be seen with extrapyramidal disorders and multiple sclerosis. Vascular, infectious, toxic, metabolic, hydrocephalic, traumatic, neoplastic, and enzymatic etiologies are also considered in detail (with wonderful tables).

42. **Reichman WE, Cummings JL:** Diagnosis of rare dementia syndromes: an algorithmic approach. *J Geriatr Psychiatry Neurol* 3:73–84, 1990

Some of the less common dementia syndromes may present with early personality and mood changes. This article outlines an approach to the diagnosis of such syndromes after the usual dementia workup has been unrevealing. The algorithm makes use of neuroimaging results to guide biochemical, enzymatic, immunologic, and biopsy studies.

Neuropsychology and Cognitive Neuroscience

43. **Heilman KM, Valenstein E** (eds): *Clinical Neuropsychology*, 3rd Edition. New York, Oxford University Press, 1993

This is a well-known work with instructive chapters on aphasia, alexia, agraphia, acalculia, body schema changes, apraxia, visuospatial agnosia, neglect, callosal syndromes, frontal syndromes, emotional disorders resulting from central nervous system disease, amnesia, dementia, and treatment and recovery.

44. **LeDoux JE, Hirst W** (eds): *Mind and Brain: Dialogues in Cognitive Neuroscience.* Cambridge, MA, Cambridge University Press, 1986

This book provides informative and fascinating dialogues between a neurobiologist and a cognitive psychologist about perception, attention, memory, and emotion. It is an excellent review and integration of animal and human research concerning these neuropsychological processes.

45. **Lezak MD:** Neuropsychological assessment, in *Clinical Neuropsychology, Handbook of Clinical Neurology*, Vol. 45. Edited by Vinker PJ, Bruyn GW, Klawans HL, Frederiks JAM. New York, Elsevier Science Publishing, 1985, pp. 515–530

This is a concise description of the indications for, and implications of, neuropsychological testing by the author of the classic text on the same subject. That textbook (*Neuropsychological Assessment*, New York, Oxford University Press, 1983) and the rest of the volume in which this chapter appears are also recommended.

Brain Imaging and Electrophysiology

46. Andreasen NC (ed): *Brain Imaging, Applications in Psychiatry.* Washington, DC, American Psychiatric Press, 1989

This is a review of structural and functional imaging techniques and findings in psychiatric disorders and normal cognition. The explanation of neuroreceptor studies with positron-emission tomography and the chapter on brain electrical activity mapping are worth noting.

47. *Bench CJ, Dolan RJ, Friston KJ, Frackowiak RSJ: Positron emission tomography in the study of brain metabolism in psychiatric and neuro-psychiatric disorders. *Br J Psychiatry* 157 (suppl 9):82–95, 1990

This article is a good review of the significant contribution of positron-emission tomography to our understanding of in vivo brain function abnormalities in patients with schizophrenia, affective disorders, obsessional disorders, anxiety disorders, and dementias.

48. Guze BH: Magnetic resonance spectroscopy: a technique for functional brain imaging. *Arch Gen Psychiatry* 48:572–574, 1991

Magnetic resonance spectroscopy permits the imaging of specific chemical compounds in the brain. This article provides a brief introduction to this new technology, which is making its way into the psychiatric research literature.

49. Hughes JR, Wilson WP (eds): *EEG and Evoked Potentials in Psychiatry and Behavioral Neurology.* Boston, MA, Butterworths, 1983

This is a valuable guide to electrophysiological findings in patients with organic mental syndromes, schizophrenia, affective disorders, alcohol abuse, sleep disturbances, child psychiatric problems, and mental retardation. There are also descriptions of findings associated with psychotropic medication and electroconvulsive therapy.

50. Kwong KK, Belliveau JW, Chesler DA, Goldberg IE, Weisskoff RM, Poncelet BP, Kennedy DN, Hoppel BE, Cohen MS, Turner R, Cheng H-M, Brady TJ, Rosen BR: Dynamic magnetic resonance imaging of human brain activity during primary sensory stimulation. *Proc Natl Acad Sci U S A* 89:5675–5679, 1992

This article is an example of recent work in the rapidly developing field of magnetic resonance functional brain imaging. This technology will play an increasing role in the study of the brain and mind in health and illness.

51. **Mazziotta JC, Gilman S** (eds): *Clinical Brain Imaging: Principles and Applications.* Philadelphia, PA, FA Davis, 1992

The chapters on computed tomography, magnetic resonance imaging, single photon emission tomography, and positron-emission tomography (PET) imaging modalities give comprehensible explanations of these important technologies. The clinical applications sections focus on neurologic disease categories. Although primary psychiatric disorders are not covered in detail, there is a chapter on imaging in the diagnosis and management of dementing illnesses and a section on the value of PET in psychiatric disorders.

Neurobiological Models of Psychiatric Disease

52. **Bachneff SA:** Positron emission tomography and magnetic resonance imaging: a review and a local circuit neurons hypo(dys)function hypothesis of schizophrenia. *Biol Psychiatry* 30:857–886, 1991

This is a review of functional and structural brain-imaging studies of schizophrenia and a proposed pathophysiologic model of the positive and negative symptoms based on the integration of the imaging data with data from transmitter neurocircuitry, neurophysiology, neuropathology, and neuropsychology.

53. **Trimble MR:** The neurology of anxiety. *Postgrad Med J* 64 (suppl 2):22–26, 1988

This article is a discussion of central and peripheral nervous system involvement in, and genetic contributions to, the pathogenesis of anxiety.

54. **Voeller KK:** What can neurological models of attention, intention, and arousal tell us about attention-deficit hyperactivity disorder? *Journal of Neuropsychiatry and Clinical Neuroscience* 3:209–216, 1991

This article reviews the three interrelated neuronal systems with a suggestion of a model for the neural basis of attention-deficit/hyperactivity disorder.

Biological Theories of Mind

55. **Black IB:** *Information in the Brain.* Cambridge, MA, MIT Press, 1991

This is a scholarly yet innovative approach to the mind-brain problem that breaks down the dichotomy between the "hardware" and "software" of the nervous system. Black, a molecular neuroscientist and neurologist, explains how the biological properties of, and connections between, neurons enable them to communicate with each other and to change with experience. The emergence of symbolic functions and subjective experience are discussed within this context.

56. **Dennett DC:** *Consciousness Explained.* Boston, MA, Little, Brown, 1991

A leading philosopher of mind combines neuroscientific and experimental psychological findings with a rigorous philosophical approach to produce a theory that attempts to explain our subjective experience. The book is highly entertaining and thought provoking.

57. **Edelman GM:** *The Remembered Present.* New York, Basic Books, 1989

A biological theory of consciousness put forward by a leading theoretical and computational neuroscientist, this book is a brilliant, if controversial, synthesis of evolutionary theory and neural network systems analysis in an attempt to explain the mechanisms that constitute unconscious states, conscious experience, and psychiatric disorders of consciousness.

35

Novel Approaches to Diagnostic Assessment in Neuropsychiatry

John A. Sweeney, Ph.D.
Kevin M. Malone, M.D.

Although the mental status examination remains the essential diagnostic process in clinical psychiatry, recent advances in basic neurosciences and in in vivo electrophysiologic, biochemical, and neuroimaging technology should enhance our clinical findings over the coming decade.

Neuroimaging has probably been the most proliferative area of such developments. For the differential diagnosis of dementias in the elderly, and to rule out occult neurological causes of psychiatric symptomatology in younger patients, there is a clear-cut and established role for functional and structural diagnostic neuroimaging procedures.

Beyond this purpose of diagnosing neurologic disorders, a growing body of evidence now indicates that distinctive physiologic and anatomic brain abnormalities are relatively common in severe psychiatric illnesses. Most studies suggest that these abnormalities predict poor prognosis in a range of disorders, including schizophrenia and affective disorders.

The validity of using neuroimaging procedures for the differential clinical diagnosis of psychiatric disorders is not yet well established. Comparisons of different diagnostic groups in terms of neuroimaging findings have generally not identified pathological features with high sensitivity and specificity for different psychiatric disorders. This pattern of findings raises the possibility that current diagnostic categorizations based on clinical symptomatology might not map perfectly well with clinically relevant patterns of pathophysiological disturbances in the brain.

As we develop a better understanding of the biological bases of severe psychiatric disorders, and as relationships between brain abnormalities and clinical symptomatology are clarified, there may need to be a basic reconceptualization of the psychiatric diagnostic process. This would likely involve a combined emphasis on identifying both types of brain dysfunction and types of clinical psychopathology. As the pathophysiological mechanisms of different forms of psychopathology are clarified and as the treatment-relevance of abnormal findings in brain structure, metabolism, and receptor biochemistry are established, the clinical use of neuroimaging and other special testing procedures is likely to expand dramatically in coming years.

Advances also continue to be made in neuroendocrine challenge studies. Research using challenge paradigms in schizophrenia, depression, obsessive-compulsive disorder, and eating disorders have explored putative abnormalities in neurotransmitter systems that may play a major role in the etiology of these illnesses. These tests may have clinical potential in the early detection of patients likely to be nonresponders to standard treatments and in guiding the selection of the type and duration of pharmacologic treatment strategies most likely to have the greatest clinical benefit.

Electrophysiological studies continue to provide an approach for studying disorders of information processing that are central to major psychiatric disorders. Electroencephalographic (EEG) studies, including standard clinical studies, event-related potentials, and brain electrical activity monitoring, offer important diagnostic information in the evaluation of many neuropsychiatric disorders. A number of studies indicate that specific EEG abnormalities may identify individuals at increased genetic risk for substance abuse and schizophrenia.

Depressed patients have well-documented EEG sleep architecture abnormalities, in particular rapid eye movement abnormalities in the first 90 minutes of sleep. There is now evidence emerging that certain sleep abnormalities may have clinical value in terms of predicting antidepressant treatment response. In this increasingly sophisticated field of research, it is likely that technological refinements and ongoing research will bring this procedure more and more into the clinical arena.

Eye movement studies also have the potential to become an important noninvasive diagnostic testing procedure in psychiatry. Spurred by data from monkey and human clinical studies indicating important roles for specific neocortical regions in the regulation of particular forms of eye movement activity, and data indicating that pursuit eye movement abnormalities may be a marker for genetically mediated risk for schizophrenia, clinical use of eye movement studies in psychiatry may grow considerably in coming years.

Postmortem brain studies may at some point come to play a confirmatory role for diagnosis in psychiatry, as they now do in some neurologic disorders such as Alzheimer's disease. Studies of brain tissue from suicide victims indicate that prominent changes in the serotonergic and perhaps adrenergic systems appear to be pronounced in areas of prefrontal cortex. In schizophrenia, several reports of degenerative changes in left temporal/limbic and parahippocampal areas have recently been published. This latter finding is consistent with some magnetic resonance imaging studies that also show atrophic changes in this brain region.

In the years to come, specialized diagnostic tests such as those described here have the potential to aid in differential clinical diagnosis, in treatment planning, and in identifying individuals at high genetic risk for psychiatric disorders. The growing integration of the basic neurosciences with clinical psychiatric research offers promise that the brain mechanisms of different severe psychiatric disorders will become better understood, and this knowledge will probably lead to the expanded use of biological testing procedures in clinical practice. However, for most of these still novel procedures, further research validation, technological advances, and cost reduction are needed before they will have a prominent influence on clinical practice.

Overview

1. **Andreasen NC** (ed): *Brain Imaging: Applications in Psychiatry.* Washington, DC, American Psychiatric Press, 1989

   This text presents a solid overview of the major approaches for structural and functional neuroimaging that are currently used in psychiatric research. The text also summarizes major findings in neuroimaging studies of psychiatric disorders.

2. *Meltzer HY (ed): *Psychopharmacology: The Third Generation of Progress.* New York, Raven, 1987

   This very systematic and thorough text, written in association with the American College of Neuropsychopharmacology, offers a detailed review of neuroendocrine challenge tests and other biochemical studies used widely in investigations of affective disorders and schizophrenia. It also provides an understanding of the function of drugs and chemical agents used to prevent and treat mental illness, drug abuse, and alcoholism.

3. **Steinhauer SR, Gruzelier JH, Zubin J** (eds): *Handbook of Schizophrenia, Vol. 5: Neuropsychology, Psychophysiology, and Information Processing.* Amsterdam, Netherlands, Elsevier, 1991

   This edited review presents a comprehensive presentation of electrophysiological and cognitive approaches used in neuropsychiatric research, particularly procedures that have been used in the study of schizophrenia.

Functional Brain-Imaging Studies

4. **Agren H, Reibring L, Hartvig P, Tedroff J, Bjurling P, Hornfeldt K, Andersson Y, Lundqvist H, Langstrom B:** Low brain uptake of L-[^{11}C]5-hydroxytryptophan in major depression: a positron emission tomography study on patient and healthy volunteers. *Acta Psychiatr Scand* 83:449–455, 1991

   This research used positron-emission tomography to demonstrate that there may be a deficient transfer of 5-hydroxytryptamine (5-HT) across the blood-brain barrier in major depression. Such an abnormality might be a cause of reduced central serotonergic function in depression that may play a role in the etiology of the disorder.

5. **Benkelfat C, Nordahl TE, Semple WE, King C, Murphy DL, Cohen RM:** Local cerebral glucose metabolic rates in obsessive-compulsive disorder. *Arch Gen Psychiatry* 47:840–848, 1990

   This article is one of several neuroimaging studies of obsessive-compulsive disorder indicating increased metabolic activity in regions of prefrontal cortex. This pattern, which has also been reported to occur in caudate/putamen, appears to be a state-related correlate of obsessive-compulsive disorder.

6. **Kumar A, Schapiro MB, Grady C, Haxby JV, Wagner E, Salerno JA, Friedland RP, Rapoport SI:** High-resolution PET studies in Alzheimer's disease. *Neuropsychopharmacology* 4:35–46, 1991

   This positron-emission tomography study of Alzheimer's disease demonstrates diffuse reductions of resting metabolic activity in most major neocortical and subcortical gray matter regions. Of importance, these disease-related effects were evident even very early in the course of the illness.

7. **Pettegrew JW, Keshavan MS, Panchalingam K, Strychor S, Kaplan DB, Tretta MG, Allen M:** Alterations in brain high-energy phosphate and

membrane phospholipid metabolism in first-episode, drug-naive schizophrenia. *Arch Gen Psychiatry* 48:563–568, 1991

This is the first major study to use nuclear magnetic resonance spectroscopy to study schizophrenia. The results demonstrated abnormalities of phosphate and membrane phospholipid metabolism in never-medicated first-episode schizophrenic patients. These findings indicate disturbances in metabolic function, and suggest that there may be a loss of neuronal cell membranes early in the course of schizophrenia.

8. *Sedvall G: The current status of PET scanning with respect to schizophrenia. *Neuropsychopharmacology* 7:41–54, 1992; **Murphy D, Rapoport SI:** PET scanning in schizophrenia: a critical evaluation. *Neuropsychopharmacology* 7:59–61, 1992

This overview provides an update on findings from positron-emission tomography studies of metabolic activity and receptor binding in schizophrenia.

Sleep

9. **Reynolds CF III, Hoch CC, Buysse DJ, George CJ, Houck PR, Mazumdar S, Miller M, Pollock BG, Rifai H, Frank E, Cornes C, Morycz RK, Kupfer DJ:** Sleep in late-life recurrent depression changes during early continuation therapy with nortriptyline. *Neuropsychopharmacology* 5:85–96, 1991

This study provides a recent account of methodological and theoretical considerations involved in evaluating sleep abnormalities in depression. The findings indicate that continuation therapy with nortriptyline was associated with improvement in several sleep parameters.

10. **Thase ME, Kupfer DJ:** Current status of EEG sleep in the assessment and treatment of depression, in *Advances in Human Psychopharmacology.* Edited by Burrows GD, Werry JS. Greenwich, CT, JAI Press, 1987, pp. 93–148

This chapter reviews major aspects of sleep research in depression through the life cycle, including sleep abnormalities, prediction of treatment response, implications of electroencephalographic sleep abnormalities for the pathophysiology of depression, and future directions and limitations of sleep research.

Neuroendocrine Studies

11. **Arana GW, Baldessarini RJ, Ornsteen M:** The dexamethasone suppression test for diagnosis and prognosis in psychiatry. *Arch Gen Psychiatry* 42:1193–1204, 1985

    The dexamethasone suppression test (DST) is a laboratory marker for disturbances in the hypothalamic-pituitary-adrenal axis that are associated with endogenous depression, and evidence for its state-relationship to depression is fairly strong. This article provides a useful review of the advantages and limitations of the DST in research and clinical psychiatry.

12. **Bartalena L, Placidi GF, Martino E, Falcone M, Pellegrini L, Dell'Osso L, Pacchiarotti A, Pinchera A:** Nocturnal serum thyrotropin (TSH) surge and the TSH response to TSH releasing hormone: dissociated behavior in untreated depressives. *J Clin Endocrinol Metab* 71:650–655, 1990

    One of the most frequent abnormalities in major depression is a blunted thyroid-stimulating hormone (TSH) response to thyroid-releasing hormone (TRH) infusion. Depressed patients whose TRH tests fail to normalize after treatment are at greater risk for relapse. This elegant study examines TSH in untreated depressed patients versus healthy control subjects and reports an abolition of nocturnal TSH surge in 14 of 15 cases. The authors conclude that although baseline morning TSH evaluation and TSH response to TRH may not reveal differences in depression, measurement of nocturnal TSH surge may be a more sensitive indicator of TSH abnormalities in endogenous depression.

13. **Delgado PL, Charney DS, Price LH, Aghajanian GK, Landis H, Heninger GR:** Serotonin function and the mechanism of antidepressant action. *Arch Gen Psychiatry* 47:411–418, 1990

    The authors report a reversal of antidepressant-induced clinical remission by rapid depletion of plasma tryptophan in depressed patients and conclude that the therapeutic effects of some antidepressant drugs may be dependent on serotonin bioavailability.

14. **Lieberman JA, Kane JM, Sarantakos S, Gadaleta D, Woerner M, Alvir J, Ramos-Lorenzi J:** Prediction of relapse in schizophrenia. *Arch Gen Psychiatry* 44:597–603, 1987

    This study involved conducting a neuroendocrine challenge test in schizophrenic patients. The results indicate that response to methylphenidate challenge predicted early relapse in unmedicated schizophrenic patients.

15. *Mann JJ: Neurobiologic models, in *Models of Depressive Disorders*. Edited by Mann JJ. New York, Plenum, 1989, pp. 143–177

    This book chapter provides a review of the psychobiology of depression. It reviews data relevant to the catecholamine hypothesis of the disorder.

16. Meltzer HY, Lowy MT: The serotonin hypothesis of depression, in *Psychopharmacology: The Third Generation of Progress*. Edited by Meltzer HY. New York, Raven, 1987, pp. 513–526

    This chapter presents an excellent review of various neuroendocrine paradigms that have been used in psychiatric research. It provides an extensive bibliography for further reading in this area.

17. Siever LJ, Trestman RL, Coccaro EF, Bernstein D, Gabriel SM, Owen K, Moran M, Lawrence T, Rosenthal J, Horvath TB: The growth hormone response to clonidine in acute and remitted depressed male patients. *Neuropsychopharmacology* 6:165–177, 1992

    This study reports that a blunted growth hormone response to clonidine may represent a state-independent noradrenergic abnormality in some forms of severe depression.

Electrophysiology

18. Holzman PS: Recent studies of psychophysiology in schizophrenia. *Schizophr Bull* 13:49–75, 1987

    This review article presents an overview of psychophysiology research in schizophrenia.

19. Malloy P, Rasmussen S, Braden W, Haier RJ: Topographic evoked potential mapping in obsessive-compulsive disorder: evidence of frontal lobe dysfunction. *Psychiatry Res* 28:63–71, 1989

    This study provides an example of the use of electroencephalographic research paradigms to test hypotheses about localized brain dysfunction. Specifically, the study indicated that there is a disturbance of prefrontal cortex associated with obsessive-compulsive disorder.

20. *McCarley RW, Faux SF, Shenton ME, Nestor PG, Adams J: Event-related potentials in schizophrenia: their biological and clinical correlates and a new model of schizophrenic pathophysiology. *Schizophr Res* 4:209–231, 1991

This research represents an effort to link evoked potential abnormalities in schizophrenia to aspects of clinical phenomenology and neuroanatomic abnormalities. The results support a model that psychobiological changes occurring during acute psychosis may cause cell death in left temporal limbic cortex via excitotoxicity.

21. **Shagass C:** Deviant cerebral functional topography as revealed by electrophysiology, in *Biological Perspectives of Schizophrenia.* Edited by Helmchen H, Henn FA. New York, Wiley, 1987, pp. 237–253

This chapter provides a thorough review of recent research using electroencephalography and event-related potential methodologies in psychotic disorders by an investigator who has long been one of the leading figures in this area of research.

Eye Movement Studies

22. **Clementz B, Sweeney JA:** Is eye movement dysfunction a biological marker for schizophrenia? a methodological review. *Psychol Bull* 108:77–92, 1990

This review of pursuit eye movement studies in schizophrenia discusses the evidence relevant to the hypothesis that the abnormality is a familial marker for the illness. The article provides extensive discussion of major methodological issues that are important for interpreting results from eye movement studies.

23. **Holzman PS, Kringlen E, Levy DL, Haberman SJ:** Deviant eye tracking in twins discordant for psychosis. *Arch Gen Psychiatry* 37:627–631, 1980

These results from a major twin study support the hypothesis that abnormal eye tracking is an indicator of familially transmitted risk for schizophrenia.

24. **Siever LJ, Coursey RD:** Biological markers for schizophrenia and the biological high-risk approach. *J Nerv Ment Dis* 173:4–16, 1985

This article presents the conceptual rationale for the high-risk approach in studies of the etiology of major psychiatric disorders. It also provides new data on platelet monoamine oxidase and eye movement studies as markers of risk for schizophrenia in a community population.

Postmortem Studies

25. *Arango V, Mann JJ:** Relevance of serotonergic postmortem studies to suicidal behavior. *International Review of Psychiatry* 4:131–140, 1992

This article reviews biochemical postmortem studies of suicide victims. It nicely summarizes data indicating that there is a disturbance in serotonergic function in brains of suicide victims and that this disturbance appears to be particularly pronounced in prefrontal cortex.

26. **Bogerts B, Hantsch J, Herzer M:** A morphometric study of the dopamine-containing cell groups in the mesencephalon of normals, Parkinson patients, and schizophrenics. *Biol Psychiatry* 18:951–969, 1983

This article contrasts the pathology of dopaminergic neurons of the nigrostriatal and mesolimbic systems in Parkinson's disease and schizophrenia.

27. **Bogerts B, Meertz E, Schonfeldt-Bausch R:** Basal ganglia and limbic system pathology in schizophrenia. *Arch Gen Psychiatry* 42:784–791, 1985

This study presents results from a gross histological postmortem study of brains from schizophrenic individuals. The findings suggest reduced volume of medial temporal/limbic structures in schizophrenia.

IV

Treatment

36

Psychopharmacology

Carl Salzman, M.D.

O ver the past 30 years, therapeutic efficacy of psychotropic drugs has been repeatedly demonstrated for symptom reduction in schizophrenia, affective disorder, and anxiety-related disorders. Although available drugs are imperfect as therapeutic agents with response rates and side-effect profiles varying from person to person, they nevertheless have revolutionized psychiatric treatment. The literature describing research and clinical practice with these drugs is enormous, and any list of recommended readings that is limited by length must, by its very nature, eliminate articles that some readers would consider to be essential. The following list is not meant to be inclusive nor exclusive but simply represents an attempt to gather past as well as recent articles portraying the range of psychopharmacologic information available to the clinician. Most of the articles were selected for having direct therapeutic application as opposed to theoretical research data. All articles selected have comprehensive bibliographies that should enable the reader to explore further a particular psychopharmacologic topic. The articles were also selected for their readability, for a particular clinical point that is made, for historical perspective, or to illustrate current problems in both clinical practice and research methodology in psychopharmacology.

General Reviews of Psychopharmacology

1. **Cooper JR, Blum FE, Roth RH:** *The Biochemical Basis of Neuropharmacology,* 6th Edition. New York, Oxford, 1991

   This book is a time-honored summary of the relationship between neurotransmission, psychopathology, and psychopharmacologic treatment. Now in its 6th edition, it is exceptionally readable and comprehensive.

2. **Gelenberg AJ, Basssuk EL, Schoonover SC:** *The Practitioner's Guide to Psychoactive Drugs.* New York, Plenum Medical, 1991

   Among the many spiral-bound handbooks available to the clinician, this volume is noteworthy for its comprehensive yet lucid approach to use of psychotropic drugs. Clear clinical prescribing suggestions are provided and are balanced nicely with a theoretical perspective that is lacking in many other handbooks.

3. **Goodwyn FK, Jamison KR:** *Manic-Depressive Illness.* New York, Oxford University Press, 1990

   This is an extraordinary volume that every psychiatrist should own. It is a lucid, comprehensive encyclopedia of this disorder. It is indispensable for researchers, but is equally essential for clinicians. Five chapters are focused specifically on the treatment of manic episodes, bipolar depression, maintenance medical treatment, the use of psychotherapy, and problems in medication compliance. In addition, there are two chapters on treatment of substance-abusing, manic-depressive patients and suicidal manic-depressive patients. The information is most comprehensive, up-to-date, and accessible to the average reader.

4. **Hyman SE, Nestler EJ:** *The Molecular Foundations of Psychiatry.* Washington, DC, American Psychiatric Press, 1993

   Hyman and Nestler have taken the latest information on neurobiology, molecular biology, and fundamental psychopharmacology and woven it into a tapestry of exceptional clarity. Readers who have been intimidated by the neurobiologic revolution will welcome this volume as a clear step-by-step guide to central nervous system function. The use of psychotropic drugs is then presented using the neurobiological and molecular biological foundation provided.

5. **Jefferson JW, Greist JH, Ackerman DL, Carol JA:** *Lithium Encyclopedia for Clinical Practice,* 2nd Edition. Washington, DC, American Psychiatric Press, 1987

This is an indispensable overall reference on lithium for all practicing psychiatrists. Topics are listed alphabetically, and comprehensive reference lists are provided at the end of each section. Although this book is not meant to be read cover to cover, it is essential as a reference.

6. **Kane JM, Lieberman JA:** *Adverse Effects of Psychotropic Drugs.* New York, Guilford, 1992

It is surprising that a book on psychotropic drug side effects has not been published for more than 25 years. Kane and Lieberman have sought to correct that by providing an up-to-date review of the etiology and treatment of common psychotropic drugs side effects. Not all categories of side effects are represented, and movement disorders from neuroleptics are overly represented. However, the information that is available in this book is accessible, complete, and highly useful.

7. **Meltzer HY** (ed): *Psychopharmacology: The Third Generation of Progress.* New York, Raven, 1987

This book is the definitive review of the neurobiologic theories and treatment of psychiatric disorder and of the use of psychotropic medication. It is weighty, very scholarly, and research oriented. Clinicians will find only some of the information useful, but it is the standard reference on which all other psychopharmacology texts are based. It should certainly be in the library of any psychiatrist with research interest in psychopharmacology or neurobiology.

8. **Salzman C:** *Clinical Geriatric Psychopharmacology,* 2nd Edition. Baltimore, MD, Williams & Wilkins, 1992

This is both a scholarly as well as a clinically oriented state-of-the-art volume on prescribing psychiatric drugs to elderly patients. Case vignettes are included, and the bibliographies are extensive.

9. **Schatzberg AF, Cole JO:** *Manual of Clinic Psychopharmacology,* 2nd Edition. Washington, DC, American Psychiatric Press, 1991

This clinically oriented, spiral-bound handbook is an excellent overall guide for psychopharmacology. Written by two well-known psychopharmacologists, it is unique in providing the personal clinical experiences of the authors as well as reviewing published reports.

Schizophrenia: Historical Treatment

10. **Cole JO, Klerman GL, Goldberg SC:** Phenothiazine treatment in acute schizophrenia. *Arch Gen Psychiatry* 10:246–261, 1964

Multisite collaborative psychopharmacology studies are now common-place in psychopharmacology research. Among the earliest were the multisite collaborative studies of neuroleptics in acute schizophrenia under the direction of Jonathan O. Cole at the National Institute of Mental Health. This article illustrates an early model of a collaborative study and serves as a forerunner of contemporary collaborative psychopharmacology studies. The data presented on the therapeutic efficacy of these drugs in acute schizophrenia are still applicable today.

11. **Creese I, Burt DR, Snyder SH:** Dopamine receptor binding predicts clinical and pharmacologic potencies of antischizophrenic drugs. *Science* 192:481–483, 1976

The effect of neuroleptics on central nervous system dopamine func-tion has led to the dopamine hypothesis of schizophrenia. This article is one of the basic and most-often quoted pharmacologic studies of differential dopamine binding of neuroleptic drugs.

12. **Davis JM:** Overview: maintenance therapy in psychiatry, I: schizophre-nia. *Am J Psychiatry* 132:1237–1245, 1975

This article was one of the first and still best examples of "meta-analy-sis," the statistical technique of combining the results of many studies to draw an overall conclusion. The data clearly demonstrate over 90% relapse rate when neuroleptic drugs are discontinued over a 12-month period.

13. **Delay J, Deniker P, Harl J:** Utilization therapeutique psychiatrique d'une phenothiazine d'action centrale elective (4560 RP). *Ann Med Psychol (Paris)* 110:112–117, 1952

The first observation that the class of compounds now known as neuro-leptics had therapeutic efficacy in schizophrenia and other psychotic states that was independent of central nervous system sedation was made by these French workers. This article includes a marvelous de-scription of the "neuroleptic triad" of behavioral quieting, affective blunting, and cognitive tightening that remains the hallmark of these drugs' effect.

14. **Donlon PT, Tupin JP:** Rapid "digitalization" of decompensated schizo-phrenic patients with antipsychotic agents. *Am J Psychiatry* 132:1023–1026, 1975

In the 1970s, several groups of researchers studied the effects of high-dose rapid treatment for acute schizophrenia. Rapid neuroleptization became extremely popular until it was realized that the long-term effects were not superior to slower treatment using more modest doses;

extrapyramidal and cardiovascular side effects were also more frequent and serious. This article describes one such treatment strategy.

15. **May PRA, Tuma AH, Yale C, Potepan P, Dixon WJ:** Schizophrenia—a follow-up study of results of treatment, II: hospital stay over two to five years. *Arch Gen Psychiatry* 33:481–486, 1976

May et al. performed a pioneering comparative study of pharmacologic and other treatments of schizophrenia in hospitalized patients. This article is one of many that culminated in a book clearly indicating the necessity for neuroleptic treatment for seriously ill schizophrenic patients. The study also indicated that reducing periods of acute psychosis may result in a better long-term prognosis.

16. **Salzman C:** The use of ECT in the treatment of schizophrenia. *Am J Psychiatry* 137:1032–1041, 1980

In the 1940s and 1950s, electroconvulsive therapy (ECT) was widely used to treat schizophrenia. This article reviews all research as well as clinical reports on the effect of ECT in schizophrenia, concluding that this treatment, at best, produces only a transitory therapeutic effect.

Schizophrenia: Contemporary Treatment

17. **Baldessarini RJ, Cohen BM, Teicher MH:** Significance of neuroleptic dose and plasma level in the pharmacological treatment of psychoses. *Arch Gen Psychiatry* 45:79–91, 1988

Dose and blood levels of neuroleptics have always been an uncertain matter clinically. Both high doses and low doses have been suggested, and a variety of studies have produced contradictory data regarding correlation of blood levels with therapeutic and toxic effects. This article is a superb review of these subjects.

18. **Herz MI, Szymanski HV, Simon JC:** Intermittent medication for stable schizophrenic outpatients. *Am J Psychiatry* 139:918–922, 1982

As an alternative to high-dose neuroleptic treatment strategies for acute schizophrenia, several investigators have been focusing on the use of low-dose treatment strategies for maintenance of chronic schizophrenic outpatients. This article represents one of the low-dose treatment strategies, the restriction of neuroleptic treatment to intermittent periods of psychosis. After recompensation, the patient is gradually weaned from the neuroleptic and then followed in a neuroleptic-free state. When early-warning signs of psychosis reappear (e.g., anxiety, change in sleep pattern), then neuroleptics are restarted.

19. **Kane J, Honigfeld G, Singer J, Meltzer H:** Clozapine for the treatment resistant schizophrenic: a double-blind comparison with chlorpromazine. *Arch Gen Psychiatry* 45:789–796, 1988

The most recent collaborative psychopharmacologic study in schizophrenia has been the multisite study of clozapine. This article is both a model of outstanding careful collaborative research, as well as the seminal article on the antipsychotic efficacy of clozapine.

20. **Rosebush PI, Hildebrand AM, Furlong BG, Mazurek MF:** Catatonic syndrome in a general psychiatric inpatient population: frequency, clinical presentation, and response to lorazepam. *J Clin Psychiatry* 51:357–362, 1990

Catatonia is a striking syndrome that is still searching for a place in psychiatric classification, for a pathogenesis, and for a specific treatment. Over the past two decades, it has been considered a subform of schizophrenia; treatments have included standard neuroleptics and electroconvulsive therapy. This article illustrates that catatonia is more properly considered a syndrome than a disease and that treatment with parenteral lorazepam produces a dramatic response within 1–3 hours. This treatment approach should now be considered for rapid resolution of this potentially lethal syndrome.

21. **Salzman C, Solomon D, Miyawaki E, Glassman R, Rood L, Flowers E, Thayer S:** Parenteral lorazepam vs parenteral haloperidol for the control of psychotic disruptive behavior. *J Clin Psychiatry* 52:177–180, 1991

Several anecdotal publications have suggested the usefulness of using parenteral benzodiazepines as adjunctive therapy for behavioral control in psychotic disruptive states. This is a prospective double-blind study that followed up on earlier retrospective data, both reporting the usefulness of combined therapy. Combining neuroleptics and benzodiazepines for the control of severe agitation and disruptive behavior has now become standard treatment.

22. **Siris SG, Morgan V, Fagerstrom R, Rifkin A, Cooper TB:** Adjunctive imipramine in the treatment of post-psychotic depression: a controlled trial. *Arch Gen Psychiatry* 42:533–539, 1987

Depression following resolution of an acute psychotic state is very frequent and often debilitating. This group has done much of the work in antidepressant treatment of postpsychotic depression and has reported on the positive therapeutic benefits of such treatment.

Schizophrenia: Side Effects

23. **American Psychiatric Association:** *American Psychiatric Association Task Force Report No. 18: Tardive Dyskinesia.* Washington, DC, American Psychiatric Association, 1980

Although somewhat out of date, this very thoughtful and comprehensive review of tardive dyskinesia is am important reference for all psychiatrists. It is a superb and comprehensive review of the clinical manifestations of this disorder, the presumed etiology and pathogenesis, prevalence, and treatment. The thoughtful conclusions are drawn by outstanding clinicians and researchers; the bibliography is comprehensive.

24. **Cohen WJ, Cohen NH:** Lithium carbonate, haloperidol, and irreversible brain damage. *JAMA* 230:1283–1287, 1974

For nearly 30 years, clinicians have been concerned about potential neurotoxicity when combining neuroleptics with lithium. This article is the initial report of serious irreversible neurologic damage that was linked to the combination of drugs.

25. **Levenson J:** Neuroleptic malignant syndrome. *Am J Psychiatry* 142:1137–1145, 1985

It is essential for all psychiatrists to understand the diagnosis and treatment of neuroleptic malignant syndrome thoroughly. Many excellent articles on this syndrome have been published; this is one of the best.

26. **Lipinski JF Jr, Zubenko GS, Cohen BM, Bareira PJ:** Propranolol in the treatment of neuroleptic-induced akathisia. *Am J Psychiatry* 141:412–415, 1984

Traditionally, neuroleptic-induced extrapyramidal symptoms have been treated with anticholinergic substances. These drugs are only moderately effective for akathisia, however, and also produce considerable toxicity. This article suggests the usefulness of propranolol to relieve this side effect.

27. **Rifkin A, Quitkin F, Klein DF:** Akinesia: a poorly recognized drug induced extrapyramidal behavior disorder. *Arch Gen Psychiatry* 32:672–674, 1975

Akinesia, one of the extrapyramidal symptoms, may be confused with depression and may also contribute to poor drug compliance. This is the first, and still the clearest, review of the topic.

28. **Van Putten T, Mutalipassi LR, Malkin MO:** Phenothiazine-induced decompensation. *Arch Gen Psychiatry* 30:102–105, 1974

   Van Putten has been one of the leaders in pointing out that neuroleptic side effects, particularly akathisia, may interfere with the therapeutic effect of medication. This is one of the earliest, and still best, reviews.

29. **Van Putten T, Marder SR, Mintz J, Poland RE:** Haloperidol plasma levels and clinical response: a therapeutic window relationship. *Am J Psychiatry* 149:500–505, 1992

   Pharmacokinetic studies of neuroleptics have been relatively few in number compared with kinetic studies of tricyclic antidepressants and benzodiazepines. The correlation between blood level and therapeutic response of most neuroleptics has been inconclusive. There appears to be a curvilinear relationship for haloperidol. This carefully controlled study suggests that the optimal therapeutic response to haloperidol in newly admitted schizophrenic men is in the range of 5–12 ng/ml.

Depression: Historical

30. **Charney DS, Menkes DB, Heninger GR:** Receptor sensitivity and the mechanism of action of antidepressant treatment. *Arch Gen Psychiatry* 38:1160–1180, 1981

   Since the advent of the catecholamine hypothesis of affective disorder, researchers have focused on the effect of antidepressant drugs on monoamine neurotransmission and their receptors. This article is one of the more comprehensive and lucid reviews of these relationships.

31. **Kuhn R:** The treatment of depressive states with G22355 (imipramine hydrochloride). *Am J Psychiatry* 115:459–464, 1958

   This is the original report on the therapeutic effectiveness of imipramine. Contemporary readers will be startled at the extraordinary clinical acumen of the author. He describes the therapeutic efficacy of imipramine as well as or better than authors of more complicated studies 30 years later.

32. **Greenblatt M, Grosser GH, Wechsler H:** Differential response of hospitalized depressed patients to somatic therapy. *Am J Psychiatry* 120:935–943, 1964

   Most clinicians would agree that electroconvulsive therapy (ECT) remains the most rapid and most effective treatment for the most severely ill depressed patients. It is noteworthy, however, that there have been no recent comparative controlled studies of ECT and other antidepressants. This is the best comparative article, dating back to 1964, comparing ECT, imipramine, phenelzine, and placebo, in patients with major depressive disorder, clearly indicating the superior efficacy with ECT.

33. **Prange AJ Jr, Wilson IC, Rabon AM, Lipton MA:** Enhancement of imipramine antidepressant activity by thyroid hormone. *Am J Psychiatry* 126:457–469, 1969

Among the augmenting strategies used for enhancement of partial antidepressant therapeutic response has been the addition of thyroid hormone. Much of the work on thyroid hormone comes from this group of workers.

Depression: Contemporary Treatment

34. **Akiskal HS:** Toward a definition of dysthymia: boundaries with personality and mood disorders, in *Dysthymic Disorder.* Edited by Burton SW, Akiskal HS. London, Gaskell, 1990, pp. 1–12

Akiskal has led the field in proposing that depressions that were previously considered characterologic were actually a variant of affective disorder. His work has defined the relationship between these depressions, personality disorder, the current definitions of dysthymia, and certain forms of bipolar disorder. His work also encourages the use of psychotropic drugs to treat these patients, many of whom suffer considerably for extended periods of their lives.

35. **Baldessarini RJ:** Current status of antidepressants: clinical pharmacology and therapy. *J Clin Psychiatry* 50:117–126, 1989

Numerous articles have reviewed the pharmacology and therapeutic effects of antidepressants. This author has been long known for his scholarly and thoughtful pharmacologic reviews.

36. **De Montigny C, Cournoyer G, Morissette R, Langlois R, Caillie G:** Lithium carbonate addition to tricyclic antidepressant-resistant unipolar depression. *Arch Gen Psychiatry* 40:1327–1334, 1983

Current clinical practice suggests the addition of lithium carbonate to antidepressants in patients who have only a partial therapeutic response. This suggestion is derived from early work by this group, as illustrated in this article.

37. **Elkin I, Shay T, Watkins JT, Imber SD, Collins JF, Glass DR, Pilkonis PA, Leber WR, Docherty JP:** National Institute of Mental Health Treat-

ment of Depression Collaborative Research Program. *Arch Gen Psychiatry* 46:971–982, 1989

Should major depression be treated with antidepressants alone, with psychotherapy alone, or with some combination? An extremely carefully planned and well-executed study of the use of antidepressants and psychotherapy in the treatment of schizophrenia was sponsored by the National Institute of Mental Health. This report of the study, one of many, illustrates the extraordinary complexity of these seemingly simple questions. The study concludes that both psychotherapy and pharmacotherapy are useful for the treatment of depression, but that each has its own unique role in the overall treatment program. In the treatment phase, no significant differences were found between either of two forms of psychotherapy and imipramine plus standard clinical management, although imipramine had more rapid effect. Imipramine also seemed better for more severely ill patients.

38. **Glassman AH, Kantor SJ, Shostak M:** Depression, delusion, and drug response. *Am J Psychiatry* 132:716–719, 1975

Delusionally depressed patients (psychotic depression) often do not respond to traditional monotherapy with chemical antidepressants. These authors' results as well as subsequent data led to the current clinical practice of combining antidepressants and neuroleptics for the treatment of delusional depression as an alternative to electroconvulsive therapy.

39. **Glassman AH, Perel JM, Shostak M, Kantor SJ, Fleiss JL:** Clinical implications of imipramine plasma levels for depressive illness. *Arch Gen Psychiatry* 34:197–204, 1977

Measurement of plasma levels of antidepressants has become commonplace in contemporary psychiatry. This article describes the classic sigmoidal curve relationship between therapeutic response to imipramine.

40. **Keller MB, Lavori PW, Endicott J, Coryell W, Klerman GL:** Double depression: two-year follow-up. *Am J Psychiatry* 140:689–694, 1983

Many patients who suffer from major depression and who respond well to antidepressant treatment still have residual feelings of discontent, low self-esteem, and high self-criticism. This article introduced the term *double depression* to describe patients who suffered both a lifelong chronic state of dysphoria and who also developed a superimposed major depressive disorder.

41. **Kupfer DJ, Frank E, Perel JM, Cornes C, Mallinger AG, Thase ME, McEachran AB, Grochocinski VJ:** Five-year outcome for maintenance therapies in recurrent depression. *Arch Gen Psychiatry* 49:769–773, 1992

This article reports an extraordinary longitudinal study of the pharmacologic and psychotherapeutic treatment of major depression. After
5 years, a highly significant prophylactic effect for active imipramine
maintained at an average dose of 200 mg was demonstrated. These data
strongly support the necessity for ongoing pharmacologic maintenance
in patients who have had recurrent major depression.

42. **Liebowitz MR, Quitkin FM, Stewart JW, McGrath PJ, Harrison WM,
Markowitz JS, Rabkin JG, Tricamo E, Goetz DM, Klein DF:** Antidepressant
specificity in atypical depression. *Arch Gen Psychiatry* 45:129–137, 1988

There is a recently emerging recognition that one form of serious
depressive illness may be atypical in its symptom pattern and response
to antidepressants. This is one of the earliest and best articles to date on
the treatment of atypical depression.

43. **Prien RF, Kupfer DJ, Mansky PA, Small JG, Tuason VB, Voss CB,
Johnson WE:** Drug therapy in the prevention of recurrences in unipolar
and bipolar affective disorders: report of the NIMH Collaborative Study
Group Comparing Lithium Carbonate, Imipramine, and a Lithium Carbonate Imipramine Combination. *Arch Gen Psychiatry* 41:1096–1104, 1984

This study was a classic demonstration of the prophylactic efficacy of
pharmacologic treatment in affective disorders. With bipolar patients,
lithium carbonate alone or in combination with imipramine was the
best prophylactic treatment for bipolar patients, but imipramine alone
was as effective as lithium or the combination in unipolar patients.
Thus, "lithium carbonate is an effective treatment for acute mania and
is also effective in preventing or dampening manic recurrences. Imipramine is not an effective treatment for acute mania or for preventing
its recurrence, but is a standard treatment for acute unipolar depression and is also an effective preventive treatment for recurrent unipolar
depression" (p. 104).

44. **Quitkin F, Rabkin A, Klein DF:** Monoamine oxidase inhibitors. *Arch Gen
Psychiatry* 36:749–760, 1979

Although monoamine oxidase inhibitors have been in use for more
than 30 years, and their pharmacology is reasonably well understood,
careful clinical guidelines still need to be developed. This article comes
from one of the American research groups that has most studied this
class of antidepressants.

45. **Quitkin FM, Rabkin JG, Ross D, McGrath PJ:** Duration of antidepressant drug treatment: what is an adequate trial? *Arch Gen Psychiatry*
41:238–245, 1984

It has become standard practice to assume that tricyclic antidepressant therapeutic effect may take 4–6 weeks to develop. This article carefully demonstrates that even longer periods of treatment may be associated with improved outcome and makes the point that many depressed patients may continue to be undermedicated or wrongly discontinued from treatment before therapeutic efficacy can be adequately established.

46. **Rosenthal NE, Sack DA, Carpenter CJ, Parry BL, Mendelson WB, Wehr TA:** Antidepressant effects of light in seasonal affective disorder. *Am J Psychiatry* 142:163–170, 1985

Seasonal affective disorder has emerged as a verifiable syndrome that, in some cases, responds to light therapy. This report from a group from the National Institute of Mental Health reports on some of the pioneering work using bright light treatment.

47. **Sackheim HA, Prudic J, Devanand DP, Kiersky JE, Fitzsimons L, Moody DJ, McElhiney MC, Colman EA, Settembrino JM:** Effects of stimulus intensity and electrode placement on the efficacy and cognitive effects of electroconvulsive therapy. *N Engl J Med* 328:839–846, 1993

Controlled studies of electroconvulsive therapy (ECT) have not been frequently reported for almost 20 years. This group is one of the leaders of a new generation of ECT researchers, and this article demonstrates the high quality of their work. It is now possible to draw meaningful conclusions regarding the therapeutic and toxic effects of increasing electrical dosage, as well as placement of the electrodes themselves. The article also provides a more up-to-date ECT bibliography than is usually available.

48. **Spiker DG, Perel JM, Hanin I, Dealy RS, Griffin SJ, Soloff PH, Weiss JC:** The pharmacological treatment of delusional depression: part II. *J Clin Psychopharmacol* 6:339–342, 1986

This article reports the first clear therapeutic efficacy in delusional depressed patients of combining neuroleptics with tricyclic antidepressants. It is clear that for these patients the combined drug program is superior to either drug individually for these patients, and these findings have led to the acceptance of dual pharmacologic treatment for delusional depressed patients.

49. **Teicher MH, Glod C, Cole JO:** Emergence of intense suicidal preoccupation during fluoxetine treatment. *Am J Psychiatry* 147:207–210, 1990

All psychiatrists are aware of the recently emerging controversy regarding the effect of fluoxetine in producing and increasing suicidal or aggressive behavior. Much of the focus of this controversy began with the publication of this article, which describes increased intense suicidality in six psychiatric inpatients who received fluoxetine.

Treatment of Mania

50. **Ballenger JC, Post RM:** Carbamazepine in manic-depressive illness: a new treatment. *Am J Psychiatry* 137:782–790, 1980

Following these authors' hypothesis that cycling mood disorder may be analogous to a neurophysiologic state of kindling, anticonvulsant drugs that inhibit kindling were introduced as a possible treatment for mania and bipolar disorder. Since the publication of this article, anticonvulsant drugs have become accepted as second-line treatments or adjunctive treatments for this disorder.

51. **Carlson GA, Goodwyn FK:** The stages of mania: a longitudinal analysis of the manic episode. *Arch Gen Psychiatry* 28:221–228, 1973

This classic article defines mania in three stages: 1) hypomanic; 2) classic mania (extremely labile, suspicious, disoriented, and very angry; and 3) psychotic. Such a description is clinically useful and also helps the clinician to gauge the course of treatment.

52. **Chouinard G:** Antimanic effects of clonazepam. *Psychosomatics* 26 (suppl):7–11, 1985

It is controversial whether benzodiazepines are effective in treating mania. Clonazepam, however, has been used with increasing frequency as a treatment for control of acute manic disruptive behavior. This article, one of the earliest reports of the clonazepam antimanic effect, illustrates the usefulness as well as potential methodological difficulties in interpreting the data presented in this article, suggesting the need for a careful prospective double-blind, placebo-controlled study.

53. **Gelenberg AJ, Kane JM, Keller MB, Lavori P, Rosenbaum JF, Cole K, Lavelle J:** Comparison of standard and low serum levels of lithium for maintenance treatment of bipolar disorder. *N Engl J Med* 321:1489–1493, 1989

Since the introduction of lithium as a treatment and prophylactic agent for mania and bipolar disorder, there has been clinical controversy regarding appropriate therapeutic and maintenance plasma levels. This article demonstrates the importance of adequate serum levels of lithium for maintenance treatment (at least 0.8 mEq/L) as opposed to the lower levels that had been advocated in earlier years.

54. **Himmelhoch JM, Forest J, Neil JF, Detre TP:** Thiazide-lithium synergy in refractory mood swings. *Am J Psychiatry* 134:149–152, 1977

Not all bipolar patients are responsive to lithium, and many strategies have been employed to improve therapeutic response. One of the earliest and still most effective is the combination of lithium with thiazide diuretics.

55. **Himmelhoch JM, Thase ME, Mallinger AG, Houck P:** Tranylcypromine versus imipramine in anergic bipolar depression. *Am J Psychiatry* 148:910–916, 1991

In a series of studies, this group of researchers has demonstrated that the monoamine oxidase inhibitor tranylcypromine is superior to imipramine in the treatment of the anergic depression associated with bipolar disorder. Although not placebo controlled, the data favoring tranylcypromine are striking. The authors also point to the clinical similarity of this type of depression, and atypical depression; both respond to monoamine oxidase inhibitors.

56. **Janowsky DS, Leff M, Epstein RS:** Playing the manic game: interpersonal maneuvers of the acutely manic patient. *Arch Gen Psychiatry* 22:252–261, 1970

This classic article marvelously describes the clinical behavior of a manic patient on an inpatient unit. The description still serves clinicians today. Understanding the interpersonal maneuvers can help a psychopharmacologist more effectively approach a manic patient and form a therapeutic alliance.

57. **Kocsis JH, Sutton BM, Frances AJ:** Long-term follow-up of chronic depression treated with imipramine. *J Clin Psychiatry* 52:56–59, 1991

This study illustrates the importance of maintaining patients on medication to which they responded. The data suggest clearly that ongoing imipramine treatment, or maintenance therapy in general, may be indicated and effective for chronically depressed patients.

58. **Pope HG, McElroy SL, Keck PE Jr, Hudson JI:** Valproate in the treatment of acute mania: a placebo-controlled study. *Arch Gen Psychiatry* 48:62–68, 1991

Following carbamazepine, valproate was introduced as part of the treatment program for bipolar disorders and was rapidly accepted into clinical practice. This well-designed, placebo-controlled study clearly demonstrates substantial antimanic effects of therapeutic serum valproate concentrations and the lack of serious or common side effects at these levels.

59. **Prien RF, Kupfer DJ, Mansky PA, Small JG, Tuason VB, Voss CB, Johnson WE:** Drug therapy in the prevention of recurrences in unipolar and bipolar affective disorders. *Arch Gen Psychiatry* 41:1096–1104, 1984

Because of the recurring nature of affective disorders, considerable research efforts have been directed toward studying the prevention of such recurrence. Some of the most exciting and clinically relevant work has come from this group, emphasizing the use of lithium for bipolar patients and antidepressants and/or lithium for unipolar patients to prevent recurrences.

60. **Suppes T, Baldessarini RJ, Faedda GL, Tohen M:** Risk of recurrence following discontinuation of lithium treatment in bipolar disorder. *Arch Gen Psychiatry* 48:1082–1088, 1991

This article is the first and still one of the best raising alarm about the consequences of discontinuing lithium from a bipolar patient who has been successfully maintained on lithium. Risk of early recurrence of bipolar illness, especially of mania, is increased following discontinuation of lithium despite years of prior stabilization. These findings strongly indicate the need for bipolar patients to remain on lithium maintenance treatment even after years of stability. What is most alarming about these findings, however, is that when these patients are placed back on lithium, they do not seem to achieve the same level of stability that they had prior to discontinuation.

61. **Wehr TA, Goodwin FK:** Can antidepressants cause mania and worsen the course of affective illness? *Am J Psychiatry* 144:1403–1411, 1987

Although antidepressants are commonly used in the treatment and prophylaxis of bipolar mood disorder patients, some questions have been raised regarding the possible deleterious effects of antidepressants on the course of bipolar illness. Although still controversial, the possibility that antidepressants may worsen the life course of these patients is most serious.

62. **Wehr TA, Sack DA, Rosenthal NE, Cowdry RW:** Rapid cycling affective disorder: contributing factors and treatment responses in 51 patients. *Am J Psychiatry* 145:179–184, 1988

Although bipolar disorders in general tend to respond well to standard treatments, patients whose episodes come more frequently, known as rapid-cycling patients, tend to have a much poorer response. Many strategies have been employed to improve the treatment response in these patients as illustrated in this article.

Anxiety Disorders

63. **Greenblatt DJ, Shader RI, Abernethy DR:** Current status of benzo-diazepines, part 1. *N Engl J Med* 309:354–359, 1983; **Greenblatt DJ, Shader RI, Abernethy DR:** Current status of benzodiazepines, part 2. *N Engl J Med* 309:410–415, 1983

These two articles, although a decade old, still represent the most concise and lucid information on the pharmacology and therapeutic uses of benzodiazepines.

64. **Klein DF, Fink M:** Delineation of two drug-responsive anxiety syndromes. *Psychopharmacologia* 5:397–408, 1964

This is one of the original and most insightful of the author's articles identifying panic disorder as a discrete syndrome with distinct drug response.

65. **Salzman C, Shader RI, Greenblatt DJ, Harmatz JS:** Long versus short half-life benzodiazepines in the elderly: kinetics and clinical effects of diazepam and oxazepam. *Arch Gen Psychiatry* 40:293–297, 1983

Clinical relevance of benzodiazepine half-lives is especially important in the elderly. This double-blind study demonstrates the prolongation of half-life by age in some benzodiazepines and the lack of effect of age in others; clinical suggestions are offered based on these differences.

66. **Salzman C, Shader RI, Greenblatt DJ, Harmatz JS:** *Benzodiazepine Dependence, Toxicity, and Abuse: A Task Force Report of the American Psychiatric Association.* Washington, DC, American Psychiatric Press, 1990

This report, edited by Salzman with contributions from the world's leading experts on benzodiazepines, is essential reading for all clinicians. The reference list of more than 800 articles is comprehensive.

Panic Disorder and Agoraphobia

67. **Ballenger JC, Burrows GD, DuPont RL Jr, Lesser IM, Noyes R Jr, Pecknold JC, Rifkin A, Swinson RP:** Alprazolam in panic disorder and agoraphobia: results from a multicenter trial, I: efficacy in short-term treatment. *Arch Gen Psychiatry* 45:413–422, 1988

The efficacy of alprazolam in treating panic disorder was demonstrated through a large worldwide multisite collaborative center. This is the first of three articles describing the therapeutic effects, side effects, and consequences of drug discontinuation from this study.

68. Fyer AJ, Liebowitz MR, Gorman JM, Campeas R, Levin A, Sandberg D, Fyer M, Hollander E, Papp L, Goetz D, Klein D: Discontinuation of alprazolam treatment in panic patients. *Am J Psychiatry* 144:303–308, 1987

Questions have been raised whether it is more difficult to discontinue patients from alprazolam than other benzodiazepines with a short half-life or other high-potency benzodiazepines. This study demonstrates some of the difficulties associated with alprazolam discontinuation.

69. Herman JB, Rosenbaum JF, Brotman AW: The alprazolam to clonazepam switch for the treatment of panic disorder. *J Clin Psychopharmacol* 7:175–178, 1987

Some patients who were treated for their panic disorder with alprazolam experienced interdose rebound symptoms or have difficulty with discontinuation. One strategy for this problem has been to switch to a long half-life, high-potency benzodiazepine clonazepam, and this has been utilized with considerable success.

70. Liebowitz MR: Antidepressants in panic disorders. *Br J Psychiatry* 155 (suppl 6):46–52, 1989

Antidepressants were the first drugs demonstrated to be effective in panic disorder (tricyclics), and currently most antidepressants have been shown to be therapeutically effective. Some authors believe that antidepressants still should be used as the first-choice treatment for panic disorder. This is an excellent overview of the therapeutic efficacy of antidepressants in panic disorder.

71. Rosenbaum JF (ed): New uses of clonazepam in psychiatry. *J Clin Psychiatry* 48:3S–56S, 1987

Clonazepam, a high-potency antidepressant like alprazolam only with a long half-life, also has demonstrated efficacy in the treatment of panic disorder. Some authors believe it to be superior because it lacks interdose rebound, although others note its high level of sedation at therapeutic doses.

72. Schweizer E, Rickels K, Weiss S, Zavodnick S: Maintenance drug treatment of panic disorder, I: results of a prospective, placebo-controlled comparison of alprazolam and imipramine. *Arch Gen Psychiatry* 50:61–68, 1993

There are many current clinical opinions, sometimes passionate, about the risks versus benefits of different pharmacologic approaches for the treatment of panic disorder. This prospective, placebo-controlled study demonstrates that alprazolam was superior to imipramine in the acute treatment of panic disorder. In the maintenance phase, both treatments were effective, but imipramine was less well accepted by the patients. It is important to have data like these in addition to clinical and anecdotal experience; concern over adverse drug effects is legitimate and certainly appropriate, but must be balanced with carefully obtained research data.

Personality Disorder

73. **Cowdry R, Gardner D:** Pharmacotherapy of borderline personality disorder: alprazolam, carbamazepine, trifluoperazine and tranylcypromine. *Arch Gen Psychiatry* 45:111–119, 1988

Borderline personality disorder has been treated with a variety of psychotropic drugs with mixed successes. This article is an excellent review of a number of these treatments.

74. **Markovitz PJ, Calabrese JR, Schulz SC, Meltzer HY:** Fluoxetine in the treatment of borderline and schizotypal personality disorders. *Am J Psychiatry* 148:1064–1067, 1991

Recent unpublished research has suggested that selective serotonin reuptake inhibitors are useful in the treatment of borderline personality disorder. This article is one of the earliest and best of the published nondouble-blind studies illustrating the efficacy of fluoxetine in borderline patients. A particular value of the study was its 12-week treatment phase, which is necessary when studying fluoxetine.

75. **Rifkin A, Quitkin F, Carrillo C, Blumberger AG, Klein DF:** Lithium carbonate in emotionally unstable character disorder. *Arch Gen Psychiatry* 28:519–523, 1972

One of the earliest approaches to patients now called borderline was to subtype them and treat different subtypes with different classes of psychotropic drugs. Among the more prominent of the subtypes was the so-called emotionally unstable character disorder. This early pioneering work has led to some of the more recent attempts to use psychotropic drugs to treat this difficult class of patients.

76. **Sheard MH, Marini JL, Bridges CI, Wagner E:** The effect of lithium on impulsive aggressive behavior in man. *Am J Psychiatry* 133:1409–1413, 1976

Control of aggressive and dangerous violent behavior is exceedingly difficult unless one heavily sedates the patient. Searches for nonsedating drugs that are reliably effective have explored many different classes of compounds. Among the more successful have been lithium and other mood stabilizers, as indicated in this early pioneering study.

Eating Disorders

77. **Walsh BT, Hadigan CM, Devlin MJ, Gladis M, Roose SP:** Long-term outcome of antidepressant treatment for bulimia nervosa. *Am J Psychiatry* 148:1206–1212, 1991

Antidepressants of all kinds are effective in treating the binges and purges associated with bulimia syndromes. This study convincingly demonstrates the superiority of desipramine over placebo in the short-term treatment of bulimia nervosa. The study illustrates, however, the problems using an antidepressant as the only treatment for this disorder. Bingeing continues, albeit at a reduced frequency, even while on treatment, and relapse rates are extraordinarily high. Associated psychotherapy is strongly suggested.

Obsessive-Compulsive Disorders

78. **Goodman WK, McDougle CJ, Price LH:** Pharmacotherapy of obsessive compulsive disorder. *J Clin Psychiatry* 53 (suppl):29–37, 1992

This is an outstanding review of the current pharmacologic strategies for treating obsessive-compulsive disorder. The article goes beyond current treatments, however, and proposes an algorithm for those patients with obsessive-compulsive disorder who fail to respond to an adequate trial with standard medications. Pharmacologic augmentation with standard drugs such as lithium and buspirone and more experimental approaches are reviewed as well.

79. **Rapoport JL:** Recent advances in obsessive-compulsive disorder. *Neuropsychopharmacology* 5:1–10, 1991

Among the more dramatic advances in psychopharmacology has been the treatment of obsessive-compulsive disorder with serotonergic drugs. Although the overall therapeutic effect is modest, the use of these drugs has improved life for many patients and opened new directions for research, as demonstrated by pioneering by this author.

Pregnancy

80. **Cohen LS, Heller VL, Rosenbaum JF:** Psychotropic drug use in pregnancy: an update, in *Medical Psychiatric Practice*, Vol. 1. Edited by Stoudemire A, Fogel BS. Washington, DC, American Psychiatric Press, 1991, pp. 615–634

These authors are leaders in gathering and disseminating information regarding the effect of psychotropic drugs in pregnancy, at the time of delivery, and during nursing. This chapter is an update of many of their previous publications and is a clearly written and accessible review of the subject. The bibliography is comprehensive. This chapter is an excellent first reference on the topic of psychotropic drugs in pregnancy; it also provides a starting point for a more exhaustive literature review.

Use of Psychotropic Drugs for Medically Ill

81. **Cummings JL:** Depression in Parkinson's disease: a review. *Am J Psychiatry* 149:443–454, 1992

The relationship between Parkinson's disease and depression has been well known. This excellent review article summarizes studies of pharmacotherapeutic efficacy as part of an overall review of the association. The author points out that most studies indicate that depression in Parkinson's disease is undertreated. He notes, however, that well-controlled studies are lacking. Electroconvulsive therapy has also been reported to be effective, but well-controlled studies of this treatment are also lacking.

82. **Lipsey JR, Robinson RG, Parlson GD, Rao K, Price TR:** Nortriptyline treatment for post-stroke depression: a double-blind study. *Lancet* 1:297–300, 1984

Robinson and co-workers have been the leaders in studying the effect of stroke on affective functioning and the treatment of poststroke depression. This article is an early and convincing demonstration that antidepressants are safe and therapeutic for treating poststroke depressions and that suffering from depression is not an inevitable consequence of having had a stroke.

83. **Stoudemire A, Fogel BS, Gulley LR:** Psychopharmacology in the medically ill: an update, in *Medical Psychiatric Practice*, Vol. 1. Edited by Stoudemire A, Fogel BS. Washington, DC, American Psychiatric Press, 1991, pp. 29–97

This chapter, part of an outstanding volume on the interface between medical illness and psychiatric syndromes, is a clearly presented review of the use of psychotropic drugs in patients with serious medical illness. The chapter is organized according to drug class and use rather than by specific disorder, although specific disorders (e.g., renal transplantation, diabetes, epilepsy, pulmonary disease, cardiovascular illness, Parkinson's disease) are considered. The information is up-to-date and clinically practical; the bibliography is extensive and extremely useful. For readers who are interested in the use of psychotropic drugs in medically ill patients, this is an excellent starting point for a literature review.

Posttraumatic Stress Disorder

84. **Frank JB, Kosten TR, Giller EL, Dan E:** A randomized clinical trial of phenelzine and imipramine for PTSD. *Am J Psychiatry* 145:1289–1291, 1988

Although posttraumatic stress disorder has been increasingly recognized as an important psychiatric syndrome, studies about the psychopharmacologic treatment of its various symptoms have been relatively sparse. Most studies are either uncontrolled, have small numbers of subjects, or have poorly defined inclusion or outcome criteria. Sifting through the various studies, it is apparent that various antidepressants may have some usefulness in treating some but not all of the symptoms of this disorder and probably are the first choice. This article is a well-controlled study comparing two of the common antidepressants that are used for this syndrome.

Psychotherapy and Psychopharmacology

85. **Gutheil TG:** The psychology of psychopharmacology, in *Psychotherapy and Medication: A Dynamic Integration.* Edited by Schachter M. North Vale, NJ, Jason Aronson, 1993, pp. 3–10

Gutheil is well known for his writings on the psychodynamic aspects of psychotropic drug prescribing. This brilliant chapter lucidly and humorously captures many of the important psychological issues that attend the psychotropic drug-treatment process. Although brief, it is illustrated with helpful clinical vignettes, and the bibliography points the reader to seminal articles in this field.

86. **Salzman C, Bemporad J:** Combined psychotherapeutic and psycho-
    pharmacologic treatment of depressed patients: clinical observations,
    in *Combination Psychiatry and Psychotherapy in Depression.* Edited by Man-
    ning DW, Francis AJ. Washington, DC, American Psychiatric Press,
    1990, pp. 152–181

    This chapter details the process, benefits, and problems of combining
    analytically oriented psychotherapy with pharmacotherapy for the
    treatment of major depressive disorders. The authors stress the positive
    interaction and make specific suggestions for some of the problems
    that arise, especially when psychotherapy and pharmacotherapy are
    administered by separate clinicians.

87. **Sotsky SM, Glass DR, Shea T, Pilkonis PA, Collins JF, Elkin I, Watkins
    JT, Imber SD, Leber WR, Moyer J, Oliveri ME:** Patient predictors of
    response to psychotherapy and pharmacotherapy: findings in the
    NIMH treatment of depression collaborative research program. *Am J
    Psychiatry* 148:997–1008, 1991

    This pioneering study of various forms of psychotherapy, as well as
    pharmacotherapy for major depressive disorder, has had far-reaching
    implications for the treatment of depression. This particular article,
    one of many, demonstrates differential patient profiles as predictors to
    various forms of treatment. Response to nonpharmacologic treatments
    was predicted best by low social and cognitive dysfunction, whereas
    high work dysfunction and high depression severity predicted superior
    response to imipramine as well as to interpersonal psychotherapy. As
    important as the specific findings are the general findings confirming
    the efficacy of pharmacotherapy for major depression, but also con-
    firming the common clinical observation that psychotherapy (in its
    various forms) is efficacious and should be an essential part of contem-
    porary treatment of major depressive disorder.

37

Electroconvulsive Therapy and Psychosurgery

John C. Markowitz, M.D.
James H. Kocsis, M.D.

Electroconvulsive therapy (ECT), one of the few psychiatric treatment procedures, is a somatic treatment with a long and checkered history. ECT remains among the most effective of psychiatric treatments and the treatment of choice for certain disorders, such as major depression with psychotic features. Yet it has long been underused as the result of irrational public fears and reaction against an electrified, seizure-inducing treatment that is frequently depicted as a barbarism or form of torture in the entertainment media.

Once nearly eclipsed by psychopharmacology, ECT has experienced a renewal in recent years. The limited efficacy and adverse effects of psychotropic medications have become more apparent, whereas ECT is now delivered with increasing sophistication and in new treatment settings (e.g., as a maintenance outpatient therapy for patients who have failed to respond to antidepressant medication prophylaxis). Since the previous edition of this volume, interest in unilateral ECT grew and waned, but overall research on ECT increased. Among important new works on ECT is the American Psychiatric Association Task Force Report (1990), an updating of its 1978 volume. The reader seeking more specialized reports may wish to consult the journal *Convulsive Therapy*.

Like ECT, psychosurgery is a treatment with a venerable history and a highly stigmatized reputation. The gross surgery of prefrontal lobotomy long ago gave way to more precise techniques such as stereotactic cingulotomy. Psychosurgery is a treatment of last resort for patients otherwise refractory to treatment, but in this compromised population often results in significant improvement and still serves a limited but useful role. We include a small number of references to acquaint readers with clinical, ethical, and scientific controversies in this area.

Electroconvulsive Therapy

General Reviews and Monographs

1. **Abrams A:** *Electroconvulsive Therapy.* New York, Oxford University Press, 1988

   This is a compact, readable, well-organized general guide to ECT.

2. *American Psychiatric Association Task Force:* *The Practice of Electroconvulsive Therapy: Recommendations for Treatment, Training, and Privileging.* Washington, DC, American Psychiatric Association, 1990

   As its title suggests, this is a definitive, succinct, and current description of all the basic information necessary to practice ECT. It constitutes essential reading, describing indications, treatment techniques, side effects, and ethical and legal issues. The bibliography is extensive, making it a helpful source book for the general reader.

3. **Fink M:** *Convulsive Therapy: Theory and Practice.* New York, Raven, 1979

   Once the authoritative texts on ECT, this book is still worth reading for its history of ECT, its historic impact, and its intelligent prose.

4. **National Institutes of Health:** *Electroconvulsive Therapy: Consensus Development Conference Statement,* Vol. 5, No. 11. Washington, DC, Department of Health and Human Services, 1985

   This is an important public document supporting the efficacy and relative safety of ECT. This conference reflected and further accelerated the resurrection of ECT as an important psychiatric treatment and attempted to reduce its public stigma.

Efficacy in Depression and Other Disorders

5. **Folstein MF, Folstein SE, McHugh PR:** Clinical predictors of improvement after electroconvulsive therapy of patients with schizophrenia, neurotic reactions, and affective disorders. *Biol Psychiatry* 7:147–152, 1973

This article reports on a study of predictors of response to ECT in 110 consecutive inpatients with various diagnoses. A notable result was that schizophrenic patients who responded to ECT tended to have affective symptoms and to respond to a brief course of treatment.

6. **Friedel RO:** The combined use of neuroleptics and ECT in drug resistant schizophrenic patients. *Psychopharmacol Bull* 22:928–930, 1986

This article provided a provocative suggestion of the benefits of combined treatment. Eleven patients with DSM-III schizophrenia who had not responded to thiothixene alone received an open trial of thiothixene plus unilateral or bilateral ECT. Eight achieved complete remission of symptoms.

7. **May PRA, Tuma AH, Yale C, Potepan P, Dixon WJ:** Schizophrenia— a follow-up study of results of treatment, II: hospital stay over two to five years. *Arch Gen Psychiatry* 33:481–486, 1976

This report addresses the relative efficacy of medications and ECT and the possible existence of a drug-resistant, ECT-responsive population.

8. **Medical Research Council:** Clinical trial of the treatment of depressive illness. *BMJ* 1:881–886, 1965

This article is the best of the nine studies reviewed in Rifkin (1988) below, but obviously dated and also methodologically flawed.

9. *Rifkin A:** ECT versus tricyclic antidepressants: a review of the evidence. *J Clin Psychiatry* 49:3–7, 1988

This brief, well-written article reviews outcome findings of nine randomized controlled studies comparing ECT with antidepressant medication. Although the popular conclusion is that these studies demonstrate the superiority of ECT, Rifkin indicates that their methodological weaknesses preclude such a decision. This is a good introduction to the literature on the efficacy of ECT.

10. **Small JG, Klapper MH, Kellams JJ, Miller MJ, Milstein V, Sharpley PH, Small IF:** Electroconvulsive treatment compared with lithium in the management of manic states. *Arch Gen Psychiatry* 45:727–732, 1988

In this only prospective controlled trial of ECT in mania, 34 manic inpatients were randomized to treatment with either lithium carbonate or with ECT followed by lithium maintenance. ECT showed an advantage on blind ratings during the first 8 weeks, but the two groups did not differ thereafter.

Complications and Adverse Effects

11. **Coffey CE, Figiel GS, Djang WT, Sullivan DC, Herfkens RJ, Weiner RD:** Effects of ECT on brain structure: a pilot prospective magnetic resonance imaging study. *Am J Psychiatry* 145:701–706, 1988

     This study found no acute structural changes on magnetic resonance imaging scans in nine patients with major depression following a course in ECT.

12. **Devanand DP, Verma AK, Tirumalasetti F, Sackheim HA:** Absence of cognitive impairment after more than 100 lifetime ECT treatments. *Am J Psychiatry* 148:929–932, 1991

     Countering concerns about cognitive impairment due to ECT, this report on a series of eight patients who had each received more than 100 treatments with bilateral modified sine wave ECT found that cognitive function scores and memory complaints were equivalent to matched patients who had never received ECT.

13. **Gerring JP, Shields HM:** The identification and management of patients with a high risk for cardiac arrhythmias during modified ECT. *J Clin Psychiatry* 43:140–143, 1982

     This article is a widely quoted report addressing the important issues of identifying and managing high-risk cardiac patients during general anesthesia and ECT. Loose study criteria that include cardiac events without clinical significance, together with the evolution of ECT delivery since this report, make the study's findings seem overblown.

14. *Squire LR, Chace PM:** Memory functions six to nine months after electroconvulsive therapy. *Arch Gen Psychiatry* 32:1557–1564, 1975

     Memory functions were tested 6–9 months after either unilateral or bilateral ECT and compared with a control group treated without ECT. No significant differences were found, although patients receiving bilateral ECT reported more subjective memory complaints.

15. **Zielinski RJ, Roose SP, Devanand DP, Woodring S, Sackeim HA:** Cardiovascular complications of ECT in depressed patients with cardiac disease. *Am J Psychiatry* 150:904–909, 1993

     This more current study assessed adverse cardiovascular events in 40 depressed patients with major depression, comparing them with 40 depressed patients without cardiac disease. The former group had more complications, but most were brief and did not prevent completion of ECT: 38 of the 40 did complete treatment. Of 21 of these 40 who had previously taken tricyclic antidepressants, 11 had discontinued them because of cardiovascular side effects.

Mechanisms of Action

16. **Milstein V, Small JG, Miller MJ, Sharpley PH, Small IF:** Mechanisms of action of ECT: schizophrenia and schizoaffective disorder. *Biol Psychiatry* 27:1282–1292, 1990

    This article provides a different and more recent perspective on the still uncertain biological explanation for ECT response than Sackeim et al. (1983) below.

17. **Sackeim HA, Decina P, Prohovnik I, Malitz S, Resor SR:** Anticonvulsant and antidepressant properties of electroconvulsive therapy: a proposed mechanism of action. *Biol Psychiatry* 18:1301–1310, 1983

    This article is a useful discussion of potential explanations for the efficacy of ECT.

Treatment Issues

18. *Sackeim HA, Prudic J, Devanand DP, Decina P, Kerr B, Malitz S:** The impact of medication resistance and continuation pharmacotherapy on relapse following response to electroconvulsive therapy in major depression. *J Clin Psychopharmacol* 10:96–104, 1990

    This retrospective study raises the important point that depressed patients who fail adequate medication trials prior to ECT are more likely to relapse despite prophylaxis medication after ECT.

19. **Shapira B, Lerer B, Gilboa D, Drexler H, Kugelmass S, Calev A:** Facilitation of ECT by caffeine pretreatment. *Am J Psychiatry* 144:1199–1202, 1987

    This article considers an important advance in eliciting therapeutic seizures in patients with high seizure thresholds.

20. **Tandon R, Grunhaus L, Haskett RF, Krugler T, Greden JF:** Relative efficacy of unilateral and bilateral electroconvulsive therapy in melancholia. *Convulsive Therapy* 4:153–159, 1988

    Bilateral ECT treatment was more acutely effective and required fewer treatments than unilateral ECT in nonrandomly assigned depressed patients who were medication free.

Psychosurgery

21. *Bridges P: Psychosurgery revisited. *Journal of Neuropsychiatry and Clinical Neuroscience* 2:326–330, 1990

    This article is a reasonable discussion of the limited, but still marginally important use of modern psychosurgical techniques as a last resort in treatment-refractory cases. The perspective comes from Great Britain, where psychosurgery is more prevalent than in the United States.

22. **Jenike MA, Baer L, Ballantine HT, Martuza RL, Tynes S, Giriunas I, Buttolph ML, Cassem NH:** Cingulotomy for refractory obsessive-compulsive disorder: a long-term follow-up of 33 patients. *Arch Gen Psychiatry* 48:548–555, 1991

    Jenike et al. evaluated records of all 35 patients with severe and intractable obsessive-compulsive disorder who had been treated with cingulotomy at Massachusetts General Hospital over the previous quarter century. Four were suicides; two others had also died. Sixteen patients agreed to telephone interviews, whose results conservatively suggested that at least 25%–30% of patients benefited substantially from the surgery. Side effects were rare and easily controlled.

23. **Stuss DT, Benson DF, Kaplan EF, Weir WS, Della Malva C:** Leucotomized and nonleucotomized schizophrenics: comparison on tests of attention. *Biol Psychiatry* 16:1085–1100, 1981

    This article is a 25-year follow-up of a sample of 16 schizophrenic patients who had undergone prefrontal leukotomy (lobotomy). The authors found no significant differences on tests of attention between the patients who had had psychosurgery and nonschizophrenic control subjects. Surprisingly, both groups outperformed patients with schizophrenia who had not had surgery.

38

Psychoanalytic
Psychotherapy

Howard B. Levine, M.D.

The readings for this chapter have been chosen to address the pragmatic needs of the student therapist. They emphasize clinical theory rather than metapsychology and are organized around key concepts related to the process of therapy, the doctor-patient relationship, and psychotherapeutic technique. They cover such topics as resistance; transference and countertransference; therapeutic and working alliances; interventions; curative factors; the dynamics of the opening and termination phases; and the analysis of resistance, transference, and dreams. I have attempted to include articles that are classics, whose ideas travel well from psychoanalysis to psychotherapy, and in which the case material presented can serve as a model for psychotherapeutic technique. In addition, since there is often a preponderance of more disturbed patients in the caseloads of student therapists, I have cited a number of references that are specifically relevant to the understanding and treatment of psychotic, narcissistic, and borderline personalities. Above all, I have tried to select material that will bear rereading over time and that can serve not only as points of reference, but as points of departure for further discussion and exploration. Since the last edition of this volume, there has been an increased concern among analytic psychotherapists with dual treatment, ethics, and the long-term consequences of childhood sexual abuse and incest. These concerns are reflected in the current choice of articles.

Theoretical Perspectives and Overviews

1. *Freud A: *The Ego and the Mechanisms of Defense.* New York, International Universities Press, 1936; **Freud A:** *The Writings of Anna Freud,* Vol. 2. New York, International Universities Press, 1966

    This is a landmark contribution to ego psychology that remains as fresh, clear, and relevant to current psychotherapeutic practice as when it first appeared.

2. **Jacobs TJ:** *The Use of the Self: Counter-Transference and Communication in the Analytic Situation.* Madison, CT, International Universities Press, 1991

    This book contains a richly illustrated, well-written set of papers dealing with fundamental clinical concepts, such as transference, countertransference, enactments, and empathy.

3. **McDougall J:** *Theatres of the Mind.* New York, Basic Books, 1985

    McDougall's unique gifts as a writer and clinician allow her to communicate the affective immediacy of the analytic process to her readers in a way that makes analytic clinical theory come alive as a series of human encounters between analyst and patients along a broad spectrum of pathologies.

4. *Schafer R: On becoming a psychoanalyst of one persuasion or another. *Contemporary Psychoanalysis* 15:345–360, 1979; **Schafer R:** On becoming a psychoanalyst of one persuasion or another, in *The Analytic Attitude.* Edited by Schafer R. New York, Basic Books, 1983, pp. 281–296

    Although not strictly an article on psychotherapy per se, no student should graduate from a training program without the benefit of reading this. Originally intended for a graduating class of psychoanalytic candidates, this article considers issues of orthodoxy and sectarianism in so thoughtful a way that the reader cannot help but come away from it feeling more open minded, humble, and intellectually curious about the competing claims of the various schools and orientations of psychoanalysis and psychotherapy.

5. *Winnicott DW: *The Maturational Processes and the Facilitating Environment: Studies in the Theory of Emotional Development.* New York, International Universities Press, 1965

    This is a broad-ranging collection of chapters that deal with issues of dependence, object relations theory, personality formation, and their implications for psychotherapy. It includes many thought-provoking, classic contributions that are particularly relevant to the treatment of primitive personality disorders. A must reading is "Hate in the Countertransference."

6. *Zetzel ER: *The Capacity for Emotional Growth.* New York, International Universities Press, 1970

   This volume is a major developmental and ego-psychological contribution to a number of clinical and theoretical problems that lie at the heart of the therapeutic encounter. The essays on anxiety, depression, and the doctor-patient relationship; transference; therapeutic alliance; and the so-called good hysteric are classics in the field.

The Unconscious and the Concept of Conflict

7. **Arlow JA:** Unconscious fantasy and disturbance of conscious experience. *Psychoanal Q* 38:1–27, 1969

   This article discusses the structure, formation, and defensive function of unconscious fantasy as well as its relationship to metaphor, déjà vu, depersonalization experiences, identity maintenance, self-representation, and the self. It is an excellent, experientially oriented, advanced article on the unconscious.

8. *Deutsch H:** The part of the actual conflict in the formation of neurosis (1930), in *Neuroses and Character Types.* Edited by Deutsch H. New York, International Universities Press, 1965, pp. 3–13

   This chapter examines the relationship between the actual (conscious, manifest) conflict in the patient's current reality and the underlying (unconscious, latent) conflicts from the patient's past. It is a very useful chapter for introducing the dynamic unconscious and the classic view of neurosis and for strengthening beginning therapists' appreciation of the intrapsychic, subjective reality of their patients' experiences.

9. **Freud S:** The forgetting of proper names and the forgetting of foreign words (1901), in the Psychopathology of everyday life, in *The Standard Edition of the Complete Psychological Works of Sigmund Freud,* Vol. 6. Translated and edited by Strachey J. London, Hogarth Press, 1960, pp. 1–14; **Freud S:** The forgetting of foreign words (1901), in the Psychopathology of everyday life, in *The Standard Edition of the Complete Psychological Works of Sigmund Freud,* Vol. 6. Translated and edited by Strachey J. London, Hogarth Press, 1960, pp. 8–14

   These two chapters illustrate the relationship between unconscious motivations, conflict, and repression ("forgetting"). They serve as a valuable introductory demonstration of unconscious mental processes, as well as an opportunity to introduce the concepts of associative links between chains of thought and psychic determination.

10. **Freud S:** (1909) Analysis of a phobia in a five-year old boy (1909), *The Standard Edition of the Complete Psychological Works of Sigmund Freud*, Vol. 10. Translated and edited by Strachey J. London, Hogarth Press, 1955, pp. 3–149

This paper is a delightful and engaging case history that acquaints students with the psychodynamics of neurosis, including sexual and aggressive wishes, the Oedipus and castration complexes, mechanisms of defense, primary and secondary process modes of thought, and the relationship between conflict and symptom formation. It also illustrates an early use of child observation data to support inferences about unconscious mental processes derived from the clinical setting.

Transference and Alliance

11. *****Bird B:** Notes on transference: universal phenomenon and hardest part of analysis. *J Am Psychoanal Assoc* 20:267–301, 1972

This article is a profound essay on transference and transference neurosis, which considers the relationship of transference to ego functioning, reality, negative therapeutic reactions, and the psychoanalytic process.

12. **Brenner C:** Working alliance, therapeutic alliance, and transference. *J Am Psychoanal Assoc* 27 (suppl):137–157, 1979

This is an exceptionally clear, well-reasoned article that reexamines the original descriptions of the therapeutic and working alliance and attempts to demonstrate that they are not discrete entities, but simply aspects of the transference.

13. **Corwin HA:** The narcissistic alliance and progressive transference neurosis in serious regressive states. *International Journal of Psychoanalysis and Psychotherapy* 3:299–316, 1974

This article explores the nature of the attachment that exists between nonclassically analyzable (borderline, narcissistic, and psychotic) patients and their therapists and how that attachment can be used to foster a workable treatment situation.

14. *****Friedman L:** The therapeutic alliance. *Int J Psychoanal* 50:139–153, 1969

A profound essay on the problems and sources of the patient's motivation for treatment, this article includes a historical evaluation of the concept of the therapeutic alliance and its relationship to the transference.

15. *Gill MM: *Analysis of Transference, Vol. 1, Theory and Technique.* New York, International Universities Press, 1982

This volume examines the evolution of the concept of transference and critically reviews the literature on the relationship of transference analysis to the theory of technique and therapeutic change.

16. **Greenacre P:** Certain technical problems in the transference relationship. *J Am Psychoanal Assoc* 7:474–502, 1959

This article is a classic essay concerning therapist activity, patient autonomy, and the impact of the reality situation on the balance between therapeutic alliance and transference.

17. **Loewald HW:** The transference neurosis: comments on the concept and the phenomenon. *J Am Psychoanal Assoc* 19:54–66, 1971; **Loewald HW:** The transference neurosis: comments on the concept and the phenomenom, in *Papers on Psychoanalysis.* Edited by Loewald HW. New Haven, CT, Yale University Press, 1980, pp. 301–314

Loewald reexamines the transference neurosis in the light of advances in ego psychology and the understanding of pre-Oedipal development and character neuroses, emphasizing the creative, adaptive dimension to this phenomenon.

Countertransference

18. **Adler G:** Helplessness in the helpers. *Br J Med Psychol* 45:315–326, 1972

Adler examines the vicissitudes of intense feelings of helplessness and hopelessness that are inevitably stirred up in the therapists who work with patients with borderline, narcissistic, and other primitive personality disorders. Negative countertransference reactions stimulated by oral ambivalence and rage, defenses against such reactions, and their sources in the patient-therapist relationship are discussed.

19. **Gutheil TG, Gabbard GO:** The concept of boundaries in clinical practice: Theoretical and risk-management dimensions. *Am J Psychiatry* 150:188–196, 1993

This is an examination of boundaries and boundary violations in psychotherapy, including issues of role, time, place, money, gifts, clothing, language, self-disclosure, and physical contact.

20. **Heimann P:** On countertransference. *Int J Psychoanal* 31:81–84, 1950

This article is a classic (Kleinian) statement of the view that the therapist's countertransference is at least partly produced by the unconscious attempt of patients to actualize some aspect of their unconscious, inner world. This article is the foundation for the conceptualization of countertransference as a potential contribution to therapeutic technique.

21. *Maltsberger JT, Buie DH:** Counter-transference hate in the treatment of suicidal patients. *Arch Gen Psychiatry* 30:625–633, 1974

This article is an excellent clinical discussion of the various types of overt and defensively disguised angry and rejecting responses likely to be elicited in therapists by suicidal, sadomasochistic, borderline, and other hard-to-treat character-disordered patients.

22. **Sandler J:** Countertransference and role responsiveness. *International Review of Psychoanalysis* 3:43–48, 1976

This is a contemporary elaboration of Heimann's (1950) above work on countertransference that further illustrates the ways in which patients unconsciously communicate aspects of their internal worlds and conflicts to their therapists and pressure the latter toward actualization and enactment of core conflicts and significant, past relationships.

23. **Tower LE:** Countertransference. *J Am Psychoanal Assoc* 4:224–255, 1956

This article is a lucid discussion of countertransference and other affective responses of therapists, which the author believes are ubiquitous in treatment situations.

Psychotherapeutic Technique

24. **Blanck G, Blanck R:** Descriptive developmental diagnosis, in *Ego Psychology: Theory and Practice.* Edited by Blanck G, Blanck R. New York, Columbia University Press, 1974, pp. 91–118

This chapter attempts to address the problem of the relationship between traditional psychiatric classification and treatment by proposing a diagnostic scheme based on personality development. It is clinically illustrated, usefully addresses some therapeutic problems of the evaluation phase, and is especially helpful for introducing the concepts of "lines of development," "intact versus modified ego," "ego distortion," "ego deviation," "ego defect," and "ego regression."

25. **Fleming J:** Early object deprivation and transference phenomena: the working alliance. *Psychoanal Q* 41:23–49, 1972

Through a study of the therapeutic process in adults who experienced developmental disruptions due to object loss in childhood or adolescence, the author examines the persistence of immature ego organization into adult life and its implications for treatment.

26. **Fleming J:** Some observations on object constancy in the psychoanalysis of adults. *J Am Psychoanal Assoc* 23:743–759, 1975

This is a masterful case presentation illustrating the application of Mahler's work on separation-individuation to psychotherapeutic technique.

27. *Freud S:** Papers on technique (1911–1915), in *The Standard Edition of the Complete Psychological Works of Sigmund Freud*, Vol. 12. Translated and edited by Strachey J. London, Hogarth Press, 1958, pp. 85–173

This group of papers encompasses a wealth of clinical wisdom about many issues, including the interpretation of dreams, the beginning phase of treatment, transference, acting out, and the repetition compulsion.

28. *Greenson RR:** *The Technique and Practice of Psychoanalysis.* New York, International Universities Press, 1967

This is a marvelous source book on clinical technique that applies equally well to psychoanalytic psychotherapy as it does to psychoanalysis. The sections on the analysis of resistance, the working alliance, and transference are clear, pragmatic, and abundantly illustrated.

29. **Hoffer A:** Towards a definition of psychoanalytic neutrality. *J Am Psychoanal Assoc* 33:771–796, 1985

This article is a contemporary examination of a fundamental concept that is one of the defining criteria of technique and stance within classic psychoanalysis.

30. **Lichtenberg JD:** The empathic mode of perception and alternative vantage points for psycho-analytic work. *Psychoanalytic Inquiry* 1:329–355, 1981

This article is an excellent, clinically illustrated account of empathy and its use as a tool for listening and understanding patients in psychotherapy.

31. *Myerson PG:** Issues of technique where patients relate with difficulty. *International Review of Psychoanalysis* 6:363–375, 1979

This article is a major contribution to the understanding of the therapeutic process in the treatment of patients with impaired capacities for
object relations. Problems of the patient's unrelatedness to the analyst,
unrealistic expectations of the analyst, and incapacity to understand
interpretations and adopt a reflective stance are discussed in terms of
technique and pathogenesis.

32. **Roose S:** The use of medication in combination with psychoanalytic
    psychotherapy or psychoanalysis, in *Psychiatry: The Personality Disorders
    and Neuroses,* Vol. 1. Edited by Michaels R. Philadelphia, PA, JB
    Lippincott, 1990

    This chapter is a thoughtful discussion of the issues of technique raised
    by the introduction of medication into an analytic psychotherapy.

33. **Spence DP:** Discussion of "The misuse of empathy in psychoanalysis" by
    Ira Moses. *Contemporary Psychoanalysis* 24:594–598, 1988

    This article is a thoughtful counterpoint to the many articles that extol
    the unquestioned capacity for empathy as the therapist's ideal position
    in an analytic treatment.

34. **Wolf E:** Ambience and abstinence. *Annual of Psychoanalysis* 4:101–115,
    1976

    Wolf examines the consequences of misapplying Freud's "rule of absti-
    nence" on the evolving ambience of the therapeutic situation, particu-
    larly in the treatment of neurotic patients with narcissistic defenses or
    patients with narcissistic personality disorders.

Dreams and Dream Analysis

35. **Erikson EH:** The dream specimen of psycho-analysis. *J Am Psychoanal
    Assoc* 2:5–56, 1954

    Erikson draws on biographical, cultural, and historical data relevant to
    Freud's life to expand brilliantly on the analysis of the famous Irma
    dream. The intimate connections between manifest dream content and
    the dreamer's creativity, conscience, stage of adult development, and
    identity maintenance are discussed.

36. **Freud S:** The method of interpreting dreams: an analysis of a specimen
    dream (1900), Chapter 2: The Interpretation of Dreams, *The Standard
    Edition of the Complete Psychological Works of Sigmund Freud,* Vol. 4. Trans-
    lated and edited by Strachey J. London, Hogarth Press, 1958, pp. 96–121

Freud's "Interpretation of Dreams" remains one of his most profound and major contributions to psychological understanding. This section, which contains his analysis of the famous Irma dream, also includes his analogy between the structure of the dream and the structure of the neurotic symptom and his famous pronouncement that the dream is a fulfillment of a wish.

37. *Greenson RR: The exceptional position of the dream in psychoanalytic practice. *Psychoanal Q* 39:519–549, 1970

Following Freud, Greenson argues that dreams possess a special proximity to childhood memories and affects in the unconscious. As such, their analysis offers both patient and therapist a unique, convincing, and immediate experience of access to the dreamer's unconscious mind and conflicts.

Masochism and Negative Therapeutic Reaction

38. **Asch SS:** Varieties of negative therapeutic reaction and problems of technique. *J Am Psychoanal Assoc* 24:383–407, 1976

Asch expands Freud's original descriptions of the negative therapeutic reaction to include contributions from difficulties in separation-individuation and offers recommendations for treatment.

39. **Cooper AM:** Psychotherapeutic approaches to masochism. *Journal of Psychotherapy Practice and Research* 2:1–12, 1993

This is a lucid account of the problems and techniques encountered in the analytic psychotherapy of masochism and self-defeating personality disorders.

40. **Valenstein AF:** On attachment to painful feelings and the negative therapeutic reaction. *Psychoanal Study Child* 28:365–392, 1973

Valenstein explores issues of masochism and the negative therapeutic reaction in the light of early development and the persistence of residues of archaic ego states in adult patients.

Psychotherapy of Adults Who Were Sexually Abused as Children

41. *Levine HB (ed): *Adult Analysis and Childhood Sexual Abuse*. Hillsdale, NJ, Analytic Press, 1990

The essays in this book follow a case study approach organized around the treatment process to explore the clinical issues that arise in the analytic therapy of adult patients who were sexually abused or involved in incest during childhood and adolescence.

42. **Margolis M:** Parent child incest: analytic treatment experiences with follow-up data, in *The Trauma of Transgression.* Edited by Kramer S, Akhtar S. Northvale, NJ, Jason Aronson, 1991, pp. 57–92

One of the two cases that form the clinical core of this work is a remarkable account of the long-term, intensive, analytic therapy of a man who had consummated an incestuous relationship with his mother during adolescence. It is a unique and important contribution to the literature on childhood sexual abuse in men.

43. *Shengold L: *Soul Murder.* New Haven, CT, Yale University Press, 1989

This is an eloquent description of the consequences of childhood abuse (sexual and otherwise) and the clinical problems to which they can give rise.

Primitive Personality Disorders, Self Psychology, and Disorders of Narcissism

44. *Buie DH, Adler G: The uses of confrontation with borderline patients. *International Journal of Psychoanalysis and Psychotherapy* 1:90–108, 1972

This article is a succinct and lucid description of the subjective experiences of borderline patients and the drives, defenses, and object needs that underlie these phenomena. It includes a useful description of the place of confrontation as a therapeutic technique.

45. *Kernberg O: *Borderline Conditions and Pathological Narcissism.* New York, Jason Aronson, 1975

Several chapters in this collection are classics that helped establish a standard in psychoanalytic thinking about the psychopathology and treatment of primitive personality disorders. In particular, the chapters on the borderline syndrome, its treatment and prognosis, and the treatment and clinical problems of narcissistic personality disorder, which Kernberg views as a variant of borderline personality, are of special relevance and value.

46. *Kohut H: The psychoanalytic treatment of narcissistic personality disorders: outline of a systematic approach. *Psychoanal Study Child* 23:86–113, 1968

Kohut introduces the concepts of the idealizing and mirror transferences, central to the clinical contribution of Kohut and the self psychologists, and examines issues of technique, transference, and countertransference in the treatment of narcissism personality disorders.

47. **Kohut H:** Thoughts on narcissism and narcissistic rage. *Psychoanal Study Child* 27:360–400, 1972

Kohut examines manifestations of narcissistic rage in relation to problems in the vulnerability of underlying personality structures to narcissistic injury.

48. **Kohut H:** The two analyses of Mr. Z. *Int J Psychoanal* 60:3–27, 1979

This is a landmark contribution illustrating Kohut's clinical position regarding the treatment of narcissistic personality disorders. It is very useful in helping to conceptualize the differences in formulation and technique that arise from a self psychological, as opposed to a classic ego-psychological, approach to patients.

49. **Levine HB:** Some implications of self psychology. *Contemporary Psychoanalysis* 19:153–171, 1983

Levine discusses clinical concepts embodied in Kohut's self psychology that are generalizable to the practice of psychotherapy, including empathy, the self object concept, the narcissistic (self object) transferences, and the application of self psychology to supportive psychotherapy.

50. *Modell AH:** A narcissistic defense against affects and the illusion of self-sufficiency. *Int J Psychoanal* 56:275–282, 1975

Modell conceptualizes the central problem in narcissistic personality disorders as a pseudoindependent defensive stance vis-à-vis later relationships, which stems from various forms of early object disturbance and gives rise to a pathognomonic transference relationship, "the cocoon transference," based on the defense of affect blocking.

51. **Modell AH:** "The holding environment" and the therapeutic action of psychoanalysis. *J Am Psychoanal Assoc* 24:285–307, 1976

The function of the analytic situation as "holding environment" is contrasted in the treatment of neurotic and narcissistic personality disorders.

52. **Morrison A:** *Shame: The Underside of Narcissism.* Hillsdale, NJ, Analytic Press, 1989

This is a thorough contribution to the understanding and treatment of a long-neglected topic, the understanding of which is crucial to many clinical situations.

53. **Plakun EM:** Psychotherapy with the self-destructive borderline patient, in *Clinical Challenges in Psychiatry*. Edited by Sledge WH, Tasman A. Washington, DC, American Psychiatric Press, 1993, pp. 129–155

This chapter provides a clear and richly illustrated clinical discussion of the application of limit setting in the analytic therapy of self-destructive, borderline patients.

54. **Reich A:** Pathologic forms of self-esteem regulation. *Psychoanal Study Child* 15:215–232, 1960

This article is a classic, ego-psychoanalytic contribution to problems of self-esteem regulation. It raises crucial questions concerning the places of aggression, pregenital trauma, and concerns about annihilation and bodily intactness in the pathogenesis of narcissistic imbalances.

55. **Stolorow RD, Lachmann FM:** *Psychoanalysis of Developmental Arrests: Theory and Treatment.* New York, International Universities Press, 1980

This is an innovative book that explores and contrasts pre-Oedipal pathologic formations that arise from conflict with those that arise from developmental arrest.

56. **Volkan VD:** *Primitive Internalized Object Relations: A Clinical Study of Schizophrenic, Borderline and Narcissistic Patients.* New York, International Universities Press, 1976

This is an excellent clinical contribution to the psychoanalytic psychotherapy of schizophrenic, borderline, and narcissistic patients. Of particular merit are the chapters illustrating transitional objects, the use of real relationships as substitutes for internal psychic structure, and the mechanism of structural change in psychotherapy. Also included are useful discussions and illustrations of the work of Kernberg, Winnicott, and Strachey.

The Psychotherapeutic Process (Including Opening Phase and Termination)

57. **Firestein SK:** Termination of psychoanalysis of adults: a review of the literature. *J Am Psychoanal Assoc* 22:873–894, 1974

Firestein summarizes indications for termination, issues of technique, and the justification for designating termination as a separate and distinct phase of treatment.

58. **Langs R:** The framework for understanding the communications from patients in psychotherapy, in *The Technique of Psychoanalytic Psychotherapy*, Vol. 1. Edited by Langs R. New York, Jason Aronson, 1973, pp. 279–326

This chapter is an elegant conceptual framework for listening to and understanding the structure of a psychotherapy session, in terms of manifest and latent content and its important roots in the adaptive stresses presented by the patients' current life experiences, especially the therapeutic relationship.

59. *Loewald HW: The waning of the Oedipus complex. *J Am Psychoanal Assoc* 27:751–755, 1979; **Loewald HW:** The waning of the Oedipus complex, in *Papers on Psychoanalysis*. Edited by Loewald HW. New Haven, CT, Yale University Press, 1980, pp. 384–404

This work is a masterful essay on the place of the Oedipus complex in contemporary psychoanalytic practice and theory.

60. **Stone L:** *The Psychoanalytic Situation: An Examination of its Developmental and Essential Nature.* New York, International Universities Press, 1961

Stone explores the affective essence of the psychoanalytic relationship by examining the tensions inherent in the basic emotional ties existing between patient and analyst and the psychobiological developmental structures that underlie them.

Curative Factors in Psychotherapy and Psychoanalysis

61. **Alexander F:** The principle of flexibility and the principle of corrective emotional experience, in *Psychoanalytic Therapy: Principles and Application.* Edited by Alexander F, French T. New York, Ronald Press, 1946, pp. 25–70

Alexander's attempts to shorten analytic treatment through the use of active role-playing techniques designed to counterbalance patients' early pathogenic object relations remains the bête noire of contemporary psychoanalytic clinical theory and should be read as an important point of contrast and departure for understanding the theory of how analysis produces change.

62. *Loewald HW: On the therapeutic action of psychoanalysis. *Int J Psychoanal* 41:16–33, 1960; Loewald HW: On the therapeutic action of psychoanalysis, in *Papers on Psychoanalysis*. Edited by Loewald HW. New Haven, CT, Yale University Press, 1980, pp. 221–256

This is a classic formulation of the therapeutic action of psychoanalysis as arising from the integrative impact of the therapeutic relationship. It draws a parallel between the treatment process and the early mother-child relationship.

63. *Strachey J: The nature of the therapeutic action of psychoanalysis. *Int J Psychoanal* 15:127–159, 1934

The classic statement of how psychoanalytic treatment produces change, Strachey's description of the dynamics of the mutative transference interpretation remains the benchmark of the theories of technique and therapeutic factors in psychoanalysis.

39

Psychoeducation

Carol M. Anderson, Ph.D.

Psychoeducation is a model of treatment that employs educational interventions as part of a larger series of treatment strategies for patients and their families. Originally developed for use with schizophrenic patients and their families, psychoeducational models have since been applied to the treatment of an increasingly wide range of both psychiatric and medical illnesses. Today, numerous specific models of psychoeducational treatment exist. Although these models differ in important respects, there are three basic assumptions common to all psychoeducational models.

First, psychoeducational models assume that most serious and chronic illnesses have a biological or genetic component that interacts with the psychosocial and family environment of the patient to influence coping. Most models thus work in conjunction with chemotherapy for the illness. Second, psychoeducational models assume that the environment does not cause illness, but can strongly influence its course. These models, therefore, strongly emphasize the importance of working collaboratively with families as partners in the treatment process. By emphasizing the role of the family as a resource, psychoeducational models depart significantly from earlier professional attitudes toward families, which instead stressed family dysfunction and family etiology. Third, psychoeducational models assume that possessing concrete and practical knowledge increases the ability of both patients and families to cope with chronic illness. Therefore, these models contend that it is in the best interests of patients, families, and professionals to provide patients and families with information about the patient's illness and to teach practical strategies for its proper management.

Overall, the use of psychoeducational models has represented a significant step forward in the treatment of serious and chronic illness. Feedback from families and research conducted on the use of these models, primarily with schizophrenic patients and their families, have suggested that they are not only more effective, but more humane, than models of treatment utilized in the past.

The readings collected in this bibliography have been organized into four primary sections. The first section of annotations are selected from the two bodies of literature that have served as a background to the development of psychoeducational models. The first body of literature includes early research studies that led to psychoeducation's dual emphasis on working with families and providing education. The second body of literature is nonempirical and includes examples from both the professional and popular literature that have worked to increase the awareness of and sensitivity to the needs and strengths of the families of mentally ill persons. The second section presents four readings that provide excellent overviews of the basic models of psychoeducational treatment. The third section provides annotations that explicate the most extensively researched and documented models of psychoeducational treatment. Because each of these models was developed for use with schizophrenic patients and their families, the final section provides examples of psychoeducational models as applied to other psychiatric and medical disorders.

Background

Empirical Background

1. *Brown GW, Birley JLT, Wing JK:* Influence of family life on the course of schizophrenic disorders: a replication. *Br J Psychiatry* 121:241–258, 1972

   This article reports one of the first sophisticated investigations into the relationship between "expressed emotion" (attitudes and behavior of family members toward mentally ill relatives) and patient relapse. This study and future studies that replicated its results had a significant influence on working with families using a psychoeducational approach.

2. **Hatfield AB:** Psychological costs of schizophrenia to the family. *Social Work* 23:355–359, 1978

This article describes one of the earliest studies to focus on the stressful impact of caring for a family member with schizophrenia. Hatfield's findings laid the groundwork for the development of psychoeducational models by describing families' urgent needs for education about schizophrenia and its daily management.

3. **Hogarty GE:** Depot neuroleptics: the relevance of psychosocial factors. *J Clin Psychiatry* 45 (sec 2):36–42, 1984

This article provides a succinct overview of much of the research that helped lay the foundation for the development of psychoeducational models. It summarizes the clinically relevant implications of studies conducted on the relationship between relapse and medication non-compliance, on the impact of environmental and family stress, and on the effectiveness of psychosocial interventions with schizophrenia.

4. ***Hooley JM:** Expressed emotion: a review of the critical literature. *Clinical Psychology Review* 5:119–139, 1985

This article provides a comprehensive review of the research conducted on expressed emotion. An understanding of this work is critical to an understanding of the theoretical basis of psychoeducational interventions, because it was research on expressed emotion that empirically confirmed long-held clinical assumptions that patients' environments have an impact on the course of their illnesses.

5. **Pearlin LI, Schooler C:** The structure of coping. *J Health Soc Behav* 19:2–21, 1978

This article represents a critical examination and comparison of the effectiveness of individual coping strategies and styles. This literature heavily influenced psychoeducation's emphasis on the importance of providing education as a means to augment the coping abilities of patients and families.

6. ***Vaughn CE, Leff JP:** The influence of family and social factors on the course of psychiatric illness. *Br J Psychiatry* 129:125–137, 1976

This classic article presents a clear and succinct account of the first replication of Brown et al.'s (1972) earlier work above on expressed emotion, providing additional evidence that patients from households characterized by high levels of expressed emotion are at greater risk for relapse.

Non-Empirical Background

7. **Appleton WS:** Mistreatment of patients' families by psychiatrists. *Am J Psychiatry* 131:655–657, 1974

   This excellent, inspiring article illustrates the vicious cycle that can ensue when families' needs for information and support are ignored, dismissed, and even distorted by "helping professionals." It presents a call from within the field to begin treating families with greater respect and compassion.

8. **Bernheim KF, Lewine RRJ, Beale CT:** *The Caring Family: Living With Chronic Mental Illness.* New York, Random House, 1982

   This popular book has helped to provide families with useful information about a wide range of chronic mental illnesses and has also been helpful in increasing the public awareness of common emotional responses families have to such illnesses.

9. **Sheehan S:** *Is There No Place on Earth for Me?* Boston, Houghton Mifflin, 1982

   This book presents in detail the story of a young woman diagnosed with schizophrenia; it includes a painfully accurate portrayal of the (at-best) inadequate treatment available to her and her family.

10. *****Torrey EF:** *Surviving Schizophrenia: A Family Manual.* New York, Harper & Row, 1983

    This classic book for families provides a wealth of practical information about schizophrenia, its course, treatment, and their role in its management. It delivers an empathic message encouraging families to advocate for their own rights and those of their relatives with schizophrenia.

11. **Vine P:** *Families in Pain: Children, Siblings, Spouses, and Parents of the Mentally Ill Speak Out.* New York, Pantheon Books, 1982

    This book presents the stories of families with mentally ill relatives and details their efforts to cope with both the challenges of the illness and mental health systems. This important book has worked to increase awareness of the needs of families and their contributions to the care of mentally ill persons.

12. **Wasow M:** *Coping With Schizophrenia: A Survival Manual for Parents, Relatives, and Friends.* Palo Alto, CA, Science & Behavior Books, 1982

    This book is particularly valuable for its moving account of the author's own struggle and the overwhelming obstacles she faced as she tried to

obtain basic and reliable information for herself and effective treatment for her son, who was diagnosed with schizophrenia.

Overviews of Basic Models of Psychoeducational Treatment

13. **Anderson CM, Reiss DJ:** Approaches to psychoeducational family therapy. *International Journal of Family Psychiatry* 3:501–517, 1983

This introduction to psychoeducation clearly describes the historical
background and underlying assumptions of psychoeducational models
and presents a comprehensive but succinct summary of the major
models of psychoeducational treatment, with an emphasis on the
model developed by Anderson, Hogarty, Reiss, and colleagues.

14. *Goldstein MJ* (ed): *New Developments in Interventions With Families of
Schizophrenics.* San Francisco, CA, Jossey-Bass, 1981

This highly recommended volume is one of the best collections containing early articles from each of the original architects of the major
models of psychoeducational, family-oriented treatment. Chapters are
concise but comprehensive.

15. **Goldstein MJ:** Psychosocial (nonpharmacologic) treatments for schizophrenia, in *American Psychiatric Press Review of Psychiatry*, Vol. 10. Edited
by Tasman A, Goldfinger SM. Washington, DC, American Psychiatric
Press, 1991, pp. 116–135

This excellent chapter provides a valuable overview of the basic assumptions, principles, and objectives of psychoeducational models as well as
a concise review of the research on the efficacy of these models. The
chapter helps to define the term *psychoeducation* and discusses the
important distinction between family education and psychoeducational
models.

16. **McFarlane WR** (ed): *Family Therapy in Schizophrenia.* New York, Guilford,
1983

Although this volume does not focus exclusively on psychoeducation, it
does contain a series of chapters that provide an excellent overview of
the field of psychoeducation. It is also useful for contrasting the psychoeducational models to other family-oriented approaches to the
treatment of schizophrenia.

Specific Models of Psychoeducational Treatment

Anderson, Hogarty, and Reiss

17. *Anderson CM, Hogarty GE, Reiss DJ:** Family treatment of adult schizophrenic patients: a psycho-educational approach. *Schizophr Bull* 6:490–505, 1980

> This classic article, which coined the term *psychoeducation,* was the first published account of the Anderson, Hogarty, and Reiss model of psychoeducation. The original model included four (later expanded to five) phases of treatment: connection with the family, survival skills workshops (focus on education and concrete caretaking challenges), reentry and application, and maintenance. The model combined behavioral, structural, dynamic, and information-sharing aspects.

18. **Anderson CM, Reiss DJ, Hogarty GE:** *Schizophrenia and the Family.* New York, Guilford, 1986

> This text presents the most complete description of the Anderson, Hogarty, and Reiss model of psychoeducation. It also includes practical information on how to implement psychoeducational models in mental health settings. It is a useful tool for teaching about the basic components of psychoeducation and the attitudes about families and chronically mentally ill persons that underlie such an approach.

19. *Hogarty GE, Anderson CM, Reiss DJ, Kornblith SJ, Greenwald DP, Ulrich RF, Carter M:** Family psychoeducation, social skills training, and maintenance chemotherapy in the aftercare treatment of schizophrenia: two-year effects of a controlled study on relapse and adjustment. *Arch Gen Psychiatry* 48:340–347, 1991

> This article presents 2-year follow-up results on the Anderson, Hogarty, and Reiss (and colleagues) model of psychoeducation that suggest that family intervention helps to delay but does not prevent relapse. Follow-up articles such as this and the others cited below are essential to a continuing understanding of the efficacy of psychoeducational models.

Falloon and Colleagues

20. **Falloon I, Boyd JL, McGill C:** *Family Care of Schizophrenia.* New York, Guilford, 1984

> This text provides the most detailed discussion of the model of psychoeducation of Falloon and colleagues. Their model is a home-based

program that devotes the first two family sessions to education and utilizes the remaining sessions for behavioral intervention. Unlike other models, their model has been researched with a population including a large percentage of African American and Hispanic subjects.

21. *Falloon IR, Boyd JL, McGill CW, Williamson W, Razoni J, Moss HB, Gilderman AM, Simpson GM: Family management in the prevention of morbidity of schizophrenia: clinical outcome of a two-year longitudinal study. *Arch Gen Psychiatry* 42:887–896, 1985

This article presents the 2-year follow-up results on the authors' controlled 9-month study comparing the effectiveness of their home-based, family psychoeducational model to a more traditional clinic-based, individual model.

Goldstein

22. *Goldstein MJ, Rodnick EH, Evans JR, May PRA, Steinberg MR: Drug and family therapy in the aftercare treatment of acute schizophrenics. *Arch Gen Psychiatry* 35:1169–1177, 1978

This classic article reports the results of the first controlled study to provide empirical data on the effectiveness of teaching patients and families about schizophrenia and its management. The Goldstein model of psychoeducation utilized in this study was brief (six sessions), concrete, and problem focused.

Leff, Berkowitz, and Colleagues

23. *Leff J, Kuipers L, Berkowitz R, Eberlein-Vries R, Sturgeon D: A controlled trial of social intervention in the families of schizophrenic patients. *Br J Psychiatry* 141:121–134, 1982

The Leff, Berkowitz, and colleagues model of intervention combines education (provided in four lectures), individual sessions between patient and family, and multiple-family groups. Their model aims to reduce patient relapse by decreasing the family's level of expressed emotion and the face-to-face contact between patient and family. This article describes their model and the results of a 9-month controlled study comparing its effectiveness to more traditional outpatient care.

24. Leff J, Kuipers L, Berkowitz R, Sturgeon D: A controlled trial of social intervention in the families of schizophrenic patients: two year follow-up. *Br J Psychiatry* 146:594–600, 1985

This article presents the 2-year follow-up results on the study reported in the above-cited article.

Psychoeducational Models Applied to Disorders Other Than Schizophrenia

25. **Daley D:** A psychoeducational approach to relapse prevention. *Journal of Chemical Dependency Treatment* 2:105–124, 1989

    This article describes a structured, eight-session relapse prevention psychoeducational program designed for use with chemically dependent patients in a 28-day rehabilitation program. Although initially developed for use on an inpatient basis, information is also included on ways in which the program can be adapted for outpatient and family treatment.

26. *Daley D, Bowler K, Cahalane H:** Approaches to patient and family education with affective disorders. *Patient Education and Counseling* 19:163–174, 1992

    This article presents a strong rationale for the importance of education and psychoeducation interventions with affective disorders and provides an excellent overview of a wide range of such interventions applicable to both individual and family treatment.

27. *Gonzalez BA, Steinglass P, Reiss D:** Putting the illness in its place: discussion groups for families with chronic medical illness. *Fam Process* 28:69–87, 1989

    This article is one of the better illustrations of the use of psychoeducation with nonpsychiatric populations. It describes the components of a short-term, psychoeducational, multiple-family group approach to working with families and patients in the chronic stage of a wide range of medical illnesses.

28. **Holder D, Anderson CM:** Psychoeducational family interventions for depressed patients and their families, in *Depression and Families: Impact and Treatment.* Edited by Keitner GI. Washington, DC, American Psychiatric Press, 1990, pp. 159–184

    This chapter is particularly useful as a demonstration of the ways in which psychoeducational models can be applied to major psychiatric disorders other than schizophrenia. It describes the application of the Anderson, Hogarthy, and Reiss model of psychoeducation to families with patients diagnosed with affective disorders and includes separate discussions of the use of psychoeducation with children, adolescents, and the elderly with affective disorder diagnoses.

29. **Livingston-Van Noppen B, Rasmussen SA, Eisen J, McCartney L:** Family function and treatment in obsessive-compulsive disorder, in *Obsessive-Compulsive Disorders: Theory and Management.* Edited by Jenike MA, Baer L, Minichiello WE. Chicago, IL, Year Book Medical Publishers, 1990, pp. 325–340

This chapter presents the authors' preliminary results from their study evaluating the efficacy of an eight-session, multiple-family psychoeducational support group for obsessive-compulsive disorder. The chapter includes excellent clinical illustrations of the impact of obsessive-compulsive disorder on patients and families as well as a detailed description of topics and process issues covered in each multiple-family group session.

30. **Miklowitz DJ, Goldstein MY:** Behavioral family treatment for patients with bipolar affective disorder. *Behav Modif* 14:457–489, 1990

This article is another excellent example of how to adapt psychoeducational models developed for schizophrenia to the unique needs of other psychiatric disorders. The authors discuss in detail the specific needs and characteristics of families of patients with bipolar disorder and present an educational, skill-building model based on the work of Falloon and colleagues with patients with schizophrenia.

40

Cognitive Psychotherapy

Aaron T. Beck, M.D.
Deborah Clark, B.A.

The following readings provide a comprehensive introduction to the therapy and practice of cognitive therapy. Cognitive psychotherapy is an active, time-limited, structured approach used to treat a variety of psychiatric problems (e.g., depression, anxiety, phobias, personality disorders, and substance abuse). It is based on the cognitive model of psychopathology. The key assumption is that individuals' affect and behavior are largely determined by the way in which they structure their experiences. The thesis of this model of psychopathology is that emotional disorders are related to cognitive distortions (or systematic errors in thinking) and dysfunctional beliefs. For example, the thinking of depressed patients is dominated by a negative view of themselves, their experiences, and their future that is maintained by errors in the way they infer, recollect, and generalize information.

A variety of cognitive, behavioral, and experiential strategies are utilized in cognitive therapy. The cognitive techniques are aimed at delineating and testing the individual's specific misconceptions and dysfunctional beliefs. This approach consists of highly specific learning experiences designed to teach patients the following operations: 1) to monitor their negative or distorted thoughts; 2) to recognize the connection between cognition, affect, and behavior; 3) to examine the evidence, for and against, and to test misinterpretations empirically; 4) to substitute more reality-oriented interpretations for these biased cognitions; and 5) to learn to identify and alter the dysfunctional beliefs that predispose them to distort their experiences. The therapy focuses on specific "target symptoms" (e.g., suicidal impulses). The beliefs supporting these symptoms are identified (e.g., "My life is worthless and I can't change it.") and then subjected to logical and empirical investigation. Experiential strategies include imaging, role playing, and recreating traumatic childhood incidents.

In addition to texts that provide a clear account of the above-outlined cognitive theory and treatment procedures, the bibliography includes readings on the application of cognitive therapy to suicide, depression, anxiety, personality disorders, and stress as well as readings comparing cognitive psychotherapy to pharmacotherapy and behavior therapy.

1. **Beck AT:** *Depression: Causes and Treatment.* Philadelphia, PA, University of Pennsylvania Press, 1970

   This classic work elegantly describes depression both theoretically and clinically and provides experimental corroboration. It not only outlines cognitive therapy but also reviews other influential theories of depression. Finally, the cognitive treatment for depression is introduced and compared and contrasted with therapies based on the other models.

2. **Beck AT:** *Cognitive Therapy and the Emotional Disorders.* New York, International Universities Press, 1976

   The philosophical and theoretical basis of cognitive therapy is established and then applied to a wide range of specific disorders: depression, anxiety neurosis, phobias, obsessions, compulsions, hysteria, and psychosomatic disorders. This is an excellent general introduction to cognitive therapy.

3. **Beck AT:** Cognitive approaches to panic disorder: theory and therapy, in *Panic: Psychological Perspectives.* Edited by Rochman S, Maser J. Hillsdale, NJ, Lawrence Erlbaum, 1987, pp. 91–109

   In this chapter, Beck describes the cognitive model of panic disorder. This model is based on the clinical observation that panic-prone patients are highly sensitive to the experience of any physical sensation or mental state that cannot be dismissed as normal. The cognitive model helps these patients to use their reason or prior information to correct the misinterpretations of their sensations. Beck describes the different steps that are involved in the cognitive treatment of panic disorder.

4. **Beck AT:** *Love Is Never Enough.* New York, Harper & Row, 1988

   Beck analyzes actual dialogue to illuminate the most common problems experienced by couples: the power of negative thinking, disillusionment, rigid rules and expectations, and miscommunication. This book is the first to make the insights and techniques of cognitive therapy applied to relationship problems available to the general reader.

5. **Beck AT:** Cognitive therapy: a 30-year retrospective. *Am Psychol* 46:299–307, 1991

In this article, Beck returns to answer his question from 1976: "Can a fledgling psychotherapy challenge the giants in the field—psychoanalysis and behavior therapy?" A large number of studies have been conducted in the past three decades to test the cognitive model of depression and other disorders. The cognitive model of depression has led to the development of treatments for a wide variety of disorders.

6. **Beck AT:** Cognitive approaches to stress, in *Principles and Practice of Stress Management,* 2nd Edition. Edited by Woolfolk R, Lehrer P. New York, Guilford, 1993, pp. 333–372

In this excellent, comprehensive chapter for theoretical understanding and practical management of stress, Beck conceptualizes a clinical case in terms of the outlined principles and uses it to illustrate specific therapeutic strategies and techniques.

7. **Beck JS:** *Cognitive Therapy: Basics and Beyond.* New York, Guilford (in press)

This is an outstanding primer for novice cognitive therapists.

8. **Beck AT, Freeman A (and associates):** *Cognitive Therapy of Personality Disorders.* New York, Guilford, 1990

This ground-breaking work effectively brings cognitive therapy to bear on a most difficult clinical problem: the treatment of personality disorders. Regardless of primary orientation, all clinicians who work with personality-disordered clients will be well served by this volume. Researchers will find this work interesting; graduate-level courses will be enhanced by its use as a text.

9. **Beck AT, Rush AJ:** Cognitive therapy, in *Comprehensive Textbook of Psychiatry/VI,* 6th Edition. Edited by Kaplan HI, Sadock BJ. Baltimore, MD, Williams & Wilkins (in press)

This chapter discusses the basic premises of cognitive therapy and the theories on which it is based. Beck and Rush present the theory that cognitive therapy is based on a conceptualization of psychopathology that draws from cognitive and social psychology, information-processing theory, and psychoanalytic theory. The authors have found that cognitive therapy can be considered, either alone or in combination with pharmacotherapy, for a variety of psychological conditions.

10. **Beck AT, Rush AJ, Shaw BF, Emery G:** *Cognitive Therapy of Depression.* New York, Guilford, 1979

This definitive volume on the cognitive therapy of depression proceeds from a clear, succinct explication of cognitive therapy to a step-by-step demonstration of cognitive techniques—from initial session to termination. A full range of patient problems is discussed, and numerous case examples illustrate scenarios and strategies. The work is completed by valuable appendixes, including copies of many widely used diagnostic scales.

11. **Beck AT, Emery G, Greenberg RL:** *Anxiety Disorders and Phobias: A Cognitive Perspective.* New York, Basic Books, 1985

This comprehensive work lays the groundwork for the cognitive therapy of anxiety disorders. In part 1, Beck outlines an explanatory model, demonstrating how specific nonadaptive cognitive patterns lead to the complex symptoms of generalized anxiety disorder, simple phobias, and agoraphobia. In part 2, Emery presents a program for treating these disorders based on the cognitive model.

12. **Beck AT, Resnick HLP, Lettieri DJ:** *The Prediction of Suicide.* Philadelphia, PA, Charles Press, 1986

This book focuses on crucial issues for the therapist, such as how to determine whether a person is suicidal and when and how the mental health professional should intervene. Topics include prediction models, variables for assessing suicidal risk, depression and suicide, and development of suicidal intent scales.

13. **Beck AT, Brown GK, Berchick RJ, Stewart B, Steer RA:** Relationship between hopelessness and ultimate suicide: a replication with psychiatric outpatients. *Am J Psychiatry* 147:190–195, 1990

This study identifies a number of variables that may prove to be predictors of eventual suicide, including previous suicide attempts, previous psychiatric hospitalizations, a high level of depression, a diagnosis of major affective disorder, and the presence of suicidal ideation. Hopelessness, depression, and suicidal ideation are subject to modification through cognitive psychotherapy.

14. **Beck AT, Wright FD, Newman CF:** Cocaine abuse, in *Comprehensive Casebook of Cognitive Therapy.* Edited by Freeman A, Dattilio FM. New York, Plenum, 1992, pp. 185–192

This chapter outlines the cognitive model of drug use and explains how this model can be used to change the beliefs of the patient using cocaine. The chapter also explains how these beliefs can become more complex over prolonged cocaine use; treatment is aimed at modifying each separate category of beliefs: anticipatory, craving, and permissive/facilitating.

15. **Beck AT, Sokol L, Clark DA, Berchick R, Wright F:** A crossover study of focused cognitive therapy for panic disorder. *Am J Psychiatry* 149:778–783, 1992

   This crossover study for panic disorder showed that focused cognitive therapy offers a nonpharmacological alternative for panic disorder. This is important because although panic disorder has been shown to be effectively treated pharmacologically, there are certain problems such as resistance to medication, side effects, and relapse. At 1-year follow-up, 87% of the group who received cognitive therapy remained free of panic attacks.

16. **Beck AT, Wright FD, Newman CF, Liese BS:** *Cognitive Therapy of Substance Abuse.* New York, Guilford, 1993

   This volume covers rationale for therapy, therapist guidelines, techniques and their applications, symptom relief, management of substance abuse and dependency, resocialization, dysfunctional addictive beliefs, special problems, strategies for the modification of antisocial behavior, and how to counteract therapist "burnout."

17. **Dobson KS:** A meta-analysis of the efficacy of cognitive therapy for depression. *J Consult Clin Psychol* 57:414–419, 1989

   This article reviews the effectiveness of Beck's cognitive therapy for depression using the meta-analysis format. Dobson identifies 28 studies that used a common outcome measure of depression and compares cognitive therapy with other therapeutic modalities. Dobson's results show a greater degree of improvement among cognitive therapy patients compared with a waiting list or no-treatment control group as well as other psychotherapies. Dobson also discusses the implications for further outcome and process studies in cognitive therapy.

18. **Haaga DAF, Dyck MJ, Ernst D:** Empirical status of cognitive theory of depression. *Psychol Bull* 110:215–236, 1991

   This article reviews studies that test the cognitive theory of depression and define depression as a clinical syndrome. Haaga et al. describe that depressive persons have a particular way of thinking that has been substantiated empirically. However, they raise the point that the theory that depressive thinking is illogical or inaccurate lacks evidence.

19. **Layden M, Newman CF, Freeman A, Morse SB:** *Cognitive Therapy of Borderline Personality Disorder.* Des Moines, IA, Allyn & Bacon, 1993

This book is written by four associates of Beck and provides the first comprehensive practitioner's guide to using cognitive therapy techniques for patients diagnosed with borderline personality disorder. It skillfully covers all the important facets of advanced cognitive therapy in detail. It is the first text in cognitive-behavioral literature to integrate Eriksonian and Piagetian developmental theories into the understanding of the etiology of this population. This informative text includes a discussion of pharmacological therapy and a proposal of three borderline personality disorder subtypes to aid in case conceptualization and treatment. It also provides five extensive illustrative case studies.

20. **Shea MT, Elkin I, Imber SD, Sotsky SM, Watkins JT, Collins JF, Pilkonis PA, Beckham E, Glass DR, Dolan RT, Parloff MB:** Course of depressive symptoms over follow-up: findings from the National Institute of Mental Health treatment of depression collaborative research program. Arch Gen Psychiatry 49:782–787, 1992

Shea et al. report on the course of depressive symptoms over an 18-month naturalistic, follow-up period for outpatients with major depressive disorder treated in the National Institute of Mental Health Treatment of Depression Collaborative Research Program. The treatment consisted of 16 weeks of cognitive-behavioral therapy, interpersonal therapy, imipramine plus clinical management, or placebo plus clinical management. Most importantly, this work highlights the fact that 16 weeks of these types of treatment are not sufficient for most patients to achieve and maintain full recovery.

21. **Weishaar ME, Beck AT:** Clinical and cognitive predictors of suicide, in *Assessment and Prediction of Suicide.* Edited by Maris RW, Berman AL, Maltsberger JT, Yufit RI. New York, Guilford, 1992, pp. 467–483

In this chapter, Weishaar and Beck identify the clinical risk factors that may help avert suicide in the individual patient. They also discuss some of the cognitive characteristics of suicidal individuals. Beck presents his model of suicidal behavior, which includes hopelessness as the key psychological variable. The majority of the chapter is based on cognitive therapy research.

22. **Wright JH, Thase ME, Beck AT, Ludgate JW** (eds): *Cognitive Therapy With Inpatients: Developing a Cognitive Milieu.* New York, Guilford, 1992

This book is specifically devoted to applying Beck's cognitive model of depression to the treatment of the inpatient population. An overview of Beck's model of depression is presented. The historical background of cognitive therapy is discussed as well as the fundamental principles of cognitive therapy. The relevant treatment data from outpatient studies of clinical depression will be summarized and applied to the cognitive therapy in inpatient settings. The theory is presented that the features of cognitive therapy make it well suited for hospitalized patients.

41

Brief Psychotherapy

Deborah Fried, M.D.

In medicine, politics, the media, and fashion, brevity is the current zeitgeist. Psychotherapy is no exception, and not only for the financial constraints that mitigate against time-unlimited treatments. There are powerful therapeutic advantages to time-limited or brief psychotherapy, benefits well described by the literature annotated below.

Two features render brief therapy a discrete treatment modality: an a priori time limit and a focus for the psychotherapy. Both time and focus allow therapist and patient to harness their skills and collaborate actively to increase understanding and ameliorate pain. The time limit is generally in the range of 6–40 sessions. Treatment foci vary according to the school of brief therapy. Major depression, Oedipal conflict, and obsessional rituals have all been considered proper targets for brief therapy strategies.

The literature on brief therapy is a pleasure; it exemplifies some of the clearest and most persuasive writing in psychiatry. This chapter includes some more recent writing, especially in the area of individual supportive psychotherapy. As the literature on family and group brief therapy has expanded, so has this listing of contributions. The writings of Malan, Mann, Sifneos, and Davanloo continue to be included, because they remain the bedrock of dynamic brief therapy. Beck, represented elsewhere in this volume (Beck and Clark, Chapter 40), has a place in this chapter, given that cognitive therapy is a time-limited effort.

This chapter is divided into six sections. The first includes research studies and historically based overviews of brief therapy. Individual treatments are next considered and are divided into dynamic, supportive, and other types (including cognitive-behavioral therapies). A section on couples and family treatment is included, following readings on brief group therapies.

Overview and Research

1. *Budman SH, Gurman AS: The practice of brief therapy: an introduction, in *Theory and Practice of Brief Therapy*. Edited by Budman SH, Gurman AS. New York, Guilford, 1988, pp. 1–25

This is one of the best historical reviews of the brief psychotherapy literature from Freud through Ferenczi and Rank, Alexander and French, Lindemann, the 1960s community mental health center laws, and the current wave of time-limited psychotherapy. It is helpful to trainees for its delineation of long-term versus short-term therapy techniques, treatment goals, and patient selection.

2. Crits-Christoph P: The efficacy of brief dynamic psychotherapy: a meta-analysis. *Am J Psychiatry* 149:151–158, 1992

A carefully prepared analysis of the more thoroughly researched brief dynamic therapies, this study demonstrates large effect sizes when dynamic brief therapies are compared with "no-treatment" but only slight superiority of the dynamic brief treatments over nondynamic interventions such as clinical management.

3. Freud S: Analysis terminable and interminable (1937), in *The Standard Edition of the Complete Psychological Works of Sigmund Freud*, Vol. 23. Translated and edited by Strachey J. London, Hogarth Press, 1956, pp. 216–253

Lest brief therapy be thought of as "new," this work is included as a reminder that the issues surrounding ending treatment in a timely fashion have long been a part of psychodynamic thinking. The mutative effects of treatment are considered with caution; the chapter offers a sobering comment on the power and limitations of psychoanalysis.

4. Gustafson JP: *The Complex Secret of Brief Psychotherapy*. New York, WW Norton, 1986

The first half of this book is an in-depth history of the brief therapies. The second half offers pragmatic and theoretical details of Gustafson's own method of helping a patient remedy the persistent, painful recapitulation of the patient's own past in his or her present experience.

5. **Horowitz M:** The history of brief dynamic psychotherapy, in *Personality Styles and Brief Psychotherapy.* New York, Basic Books, 1990, pp. 3–33

   A remarkably thorough explication of each of the major schools of dynamic brief therapy plus a section on cognitive treatment, this chapter summarizes research on outcome of brief therapy.

6. **Koss M:** Research on brief psychotherapy, in *Handbook of Psychotherapy and Behavior Change,* 3rd Edition. Edited by Garfield SL, Bergin AE. New York, Wiley, 1986, pp. 627–670

   Koss offers a comprehensive overview of the major schools of brief therapy. Essential features of brief therapy are explained, and empirical studies of process and outcome are critically reviewed.

7. **Phillips EL:** *A Guide for Therapists and Patients to Short-Term Therapy.* Springfield, IL, Charles C Thomas, 1985

   Phillips offers theoretical information about the various sorts of currently practiced short-term treatments, including psychodynamic, behavioral, cognitive, Rogerian, humanistic, and rational-emotive. The book includes an interesting section on alternative approaches such as "body-therapy," bio-energetics, and Morita (a Japanese psychotherapy).

8. *Sifneos PE:** Brief psychotherapy and crisis intervention, in *Comprehensive Textbook of Psychiatry/II,* 3rd Edition, Vol. 2. Edited by Kaplan HI, Friedman AM, Saddock BJ. Baltimore, MD, Williams & Wilkins, 1980, pp. 2247–2256

   This is one of the best schemas for deciding what treatment best suits a patient: brief therapy versus crisis intervention, and anxiety-suppressive versus anxiety-provoking treatment. Never offered in subsequent revisions of the textbook, this chapter is very helpful for trainees learning the arts of triage and time-limited intervention.

9. **Sledge WH, Moras K, Hartly D, Levine M:** Effect of time-limited psychotherapy on patient dropout rates. *Am J Psychiatry* 147:1341–1347, 1990

   This article reports on a study demonstrating the fundamental efficacy of predetermined treatment time limits: patients do not leave treatment as often as they do in open-ended treatment. This lesson has yet to be heeded in the public and private sectors.

10. **Wells RA, Phelps PA:** The brief psychotherapies: a selective overview, in *Handbook of the Brief Psychotherapies.* Edited by Wells RA, Gianetti VJ. New York, Plenum, 1990, pp. 3–26

In this well-researched chapter on the varieties of brief treatments, including behavioral, family, and psychodynamic individual, emphasis is placed on the especially high level of therapist activity that, along with treatment focus and time limit, are the sine qua non of brief therapy. Attention is paid to the political and commercial aspects of brief therapy in the 1990s.

Individual Dynamic Brief Therapy

11. **Alexander F, French TM:** Efficacy of brief contact, in *Psychoanalytic Therapy: Principles and Application.* New York, Ronald Press, 1946, pp. 145–164; **Alexander F, French TM:** The principle of flexibility, in *Psychoanalytic Therapy: Principles and Application.* New York, Ronald Press, 1946, pp. 25–65; **Alexander F, French TM:** The principle of corrective emotional experience, in *Psychoanalytic Therapy: Principles and Application.* New York, Ronald Press, 1946, pp. 66–70

Three cases of very brief treatment (3 sessions) are presented. "Efficacy of Brief Contact" is important as a catalyst "to investigate the therapeutic possibilities of briefer procedures based on psychoanalytic knowledge and experience" (p. 146). Good illustrations of the possibility, with a right match between patient and therapist, for lasting work that can be accomplished in only 3 hours, are provided.

"The Principle of Flexibility" advocates that the therapist consider altering aspects of the treatment (e.g., length of treatment, frequency of sessions, intensity of emotional involvement, interruptions, and termination), with an understanding that deviations from "standard" analytic technique may be in the patient's best interest.

"The Principle of Corrective Emotional Experience" formalizes a concept that is often considered a mainstay of the therapeutic encounter: the corrective emotional experience. The vehicle is the tale of Jean Valjean, which demonstrates a man's profound change after a new interpersonal experience.

12. **Bauer GD, Kobos JC:** *Brief Therapy: Short Term Psychodynamic Intervention.* Northvale, NJ, Jason Aronson, 1987

An integration of the work of Sifneos (selection criteria), Malan (using the triangles of insight and conflict), and Davanloo ("relentless" interpretation of resistance), this book is well written and true to these pioneers of brief therapy.

13. **Bloom BL:** Focused single session therapy: initial development and evaluation, in *Forms of Brief Therapy.* Edited by Budman SH. New York, Guilford, 1981, pp. 167–216

This work offers perhaps the best remedy for brief therapy skeptics. Bloom details the considerable accomplishments rendered in one prolonged sitting with a patient. In this heavily annotated transcript, he shows us as much from his "mistakes" as from his correct moves.

14. **Davanloo HB:** A method of short-term dynamic psychotherapy, in *Short-Term Dynamic Psychotherapy*. Edited by Davanloo HB. Northvale, NJ, Jason Aronson, 1980, pp. 43–71

A pioneer of dynamic brief therapy, Davanloo's trademark lies in being "relentless." This attitude toward questioning, clarifying, and interpreting speeds the treatment along, with immediate and continual attention to transference. The Menninger triangles of conflict and person are explained and demonstrated as is his whole technique in vivid case examples.

15. **Horowitz M, Marmar C, Krupnick J, Wilner N, Kaltreider N, Wallerstein R:** Our approach to brief therapy: focused on current stressors, in *Personality Styles and Brief Psychotherapy*. New York, Basic Books, 1984, pp. 34–50

A how-to, summarizing Horowitz's 12-session approach to the treatment of acute stress reactions, this chapter offers a psychodynamic and practical guideline to how the therapist and patient experience and behave in such a treatment.

16. **Klerman GL, Weissman MM, Rounsaville BJ, Chevron ES:** *Interpersonal Psychotherapy of Depression*. New York, Basic Books, 1984

A presentation of focal, time-limited interpersonal treatment that deals nearly exclusively with the patient's current life, this book is written in a straightforward, pragmatic style, demonstrating how to put into operation the supportive elements of clarification, reassurance, and reality testing. Depression is understood to be a problem of interpersonal relations rather than a manifestation of internal conflict.

17. **Luborsky L:** *Principles of Psychoanalytic Psychotherapy*. New York, Basic Books, 1984

Deceptively simple, the richness of this text seems proportional to one's amount of clinical experience. As a training manual, the book is applicable to both time-limited and time-unlimited therapies. Supportive and expressive techniques are described. Throughout the book, the "core conflictual relationship theme" method of formulating patients' main relationship problems is discussed as a research, clinical, and educational tool.

18. ****Malan DH:** *The Frontier of Brief Psychotherapy.* New York, Plenum, 1976

One of the brief therapy classics, this book views the field from the larger picture of psychotherapy in general to the details of specific statements a brief therapist might make to a patient. It starts with an excellent historical overview, includes Malan's research on brief therapy, and offers many clinical examples.

19. **Malan DH:** *Individual Psychotherapy and the Science of Psychodynamics.* London, Butterworth, 1979

A clearly written how-to book, excellent for the novice yet not at all simple, this book is applicable to any length of treatment. Psychodynamic principles are put into action in a refreshingly lucid way.

20. ****Mann J:** *Time Limited Psychotherapy.* Boston, MA, Harvard University Press, 1973

In some circles, this book is still "the bible" of dynamic brief therapy. A poetic chapter on time sets the tone for the ensuing work that depicts 12-session treatment. Whom to treat, how to treat them, and how to teach this kind of therapy are explained and then depicted via a lengthy case report. The book demonstrates the derivation of a treatment focus, the articulation of that focus to the patient, and how adherence to the focus throughout treatment is critical. Termination is seen as a recapitulation of a patient's previous experience with loss, offering a unique opportunity for the patient to learn.

21. **Mann J, Goldman R:** *A Casebook in Time-Limited Psychotherapy.* Washington, DC, American Psychiatric Press, 1982

Coming nearly a decade after Mann's well-known first book (Mann 1973) above, this text stands on its own. Half of the 10 chapters are devoted to explaining Mann's theory of dynamic change via the treatment of a carefully chosen central issue. Five cases are presented, with excerpts of session transcripts that colorfully assist the reader in envisioning this kind of treatment process.

22. ****Schafer R:** The termination of brief psychoanalytic psychotherapy. *International Journal of Psychoanalytic Psychotherapy* 2:135–148, 1973

This article is a beautifully crafted statement of the power of analytic brief treatment, seen with special clarity during termination. The newly understood continuity and historicity of the patient's life fosters self-understanding, a main treatment goal.

23. ****Sifneos PE:** *Short-Term Dynamic Psychotherapy.* New York, Plenum, 1987

What is unique to Sifneos is his readiness to induce and then utilize patients' anxiety. Admittedly appropriate for only a select group of patients, this kind of treatment aims to resolve Oedipal difficulties. Theory and case notes are lucidly presented.

24. **Strupp H, Binder JL:** The dynamic focus, in *Psychotherapy in a New Key.* New York, Basic Books, 1984, pp. 65–109; **Strupp H, Binder JL:** Technique, in *Psychotherapy in a New Key.* New York, Basic Books, 1984, pp. 135–194

"The Dynamic Focus" explains the focus of dynamic brief therapy as a jointly (therapist and patient) derived understanding of the patient's repetitive and maladaptive interactions. Both the patient's narrative and relationship with the therapist contribute to discerning the focus. Fairly detailed clinical examples are offered.

In "Technique," the present-day, in-session recreation of outdated, faulty learning is discussed as the modus operandi for this kind of treatment. Explicit guidelines for therapist's interventions are given and exemplary cases offered.

Individual Supportive Brief Therapy

Although all psychotherapy should be experienced by the patient as generally supportive, some techniques are explicitly geared to lessen anxiety, whereas others (e.g., Sifneos, above) use increased anxiety to catalyze therapeutic work and change. Below are readings about therapies for patients considered too disturbed to benefit from the generation of anxiety as a therapeutic tool.

25. **Kernberg OK:** Supportive psychotherapy, in *Severe Personality Disorders.* New Haven, CT, Yale University Press, 1984, pp. 147–164

Not just about brief therapy, this chapter offers a refreshingly clear explanation of how a dynamically oriented therapist undertakes supportive treatment (e.g., evaluating and understanding but not interpreting transference). This work is useful for dynamically trained therapists developing their skills of supportive, time-limited work.

26. **Malan DH:** Partial foci in more disturbed patients, in *The Frontier of Brief Psychotherapy.* New York, Plenum, 1976, pp. 297–320

This chapter considers how to treat those patients we would usually not presume to treat with a time limit in mind—those with borderline, paranoid, and other types of character pathology. Detailed case notes are presented, and interpretations are explained with care. This is an excellent teaching chapter.

27. **Rockland LH:** Choosing the appropriate supportive-exploratory mix, in *Supportive Psychotherapy: A Psychodynamic Approach.* New York, Basic Books, 1989, pp. 253–273

   Rockland includes a presentation of three cases illustrative of supportive strategies in time-limited therapy and demonstrates the combination of a dynamic focus with a noninterpretive approach.

28. **Werman DS:** *The Practice of Supportive Psychotherapy.* New York, Brunner/Mazel, 1984

   This is another resource that is not specifically about brief therapy but is one of the few texts about supportive psychotherapy. The techniques described are particularly apt for the brief therapist. Sections on the treatment of distinct characterologic types are included.

Other Types of Individual Brief Therapy

29. **Beck AT, Rush AJ, Shaw BF, Emery G:** An overview, in *Cognitive Therapy of Depression.* Edited by Beck AT, Rush AJ, Shaw BF, Emery G. New York, Guilford, 1979, pp. 1–33

   This is an important resource for two reasons. First is the novelty of the central idea of cognitive therapy: that depression consists of a negative cognitive triad (i.e., idiosyncratic and exclusively negative views of the self, the future, and current experiences). Second, there is a good amount of empirical support for the efficacy of this type of brief treatment. The overview chapter articulates the basic premises of cognitive causes and treatments of depression.

30. **Garfield SL:** *The Practice of Brief Psychotherapy.* Elmsford, NY, Pergamon, 1989

   This is a manual-style book on Garfield's own melange of dynamic, cognitive, and behavioral techniques. Special attention is paid to therapist activities, the initial interview, posttherapy considerations, and research on brief psychotherapy.

31. **Winston A** (ed): *Clinical and Research Issues in Short-Term Dynamic Psychotherapy.* Washington, DC, American Psychiatric Press, 1985

   This monograph explains the Beth Israel (New York) clinical and research project on two forms of brief therapy: 1) Davanloo's model and 2) "brief adaption oriented psychotherapy," a Beth Israel model much like Sifneos' but with emphasis on cognition rather than transference.

Short-Term Group Therapies

32. **Budman SH, Bennett MJ, Wisneski MJ:** An adult developmental model of short-term group psychotherapy, in *Forms of Brief Therapy.* Edited by Budman SH. New York, Guilford, 1981, pp. 305–342

The theoretical and technical aspects of the "Harvard Community Health Plan" short-term groups are described. Three age-determined groups are conducted (20s, 30–50, over 50), each focusing on age-related issues.

33. **Garvin CD:** Short term group therapy, in *Handbook of the Brief Psychotherapies.* Edited by Wells RA, Gianetti VJ. New York, Plenum, 1990, pp. 513–536

This chapter considers how individual change comes about via patients' experimentation with different behaviors in the group, followed by transferring their successes to other situations.

34. **MacKenzie KR:** *Introduction to Time-Limited Group Psychotherapy.* Washington, DC, American Psychiatric Press, 1990

This book is written for therapists experienced in treating individuals. The approach uses systems theory, social psychology, learning theory, and interpersonal psychodynamic theory.

35. **Sabin JE:** Short-term group psychotherapy: historical antecedents, in *Forms of Brief Therapy.* Edited by Budman SH. New York, Guilford, 1981, pp. 271–282

A refreshingly candid history of T-groups and encounter groups, leading up to an introduction of dynamically oriented brief therapy groups.

36. **Yalom ID:** *The Theory and Practice of Group Psychotherapy,* 2nd Edition. New York, Basic Books, 1975

Not specifically about time-limited therapy, but important to any group therapist and the best known book about group psychotherapy, this book is replete with clinical examples. Special attention is paid to the tasks and techniques of the group therapist as facilitator of the group, which is itself the agent of change.

Short-Term Treatment for Couples and Families

37. **Epstein NB, Bishop DS, Keitner GI:** A systems therapy: problem centered systems therapy for the family, in *Handbook of the Brief Psychothera-*

pies. Edited by Wells RA, Gianetti VJ. New York, Plenum, 1990, pp. 405–436

The McMaster model of family functioning is described, where the family is seen as an open system consisting of many other interdependent systems (individual, marital, school, industrial, religious). Treatment techniques of assessment, problem clarification, contracting, task setting, and evaluation are described.

38. **Gurman AS:** Integrative marital therapy, in *Forms of Brief Therapy.* Edited by Budman SH. New York, Guilford, 1981, pp. 415–457

In this compelling discussion of three approaches to marital therapy (dynamic, behavioral, and systems), it is argued that a psychodynamic foundation can link these into an integrative approach that addresses multiple levels and domains of the marital relationship.

39. *Kinston W, Bentovim A:** Creating a focus for brief marital or family therapy, in *Forms of Brief Therapy.* Edited by Budman SH. New York, Guilford, 1981, pp. 361–386

This chapter covers one of the essential elements of brief therapy: how to determine a treatment focus. Although oriented specifically toward families and couples, the ideas are relevant also to individual treatments. David Malan is a main reference; his ideas permeate the chapter.

40. **Kreilkamp T:** *Time Limited, Intermittent Therapy With Children and Families.* New York, Brunner/Mazel, 1989

Kreilkamp explains the system of family therapy offered at the "Harvard Community Health Plan," with a theory derived from analytic, cognitive, behavioral, systems, and other schools. How theory drives clinical practice is described, emphasizing therapist activity.

41. **Minuchin S:** *Families and Family Therapy.* Boston, MA, Harvard University Press, 1974

Minuchin created "structural family therapy"—not so billed, but essentially a brief therapy because of the usual treatment length of 12 sessions. In this therapy, each individual is understood in the family context; treatment goals are basically symptom relief; and families return as needed.

42. **Sager C:** *Marriage Contracts and Couples Therapy.* New York, Brunner/Mazel, 1976

Sager introduces a compelling concept, that of the marriage contract: the overt and covert deals partners usually unwittingly make with each other. Treatment length ranges from 1 to 50 sessions, spaced weekly at first and, if indicated, at increasing intervals thereafter. The therapist and couple agree on homework assignments aimed to facilitate new ways of thinking about and behaving in the couple's relationship.

42

Crisis Intervention and Emergency Psychiatry

Howard C. Blue, M.D.

E
mergency psychiatry and crisis intervention comprise overlapping areas of clinical practice. An emotional crisis may be precipitated whenever a person is confronted with an imbalance between a perceived life difficulty and their available capacity to cope and adapt. The state of crisis that evolves from this imbalance may reach dramatic and even life-threatening proportions. Frequently, loss, stress, and trauma pose great risk for the development of a state of emotional crisis that may bring the person to the attention of mental health professionals. Events leading to the emotional changes that constitute crises are significantly varied. Some are intensely individual (e.g., rape, spousal battering), whereas others may involve entire communities (e.g., natural disasters). The suggested readings in this chapter reflect this variability. A practitioner's interventions for people in crisis must be guided by a generic set of principles that reflect an understanding of common human responses to stress and trauma, but also respect the specific nuances of an individual's experiences. Although the selection of readings on this topic cannot reflect the full range of crisis events that may bring a person to the attention of a mental health professional, these readings may help underscore some basic principles of practice and decision making that may lead to effective interventions. The readings in this chapter were selected to

provide a firm foundation in the theory, phenomenology, and clinical practice of emergency psychiatry and crisis intervention.

Definition of and Selection Criteria for Crisis Intervention

1. *Clarkin JF, Frances A:** selection criteria for the brief psychotherapies. *Am J Psychother* 36:166–180, 1982

   This article gives brief overviews of five forms of brief psychotherapy with emphasis on therapeutic indications, contraindications, and patient-enabling factors. Case examples help to illustrate the clinical rationale for specific interventions.

2. **Jacobson GF, Strickler M, Morley WE:** Generic and individual approaches to crisis intervention. *Am J Public Health* 58:338–343, 1968

   This article provides a concise definition of crisis and the role of specific kinds of therapeutic intervention. The authors use case examples to examine two different approaches to treatment intervention. The generic approach focuses on the characteristic course a particular crisis follows and the development of a treatment plan aimed toward adaptation. The individual approach focuses on the intrapsychic and interpersonal processes of the person in crisis.

3. **Klar H:** The setting for psychiatric treatment, in *Psychiatry Update: American Psychiatric Association Annual Review,* Vol. 6. Edited by Hales RE, Frances AJ, Washington, DC, American Psychiatric Press, 1987, pp. 336–352

   This chapter provides a brief overview of selection criteria, clinical considerations, and research data on a range of treatment options including crisis intervention.

Models of Practice of Crisis Intervention

4. *Ewing CP:** A model for the clinical practice of crisis intervention as psychotherapy, in *Crisis Intervention as Psychotherapy.* New York, Oxford University Press, 1978, pp. 93–118

   Ewing presents a set of guidelines for conducting crisis intervention that emphasizes six stages: problem delineation, evaluation, contracting, intervening, termination, and follow-up. Each stage is discussed, and cases are presented for further explication of the model.

5. *Glick RA, Meyerson AT: The use of psychoanalytic concepts in crisis intervention. *International Journal of Psychoanalysis and Psychotherapy* 8:171–188, 1980–1981

The authors view crises as opportunities to observe significant character patterns that contribute to and lead to the crisis situation. They suggest that an adequate view of crises consists of both the present reality and vulnerabilities to stress that are dictated by past neurotic conflicts and ego dysfunction.

6. Nichols NH: Crisis intervention through early interpretation of unconscious guilt. *Bull Menninger Clin* 53:115–122, 1989

Nichols presents an approach to crisis intervention based on the assumption that a person's crisis reconfirms pathogenic and conflictual beliefs and increases unconscious guilt. Nichols suggests and demonstrates through case examples that interpreting that unconscious guilt may lead to crisis resolution and incipient character change.

The Effects of Loss, Stress, and Trauma

7. *Caplan G: Loss, stress, and mental health. *Community Ment Health J* 26:27–48, 1990

Caplan, one of the early theorists on the nature of crises, presents an overview of the effect of loss and stress on mental health. This article gives the reader some "precise ideas about mechanisms connecting loss with changes in mental health" (p. 45) and about the rationale for techniques of crisis intervention.

8. *Flannery RB, Harvey MR: Psychological trauma and learned helplessness: Seligman's paradigm reconsidered. *Psychotherapy* 28:374–378, 1991

The authors attempt to explain the variability in individual differences arising from traumatic events and use Seligman's paradigm of learned helplessness as explanation of some of the behavioral features found in traumatized individuals.

9. *Lindeman E: Symptomatology and management of acute grief. *Am J Psychiatry* 101:141–148, 1944

In this seminal work on the processes of bereavement, Lindeman was able to define a syndrome of normal grief reaction in people who had lost loved ones in the Coconut Grove Fire as well as atypical grief responses. This work laid the foundation for the author's subsequent efforts in studying the impact of maladaptive bereavement on the development of mental disorders.

10. *__Rutter M:__ Stress, coping, and development: some issues and some questions, in *Stress, Coping, and Development in Children*. Edited by Garmezy N, Rutter M. New York, McGraw-Hill, 1983, pp. 1–41

    Rutter poses a series of questions about the nature of stress and coping and their influence on psychological development. His questions vividly illustrate the complexity of the topic and clarify elements of the discussion that require further study. This chapter is an important model for thinking about the effects of stress on human development and mental health.

11. __Sable P:__ Attachment, anxiety, and loss of a husband. *Am J Orthopsychiatry* 59:550–556, 1989

    A retrospective, self-reported study of 81 women widowed for 1–3 years found support for the hypothesis that childhood experiences of separation and loss or threats of abandonment contributed to greater anxiety and depression in bereavement.

Specific Crisis Events and Patterns of Response

12. *__Burgess AW, Holmstrom LL:__ Rape trauma syndrome. *Am J Psychiatry* 131:981–986, 1974

    In this examination of 92 victims of forcible rape, this article describes manifestations and variations of the rape trauma syndrome and describes management of the syndrome.

13. *__Green BL, Lindy JD, Grace MC, Gleser GC, Leonard AC, Korol M, Winget C:__ Buffalo Creek survivors in the second decade: stability of stress symptoms. *Am J Orthopsychiatry* 60:43–54, 1990

    This follow-up study of 120 adult survivors of the Buffalo Creek disaster provides evidence of gradual decrease in psychological symptoms and an improvement of functioning for persons suffering a traumatic event. Additionally, there was a demonstration of the late onset of posttraumatic stress disorder (PTSD) in 11% of the sample. An interesting and unexplained phenomenon was the apparent increased risk of late-onset PTSD in blacks and the decreased likelihood of their recovery from PTSD.

14. *Herman JL: Child abuse, in *Trauma and Recovery*. New York, Basic Books, 1992, pp. 96–114

This chapter gives compelling insights on the damage that child abuse can produce and the ways that childhood abuse can become manifest in adulthood. Herman explores the psychic strain faced by children who grow up in environments where they must "find a way to preserve a sense of trust in people who are untrustworthy, safety in a situation that is unsafe, control in a situation that is terrifyingly unpredictable, power in a situation of helplessness" (p. 96). Her examination of the ways such children attempt to adapt is both truly informative and arrestingly poignant.

15. *Moscarello R: Psychological management of victims of sexual assault. *Can J Psychiatry* 35:25–30, 1990

Moscarello provides an overview of the psychological sequelae of sexual assault and provides some guidelines for effectively managing persons victimized by it. The acute and long-term consequences of rape, factors influencing the severity of posttraumatic responses, and the psychodynamics of sexual assault are described.

16. *Nadelson CC: Consequences of rape: clinical and treatment aspects. *Psychother Psychosom* 51:187–192, 1989

This article describes the short-term and long-term clinical repercussions of sexual abuse and presents treatment implications that emphasize specific aspects of the approach to the victim.

17. Pynoos RS, Frederick C, Nader K, Arroyo W, Steinberg A, Eth S, Nunez F, Fairbanks L: Life threat and posttraumatic stress in school age children. *Arch Gen Psychiatry* 44:1057–1063, 1987

This study examined a sample of 159 school children after a sniper attack on their elementary school playground during which 1 child and 1 passerby were killed and 13 other children were injured. Children were examined approximately 1 month after the attack. The child "PTSD Reaction Index" was used to record a child's report of symptoms. The findings suggested that acute posttraumatic stress disorder (PTSD) symptoms do occur in children, with a correlation between proximity to the violence and the type and number of PTSD symptoms.

18. *Terr LC: Psychic trauma in children: observations following the Chowchilla school bus kidnapping. *Am J Psychiatry* 138:14–19, 1981

This article is a description of the aftermath of the kidnapping of 26 children ages 5–14. This event was a rare occurrence of purely psychological trauma. Terr describes the manifestations of psychic trauma in children and compares those findings with adult forms of traumatic stress reactions.

19. *Thompson J:** Theoretical issues in responses to disaster. *J R Soc Med* 84:19–22, 1991

Thompson proposes the development of a theoretical framework to explain human reactions to disasters. He proposes some necessary components of such a theory that must include ways to measure major stressors and methods of assessing threat and measuring loss.

20. **Titchner JL, Kapp FT:** Family and character change at Buffalo Creek. *Am J Psychiatry* 133:295–299, 1976

The authors report their findings of the psychological effects on a group of litigants who had been victims of the collapse of a dam at Buffalo Creek. The authors describe a definable clinical entity characterized by a complex of clinical symptoms and changes in character and lifestyle. The authors postulate that certain defenses used in attempts to cope with the disaster actually preserved traumatic symptoms and led to disabling character changes.

Issues in Emergency Psychiatry

21. *Anderson WH, Stern TA:** Psychiatric emergencies, in *Emergency Medicine: Scientific Foundations and Current Practice*, 3rd Edition. Edited by Wilkins EW. Baltimore, MD, Williams & Wilkins, 1989, pp. 423–443

This chapter provides a thorough compilation of important topics in the practice of emergency psychiatry. Although a range of objectively life-threatening conditions are covered (e.g., delirium, suicide, homicidal and assaultive patients), the authors also include less severe conditions that are subjectively urgent to patients and/or their families (e.g., anxiety attacks, insomnia, grief reactions). Emphasis is placed on thorough assessment and reasoned intervention.

22. *Ellison JM, Hughes DH, White KA:** An emergency psychiatry update. *Hosp Community Psychiatry* 40:250–260, 1989

The authors present a brief but comprehensive overview of trends in emergency psychiatry. They address patient populations with special needs including adolescents, the elderly, patients with substance abuse disorders, and patients with acquired immunodeficiency syndrome. There is also comment on emergency psychopharmacology, legal issues in the practice of emergency psychiatry, the assessment and prediction of violence, and the role of the psychiatric emergency room in residency training.

23. **Gaynor J, Hargreaves WA:** "Emergency room" and "mobile response" models of emergency psychiatric services. *Community Ment Health J* 16:283–292, 1980

In this examination of two different models of psychiatric care, the authors examine service response styles, staff compositions, location of services, and organizational structure of services and argue that developing a typology of emergency psychiatric programs has significant implications for evaluating the relative effectiveness of services and for planning future programs.

24. *Gerson S, Bassuk E:** Psychiatric emergencies: an overview. *Am J Psychiatry* 137:1–11, 1980

This article presents an overview of psychiatric emergency services and dispositional determinants. The authors suggest a model of emergency psychiatric care that focuses more on the "adaptive resources and competence" (p. 9) of the patient and the community and less on diagnosis and symptoms.

25. *Hawley CJ, James DV, Birkett PL, Baldwin DS, DeRuiter MJ, Priest RG:** Suicidal ideation as a presenting complaint: associated diagnoses and characteristics in a casualty population. *Br J Psychiatry* 159:232–238, 1991

This article presents a prospective study of a population of patients presenting to an emergency psychiatric service with a specific and spontaneous complaint of suicidal ideation without any accompanying act of self-harm. The study suggests that this presentation "proved less associated with depressive illness than with long standing maladjustment as evidenced by personality disorder, criminality, substance abuse, and recurrent deliberate self-harm" (p. 237).

26. *McNiel DE, Myers RS, Zeiner HK, Wolfe HL, Hatcher C:** The role of violence in decisions about hospitalization from the psychiatric emergency room. *Am J Psychiatry* 149:207–212, 1992

In this retrospective review of the charts of 321 unduplicated patients presenting to a psychiatric emergency room, the authors evaluated the relationship between the decision to hospitalize and violent behavior. They found that clinical variables such as diagnosis and the overall severity of psychiatric impairment were more important than violent behavior in predicting hospitalization decisions.

27. **Turner PM, Turner TJ:** Validation of the crisis triage rating scale for psychiatric emergencies. *Can J Psychiatry* 36:651–654, 1991

   In this study of the relationship between scores obtained on the Crisis Triage Rating Scale (CTRS) and decisions to hospitalize, the authors found statistically significant relationships between the subscales of dangerousness, support system, ability to cooperate, and total CTRS score and whether or not a person was hospitalized.

28. *Wellin E, Slesinger DP, Hollister CD:** Psychiatric emergency services: evolution, adaptation, and proliferation. *Soc Sci Med* 24:475–482, 1987

   The authors examine the development of crisis intervention and psychiatric emergency services over recent decades. Particular emphasis is placed on how these systems have evolved, how they have been influenced by policy and service demands, and how they have proliferated.

Other Topics

29. *Chu JA:** The revictimization of adult women with histories of childhood abuse. *Journal of Psychotherapy Practice and Research* 1:259–269, 1992

   This article explores clinical observations and research statistics that demonstrate that childhood abuse survivors are more vulnerable to revictimization as adults. Chu suggests that understanding this phenomenon and three influencing forces—the repetition compulsion, posttraumatic syndromes, and profound relational disturbances—may allow the therapist to provide more adequate treatment and protection.

30. *van der Kolk BA, Saporta J:** The biological response to psychic trauma: mechanisms and treatment of intrusion and numbing. *Anxiety Research* 4:199–212, 1991

   This article examines the effect of trauma on the functioning of the central nervous system with particular focus on the phenomenology of stress response syndromes. The authors present a review of biological changes associated with trauma and present implications for treatment.

43

Group Psychotherapy

Howard D. Kibel, M.D.

G roup psychotherapy has been used to treat almost every kind of psychopathology and patient population in virtually every clinical setting with a range of techniques from various theoretical orientations. No core reading list could encompass the breadth of such a field. This bibliography is focused primarily on the psychodynamic approaches, because most practitioners in the field agree that a grounding in psychodynamic group process and group dynamics must precede any venture into more select areas.

The reading list begins with several general references, follows with some on theory, and then proceeds to practice. It culminates with references on the treatment of some special patient populations. The list includes a number of classic articles, but also many recent ones that synthesize the development of thinking in the field. Two of the general references are anthologies of classic articles, some of which are also listed here.

It is difficult for the neophyte to understand the group literature because different practitioners emphasize different aspects of group life. This changing and diverse emphasis is most evident in the sections on theory and methods. Those unfamiliar with the variability may become confused when trying to differentiate one approach from another. Broadly speaking, there can be distinguished three distinct, but overlapping, dynamic systems in the group—namely, that of the individual in this context, an interactive one of member-to-member relationships, and that which encompasses the collective. With this in mind, Parloff (1968) below devised a useful classification of group practice based on therapists' focus of interventions: 1) the intrapersonalists, who transpose the theories and practice of individual psychoanalytic treatment directly into the group; 2) the transactionalists or interpersonalists, who mainly explore the diversity of the relationships among the members; and 3) the integralists (a coined term), who examine group-as-a-whole dynamics and each member's participation in them. In using this chapter, knowledge of this classification will help the reader to understand more thoroughly the various approaches found in this list.

The latter part of this reading list is easier to use. Those citations on the structure and practice of treatment address the pragmatics of organizing and conducting adult outpatient groups. There is a separate section devoted to treatment of special patient populations. Those on adolescents and children serve as introductions to these subspecialties. There is one on the treatment of patients with a history of trauma and another on self-help groups; interest in them has increased in recent years. The final section contains four articles that describe less traditional forms of group psychotherapy. In practice, there are a plethora of methods, some of which claim to be psychodynamic and some which eschew any semblance of analytic theory.

General References

1. **MacKenzie KR** (ed): *Classics in Group Psychotherapy*. New York, Guilford, 1992

   This monograph was compiled to celebrate the 50th anniversary of the founding of the American Group Psychotherapy Association. It reprints 26 classic articles that were seminal to the development of the field. Included are some listed below, namely those by Foulkes (1965), Glatzer (1970), Horwitz (1977), Parloff (1968), and Scheidlinger (1974).

2. **Rutan JS, Stone WN:** *Psychodynamic Group Psychotherapy*, 2nd Edition. New York, Guilford, 1993

   A basic text that can prove useful to the relatively experienced group psychotherapist, this book also can serve as an introduction for the novice. It is unique in that it attempts to integrate and put to therapeutic use a variety of perspectives on the group experience—namely, what happens with individuals, the interactions between members, and the dynamics of the group-as-a-whole.

3. **Scheidlinger S** (ed): *Psychoanalytic Group Dynamics: Basic Readings.* New York, International Universities Press, 1980

This book is a reprinting of classic articles on the use of group dynamics in psychotherapy. It includes Bion's original summary of his theories (whose critique by Rioch 1970 below is more lucid), its application by Ezriel (which is summarized by Heath and Bacal 1972 below), and those listed below by Foulkes (1965) and Redl (1942).

4. **Stein A, Kibel HD, Fidler JW, Spitz HI:** The group therapies, in *Treatment Planning in Psychiatry.* Edited by Lewis JM, Usdin G. Washington, DC, American Psychiatric Association, 1982, pp. 43–85

This chapter highlights notable group phenomena and dynamics; surveys the variety of groups in use; and discusses group composition, selection, and preparation of patients for referral. It reflects a consensus in the field and is designed to acquaint the generalist with the appropriate use of groups for treatment planning.

5. **Yalom ID:** *The Theory and Practice of Group Psychotherapy,* 3rd Edition. New York, Basic Books, 1985

This widely used basic source is now in its 3rd edition, a testimony to its popularity. Most of the practical aspects of treatment are covered in this textbook. The author's interpersonal method of practice has been adopted by most American clinicians.

Theory and Its Practical Applications

6. **Foulkes SH:** Group analytic dynamics with special reference to psychoanalytic concepts. *Int J Group Psychother* 7:40–52, 1957; also in *Therapeutic Group Analysis.* Edited by Foulkes SH. New York, International Universities Press, 1965, pp 147–162

Major group phenomena are described, such as mirror reactions, resonance, and the group matrix. The therapeutic emphasis here on communication within the group emanates from the view that neuroses have a social origin.

7. **Kaplan SR, Roman M:** Phases of development in an adult therapy group. *Int J Group Psychother* 13:10–26, 1963

This is a vivid clinical account of the progress of a psychotherapy group from a relatively loosely organized state into a dynamic system. Understanding this process of group development can help the clinician identify phase-specific behavior of the members.

8. **Kissen M:** General systems theory: practical and theoretical implications for group intervention. *Group* 4:29–39, 1980

   Kissen succinctly defines general systems theory concepts and describes their relevance to the practice of group psychotherapy. The author considers object relations theory to be a useful complement.

9. **Redl F:** Group emotion and leadership. *Psychiatry* 5:573–596, 1942

   A useful way to begin understanding the complexity of group dynamics is to examine the formative processes that crystallize around a member who occupies a focal position in a group. This article describes the variety of relationships to this central person and derivative emotions that develop among the group members.

10. *Rioch MJ:** The work of Wilfred Bion on groups. *Psychiatry* 33:56–66, 1970; also in *Progress in Group and Family Therapy.* Edited by Sager CJ, Kaplan HS. New York, Brunner/Mazel, 1972, pp. 18–32

    This article succinctly describes a complex theory that has had a major impact on group dynamic approaches to treatment. Bion applied Melanie Klein's theories to explain group-as-a-whole phenomena. He described the simultaneous existence of two levels of functioning in groups: one is task-oriented, whereas the other is concerned with security, aggression, or intimacy.

11. **Scheidlinger S:** On the concept of the "mother-group." *Int J Group Psychother* 24:417–428, 1974

    This seminal paper, which presents a theory of therapeutic regression, conceptually integrates group dynamics with interactional aspects of the treatment. Identification by group members with the group as an entity promotes the therapeutic alliance and the development of cohesion and provides support.

12. **Scheidlinger S:** On scapegoating in group psychotherapy. *Int J Group Psychother* 32:131–143, 1982

    Scapegoating is a ubiquitous phenomena in groups. This article traces its historical roots, describes the various ways it has been depicted as a clinical event, and proposes a theoretical and practical framework for understanding it.

13. **Stock D:** Interpersonal concerns during early sessions of therapy groups. *Int J Group Psychother* 12:14–26, 1962

    A method called "group focal conflict" analysis is used to identify shared conflicts among the members and their compromise solutions.

This approach, derived from Thomas French's work with individuals, translates the familiar analytic triad of wish, anxiety, and defense to the level of the group-as-a-whole.

Methods of Treatment

14. Durkin HE, Glatzer HT: Transference neurosis in group psychotherapy: the concept and the reality, in *Group Therapy: 1973: An Overview.* Edited by Wolberg LR, Schwartz EK. New York, Intercontinental Medical Book Corp, 1973, pp. 129–144

Durkin and Glatzer apply psychoanalytic ego psychology to group psychotherapy. Structural change is achieved through systematic interpretation in the here-and-now of a myriad of intragroup transference, along with attendant character defenses and their translation in terms of genetic origin.

15. Ganzarain R: Introduction to object relations group psychotherapy. *Int J Group Psychother* 42:205–223, 1992

Ganzarain translates Kleinian theory to the group setting but in a uniquely humanistic way. He describes how patients' mental images of the group serve as a backdrop for the emergence of primitive defenses and how members use each other to work through guilt over unconscious greed and hatred.

16. Heath ES, Bacal HA: A method of group psychotherapy at the Tavistock Clinic. *Int J Group Psychother* 18:21–30, 1968; also in *Progress in Group and Family Therapy.* Edited by Sager CJ, Kaplan HS. New York, Brunner/Mazel, 1972, pp. 33–42

This is an excellent summary of a method that was developed in England and has fallen into disuse. Reprints of the original articles can be found in Scheidlinger (1980) and Yalom (1985), both above. The unique contribution of this method is that it demonstrated the clinical relevance of the collective unconscious process within the group, which is designated as the "common group tension."

17. Horwitz L: A group-centered approach to group psychotherapy. *Int J Group Psychother* 27:423–439, 1977

Horwitz persuasively argues for viewing discrete events in a group session as part of collective reactions of the total membership. This group-centered hypothesis offers unique advantages for treatment, which can be integrated with a clinical focus on individuals and peer interactions.

18. **Parloff MB:** Analytic group psychotherapy, in *Modern Psychoanalysis.* Edited by Marmor J. New York, Basic Books, 1968, pp. 492–531

Parloff classifies the multiplicity of group psychotherapy methods according to whether the focus is on the individual in the group, subgroups, or member dyads or on the group as a unit. Although his title refers to analytic groups, this classic work provides a basic typology for the field in general.

19. **Stein A, Kibel HD:** A group dynamic peer-interaction approach to group psychotherapy. *Int J Group Psychother* 34:315–333, 1984

Stein previously translated Freud's treatise on group psychology to explain why there are specific alterations in the transference to the therapist and a rapid exposure of members' character pathology. That thesis has been adopted by many who focus on member dyads and subgroups as the essence of the therapeutic work. The unique contribution of this article is its description of how group dynamics influence the interactional process.

20. *Tuttman S:* Theoretical and technical elements which characterize the American approaches to psychoanalytic group psychotherapy. *Int J Group Psychother* 36:499–515, 1986

This article examines the evolution and practice of the psychoanalytic methods, including the pioneering works of Slavson and Wolf, who focused on the individual in the group and eschewed clinical use of group dynamics. Contemporary practices are reviewed in terms of their efforts to integrate individual- and group-level processes.

Structure and Process of Treatment

21. *Freedman MB, Sweet BS:* Some specific features of group psychotherapy and their implications for selection of patients. *Int J Group Psychother* 4:355–368, 1954

The authors provide a rich analysis of several features of groups that are relevant to treatment planning. Their bias is toward a view that group is the preferred mode of psychotherapy for many difficult-to-treat outpatients.

22. **Glatzer HT:** Working through in analytic group psychotherapy. *Int J Group Psychother* 19:292–306, 1969

Analytic group psychotherapy facilitates the working through process in several ways. Old hurts and traumas are vividly revived in group.

Because fellow members suffer from similar character problems and transference distortions, they are mutually accepting and are more receptive to peer interpretations than those that emanate from the therapist.

23. **Grunebaum H, Kates W:** Whom to refer for group psychotherapy. *Am J Psychiatry* 134:130–133, 1977

The authors present fundamental and practical indications for group therapy. Referral is advised for treatment of various characterological problems and for those individuals in whom there is a potential or existing transference that impedes individual therapy.

24. **Kauff PF:** The termination process: its relationship to the separation-individuation phase of development. *Int J Group Psychother* 27:3–18, 1977

Termination of any one group member, therapist, or patient has a profound impact on that individual and an appreciable effect on everyone else in the group. Using the paradigm of the separation-individuation process, clinical vignettes illustrate the reactivation of primitive defense mechanisms in the face of loss.

25. **McGee TF, Schuman BN:** The nature of the co-therapy relationship. *Int J Group Psychother* 20:25–36, 1970

McGee and Schuman provide practical advice and guidance for the use of co-leaders. A group conducted by co-therapists tends to replicate the original family constellation and alters the transference accordingly. The co-therapy relationship influences the group's operation and vice versa.

26. **Rabin HM:** Preparing patients for group psychotherapy. *Int J Group Psychother* 20:135–145, 1970

Adequate preparation of patients for entry into group psychotherapy is vital, because it generally takes weeks or months to be inculcated into the group culture. Several preparatory practices are described, and practical suggestions for induction are given.

27. **Rodenhauser P:** Group psychotherapy and pharmacotherapy: psychodynamic considerations. *Int J Group Psychother* 39:445–456, 1989

In a typical psychotherapy group, some patients receive medication whereas others do not. This article provides a perspective on the psychodynamics of pharmacotherapy in a group. It examines the psychological meanings of medication to those for whom it is prescribed, to those for whom it is not, for the group as a whole, and for the group leaders. Medication prescription generates issues around dependency, control, and rivalry.

28. **Scheidlinger S, Porter K:** Group therapy combined with individual psychotherapy, in *Specialized Techniques in Individual Psychotherapy*. Edited by Karasu TB, Bellak L. New York, Brunner/Mazel, 1980, pp. 426–440

The authors discuss the use of simultaneous treatment, conducted by different therapists (conjoint therapy) and by the same therapist (combined therapy). They review the literature and discuss indications and contraindications, structuring of this approach, and special issues such as confidentiality.

Special Patient Populations

29. **Ganzarain R, Buchele B:** Countertransference when incest is the problem. *Int J Group Psychother* 36:549–566, 1986

Groups are unique modalities for the treatment of patients who have a history of trauma. Notably, they reenact their experience with trauma in the group and repeat the numerous roles they learned in childhood when incest occurred. Others in the group are influenced by role suction and role reversal to play out the exciting and destructive aspects of these relationships.

30. **Horwitz L:** Group psychotherapy of the borderline patient, in *Borderline Personality Disorders*. Edited by Hartocollis P. New York, International Universities Press, 1977, pp. 399–422

This chapter provides an excellent review of the literature and discusses the special features of groups that are suited to the treatment of these patients. These include dilution of transference, a reality orientation, emotional support through belonging, unique means for the expression of hostility, the unfolding of character armor, peer confrontation, and the development of sustained identifications.

31. **Hurst AG, Gladieux JD:** Guidelines for leading an adolescent therapy group, in *Group and Family Therapy 1980*. Edited by Wolberg LR, Aronson ML. New York, Brunner/Mazel, 1980, pp. 151–164

This chapter outlines several practical strategies for forming and conducting adolescent outpatient groups. Developmental issues of adolescence necessitate specific modifications in technique. The therapist is advised to conduct the group as an authority who actively guides the members in the mutual exploration of their lives.

32. **Kibel HD:** The therapeutic use of splitting: the role of the mother-group in therapeutic differentiation and practicing, in *Psychoanalytic Group Theory and Therapy: Essays in Honor of Saul Scheidlinger.* Edited by Tuttman S. Madison, CT, International Universities Press, 1991, pp. 113–132

There are many methods proposed in the literature for the outpatient treatment of patients with severe psychopathology. This is one of the few that is a psychoanalytically informed group psychotherapy. The chapter presents theory, technique, and a way to understand the mechanisms for change.

33. *Kibel HD:** Inpatient group psychotherapy, in *Group Therapy in Clinical Practice.* Edited by Alonso A, Swiller HI. Washington, DC, American Psychiatric Press, 1993, pp. 93–111

This chapter provides a review of inpatient group psychotherapy, including its history and current practices. Practical guidelines are given on the structure of inpatient groups, selection of patients, group composition, and goals of treatment. Techniques are described that aim to clarify for the members their experience in the group and how this is relevant to their overall treatment.

34. **Lieberman MA:** A group therapist perspective on self-help groups. *Int J Group Psychother* 40:251–278, 1990

Many people in distress use groups of this sort as a primary source for help or as an adjunct to treatment. The author provides an overview of self-help groups in terms of their origins, growth, scope, and effectiveness and then compares them with professionally led psychotherapy groups. Specific ideology plays a major role in self-help groups, of which Alcoholics Anonymous, Recovery Inc., and Synanon are prime examples.

35. **Schamess G:** Group treatment modalities for latency age children. *Int J Group Psychother* 26:455–473, 1976

This excellent review of the literature categorizes the plethora of outpatient methods according to the specific patient populations for which they were designed. The author notes that children's groups must be homogeneously composed. For each type, the literature prescribes distinct approaches to treatment, including specifics for the therapist's role, the structure of the group, and the equipment employed.

36. **Stone WN, Gustafson JP:** Technique in group psychotherapy of narcissistic and borderline patients. *Int J Group Psychother* 32:29–47, 1982

Concepts from self psychology are explained and translated to group treatment. Modifications in usual technique are advised for these difficult patients. Suggestions are given and illustrated for the use of group interpretations and noninterpretative therapist activity, including empathy and benign confrontation.

37. **Yalom ID:** *Inpatient Group Psychotherapy.* Basic Books, New York, 1983

In response to the rapid turnover of patients on the modern psychiatric unit, Yalom developed a method in which problems are addressed in one session and not carried over to the next. He employs a structured technique to help patients use the group as a laboratory for learning about the interpersonal consequences of maladaptive behavior and for them to practice corrective measures there. The method is pragmatic; this book can be used as a self-teacher.

Other Methods of Group Treatment

38. **Gruen W:** Use of the leader and of the group process in gestalt therapy groups. *Group* 2:195–209, 1978

Modern, so-called innovative, group therapists use their own personality in a very active way to motivate patients, facilitate catharsis, and direct the group process. Gestalt therapy is only one of a number that use "action" techniques. In this article, Gruen, a clinical researcher, examines the role of the leader and the effect of focusing exclusively on one member while the rest of the group serves a passive function.

39. **Kipper DA:** Psychodrama: group psychotherapy through role playing. *Int J Group Psychother* 42:495–521, 1992

Jacob Moreno, the founder of psychodrama and one of the pioneers of group psychotherapy, developed this treatment apart from its traditional psychodynamic counterparts. He first created a method that dramatized patients' conflicts in a group. It then evolved into the group method he called sociodrama. This article describes the theory and procedure of psychodrama and sociodrama and provides vivid illustrations of the process.

40. **O'Hearne JJ:** How and why do transactional-gestalt therapists work as they do? *Int J Group Psychother* 26:163–172, 1976

Transactional analysis was developed by Eric Berne as a method of treatment that could be applied to individual or group therapy. Gestalt therapy, developed by Fritz Perls, has used a group format since its inception. Transactional analysis uses interpersonal behavior to analyze various ego structures that reflect aspects of identification. The gestalt therapist, in a very active way, uses confrontation to enhance the patient's awareness of concealed emotions. Today these two methods are often used in combination.

41. **Rose SD:** Coping skill training in groups. *Int J Group Psychother* 39:59–78, 1989

Although cognitive therapy and behavior therapy developed as separate modalities, they have much in common. Both employ concrete intervention strategies and use guidance to foster problem solving and the emergence of adaptive skills. Cognitive-behavioral group therapy is well illustrated by this article, which describes a time-limited treatment method.

Family and Marital Therapy

John F. Clarkin, Ph.D.
Ira D. Glick, M.D.

This is an era of differential therapeutics (American Psychiatric Association 1989; Beutler and Clarkin 1990; Frances et al. 1984)—that is, the development of decision rules helpful in matching the individual patient with the most effective and efficient treatment (or treatment package) with his or her diagnosis, personality characteristics, and support system. Family therapy is not a panacea, but rather one of the various formats of treatment (along with individual and group) that can be used in selected cases for specific reasons and takes its place in a general differential therapeutic system. The decision rules for the utilization of the family treatment format must be based on research and accumulated clinical wisdom.

The organization of this section reflects these biases. The field of family therapy can no longer afford to ignore the current methods of diagnosing the individual patient. Research on the effectiveness of family therapy is a sine qua non, and it will proceed in the present climate with a focus on isolating homogeneous samples in terms of the diagnosis or problem areas of the individual with investigation of family and marital treatment for that individual and the involved family.

This orientation has many implications. First of all, family assessment will focus on the individual and his or her individual diagnosis and a "diagnosis" of the family that relates to that individual disorder. Second, it suggests that family therapy can be seen as both a general orientation and as a specific targeted intervention when one family member has a specific disorder.

1. **American Psychiatric Association:** *Treatments of Psychiatric Disorders: A Task Force Report of the American Psychiatric Association.* Washington, DC, American Psychiatric Association, 1989

2. **Beutler LE, Clarkin JF:** *Systematic Treatment Selection: Toward Targeted Therapeutic Interventions.* New York, Brunner/Mazel, 1990

3. **Frances A, Clarkin JF, Perry S:** *Differential Therapeutics in Psychiatry: The Art and Science of Treatment Selection.* New York, Brunner/Mazel, 1984

Family Interaction and Psychopathology

4. **Haas GL, Clarkin JF:** Affective disorders and the family context, in *Affective Disorder and the Family.* Edited by Clarkin JF, Haas G, Glick ID. New York, Guilford, 1988, pp. 3–28

This chapter is a review of antecedents and sequelae of affective disorders in a family member.

5. *Hooley JM:** The nature and origins of expressed emotion, in *Understanding Major Mental Disorder: The Contribution of Family Interaction Research.* Edited by Hahlweg K, Goldstein MJ. New York, Family Process Press, 1987, pp. 176–194

This chapter is a review of the key concept of expressed emotion by one of the best researchers in the area.

6. **Jacob T, Seilhamer R:** Alcoholism and family interaction, in *Family Interaction and Psychopathology.* Edited by Jacob T. New York, Plenum, 1987, pp. 535–560

Alcohol use and abuse is rampant and has powerful effects on families. Jacob, a noted researcher in this area, and Seilhamer provide an overview.

7. *Minuchin S:** A family model, in *Families and Family Therapy.* Cambridge, MA, Harvard University Press, 1974, pp. 46–66

Minuchin's clarity and perception of the structure of the family have no equal.

8. **Yager J, Strober M:** Family aspects of eating disorders, in *Psychiatry Update: American Psychiatric Association Annual Review,* Vol. 4. Edited by

Hales RE, Frances AJ. Washington, DC, American Psychiatric Press, 1985, pp. 481–502

Yager and Strober review the family characteristics, including parent-child interactions, personality, and stress response patterns of the family, along with assessment and treatment planning guidelines.

Problem Description and Assessment

9. **Carter E, McGoldrick M:** The family life cycle and family therapy: an overview, in *The Family Life Cycle: A Framework for Family Therapy.* New York, Gardner Press, 1980, pp. 3–20

This chapter is a classic piece on placing the clinical picture of the family in time. It clearly relates the purpose of the family to the family structure to change in time and to the development of symptoms.

10. **Clarkin JF, Glick ID:** Instruments for the assessment of family malfunction, in *Measuring Mental Illness: Psychometric Assessment for Clinicians.* Edited by Wetzler S. Washington, DC, American Psychiatric Press, 1989, pp. 211–227

Clarkin and Glick review constructs and related instruments useful in the assessment of the family.

11. *Minuchin S: The initial interview: the Gordens and Braulio Montalvo, in *Families and Family Therapy.* Cambridge, MA, Harvard University Press, 1974, pp. 206–239

This chapter is a detailed description and analysis of a master at the work of initial assessment.

12. **Widiger TA, Frances AJ, Pincus HA, First M:** Family/relational issues section, in *DSM-IV Sourcebook,* Volume 3. Washington, DC, American Psychiatric Press (in press)

This chapter provides reviews of the research in family and marital problem areas that may merit special focus in DSM-IV.

Schools of Marital and Family Therapy

13. *Baucom DH, Epstein N: An integrated approach to skills-oriented marital therapy, in *Cognitive-Behavioral Marital Therapy.* Edited by Baucom DH, Epstein N. New York, Brunner/Mazel, 1990

This is a scholarly chapter that summarizes basic research and marital intervention with a cognitive-behavioral orientation.

14. *Bowen M:** Theory in the practice of psychotherapy, in *Family Therapy in Clinical Practice.* Edited by Bowen M. New York, Jason Aronson, 1978, pp. 337–387

Bowen explains his own theory, based on the central notion that the successful introduction of a significant other into a disturbed relationship system can modify that system. He also explains his key concepts of emotional tension and differentiation of self.

15. *Dicks HV:** *Marital Tensions.* New York, Basic Books, 1967

If you are going to read only one book on the psychodynamic approach to marriage, read this one. It is a true classic.

16. **Gottman JM, Notarius CI, Gonso J, Markman HJ:** *A Couple's Guide to Communication.* Champaign, IL, Research Press, 1976

This is a book that family therapists can recommend for couples (and profit from themselves).

17. **Greenberg LS, Johnson SM:** *Emotionally Focused Therapy for Couples.* New York, Guilford, 1988

If the cognitive-behavioral approach to couples slights affect, this affect-focused approach is a good corrective.

18. **Haley J, Hoffman L:** *Techniques of Family Therapy.* New York, Basic Books, 1967

One way to learn the techniques of family therapy is to observe the pioneers at work through studying actual sessions. This book provides transcripts of such leading family therapists as Charles Fulweiler, Virginia Satir, D. D. Jackson, Carl Whitaker, and Frank Pittman. The authors provide questions and expert commentary.

19. **Luepnitz D:** Part III: history and insight: toward a feminist theory of psychotherapy with families, in *The Family Interpreted: Feminist Theory in Clinical Practice.* Edited by Luepnitz D. New York, Basic Books, 1988, pp. 109–200

Placing the family in historical perspective, Luepnitz uses psychoanalytic theory to frame a feminist psychotherapy with families. This is a thoughtful critique of Bateson and cybernetics.

20. *Minuchin S:** *Families and Family Therapy.* Cambridge, MA, Harvard University Press, 1974

Still a classic, this book is clear in its structural description of the family.

21. **Scharff DE, Scharff JS:** The technique of object relations family therapy, in *Object Relations Family Therapy*. Edited by Klein RS. New York,
Jason Aronson, 1987, pp. 169–200

This chapter considers object relations as a way of working with a family:
organizing the session, giving support and advice, facilitating communication, and joining the family experience through interpretation.

22. **Stierlin H:** *Psychoanalysis and Family Therapy*. New York, Jason Aronson,
1977

Stierlin's psychoanalytic understanding of the family is outstanding and
will always be worth reading.

23. **Warburton J, Newberry A, Alexander J:** Women as therapists, trainees
and supervisors, in *Women in Families: A Framework for Family Therapy*.
Edited by McGoldrick M, Anderson C, Walsh F. New York, WW Norton,
1989, pp. 152–165

With data on the topic, the authors discuss therapeutic ways to deal with
the fact that fathers are more defensive with female therapists and that
mothers are more defensive with male therapists. Because competent
women tend to be seen as sex-role incongruent, the female therapist
must engage the male client and entire system before attempting to use
power effectively.

Marital and Family Therapy for Specific Diagnoses and Problem Areas

24. *Anderson CM, Reiss DJ, Hogarty GE:** *Schizophrenia and the Family*. New
York, Guilford, 1986

This is an excellent description of a carefully constructed approach to
the family with a schizophrenic member. It is based on years of clinical
experience and research.

25. *Beach SRH, Sandeen EE, O'Leary KD:** Overview of therapy: assessment, process and the therapist's role in marital therapy for depression,
in *Depression in Marriage: A Model for Etiology and Treatment*. Edited by
Beach SRH, Sandeen EE, O'Leary KD. New York, Guilford, 1990,
pp. 87–117

Representative of a growing trend, this is a manualized treatment for
couples where one is depressed. Not only do the empirical data support
the use of this treatment, but the manual is specific enough to be useful
to a clinician.

26. **Falloon I, Boyd JL, McGill CW:** *Family Care of Schizophrenics.* New York, Guilford, 1984

    A detailed psychoeducational and behavioral approach to families with a member suffering from schizophrenia, this approach has been researched and been shown to be effective.

27. **Glick ID, Clarkin JF:** The family, in *Inpatient Psychiatry: Diagnosis and Treatment,* 3rd Edition. Edited by Sederer L. Baltimore, MD, Williams & Wilkins, 1991, pp. 255–276

    This is a basic primer concerning the hospital treatment of the family, including new information on making the family part of the treatment team and the use of psychoeducation in conjunction with medication.

28. *Haley J:* *Problem-Solving Therapy.* San Francisco, CA, Jossey-Bass, 1976

    Any review of techniques must include the seminal ideas of Haley. This book is lucid, provocative, and practical on topics such as conducting the first family interview, delivering therapy directives to families, and the stages in family therapy.

29. **Kaplan HS:** *The New Sex Therapy.* New York, Brunner/Mazel, 1974

    Although no longer new, this book set the standard in the area of sexual difficulties.

30. **Kaplan HS:** *Sexual Aversion, Sexual Phobias, and Panic Disorder.* New York, Brunner/Mazel, 1987

    Kaplan here focuses on sexual aversion, including discussions of phobia and panic disorder.

31. *Minuchin S, Fishman HC:* *Family Therapy Techniques.* Cambridge, MA, Harvard University Press, 1981

    This book provides an excellent description in concrete and succinct language of basic structural family therapy techniques.

32. **Palazzoli MS, Cirillo S, Selvini M, Sorrentino AM:** *Family Games: General Models of Psychotic Processes in the Family.* New York, WW Norton, 1989

    In contrast to the psychoeducational and behavioral approaches, this book describes an artful approach to psychosis (in the broad sense) and family intervention.

33. **Patterson GR:** *Coercive Family Process.* Eugene, OR, Castalia Press, 1982

This book explores carefully researched understanding of family behavior when there is acting-out behavior in young children. This understanding informs an effective behavioral family intervention.

34. **Rice JK, Rice DG:** *Living Through Divorce: A Developmental Approach to Divorce Therapy.* New York, Guilford, 1986

    With background attention to object loss and self-esteem issues, the authors walk the therapist through the painful process of helping couples divorce.

35. **Sager CJ, Brown HS, Crohn H, Engel P, Rodstein E, Walker L:** Section II: treatment, in *Treating the Remarried Family.* Edited by Sager CJ. New York, Brunner/Mazel, 1983, pp. 85–272

    This is a combined systems, psychoanalytic, and learning approach to the complexities of treating the remarried family.

36. **Stanton MD, Todd TC (and associates):** *The Family Therapy of Drug Abuse and Addiction.* New York, Guilford, 1982

    This is one of the best—if not the only—descriptions of family treatment when drug abuse is a current and overriding problem.

Research: Reviews and Summaries

37. **Hahlweg K, Goldstein MJ** (eds): *Understanding Major Mental Disorder: The Contribution of Family Interaction Research.* New York, Family Process Press, 1987

    This book is an edited work with sections on high-risk studies, psychopathological groups (e.g., schizophrenia and mania, and the family), and marital interaction research. Select a few chapters of interest to get a sense of the research relating family interaction and pathology.

38. **Hazelrigg MD, Cooper HM, Borduin CM:** Evaluating the effectiveness of family therapies: an integrative review and analysis. *Psychol Bull* 101:428–442, 1987

    This is the best empirical review of family therapy outcome studies. The studies are not only described but the data are analyzed across studies, providing effect sizes.

39. **Jacobson NS, Holtzworth-Munroe A, Schmaling KB:** Marital therapy and spouse involvement in the treatment of depression, agoraphobia, and alcoholism. *J Consult Clin Psychol* 57:5–10, 1989

This is a thoughtful, up-to-date review of the effectiveness of marital treatment.

Texts and Handbooks

40. Glick ID, Clarkin JF, Kessler D: *Marital and Family Therapy*, 3rd Edition. Washington, DC, American Psychiatric Press, 1987

This book is a concise introduction to clinical work with families used as a basic text in psychiatric residencies and family therapy institutes.

41. *Gurman AS, Kniskern DP (eds): *Handbook of Family Therapy*, Vol. 2. New York, Brunner/Mazel, 1991

This is the best summary in one book of the major orientations to family and marital treatment. Editors' footnotes are informative, comparative, provocative, and delightful. In fact, the pungent and pointed footnotes are much more interesting than the text in this important but somewhat staid handbook. Its focus on schools of family therapy rather than organization around problem areas and diagnosis seems dated.

45

Milieu Therapy: Inpatient and Partial Hospitalization— Special Problems and Populations

Michael H. Sacks, M.D.
Richard L. Munich, M.D.

Over the past three decades there has been a parallel decline in the utilization of inpatient resources in psychiatry and medicine. Even in the most serious of illnesses or disturbed mental states, modal lengths of stay have shifted from months to days, while powerful arguments are made to reduce them further. Hospitalization for psychiatric illness is increasingly viewed as wasteful of limited resources, especially given the demonstrated effectiveness of partial and day hospitalization. These dramatic reductions in length of stay have led to a decreased interest in the study and teaching of milieu treatment or the therapeutics of maximizing the positive impact of the inpatient unit's social environment on patient behavior and treatment. Regardless of the time spent in a treatment setting or even of the location (e.g., day hospital, partial hospital, drop-in center, residential treatment), the social system or context in which the treatment takes place has an impact on the treatment. At its worst, an institution can foster regression and loss of personal identity (Goffman 1961); at its best, an institution can promote a belief in the efficacy of the medical-psychiatric treatment (Almond 1975) and an internalization of treatment values (Edelson 1970).

These issues had their intellectual birth in the great 18th century debates between Rousseau and Diderot about the relative preeminence of the individual and the social in determining human behavior. In this century, the social impact on psychiatric or "deviant" behavior came to fruition during and shortly after World War II in the work of Maxwell Jones at Belmont Hospital in England. He used large group methods to treat soldiers who were hospitalized with severe character disorders. Closely studied by Robert Rappaport and colleagues, Maxwell's "therapeutic community" attracted wide attention and generated such social therapeutic principles as democratization, permissiveness, communalism, and reality confrontation. The ideas quickly spread to include traditional psychiatric hospitals and other diagnostic entities. The decline of the therapeutic community movement followed the development of more efficient biological treatments, the medicalization of psychiatry, reduced lengths of stay, and a paucity of research on the efficacy of milieu treatment. However, the well-established principles of social psychiatry continue to inform the practice of that psychiatry in all settings.

We have organized this section with these historical trends and modern dilemmas and practice in mind. Beginning with a selection of the classic texts on psychopathology and milieu, we move to works on the modern perspectives and locations, then list the works on practice and milieu issues with special patient populations. We end with a section on special problems. The focus is on clinical papers and books that authors have found useful in their work as directors of inpatient units, as designers of continua of care, and as teachers of residents and junior staff. The reader is referred to other chapters in this volume for references to related areas, such as group dynamics (Munich, Chapter 7), community psychiatry (Thompson and Mullins, Chapter 57), and economic issues in psychiatry (English and McCarrick, Chapter 61).

Background (Through 1970)

1. *Cumming J, Cumming E: *Ego and Milieu: Theory and Practice of Environmental Therapy.* New York, Atherton, 1962

   This is an important book that examines the interaction of a "damaged ego" with a hospital environment that like any culture can be examined in terms of beliefs about mental illness, communication patterns, role expectations, and authority hierarchies. Read this book for its practical and thoughtful guidance in changing a hospital or unit milieu. It includes advice like having coffee with the nursing staff.

2. **Edelson M:** *Sociotherapy and Psychotherapy.* Chicago, IL, University of Chicago Press, 1970

This is a tightly articulated differentiation of psychological and milieu treatments for hospitalized schizophrenic patients in which the author develops a comprehensive theory of groups. This theory is then integrated with dynamically oriented personality theory to demonstrate how the organization as an aspect of the treatment situation both conflicts with and facilitates individual therapy.

3. *Goffman E:** *Asylums: Essays on the Social Situation of Mental Patients and Other Inmates.* Garden City, NY, Doubleday, 1961

This is a brilliant book that argues the many ways an organization works to serve itself more than those it serves. The author takes the reader inside a mental hospital and other similar "total institutions" and provides a brilliant analysis of the impact of the institution on the self-concept of the "inmate."

4. **Jones M, Baker A, Freeman T, Merry J, Pomryn BA, Sandler MA, Tuxford J:** *The Therapeutic Community: A New Treatment Method in Psychiatry.* New York, Basic Books, 1953

Jones is credited as the originator of the therapeutic community. This book reviews his early work on the concept and attempts to place it in a wider context.

5. *Main TF:** The ailment. *Br J Med Psychol* 30:129–145, 1957

This article is our favorite. Main examines the impact of what we would now call the borderline patient on the psychological state of the therapist beginning with the appeal of the patient to the therapist's therapeutic interest, the progressive isolation of the patient and the therapist from the rest of the therapeutic team (what we would now call splitting), and finally the often disastrous outcome for not only the patient but often for the therapist as well. Although the language is dated, this is an article that never ceases to be rewarding on rereading.

6. **Rapoport RN:** *Community as Doctor: New Perspectives on a Therapeutic Community.* Springfield, IL, Charles C Thomas, 1960

This is an initial effort at researching a therapeutic community that is of special interest because the unit is Maxwell Jones' original therapeutic community. It provides an excellent examination of the unit's basic principles of permissiveness, shared decision making, free communication, and a democratic egalitarian social organization. Rapoport describes a process of oscillations in the commitment to these principles depending on the state of the unit. Select the chapters describing the basic principles and their oscillations.

7. **Stanton AH, Schwartz MS:** *The Mental Hospital: A Study of Institutional Participation in Psychiatric Illness and Treatment.* New York, Basic Books, 1954

Start with Chapter 15, in which the disruptive behavior of a group of schizophrenic patients is related to covert staff disagreements. Next read Chapter 16, which provides a social analysis of incontinence on a psychiatric ward. This work is a classic.

Modern Overviews: Shifting to Short-Term Lengths of Stay

8. **Almond R:** Issues in milieu treatment. *Schizophr Bull* 13:12–26, 1975

This article is an interesting presentation of milieu concepts. Of particular interest is Almond's concept of the importance of the relatedness between staff and patients regarding the unit's therapeutic effectiveness (communitas) and the role of leaders who can transmit their healing charisma to subordinate staff who can, in turn, transmit it to patients.

9. **Glick ID, Hargreaves WA:** *Psychiatric Hospital Treatment for the 1980s: A Controlled Study of Short Versus Long Hospitalization.* Lexington, MA, DC Heath, 1979

This is a rigorous outcome study of short hospitalization (21–28 days) versus long-term hospitalization (90–120 days) that cannot be easily summarized. The primary conclusion was that, for most patients with schizophrenia (especially those with a poor premorbid history) and for all patients with neurosis and personality disorder, there is no clear advantage to a long-term hospitalization. Paradoxically, longer stays may be somewhat better for the patient with a good premorbid history.

10. **Gunderson JG, Will OA, Mosher LR** (eds): *Principles and Practice of Milieu Therapy.* New York, Jason Aronson, 1983

This is an important overview of modern milieu therapy that discusses the important functions of containment, support, structure, involvement, and validation and then provides some evidence about the nature and effectiveness of the optimal milieu conditions for chronic and actively psychotic schizophrenic patients.

11. **Henisz JE:** *Psychotherapeutic Management on the Short-Term Unit: Glimpses at Inpatient Psychiatry.* Springfield, IL, Charles C Thomas, 1981

This book provides practical and specific approaches to the short-term hospital treatment of different clinical entities, including issues pertaining to the organization of the unit itself.

12. **Moos RH:** *Evaluating Treatment Environments: A Social Ecological Approach.* New York, Wiley, 1974

This is a summary of Moos' work with the Ward Atmosphere Scale, which assesses the treatment environments of hospital-based treatment programs. There are subscales that measure involvement, support, spontaneity, autonomy, practical orientation, personal problem solving, anger and aggression, order and organization, program clarity, and staff control. The scale is valid in distinguishing different kinds of inpatient units. Moos summarizes his work regarding the relationship between the treatment environment and other dimensions of hospital programs such as staffing, program policies, and characteristics of patients. This book has not received the attention from the psychiatric profession it deserves.

13. **Sederer LI** (ed): *Inpatient Psychiatry: Diagnosis and Treatment,* 2nd Edition. Baltimore, MD, Williams & Wilkins, 1991

This is an overview of psychiatry from the narrowed focus of inpatient psychiatry. Chapters on each of the diagnostic categories discuss evaluation and treatment.

Partial Hospitalization and Supported Living

14. **Gudeman JE, Shore MF, Dickey B:** Day hospitalization and an inn instead of inpatient care for psychiatric patients. *N Engl J Med* 308:749–753, 1983

This is a description and preliminary study of the reorganization of mental health services away from inpatient care to alternative day and night modalities. The dramatic alterations in patterns of usage, especially the reduction in traditional inpatient care and direct care staff, presage current thinking about service delivery.

15. **Herz MI, Endicott J, Spitzer RL, Mesnikoff A:** Day versus inpatient hospitalization: a controlled study. *Am J Psychiatry* 127:1307–1382, 1971

This was among the first controlled studies demonstrating the efficacy of day hospitalization as compared with inpatient hospitalization for patients for whom both treatments were judged clinically feasible. The superiority of day treatment was evident on virtually every measure used to evaluate outcome.

16. **Parker S, Knoll JL:** Partial hospitalization: an update. *Am J Psychiatry* 147:156–160, 1990

   In this contemporary and comprehensive review of the history, definitions, models, staffing, referral patterns, and utilization of partial hospitalization, the authors offer several provocative suggestions about why this modality has been underutilized even in this age of deinstitutionalization and cost containment.

Practice of Milieu Treatment

17. *Gabbard GO:** Splitting in hospital treatment. *Am J Psychiatry* 146:444–451, 1989

   This is a clear conceptualization of the common situation on psychiatric units in which staff disagreements (splitting) regarding a patient reflect intrapsychic splitting in the patient's internal world. Gabbard provides a number of practical strategies for managing these "recreations" in the milieu of the patient's internal world.

18. **Munich RL:** The role of the unit chief: an integrated perspective. *Psychiatry* 49:325–336, 1986

   This is an article on leadership in general but with a specific focus on the complicated tasks of running an inpatient unit. The tasks are divided into functions that address organizational and human needs and are linked with psychological valences in leaders that enhance and inhibit their implementation. The article is laced with real-life examples.

19. **Russakoff LM, Oldham JM:** The structure and technique of community meetings: the short-term unit. *Psychiatry* 45:38–44, 1982

   This article is an exemplar of the task-oriented, patient-staff meeting held on most acute and short-term inpatient units. The description of the model is complemented by details from an actual meeting.

20. **Sacks M, Carpenter WT:** The pseudotherapeutic community: an examination of anti-therapeutic forces on psychiatric units. *Hosp Community Psychiatry* 25:315–318, 1974

A pseudotherapeutic community is a psychiatric unit that subscribes to a treatment belief while covertly functioning in a way contrary to the specific belief. The authors discuss the characteristics of such a unit.

21. **Sacks MH, Carpenter WT, Scott WH:** Crisis and emergency on the psychiatric ward. *Compr Psychiatry* 15:79–85, 1974

The authors define crisis as a group behavior that threatens or prevents a psychiatric unit from accomplishing its therapeutic task, which may result in an emergency or behavior that is grossly disruptive. The recognition and prevention of crisis are examined in detail.

22. **Swenson CR, Munich RL:** Types of large-group meetings in the therapeutic community: with special emphasis on the long-term unit. *Psychiatry* 52:437–445, 1989

This is a careful delineation of the most prevalent types of large-group, community, or patient-staff meetings practiced and referred to in the literature. The special role of this meeting in expanding participants' appreciation of how various community-relevant events and themes impact on the social fabric is demonstrated by details from an actual meeting on an extended length of stay unit.

Milieu Issues With Special Populations

23. **Bjork D, Steinberg M, Lindenmayer JP, Pardes H:** Mania and milieu: treatment of manics in a therapeutic community. *Hosp Community Psychiatry* 28:431–436, 1977

The authors describe practical principles for the treatment of hospitalized patients with manic psychoses. For clinicians struggling with non-compliant manic patients, it is especially useful to learn of the authors' important milieu modifications that are necessary to meet individual treatment needs.

24. **Munich RL:** The VIP as patient: syndrome, dynamic and treatment, in *American Psychiatric Press Review of Psychiatry*, Vol. 8. Edited by Tasman A, Hales RE, Frances AJ. Washington, DC, American Psychiatric Press, 1989, pp. 580–593

This is a summary of past literature and an update on the ubiquitous and troubling phenomenon of the special or "very important person" in the milieu and the effects on treatment in the milieu. The author highlights the dysfunctional interaction between personality and social system factors and the role of entitlement in the genesis of the syndrome.

25. **Paul GL, Lentz RJ:** *Psychosocial Treatment of Chronic Mental Patients: Milieu Versus Social-Learning Programs.* Cambridge, MA, Harvard University Press, 1977

This is a report and an analysis in depth of a clinical research study designed to assess the relative effectiveness of traditional hospital treatment, milieu therapy, and a social learning program using token economy methodology. The conclusion that social learning is far superior to milieu programs is only part of the book's value, which defines the programs meticulously and includes manuals for both programs.

26. **Selzer M:** Preparing the chronic schizophrenic for exploratory psychotherapy: the role of hospitalization. *Psychiatry* 46:303–311, 1983

An elegant description of the ways one might use listening techniques and the inpatient milieu to engage otherwise treatment-resistant patients in treatment. Although psychotherapy per se is little seen in today's hospital stays, the emphasis here is on engagement and treatment alliance.

27. **Smith TE, Munich RL:** Suicide, violence, and elopement: prediction, understanding, and management, in *American Psychiatric Press Review of Psychiatry*, Vol. 11. Edited by Tasman A, Riba MB. Washington, DC, American Psychiatric Press, 1992, pp. 535–554

The authors outline the several factors involved in various untoward events in the inpatient setting. Drawing from the literature and relevant clinical and social system factors, they construct a profile of the high-risk patient and suggest ways to predict and manage these patients and events.

28. **Swenson C:** Supportive elements of inpatient treatment with borderline patients, in *Supportive Therapy for Borderline Patients: A Psychodynamic Approach.* Edited by Rockland L. New York, Guilford, 1992, pp. 269–283

This chapter categorizes and discusses the various elements relevant to the inpatient treatments of patients with borderline personality disorder. These categories include but go beyond those enumerated by Gunderson et al. (1983) above, offering functions from which the ego of the patient can temporarily "borrow" in the service of regaining stability and control.

Special Problems in the Milieu

29. **Leibenluft E, Summergrad P, Tasman A:** Academic dilemma of the inpatient unit director. *Am J Psychiatry* 146:73–76, 1989

This article is not only about the academic dilemma of the junior faculty member, but also the implications of these strains on the clinical, research, and educational functions of the inpatient unit. The authors suggest ways of relieving the situation.

30. *Ravenscroft K:* Milieu process during the residency turnover: the human cost of psychiatric education. *Am J Psychiatry* 132:506–512, 1975

This is an informative and practically heartbreaking account of the many dysfunctional sequences and consequences of the biannual transition of residents and trainees on inpatient units. This is virtually required reading for anyone leading an inpatient unit in which the training function takes place.

31. **Van Putten T:** Milieu therapy: contraindications? *Arch Gen Psychiatry* 29:640–643, 1973

This article is a strong argument that the milieu emphasis on forced social interaction, participation, and liveliness is conceptually unsound and may contain a toxic dose of environmental stimulation for some schizophrenic patients.

46

Consultation-Liaison Psychiatry

Joel J. Wallack, M.D.
Samuel W. Perry, M.D.

S ince the publication of the first edition of this bibliography in
1984, the body of knowledge constituting consultation-liaison
psychiatry has significantly expanded. A number of distinct clinical areas have emerged, several with their own organizations, journals, and
textbooks (e.g., psycho-oncology, psychonephrology, transplant psychiatry,
acquired immunodeficiency syndrome). The works selected for this chapter
are meant to address the many problems a psychiatrist confronts when
consulting in a general hospital. Although some papers are included to
provide a theoretical and historical perspective, the selection emphasizes
the more clinical aspects—that is, the specific difficulties a psychiatrist can
anticipate in working with physically ill patients and nonpsychiatric colleagues.

Along with emphasizing the practical, the selection is based on three
other considerations. First, most of the articles have an excellent bibliography of their own and thereby provide a link toward pursuing the given area
in more detail and depth. Second, the articles are meant to complement
Luber and Viederman's selections for Chapter 27 on psychosomatic medicine, which addresses the more theoretical and investigative aspects of the
field. Third, and perhaps most important, the selection was very strongly

influenced by the responses of psychiatry residents who have found the following articles to be the most helpful and stimulating during their consultation-liaison rotations.

General Textbooks

1. *__Cassem NH__ (ed): *Massachusetts General Hospital Handbook of General Hospital Psychiatry*, 3rd Edition. St. Louis, MO, CV Mosby, 1991

   This now classic text emphasizes the crucial clinical considerations regarding such topics as delirium, pain, somatization, dialysis, surgery, burns, intensive care, and dying. It also provides sufficient background, depth, and references to be far more than a "cookbook" list of instructions.

2. __Kaufman DM:__ *Clinical Neurology for Psychiatrists*, 3rd Edition. Philadelphia, PA, WB Saunders, 1990

   Based on the well-known course of the same name, this highly readable and well-organized text provides the student with a concise guide to the major areas of clinical neurology.

3. __Sherman M__ (ed): Pediatric consultation-liaison. *Psychiatr Clin North Am* 5:2, 1982

   This article not only places under one cover many relevant issues for the consultation-liaison pediatric psychiatrist (e.g., child abuse, asthma, behavioral aspects of childhood diabetes, young leukemia patients, neonatal intensive care), but also discusses liaison issues (e.g., promoting the alliance between pediatrics and child psychiatry, setting up a pediatric consultation-liaison service, communicating with pediatricians).

4. __Stoudemire A, Fogel BS:__ *Psychiatric Care of the Medical Patient.* New York, Oxford University Press, 1993

   This superb text provides the most comprehensive reference resource currently available regarding the psychiatric aspects of medical illness. General principles of diagnosis and treatment are thoughtfully addressed, as are disease- and subspecialty-specific topics. As a whole, this book provides the reader with a truly "biopsychosocial" overview of the field of consultation-liaison psychiatry.

General Concepts and Classic Articles

5. *Engel GL: The need for a new medical model: a challenge for biomedicine. *Science* 196:129–136, 1977

After presenting the limitations of the biomedical model, Engel introduces the biopsychosocial model as a "systems approach" to the physically ill patient. The article provides a conceptual scheme that is useful to consider and discuss with nonpsychiatric colleagues.

6. *Kahana RJ, Bibring GL: Personality types in medical management, in *Psychiatry and Medical Practice in a General Hospital.* Edited by Zinberg N. New York, International Universities Press, 1964, pp. 108–123

This chapter demonstrates how therapeutic interventions can be tailored to the personality types of those who are physically ill. The examples given are specific, colorful, and easily recognizable.

7. *Meyer E, Mendelson M: Psychiatric consultations with patients on medical and surgical wards: patterns and processes. *Psychiatry* 24:197–220, 1961

Using a series of well-illustrated case examples, the role of the psychiatric consultant is carefully explored. The three steps to performing a consultation—assessing the reasons for the request, redefining the patient's situation, and enabling the system to meet the patient's needs—are fully described.

8. *Perry S, Viederman M: Adaptation of residents to consultation-liaison psychiatry, I: working with the physically ill. *Gen Hosp Psychiatry* 3:141–147, 1981; **Perry S, Viederman M:** Adaptation of residents to consultation-liaison psychiatry, II: working with the non-psychiatric staff. *Gen Hosp Psychiatry* 149–156, 1981

Part I describes the special requirements for working with physically ill patients. Part II describes the defensive reactions psychiatrists may assume when confronted with the skepticism about the value of psychiatry. The two articles are particularly helpful for introducing psychiatry residents to consultation-liaison.

9. *Strain JJ: Psychological reactions to medical illness and hospitalization, in *Psychological Care of the Medically Ill: A Primer of Liaison Psychiatry.* Edited by Strain JJ, Grossman SJ. New York, Appleton-Century-Crofts, 1975, pp. 23–36

Strain discusses why adverse psychological reactions in medically ill patients are common and provides a conceptual framework to help the reader understand the basic stresses of illness and hospitalization.

Human Immunodeficiency Virus (HIV) and Acquired Immunodeficiency Syndrome (AIDS)

10. **Fernandez F, Holmes VF, Levy JK, Ruiz P:** Consultation-liaison psychiatry and HIV-related disorders. *Hosp Community Psychiatry* 40:146–153, 1989

   The authors describe the neuropsychiatric, psychosocial, and ethical-legal problems associated with HIV infection that are frequently encountered by the consultation-liaison psychiatrist. A neuropsychological screening battery is also described to assist in the evaluation process.

11. *Holland JC, Tross S:** The psychosocial and neuro-psychiatric sequelae of the acquired immunodeficiency syndrome and related disorders. *Ann Intern Med* 103:760–764, 1985

   The authors remind us that to help AIDS patients, the frequently occurring psychological, social, psychiatric, and neurologic complications of AIDS must be addressed. Health care workers also need to recognize their own reactions to this disease.

12. **Ostrow D, Grant I, Atkinson H:** Assessment and management of the AIDS patient with neuropsychiatric disturbances. *J Clin Psychiatry* 49 (suppl):14–22, 1988

   The essential and primary role for psychiatry in the diagnosis and treatment of the neuropsychiatric disturbances associated with HIV infection are discussed in this review.

13. **Perry SW:** Organic mental disorders caused by HIV: update on early diagnosis and treatment. *Am J Psychiatry* 147:696–705, 1990

   This update explores the wide range of organic mental disorders seen with HIV infection and their presentations, frequency, evaluation, and treatments.

Cancer (Psycho-Oncology)

14. **Massie MJ, Holland JC:** Overview of normal reactions and prevalence of psychiatric disorders, in *Handbook of Psycho-Oncology: Psychological Care of the Patient with Cancer.* Edited by Holland JC, Rowland JH. New York, Oxford University Press, 1989, pp. 273–290

   This comprehensive chapter from the definitive textbook on psycho-oncology carefully reviews the normal reactions to a diagnosis of cancer as well as the types of psychological disturbances frequently seen. Guidelines for psychiatric assessment and management are provided.

Cardiac Illness

15. **Booth-Kewley S, Friedman H:** Psychological predictors of heart disease: a quantitative review. *Psychol Bull* 101:343–362, 1987

The relationships of certain personality variables to coronary heart disease are examined, with particular emphasis on the components of the "Type A" personality. The authors call for further research to help define the coronary-prone personality.

16. **Heller S, Kornfeld D:** Psychiatric aspects of cardiac surgery. *Adv Psychosom Med* 15:124–139, 1986

Psychological and psychiatric factors contributing to or resulting from the cardiac surgical process are discussed with a thorough review of the outcome literature on open-heart and coronary artery bypass graft surgery. Heart transplantation and the artificial heart are also briefly covered.

Childhood Illness

17. **Freud A:** The role of bodily illness in the mental life of children. *Psychoanal Study Child* 7:69–81, 1952

Freud describes the consequences of bodily illness intercepting, and at times impeding, different phases of childhood development.

Consultation

18. *Cohen-Cole SA:** Consultation psychiatry: a practical guide, in *Psychiatry*, Vol. 2. Edited by Michels R, Cavenar JO, Cooper A. Philadelphia, PA, JB Lippincott, 1988, pp. 1–9

This "how-to" step-by-step guide to the consultation process offers clear, pragmatic information that will assist those just beginning in consultation-liaison. The dual role of the consultant as educator and provider of expert advice to nonpsychiatrists is explored.

19. *Garrick TR, Stotland NL:** How to write a psychiatric consultation. *Am J Psychiatry* 139:849–855, 1982

This article presents a conceptual and practical scheme for making decisions about the content, style, and wording of the consultation note.

Coping

20. **Janis IL:** Adaptive personality changes, in *Stress and Coping, an Anthology.* Edited by Monat A, Lazarus RS. New York, Columbia University Press, 1977, pp. 272–284

    Included in this anthology on stress and coping, this chapter shows how too much or too little anxiety may prevent the necessary worrying and trial action before surgery.

21. *****Lipowski ZJ:** Physical illness, the individual and the coping processes. *Psychiatr Med* 1:91–102, 1970

    Lipowski presents a framework of illness behavior to explain the determinants of how patients cope with the stresses of physical illness and disability. This classic article is a favorite among students of consultation-liaison.

Death and Dying

22. *****Cassem NH, Stewart RS:** Management and care of the dying patient. *Int J Psychiatry Med* 6:293–304, 1975

    After carefully describing the psychological processes involved in the dying process, the authors provide clear and useful advice on how to speak with and manage terminally ill patients.

23. **Kubler-Ross E, Wessler S, Arioli LV:** On death and dying. *JAMA* 221:174–179, 1972

    The authors summarize their vast experience working with dying patients. The different stages of dying, although admittedly too simplified, provide a structure for discussing with staff this broad and difficult topic.

24. **Norton J:** Treatment of a dying patient. *Psychoanal Study Child* 18:541–561, 1963

    In her own personal account of an intense therapeutic involvement with a depressed, dying woman, Norton describes the psychology and phenomenology of dying.

Delirium and Dementia

25. *Lipowski ZJ: Organic mental disorders: introduction and review of syndromes, in *Comprehensive Textbook of Psychiatry/III,* 3rd Edition, Vol. 2. Edited by Kaplan HI, Freedman AM, Sadock BJ. Baltimore, MD, Williams & Wilkins, 1980, pp. 1359–1392

In his usual thorough yet readable style, Lipowski walks the reader through the classification and concepts of the various organic brain syndromes with special emphasis on delirium and dementia. Also covered are the amnestic syndromes, organic hallucinosis, organic delusional syndromes, organic affective syndromes, and organic personality syndromes.

Depression in Medically Ill Patients

26. Rodin G, Voshart K: Depression in the medically ill: an overview. *Am J Psychiatry* 143:696–705, 1986

Diagnosing depression in medically ill patients poses numerous challenges for the clinician. For example, are the usual somatic criteria valid? The authors review the epidemiology, diagnosis, clinical presentations, and treatment approaches for this important population.

27. *Viederman M, Perry S: Use of psychodynamic life narrative in the treatment of depression in the physically ill. *Gen Hosp Psychiatry* 2:177–185, 1980

The authors discuss with clinical illustrations how a succinct, supportive summary can be used therapeutically to explain to the patient the meaning of his or her depression.

Difficult Patients

28. Groves JE: Management of the borderline patient on a medical or surgical ward: the psychiatric consultant's role. *Int J Psychiatry Med* 6:337–348, 1975

After describing the disruption and disorganization caused by these most difficult patients, the author carefully details a behavioral approach to not only to manage the patient but also to help staff members control their own strong countertransferential reactions.

29. *Groves JE:** Taking care of the hateful patient. *N Engl J Med* 298:883–887, 1978

Groves discusses the difficulties of defining and dealing with "crocks" and the negative reactions they elicit in physicians.

30. **Perry S, Gilmore MM:** The disruptive patient or visitor. *JAMA* 245:755–757, 1981

This article succinctly outlines how to approach, restrain, medicate, and evaluate a patient or visitor who becomes disruptive on a medical ward. The legal considerations are also discussed.

31. **Wise TN:** Psychiatric management of patients who threaten to sign out against medical advice. *Int J Psychiatry Med* 5:153–160, 1974

By understanding what factors contribute to signing out against medical advice, the psychiatrist may be able to intercept potentially destructive behavior.

Factitious Illness

32. **Hyler SE, Sussman N:** Chronic factitious disorders with physical symptoms (the Munchausen Syndrome). *Psychiatr Clin North Am* 4:365–377, 1981

The authors review the challenging subject of factitious disorders and offer suggestions about interviewing and managing a "deceitful" patient.

33. **Reich P, Gottfried LA:** Factitious disorders in a teaching hospital. *Ann Intern Med* 99:240–247, 1983

Over a 10-year period, the authors identified 41 cases of hospitalized patients with factitious disorders. These cases are subdivided into four groups: self-induced infections, simulated illnesses, chronic wounds, and surreptitious self-medication. Patient characteristics, management, and prognosis are discussed.

Historical Background

34. **Lipowski ZJ:** Review of consultation psychiatry and psychosomatic medicine, part 1: general principles. *Psychosom Med* 29:153–171, 1967; **Lipowski ZJ:** Review of consultation psychiatry and psychosomatic medicine, part 2: clinical aspects. *Psychosom Med* 29:201–224, 1967;

Lipowski ZJ: Review of consultation psychiatry and psychosomatic medicine, part 3: theoretical issues. *Psychosom Med* 30:395–422, 1968

These three articles, although now somewhat dated, provide a scholarly historical account of liaison psychiatry.

Hypochondriasis

35. **Barsky AJ, Klerman GL:** Overview: hypochondriasis, bodily complaints and somatic styles. *Am J Psychiatry* 140:273–283, 1983

The authors summarize the confusing ways hypochondriasis has been conceptualized phenomenologically, psychodynamically, perceptually, and socially. They suggest the term *amplifying somatic style* be used for further systematic investigation.

Intensive Care

36. **Cassem NH, Hackett TP:** The setting of intensive care, in *Massachusetts General Hospital Handbook of General Hospital Psychiatry,* 3rd Edition. Edited by Cassem NH. St. Louis, MO, CV Mosby, 1991, pp. 373–399

Patient reactions to the intensive care setting and the reasons for psychiatric consultation are discussed. The causes of behavioral and psychological derangements are reviewed, with particular emphasis on delirium. The authors provide practical information on how to manage the common problems faced by the consultant.

Liaison Psychiatry

37. *Mohl PC:** The liaison psychiatrist: social role and status. *Psychosomatics* 20:19–23, 1979

The differences between liaison and consultation psychiatry are discussed, with emphasis on the important role played by the liaison psychiatrist within the ward culture, enabling the psychiatrist to achieve greater acceptance and clinical effectiveness.

38. **Torem M, Saravay SM, Steinberg H:** Psychiatric liaison: benefits of an "active" approach: *Psychosomatics* 20:598–611, 1979

By using an active liaison approach, the authors of this study were able to gain access to the many hospitalized patients whose psychiatric problems often go unnoticed and untreated.

Noncompliance

39. **Strain JJ:** Non-compliance, in *Psychological Interventions in Medical Practice.* Edited by Strain JJ. New York, Appleton-Century-Crofts, 1977, pp. 91–104

   Studies have demonstrated that perhaps as many as one-half of the patients seen in the primary care setting fail to comply with their prescribed medical regimens. The author explores the psychological and sociocultural factors involved as well as the doctor's contribution to noncompliance and offers useful advice for management of these patients.

Obstetrics and Gynecology

40. **Gise L:** Psychiatric complications of pregnancy, in *Complications of Pregnancy: Medical, Surgical, Gynecologic, Psychosocial and Perinatal,* 4th Edition. Edited by Cherry SH, Merkatz IR. Baltimore, MD, Williams & Wilkins, 1991, pp. 194–250

   The author addresses psychiatric aspects of pregnancy, birth, and the postpartum period. Biological issues and psychodynamic concepts are discussed with equal importance, and clear treatment guidelines are offered. An added bonus is the excellent reference list of nearly 500 citations.

41. **Parry BL:** Reproductive factors affecting the course of affective illness in women. *Psychiatr Clin North Am* 12:207–220, 1989

   Gender-related factors predispose women to depressive illness, especially during the reproductive years. The author carefully reviews the relationship of the female reproductive hormones to the onset of these affective episodes.

Pain

42. **Benjamin S:** Psychological treatment of chronic pain: a selective review. *J Psychosom Res* 33:121–131, 1989

   Chronic pain patients frequently suffer from both psychiatric and physical illness and therefore often require a multifaceted approach. This article discusses psychiatric diagnosis in pain patients and the various intervention strategies available. The need for more research is underscored.

43. **Engel GL:** "Psychogenic" pain and the pain prone patient. *Am J Med* 26:899–918, 1959

Despite many advances in recent years regarding the mechanisms of pain, Engel's article remains a classic in describing how the meaning of pain can influence its expression, severity, and management.

44. **Marks RM, Sachar EJ:** Undertreatment of medical inpatients with narcotic analgesics. *Ann Intern Med* 78:173–181, 1973

A survey of two teaching hospitals indicated that physicians were generally ignorant about narcotic analgesics, overconcerned about iatrogenic addiction, and unwilling to provide adequate analgesia.

Psychonephrology

45. **Levy NB:** Psychological complications of dialysis: psychonephrology to the rescue. *Bull Menninger Clin* 48:237–250, 1984

The psychological stresses and complications of renal failure and dialysis are thoroughly described, as are treatment interventions. This comprehensive overview will introduce the reader to the growing subspecialty of psychonephrology.

46. **Viederman M:** Adaptive and maladaptive regression in hemodialysis. *Psychiatry* 37:68–77, 1974

47. **Viederman M:** The search for meaning in renal transplantation. *Psychiatry* 37:283–290, 1974

In these two articles, Viederman describes how regression, fantasy, transference, and partial identifications influence the response to hemodialysis and renal transplantation.

Psychopharmacology of Medically Ill Patients

48. *Stoudemire A, Moran MG, Fogel BS:** Psychotropic drug use in the medically ill, part I. *Psychosomatics* 31:377–391, 1990; *Stoudemire A, Moran MG, Fogel BS:** Psychotropic drug use in the medically ill, part II. *Psychosomatics* 32:34–46, 1991

The use of psychotropic medication in medical or surgical patients is often problematic due to the underlying medical illness or drug interactions. This two-part article carefully reviews each of the major categories of psychotropics, with special attention to their use in elderly or medically debilitated patients.

Somatization

49. *Ford CV: *The Somatizing Disorders: Illness as a Way of Life.* New York, Elsevier, 1983, pp. 49–97 (Chapters 4, 5, 6)

Ford presents a fascinating historical perspective of our current concepts of somatization, including hysteria, conversion reactions, Briquet's syndrome, and somatization disorder.

50. *Lipowski ZJ: Somatization and depression. *Psychosomatics* 31:13–21, 1990

The association of somatization with depression is extremely common, yet many if not most of these patients go unrecognized or improperly diagnosed and treated. Lipowski reviews the current state of our understanding of this ubiquitous phenomenon and emphasizes the need for clinicians to recognize and prevent persistent somatization.

Surgery

51. *Hackett TP, Weisman AD: Psychiatric management of operative syndromes. *Psychosom Med* 22:267–282, 1960

Just as useful today as it was more than 30 years ago, this well-written article uses colorful case examples to illustrate the variety of psychiatric complications ("operative syndromes") that can develop during the course of surgical treatment.

Transplant

52. **House RM, Trzepacz PT, Thompson TL:** Psychiatric consultation to organ transplant services, in *American Psychiatric Press Review of Psychiatry,* Vol. 9. Edited by Tasman A, Goldfinger SM, Kaufmann C. Washington, DC, American Psychiatric Press, 1990, pp. 515–536

This comprehensive chapter reviews the history and current status of organ transplantation, the stresses experienced by the patient during the preoperative and postoperative and rehabilitation phases, and the psychological responses commonly seen. A reference list is included for the interested reader.

47

Behavior Therapy

Gordon G. Ball, Ph.D.

B ehavior therapy is best defined as a set of treatment procedures based on experimental results from psychology and the social sciences. The focus is on maladaptive behavior and on current rather than historical events. It prescribes treatment in operational terms and specifies target behaviors for measuring outcome. Treatment derives from a behavioral diagnosis and assessment and is directed at the problem behavior itself. Since the first edition of this book, the major new developments have been the addition of cognitive techniques to behavioral approaches. Research has shown that cognitive exercises, along with behavior therapy, can be extremely effective in reducing depression. In the anxiety disorders, behavioral treatments have improved, especially in the area of panic and obsessive-compulsive behaviors. Behavioral medicine continues to expand, and behavioral techniques with children and adolescents continue to improve. There is increasing interaction between behavior therapist and psychopharmacologist in producing integrated treatment packages for many disorders, and this multidisciplinary approach is likely to blossom with time. Behavior therapy continues to be research oriented, with the general progression being from laboratory research, to field trials, to clinical applications. The references cover the history of the development of behavior therapy, general texts, theoretical issues, and procedures for behavioral assessment and treatment of specific disorders. In addition to a knowledge of these techniques, one is advised to consult the behavior therapy journals for current modification of these procedures.

History

1. **Hersen M:** Historical perspectives in behavioral assessment, in *Behavioral Assessment: A Practical Handbook.* Edited by Hersen M, Bellack AS. Oxford, United Kingdom, Pergamon, 1976, pp. 3–22

   This chapter criticizes the reliability and validity of the disease model of mental disorders in the areas of diagnosis, assessment, and treatment. Recommendations are made for more stringent criteria for psychiatric evaluation and procedural outcome.

2. **Kazdin AE:** *History of Behavior Modification: Experimental Foundations of Contemporary Research.* Baltimore, MD, University Park Press, 1978

   This book traces the development of behavior therapy from its early beginnings. This is a good historical document of the problems faced by early pioneers.

3. **Watson JB, Rayner R:** Conditioned emotional reactions. *J Exp Psychol* 3:1–14, 1920

   This classic article describes the most famous case in the history of behavior therapy: the conditioning of Albert, an 11-month-old boy, to be afraid of a white rat. It also presents the first rudimentary approaches toward the development of behavior therapy in this country.

4. **Wolpe J:** *The Practice of Behavior Therapy,* 2nd Edition. New York, Pergamon, 1973

   This book describes in detail the basic procedures involved in systematic desensitization made famous by Wolpe. It also discusses the alternate behavioral strategies for handling the various forms of anxiety.

General Texts

5. **Bellack AS, Hersen M:** *Behavioral Assessment,* 3rd Edition. New York, Pergamon, 1988

   This book offers excellent reviews on the fundamental issues in behavioral assessment and on specific assessment strategies used in planning treatment.

6. *Bellack AS, Hersen M, Kazdin AE (eds): *International Handbook of Behavior Modification and Therapy,* 2nd Edition. New York, Plenum, 1990

   This book offers the best overview of behavior therapy to date. It covers the foundations of behavior therapy; assessment and methodology;

ethical issues; and treatment of anxiety, depression, schizophrenia, substance abuse, sexual problems, obsessive-compulsive disorders, mental conflicts, and childhood disorders.

7. **Davis M, Eshelman ER, McKay M:** *The Relaxation and Stress Reduction Workbook.* Oakland, CA, New Harbinger Press, 1988

Although advertised as a self-help book, this book is used by many professionals to teach patients the skills of relaxation, refuting irrational ideas, assertiveness training, stress reduction, thought stoppage, and many other well-established behavior techniques. This is a very practical book for the behavior therapist to keep close at hand.

8. **Rapee RM, Barlow DH:** *Chronic Anxiety.* New York, Guilford, 1991

This is a comprehensive book, covering the etiology and treatment of all the anxiety disorders, along with a discussion of the interrelationship between anxiety and depression. There is also useful information on the interactions of psychopharmacological, cognitive, and behavioral treatment strategies.

9. **Turner SM, Calhoun KS, Adams HE** (eds): *Handbook of Clinical Behavior Therapy.* New York, Wiley, 1981

As a compendium of behavioral techniques, covering the whole gamut of behavior therapy, this stands out as one of the better books. It also points the reader to important references in each of the areas discussed. It covers not only anxiety disorders, but also behavioral techniques used in treating schizophrenic behavior, substance abuse, sleep disorders, sexual dysfunction, mental retardation, and childhood behavioral problems as well as behavior medicine.

Theoretical Issues

10. *Eysenck HJ, Martin I: *Theoretical Foundations of Behavior Therapy.* New York, Plenum, 1987

This book is a sophisticated discussion of the underlying mechanisms leading to treatment procedures. The authors argue against the view that behavior therapy is solely mechanistic and cannot handle covert events. They demonstrate how specific treatments can be used in complex situations.

11. **Foa EB, Emmelcamp PMG:** *Failures in Behavior Therapy.* New York, Wiley, 1983

A series of treatment failures point to shortcomings in behavior therapy. From these failures, the authors are able to make interesting suggestions about directions that behavior therapy should take, as well as making an important plea to behavior therapists to perform thorough behavioral assessments and follow rigorous treatment programs.

12. **Gray JA:** *The Neuropsychology of Anxiety.* New York, Oxford University Press, 1982

This is an extremely important book in the development of our knowledge about anxiety. It integrates neuroanatomical, neuropharmacological, and conditioning data into a coherent theory of the mechanisms behind anxiety. This book offers a useful framework for integrating the various avenues of present and future research.

13. **Hersen M, Barlow DH:** *Single Case Experimental Designs: Strategies for Studying Behavior Change.* Oxford, United Kingdom, Pergamon, 1976

Accurate behavioral observation is the first crucial step leading to behavioral assessment and treatment. This book describes observational procedures and behavioral analysis useful for evaluating single case studies in the clinical setting.

14. **Hersen M, Bellack AS:** DSM III and behavioral assessment, in *Behavioral Assessment: A Practical Handbook,* 3rd Edition. Edited by Bellack AS, Hersen M. New York, Pergamon, 1988, pp. 67–84

This chapter presents the behavior therapist's view of the advantages and disadvantages of DSM-III. They offer some interesting suggestions on how behavioral assessments can be incorporated into this standard classification in a complementary fashion.

15. **Mackintosh NJ:** *Conditioning and Associative Learning.* New York, Oxford University Press, 1983

Conditioning theory is the backbone of behavior therapy. The research over the past 20 years has produced many changes in this area. The complex associations between stimuli now play a more significant part of the theory, rather than the association between stimuli and responses. This is still the best book on conditioning presently available, offering the behavior therapist a solid background in the principles of learning.

Specific Procedures

16. **Azrin NH, Nunn RG:** Habit reversal: a method of eliminating nervous habits and tics. *Behav Res Ther* 11:619–628, 1973

Treatment of habit disorders, such as stuttering, enuresis, encopresis, vomiting, thumb sucking, nail biting, and motor tics, has met with mixed but generally favorable success by using behavior therapy procedures. This article outlines the basic procedure employed and researched by Azrin and his co-workers.

17. **Beck AT, Rush AJ, Shaw BF, Emery G:** *Cognitive Therapy of Depression.* New York, Guilford, 1979

Cognitive-behavioral therapy was launched mainly by this book. The authors present a treatment plan, based on their careful research, for managing depression. The techniques involve challenging the maladaptive thinking patterns of depressed patients and introducing structured verbal and written exercises. Behavioral exercises in social skills training, assertiveness, increased activity, and graded exposure are an important part of the treatment.

18. **Beck AT, Emery G, Greenberg RL:** *Anxiety Disorders and Phobias.* New York, Basic Books, 1985

This is a valiant attempt to use the cognitive strategies for treating anxiety disorders. Although these strategies are useful when used in conjunction with behavioral techniques, they have not had the same impact on the treatment of anxiety disorders compared with their usefulness in the treatment of depression. However, the addition of cognitive procedures to behavioral procedures is becoming more widely used.

19. **Foa EB, Steketee GS, Ozarow BJ:** Behavior therapy with obsessive-compulsives, in *Obsessive-Compulsive Disorder.* Edited by Marissakalian M, Turner SM, Michelson L. New York, Plenum, 1985, pp. 49–129

This chapter demonstrates convincingly the need for both exposure and response prevention to treat obsessive-compulsive disorders effectively. The careful analysis of the procedures is an excellent exposition of the behavioral methods used.

20. **Hersen M, Van Hasselt VB:** *Behavior Therapy With Children and Adolescents.* New York, Wiley, 1987

Operant conditioning principles have been applied to clinical and educational problems in children for the last three decades with increasing success. Summaries of the development of the techniques, and other behavioral approaches, cover issues such as autism, mental retardation, conduct disorders, substance abuses, eating disorders, anxiety, and attention-deficit disorder.

21. **Lange AS, Jakubowski P:** *Responsible Assertive Behavior.* Champaign, IL, Research Press, 1976

The general approach to problems of interpersonal dysfunction involves a combination of assertiveness skills training to improve social functioning and cognitive coping strategies to reduce anxiety. This is an excellent book on assertiveness training.

22. **Marks IM:** *Fears, Phobias and Rituals.* New York, Oxford University Press, 1987

Marks summarizes his extensive contributions to behavior therapy. He outlines the development of clinical syndromes and compares this with the development of normal fears. He postulates on mechanisms behind these anxiety disorders, elaborates on treatment, and emphasizes the importance of follow-up data.

23. **Marlatt GA, Gordon JR:** *Relapse Prevention.* New York, Guilford, 1985

The major problem in treatment of substance-abusing persons is the high rate of relapse. Abstinence in a controlled setting is relatively easily achieved; continued abstinence without the setting is successful in only a few addicted persons. An analysis of situational factors leading to relapse, along with behavioral and cognitive interventions to prevent relapse, makes this a very important book in this very difficult area.

24. **Matarazzo JD, Weiss SM, Herd JA, Miller NE:** *Behavioral Health.* New York, Wiley, 1984

This handbook on health enhancement and disease prevention offers an overview of the many areas where behavioral management can reduce health risks through diet, exercise, smoking prevention, stress reduction techniques, education, substance abuse programs, and community activities. Many well-known authors in the behavioral medicine area have contributed excellent summaries.

25. **Matthews AM, Gelder MG, Johnston DW:** *Agoraphobia.* New York, Guilford, 1981

Theoretical issues, assessment procedures, supportive drug therapy, and behavioral intervention strategies for effectively alleviating agoraphobia are described in detail.

26. **Mavissakalian M, Barlow DH:** *Phobia: Psychological and Pharmacological Treatment.* New York, Guilford, 1981

The ability to treat fears and phobias successfully has been the hallmark of behavior therapy. This book evaluates the present behavioral and pharmacological interventions and offers a critical analysis of the state of the art.

27. **Schreibman L, Koegel RL:** A guideline for planning behavior modification programs for autistic children, in *Handbook of Clinical Behavior Therapy.* Edited by Turner SM, Calhoun KS, Adams HE. New York, Wiley, 1981, pp. 500–526

The results on the behavioral treatment of autism are extremely encouraging. This chapter outlines the basic strategy.

28. **Taylor CB, Arnow B:** *The Nature and Treatment of Anxiety Disorders.* New York, Free Press, 1988

A comprehensive approach to treatment of anxiety disorders is offered in this book. It attempts to integrate behavioral, cognitive, and pharmacological techniques into a series of systematic treatment programs.

29. **Wilson GT:** Behavior modification and the treatment of obesity, in *Obesity.* Edited by Skunkard AJ. Philadelphia, PA, WB Saunders, 1980, pp. 325–344

Wilson reviews different behavioral procedures for their efficacy in controlling obesity. The book emphasizes the complexity of the variables surrounding eating behavior.

48

Interpersonal Psychotherapy

John C. Markowitz, M.D.

Interpersonal psychotherapy (IPT) is a brief, focused psychotherapy of documented efficacy and standardization. Developed as a 12- to 16-week treatment of outpatient major depression, its use has since been expanded to other patient populations. The therapist uses the "medical model" to educate the patient about his or her diagnosis. Then, by focusing on an interpersonal problem area such as bereavement, a role dispute, a role transition, or interpersonal deficits, the therapist helps the patient both to improve interpersonal functioning and to relieve symptoms. IPT has been frequently used in comparative treatment studies and can be combined with medication.

In comparison with cognitive-behavioral therapy (CBT), its frequent competitor, IPT is closer to the dynamic psychotherapy many psychiatrists employ in private practice. IPT differs from CBT in its focus on the feelings evoked in interpersonal situations, rather than on depressogenic thoughts. It differs from dynamic psychotherapy in its focus on the here and now and in its avoidance of a transferential focus and of genetic and dream interpretations. Its efficacy has at least equaled that of CBT and approached that of antidepressant medication, in most treatment trials. To date, substance abuse is the only diagnostic area studied for which IPT has not shown utility.

General Background and Training

1. *Klerman GL, Weissman MM, Rounsaville BJ, Chevron ES: *Interpersonal Psychotherapy of Depression.* New York, Basic Books, 1984

   This book, the published version of the original treatment manual, remains the basic text for understanding IPT of depression.

2. **Rounsaville BJ, Chevron ES, Weissman MM:** Specification of techniques in interpersonal psychotherapy, in *Psychotherapy Research: Where Are We and Where Should We Go?* Edited by Williams JBW, Spitzer RL. New York, Guilford, 1984, pp. 160–172

   This is a brief chapter outlining the development of the IPT manual, training procedures, evaluation, and the characteristics important in selecting therapists. (Experience helps.)

3. **Sullivan HS:** *The Interpersonal Theory of Psychiatry.* New York, WW Norton, 1953

   An extension of the theories of Adolf Meyer, this book emphasizes the importance of the environment to psychiatric disorders. As such, it embodies the historical roots of modern IPT.

4. **Weissman MM, Rounsaville BJ, Chevron E:** Training psychotherapists to participate in psychotherapy outcome studies. *Am J Psychiatry* 139:1442–1446, 1982

   This article describes training issues surrounding the conversion of experienced psychotherapists to standardized IPT in preparation for an outcome study.

Comparative Outcome Studies in Major Depression

5. **DiMascio A, Weissman MM, Prusoff BA, Neu C, Zwilling M, Klerman GL:** Differential symptom reduction by drugs and psychotherapy in acute depression. *Arch Gen Psychiatry* 36:1450–1456, 1979

   The "New Haven–Boston" acute treatment study of 81 depressed outpatients compared IPT and amitriptyline separately and in combination against a nonscheduled psychotherapy cell. Each active treatment alone was more effective than the control, and the combined treatment cell did best. Weissman et al. (1979) below elaborate on these findings, and Weissman et al. (1981) below provide a follow-up report.

6. *Elkin I, Shea MT, Watkins JT, Imber SD, Sotsky SM, Collins JF, Glass DR, Pilkonis PA, Leber WR, Docherty JP, Fiester SJ, Parloff MB: National Institute of Mental Health Treatment of Depression Collaborative Research Program: general effectiveness of treatments. *Arch Gen Psychiatry* 46:971–982, 1989

This ambitious multicenter study, the first such psychotherapy trial sponsored by the National Institute of Mental Health, randomly assigned 250 acutely depressed outpatients to IPT, CBT, or imipramine treatment or placebo. Most subjects completed at least 15 weeks or 12 treatment sessions; IPT had the least patient attrition. All active treatments proved superior to placebo. Improvement was noted in all cells, particularly for less depressed patients. IPT outcome was superior to placebo, whereas CBT was not, for more severely depressed patients.

7. *Frank E, Kupfer DJ, Perel JM, Cornes C, Jarrett DB, Mallinger AG, Thase ME, McEachran AB, Grochocinski VJ: Three-year outcomes for maintenance therapies in recurrent depression. *Arch Gen Psychiatry* 47:1093–1099, 1990

This landmark, 3-year maintenance study of 128 subjects with recurrent major depression compared the prophylactic antidepressant effects of five treatment cells: a monthly maintenance form of IPT (IPT-M), either 1) in combination with high-dose imipramine, 2) alone, or 3) with placebo; 4) high-dose imipramine alone in a medication clinic; and 5) placebo alone in a medication clinic. Patients randomized to standard dose medication rarely relapsed; "low-dose" IPT-M also had a significantly longer survival time than did placebo. IPT-M did not add to the protective effect of imipramine alone.

8. Klerman GL, DiMascio A, Weissman MM, Prusoff BA, Paykel ES: Treatment of depression by drugs and psychotherapy. *Am J Psychiatry* 131:186–191, 1974

This study, the first systematic IPT trial, randomized 150 depressed outpatients to IPT, antidepressant medication, or their combination for 8 months. IPT had a delayed effect, but by 6–8 months was associated with differentially improved social functioning, whereas medication protected against symptomatic exacerbation and relapse. Combined treatment had the best outcome.

9. Weissman MM, Prusoff BA, DiMascio A, Neu C, Goklaney M, Klerman GL: The efficacy of drugs and psychotherapy in the treatment of acute depressive episodes. *Am J Psychiatry* 136:555–558, 1979

10. **Weissman MM, Klerman GL, Prusoff BA, Sholomskas D, Padian N:** Depressed outpatients: results one year after treatment with drugs and/or interpersonal psychotherapy. *Arch Gen Psychiatry* 38:51–55, 1981

On 1-year follow-up, the patients in the study by DiMascio et al. (1979) above and Weissman et al. (1979) generally showed sustained improvement. Patients receiving IPT functioned better than those receiving either antidepressant medication alone or the control condition. Symptom relapse and recurrence did not differ across groups.

Specific Treatment Populations

11. **Carroll KM, Rounsaville BJ, Gawin FH:** A comparative trial of psychotherapies for ambulatory cocaine abusers: relapse prevention and interpersonal psychotherapy. *Am J Drug Alcohol Abuse* 17:229–247, 1991

In this study, 42 outpatients with cocaine abuse were assigned either to IPT or behavioral treatment with the goal of drug abstinence. Although most differences did not reach statistical significance, IPT generally appeared less effective than the alternative treatment.

12. **Fairburn CG, Jones R, Peveler RC, Carr SJ, Solomon RA, O'Connor ME, Burton J, Hope RA:** Three psychological treatments for bulimia nervosa: a comparative trial. *Arch Gen Psychiatry* 48:463–469, 1991

In this study, 75 patients with bulimia nervosa were randomized either to CBT, a simplified behavioral therapy, or IPT. All three treatments reduced psychopathology, including depressive symptoms and overeating. CBT more effectively modified disturbed attitudes toward shape and weight—not surprisingly, because IPT was not directed toward eating issues.

13. **Fairburn CG, Jones R, Peveler RC, Hope RA, O'Connor M:** Psychotherapy and bulimia nervosa: longer-term effects of interpersonal psychotherapy, behavior therapy, and cognitive behavior therapy. *Arch Gen Psychiatry* 50:419–428, 1993

On 1-year follow-up, the IPT and CBT conditions proved equivalent across measures, although IPT took some time to catch up fully with CBT.

14. *Klerman GL, Weissman MM:** *New Applications of Interpersonal Therapy.* Washington, DC, American Psychiatric Press, 1993

This volume comprises chapters on various new developments of IPT: its adaptation as an antidepressant maintenance therapy for recurrent depression; as marital therapy; for depressive subgroups such as dysthymic, human immunodeficiency virus (HIV)-positive, adolescent, geriatric, and primary care patients; and for other psychiatric disorders such as substance abuse and bulimia.

15. **Markowitz JC, Klerman GL, Perry SW:** Interpersonal psychotherapy of depressed HIV-seropositive patients. *Hosp Community Psychiatry* 43:885–890, 1992

This article describes adaptation of IPT to a treatment population of depressed human immunodeficiency virus (HIV)-positive patients, most of whom were gay men. This approach emphasizes the acceptance of HIV infection itself as a role transition for these patients. Preliminary data are promising: 20 of 23 subjects improved.

16. **Moreau D, Mufson L, Weissman MM, Klerman GL:** Interpersonal psychotherapy for adolescent depression: description of modification and preliminary application. *J Am Acad Child Adolesc Psychiatry* 30:642–651, 1991

This adaptation of IPT to a population of adolescent depressed patients includes a novel problem area: the single-parent family.

17. **Rounsaville BJ, Glazer W, Wilber CH, Weissman MM, Kleber HD:** Short-term interpersonal psychotherapy in methadone-maintained opiate addicts. *Arch Gen Psychiatry* 40:629–636, 1983

Recruitment, attrition, and other methodological difficulties compromised this comparison of weekly IPT to a low-contact monthly treatment visit for 72 opiate-abusing persons on methadone maintenance, which found no added benefit for IPT.

18. **Sloane RB, Stapes FR, Schneider LS:** Interpersonal therapy versus nortriptyline for depression in the elderly, in *Clinical and Pharmacological Studies in Psychiatric Disorders.* Edited by Burrow GD, Norman TR, Dennerstein L. London, John Libbey, 1985, pp. 344–346

In a 6-week pilot study comparing IPT with nortriptyline in 30 geriatric patients, IPT showed some advantages over the tricyclic antidepressant. This was largely due to medication side effects, which led to attrition in the nortriptyline group.

19. **Stuart S, O'Hara MW:** Interpersonal psychotherapy for postpartum depression: a treatment program. *Journal of Psychotherapy Practice and Research* 4:18–29, 1995

Stuart and O'Hara describe the treatment adaptation of IPT to a target population for whom psychotherapy may often be a preferable alternative to antidepressant medication. Results of a small pilot trial are encouraging.

20. **Wifley DE, Agras WS, Telch CF, Rossiter EM, Schneider JA, Cole AG, Sifford L, Raeburn SD:** Group cognitive-behavioral therapy and group interpersonal psychotherapy for the nonpurging bulimic individual: a controlled comparison. *J Consult Clin Psychol* 61:296–305, 1993

This study replicated for group IPT the findings for individual IPT in Fairburn et al. (1991, 1993) above: 16 weekly sessions of group IPT was compared with group CBT and with a waiting list control. Fifty-six women with nonpurging bulimia nervosa randomized to these conditions significantly reduced binge eating in both of the active treatments, but not in the waiting list condition.

Prediction of Response

21. **Foley SH, O'Malley S, Rounsaville B, Prusoff BA, Weissman MM:** The relationship of patient difficulty to therapist performance in interpersonal psychotherapy of depression. *J Affect Disord* 12:207–217, 1987

This analysis based on Elkin et al. (1989) above examined factors affecting therapist performance in IPT of major depression. How "difficult" patients were, a factor related to patients' preconceived negative expectations about treatment, affected therapist performance in that treatment, whereas initial severity of patients' symptoms did not affect therapist performance.

22. **Frank E, Kupfer DJ, Wagner EF, McEachran AB, Cornes C:** Efficacy of interpersonal psychotherapy as a maintenance treatment of recurrent depression. *Arch Gen Psychiatry* 48:1053–1059, 1991

An elaboration on the results presented in Frank et al. (1990) above, this process study revealed that the degree of interpersonal focus in a session had a significant positive correlation with patient survival time. Patients whose sessions had high interpersonal specificity survived a mean 2 years before developing depression, whereas a low interpersonal focus yielded only 5 months of protection before relapse.

23. **Sotsky SM, Glass DR, Shea MT, Pilkonis PA, Collins JF, Elkin I, Watkins JT, Imber SD, Leber WR, Moyer J, Oliveri ME:** Patient predictors of response to psychotherapy and pharmacotherapy: findings in the NIMH treatment of depression collaborative research program. *Am J Psychiatry* 148:997–1008, 1991

Addressing the interesting question of treatment specificity, this off-shoot of Elkin et al. (1989) above considered patient characteristics that might predict differential outcome across therapies. Among other findings, low baseline level of social dysfunction predicted a good antidepressant response to IPT; high initial severity of depression and impairment of functioning predicted superior response to IPT and to imipramine.

Additional Readings

The following references provide additional important information.

24. **Chevron E, Rounsaville B, Rothblum ED, Weissman MM:** Selecting psychotherapists to participate in psychotherapy outcome studies: relationship between psychotherapist characteristics and assessment of clinical skills. *J Nerv Ment Dis* 171:348–353, 1983

25. **Foley SH, Rounsaville BJ, Weissman MM, Sholomskas D, Chevron E:** Individual versus conjoint interpersonal psychotherapy for depressed patients with marital disputes. *International Journal of Family Psychiatry* 10:29–42, 1990

26. **Frank E:** Interpersonal psychotherapy as a maintenance treatment for patients with recurrent depression. *Psychotherapy* 28:259–266, 1991

27. **Frank E, Kupfer DJ, Perel JM:** Early recurrence in unipolar depression. *Arch Gen Psychiatry* 46:397–400, 1989

28. **Klerman GL, Weissman MM:** Interpersonal psychotherapy: efficacy and adaptations, in *Handbook of Affective Disorders,* 2nd Edition. Edited by Paykel ES. London, Churchill Livingston, 1992, pp. 501–510

29. **Klerman GL, Budman S, Berwick D, Weissmann MM, Damico-White J, Demby A, Feldstein M:** Efficacy of a brief psychosocial intervention for symptoms of stress and distress among patients in primary care. *Med Care* 25:1078–1088, 1987

30. **O'Malley SS, Foley SH, Rounsaville BJ, Watkins JT, Sotsky SM, Imber SD, Elkin I:** Therapist competence and patient outcome in interpersonal psychotherapy of depression. *J Consult Clin Psychol* 56:496–501, 1988

From data on 35 outpatients from Elkin et al. (1989) above, multiple regression analyses were used to predict outcome based on ratings of therapist skill at the 4th session, controlling for severity of depression, social adjustment, and expectations of outcome. Therapist performance contributes to the prediction of patient-rated change and change in depressive apathy, but not social adjustment at 16 weeks.

31. **Rounsaville BJ, Kleber HD:** Psychotherapy/counselling for opiate addicts: strategies for use in different treatment settings. *Int J Addict* 20:483–490, 1985

32. **Rounsaville BJ, Gawin F, Kleber HD:** Interpersonal psychotherapy adapted for ambulatory cocaine abusers. *Am J Drug Alcohol Abuse* 11:171–191, 1985

   This adaptation of IPT to reduce cocaine use has subsequently not shown treatment benefit.

33. **Rounsaville BJ, Kosten TR, Weissman MM, Kleber HD:** A 2.5 year follow-up of short-term interpersonal psychotherapy in methadone-maintained opiate addicts. *Compr Psychiatry* 27:201–210, 1986

34. **Rounsaville BJ, Chevron ES, Weissman MM, Prusoff BA, Frank E:** Training therapists to perform interpersonal psychotherapy in clinical trials. *Compr Psychiatry* 27:364–371, 1986

35. **Wagner EF, Frank E, Steiner SC:** Discriminating maintenance treatments for recurrent depression: development and implementation of a rating scale. *Journal of Psychotherapy Practice and Research* 1:280–290, 1992

36. **Weissman MM, Rounsaville BJ, Chevron ES:** Training psychotherapists to participate in psychotherapy outcome studies: identifying and dealing with the research requirement. *Am J Psychiatry* 139:1442–1446, 1982

49

Sex Therapy

Helen Singer Kaplan, M.D., Ph.D.

Prior to the advent of the new sex therapies in the 1970s, the pathogenesis of sexual disorders was poorly understood, and treatment was largely ineffective. The past two decades, however, have witnessed dramatic improvements in our ability to diagnose and treat sexual difficulties, such that today the majority of patients suffering from sexual inadequacy respond favorably to brief courses of sex therapy.

Sex therapy was invented by Masters and Johnson, who described their successful, brief, behavioral, couples-oriented treatment for sexual disorders in their ground-breaking, highly influential book, *Human Sexual Inadequacy*, which was published in 1970 and remains a classic to this day.

A further step in the evolution of modern sex therapy that made it possible to treat a wider range of patients was the integration of Masters and Johnson's cognitive-behavioral model with psychodynamic theory and techniques. This integrated approach, which is currently in wide use, is described in *The New Sex Therapy* (Kaplan 1974).

Three further extensions of sex therapy followed in short order: the recognition of the previously overlooked sexual desire disorders, the development of more specific treatment protocols for the various sexual syndromes, and the increasing use of adjunctive physiological treatments.

The clinical features and causes of deficiencies in libido or desire, as well as some proposed treatment strategies for patients with desire disorders, were initially described in two volumes: *Disorders of Sexual Desire* (Kaplan 1979) and *Sexual Aversion, Sexual Phobias and Panic Disorders* (Kaplan

599

1987). These works were rapidly followed by a number of interesting publications on this topic, which are represented in the references.

Masters and Johnson had originally used the identical protocol to treat all the sexual dysfunctions. One of the most important improvements of Masters and Johnson's method was the development of different and specific treatment strategies for each of the eight sexual dysfunction syndromes. Accordingly, this chapter lists a number of informative publications that describe the treatment of specific sexual disorders, including premature and retarded ejaculation, impotence, anorgasmia, vaginismus, and sexual desire disorders.

The 1980s witnessed a number of significant advances in the medical aspects of sex therapy, and this chapter contains selected references to some of the most important of these new developments. Included are works on the new intracavernosal injection treatments for impotence and on the sexual side effects of commonly used medications. Sex therapy has been extended and adapted to serve the needs of certain special populations, whose sexual needs had not been sufficiently considered in the past. These include cancer patients, elderly persons, and compulsive sexual offenders; selected references on these topics are included.

Finally, many sex therapists find erotic and educational reading materials useful adjuvants to sex therapy in certain clinical situations. Assigned reading is primarily used to further the patients' deficient sex education and to probe, free-up, and heighten their suppressed sexual fantasies. Contrary to some other therapeutic approaches, which attempt to diminish the patient's erotic fantasies because these are considered an undesirable obstacle to a couple's intimacy, sex therapists often encourage the patient to fantasize and to use erotic images to "bypass" their sexual inhibitions with their partners. This chapter includes a brief list of erotic books that are frequently used by sex therapists for these purposes, selected from an extensive pool of such material.

The reader is further referred to Kaplan (Chapter 22, this volume) on sexual disorders, which also contains readings germane to the topic of sex therapy.

Basic Texts

1. **Annon JS:** *The Behavioral Treatment of Sexual Problems, Vol. 1: Brief Therapy.* Honolulu, HI, Kapiolani Health Services, 1974

   This small volume, which is based on the theory that sexual problems are learned and can therefore be extinguished or modified by procedures derived from learning theory, is quite dated in theory and practice. For one, the exclusively behavioral treatments that are recommended are now rarely used because of their poor results. Moreover, the author omits any consideration of the important biological, psychodynamic, and motivational aspects of sex.

However, despite these valid criticisms and real limitations, we nevertheless recommend this book as adjunctive reading in our sex therapy training program because it contains clear and practical descriptions, perhaps the best in the literature, of commonly used cognitive-behavioral interventions. The text, which is easy to read, is illustrated throughout by interesting, verbatim segments of clinical sessions.

2. *Bieber I: The psychoanalytic treatment of sexual disorders. *J Sex Marital Ther* 1:5–15, 1974

This is an excellent summary of the psychoanalytic theory of sexual disorders, with emphasis on the concept of castration anxiety and early difficulties with the father, as important elements in the pathogenesis of male sexual dysfunctions. Even if one rejects the universal validity of the psychoanalytic formulation of psychosexual pathology, the article is helpful for understanding the deeper psychic infrastructure of certain complex sexual dysfunctions of males and for managing resistances to the rapid modification of sexual functioning that grow out of these.

3. *Kaplan HS: *The New Sex Therapy: Active Treatment of Sexual Dysfunctions.* New York, Brunner/Mazel, 1974

This volume, which has also been published in many languages and which is still widely used, describes an integrated method of sex therapy that combines behavioral interventions in the form of therapeutic "sexual homework assignments" with psychodynamic exploration of the patient's deeper emotional problems and resistances. The book also contains descriptions of different and specific treatment protocols for the eight genital-phase dysfunctions of men and women, which represented a departure from Masters and Johnson, who had used the same therapeutic program for all forms of sexual inadequacy.

4. Kolodny RC, Masters WH, Johnson VE: *Textbook of Sexual Medicine.* Boston, MA, Little, Brown, 1979

The first textbook of sexual medicine for use in a medical school curriculum, this book is organized on a classic medical text model. The first group of chapters is devoted to the basic sciences of sexology and includes material on human sexual anatomy, embryology, physiology, gender development, and endocrinology. Chapters on clinical topics follow. These include sex and chronic illness, oncology, gynecologic and urologic illness, and cardiovascular diseases among others. The psychogenic sexual disorders and their management make up the last, and arguably the strongest and most enduring, section of the text. Although some of the material is quite dated (e.g., chapters on drugs and on endocrine factors), this volume remains a valuable resource book of physiological and psychological information that is basic to the clinical practice of sex therapy.

5. **Leiblum SR, Rosen RC** (eds): *Principles and Practice of Sex Therapy: Update for the 1990s.* New York, Guilford, 1989

A little uneven, this is nevertheless an interesting and valuable compendium of chapters on a variety of sex therapy approaches by an eclectic group of talented and innovative researchers and clinicians in the field. I especially like Bernard Apfelbaum's chapter, "Retarded Ejaculation," and Judith V. Becker's chapter, "The Impact of Sexual Abuse on Sexual Functioning."

6. *Masters WH, Johnson VE:** *Human Sexual Inadequacy.* Boston, MA, Little, Brown, 1970

This is the original description of the brief, behavioral, couples-oriented treatment of the genital dysfunctions that ushered in the era of modern sex therapy. Translated into many languages, this is one of the most influential books in the mental health field. It remains a classic and is still a useful text.

7. **Masters WH, Johnson VE, Kolodny RC:** *Heterosexuality.* New York, Harper Collins, 1994

An up-to-date compendium of basic sexology and treatment from the innovators of the field of sex therapy. This book is detailed and useful.

8. **Rosen R, Rosen LR:** *Human Sexuality.* New York, Knopf, 1981

This college and graduate school textbook is a comprehensive compendium of the biological, psychological, and social aspects of human sexuality. The scope of the book is broad and includes sections that range from the history of sexuality to the current social context of sexual relationships; from embryological development through menopause to sex and old age, and from sex hormones to sex therapy. The text is clear and illustrated with interesting photographs and graphics. Although definitely in need of revision, it remains a valuable resource book.

Treatment of Specific Disorders and Populations

9. **Barbach LG:** *Women Discover Orgasm: A Therapist's Guide to a New Treatment Approach.* New York, Free Press, 1980

This book describes a useful, practical approach to the treatment of inhibited female orgasm (female orgasm disorder) by one of the foremost innovators and specialists in this area. More specifically, the author details, step by step, her highly successful method of treating anorgastic women in a group setting. The causes of female anorgasmia are reviewed, and the material is linked with specific treatment strategies. Although this book is essentially a manual for a group-therapy treatment approach, the methods and principles are equally applicable to the treatment of individual anorgastic women and/or couples.

10. *Green R, Wagner G:** *Impotence: (Erectile Failure:) Physiological, Psychological and Surgical Diagnosis and Treatment.* New York, Plenum, 1981

Although in need of updating on some of the new physiological data that have recently emerged in this burgeoning field, this superb volume by two of the leading experts in their respective disciplines, sexual physiology and psychiatric sexology, is still the best comprehensive work on erectile dysfunction that I have found.

11. **Kaplan HS:** *Disorders of Sexual Desire and Other New Concepts and Techniques in Sex Therapy.* New York, Simon & Schuster, 1979

Impairments of sexual desire or motivation are introduced in this book, which also contains an overview of the disorders and treatments of the orgasm and excitement phases of men and women.

12. **Kaplan HS:** *Sexual Aversion, Sexual Phobias, and Panic Disorder.* New York, Brunner/Mazel, 1987

This book describes the clinical features of sexual aversion disorders and discusses their causes and treatment. A strategy for combining antianxiety medication and integrated sex therapy for the treatment of sexual anxiety disorders is presented. The didactic material is illustrated by a number of clinical vignettes, representing treatment successes and failures. Of special interest is Donald Klein's informative chapter on the sexual side effects of psychoactive medication, which is an important issue in the treatment of sexually dysfunctional patients.

13. **Kaplan HS:** *PE: How to Overcome Premature Ejaculation.* New York, Brunner/Mazel, 1989

This small volume is a practical guide for patients and also provides an update for therapists on some new conceptual and technical developments in the sex therapy approach to the treatment of premature ejaculation.

14. **Kaplan HS:** *The Sexual Desire Disorders: Dysfunctional Regulation of Sexual Motivation.* New York, Brunner/Mazel, 1995

This volume conceptualizes hypoactive sexual desire as the normal controls of sexual motivation gone awry. Novel treatment strategies based on our experience with more than 2,000 patients with desire disorders are presented and illustrated with case vignettes.

15. **Leiblum SR, Rosen RC** (eds): *Sexual Desire Disorders.* New York, Guilford, 1988

This is an uneven, eclectic multiauthored compendium of interesting chapters by leading sex therapists who present their different treatment approaches to the treatment of desire disorders. The material is illustrated with pertinent case vignettes. Four chapters are outstanding: Schwartz and Masters' piece on the Masters and Johnson treatment model applied to desire disorders, Scharff's object-relation approach to the treatment of inhibited sexual desire, and two chapters by Segraves on hormones and on drugs.

16. *Leiblum SR, Previn LA, Campbell EH:** The treatment of vaginismus: success and failure, in *Principles and Practice of Sex Therapy.* Edited by Leiblum SR, Rosen RL. New York, Guilford, 1989, pp. 114–137

This excellent chapter reviews various current theories of the pathogenesis and the treatment of vaginismus. The approach centers around the gradual systematic dilation of the patient's spastic vaginal muscles, within a therapeutic context. The didactic material is illustrated by interesting case vignettes of patients whose treatment was successful or partially successful and who failed to improve.

17. *LoPiccolo J, Lobitz WC:** The role of masturbation in the treatment of orgasmic dysfunction, in *Handbook of Sex Therapy.* Edited by LoPiccolo J, LoPiccolo L. New York, Plenum, 1978, pp. 187–195

This is an excellent, well-researched chapter that has served as the model for most contemporary, behaviorally oriented therapeutic approaches to this common disorder of women. The authors present convincing evidence that self-stimulation is the most reliable way for a woman to reach orgasm. On that premise, they describe in detail a sensible treatment method that incorporates masturbation training into the Masters and Johnson's couples-oriented sex therapy model.

18. **Munjack DJ, Kanno PH:** Retarded ejaculation: a review. *Arch Sex Behav* 8:139–150, 1979

This article consists of an excellent and still timely review of various theories and treatments of ejaculatory inhibitions. The authors review the physiology of ejaculation and the organic causes of retarded or absent ejaculation. In addition, theories of psychopathogenesis are reviewed, ranging from the psychoanalytic, which regards this symptom as a product of castration anxiety and unconscious hostility toward women, through the behavioral position that these patients suffer from learned ejaculatory inhibitions, to the couple-oriented sex therapy view that adds consideration of the dynamics of the relationship with the partner. The authors also review outcomes reported by clinicians with various treatment approaches.

19. **Rosen RC, Leiblum SR** (eds): *Erectile Disorders.* New York, Plenum, 1992

This multi-authored volume by leading experts in the impotence field provides a good overview of current work in this area.

20. **Wagner G, Kaplan HS:** *The New Injection Treatment for Impotence: Medical and Psychological Aspects.* New York, Brunner/Mazel, 1993

This volume details the physiology, pharmacology, methods of administration, clinical indications, contraindications, side effects, and limitations of the new intracavernosal injections of vasodilating substances that can produce excellent erections in many impotent men. The book emphasizes the clinical strategies that are needed to translate the pharmacologically induced erections into increased sexual pleasure for the couple. Especially valuable are Wagner's chapters on recent research on the biology of erection and erectile failure, which contain the latest data in these areas—areas that are virtually exploding with new information.

Sex Therapy for Special Populations

21. **Auchincloss S:** Sexual problems in cancer patients: evaluation and management issues, in *Psycho-Oncology: The Psychological Care of Patients With Cancer.* Edited by Holland JC, Rowland JH. New York, Oxford Press, 1989, pp. 383–413

This chapter is an excellent, clear exposition of this much-neglected aspect of cancer care. The author, who is trained as a surgeon as well as a psychiatrist, describes the application of sex therapy techniques to physically ill and disabled cancer patients with sensitivity to their sexual needs.

22. **Davidson JM, Rosen RC:** Hormonal determinants of erectile function, in *Erectile Disorders: Assessment and Treatment.* Edited by Rosen RC, Leiblum SR. New York, Plenum, 1992, pp. 72–95

    This is the best summary on this complex subject that I have found in the literature.

23. **Kaplan HS:** Sex therapy with older patients, in *New Techniques in the Psychotherapy of Older Patients.* Edited by Myers WA. Washington, DC, American Psychiatric Press, 1991, pp. 21–37

    The biological effects of the aging process on the sexual desire, excitement, and orgasm phases of men and women are detailed, and the potential emotional impact of these changes are discussed. The chapter also describes some sex therapy strategies and tactics that exploit the older couple's remaining sexual reserves and compensate for their deficits. The treatment approach is illustrated by case studies.

24. **Money J:** Treatment guidelines: anti-androgens and counseling of paraphillic sex offenders. *J Sex Marital Ther* 13:219–223, 1987

    This is a brief, excellent discussion of the combined use of anti-androgen medications, which suppress the compulsive sex offender's overwhelming sexual urges on a physical basis (presumably by acting on central nervous system sex-regulatory centers), and psychosexual counseling to help these patients integrate their sexual feelings into their lives in a more controlled and constructive manner.

25. **Sager JC:** The role of sex therapy in marital therapy. *Am J Psychiatry* 133:555–558, 1976

    This article contains an excellent discussion on the interface between marital and sexual therapy and describes the interesting concept of broken "marriage contracts" as a hidden etiological element in marital and sexual problems.

26. **Segraves RT:** Pharmacologic agents causing sexual dysfunctions. *J Sex Marital Ther* 3:157–176, 1977

27. **Segraves RT:** Drugs and desire, in *Sexual Desire Disorders.* Edited by Leiblum SR, Rosen RC. New York, Guilford, 1988, pp. 271–313

    Drugs and medications are playing an ever-increasing role in the sexual complaints of our patients, and clinicians need to keep abreast with the new drugs that are constantly coming on the market, as well as with their potential sexual side effects. The author is a well-known expert in this field, and the 1977 article is a comprehensive review of commonly used medications that can cause sexual side effects. This well-organized article is still valid and useful, albeit since it was written many new drugs with sexual side effects have become available. For an update on this topic, the reader is referred to the author's more recent work, the 1988 reference.

Reading Material for Patients

28. **Barbach LG:** *For Yourself: The Fulfillment of Female Sexuality.* New York, Doubleday, 1975

This is a superb, informative, helpful book for women who suffer from orgasm disorders. Written in a constructive and sane "voice," it is also good reading for therapists. One note of caution: the lengthy "exercises" that are suggested are not for everyone, and patients should be apprised of this.

29. **Cleland J:** *Fanny Hill: Memoirs of a Woman of Pleasure.* New York, Dell/Putnam, 1963

This Victorian novel contains a panoply of sexual fantasies and has something for everyone.

30. **Friday N:** *My Secret Garden.* New York, Simon & Schuster, 1973

31. **Friday N:** *Forbidden Flowers.* New York, Simon & Schuster, 1975

32. **Friday N:** *Women on Top.* New York, Star Pocket Books, 1992

Although the author's nonprofessional and less-than-illuminating commentary detracts from these books somewhat, the wide array of superb male and female erotic fantasies that are beautifully described in all three books can be extremely helpful for uncovering patients' buried fantasies.

33. **Nin A:** *The Delta of Venus* (1969). New York, Harcourt Brace Jovanovich, 1977

34. **Nin A:** *Little Birds.* New York, Harcourt Brace Jovanovich, 1979

These books contain collections of brief, erotic stories by Anaïs Nin and Henry Miller that were originally commissioned for a wealthy male client. These books are essentially interesting and arousing compendiums of sexual fantasies. Beautifully written, these books are suitable for more literary, sophisticated patients who are often put off by more vulgar materials. The stories appeal to men and to women.

35. **Reage P:** *The Story of "O."* New York, Ballantine Press, 1965

   This story is an excellent probe to access hidden sadomasochistic fantasies.

36. **Zilbergeld B:** *The New Male Sexuality: The Truth About Men, Sex and Pleasure.* New York, Bantam, 1992

   This informative, reassuring volume "normalizes" common male sexual difficulties and is extremely useful for men with performance-anxiety–related sexual problems. The book is also valuable reading for clinicians who treat these patients.

50

Geriatric Psychiatry

Gerard Addonizio, M.D.
George Alexopoulos, M.D.

Over the past several years, geriatric psychiatry has been experiencing a rapid growth in knowledge and consequently is receiving wider recognition as a specialized area within our field. Many investigators have made numerous important contributions. We have made great strides in understanding significant differences between late-onset and early-onset geriatric depression. Utilizing imaging techniques such as magnetic resonance imaging has led to the discovery of differences in brain morphology in late-onset geriatric depressive patients. Our understanding of the interface of degenerative dementia and depression has shed new light on the course of both illnesses as well as the way in which each disorder can affect clinical presentation. Studies of neuroendocrine physiology offer the potential for being able to predict early relapse of depression. Research on monoamine oxidase activity has raised the interesting hypothesis that elevated monoamine oxidase is related to an underlying degenerative process. Pharmacologic studies have clearly shown the efficacy and potential pitfalls of antidepressants in the elderly population as well as the potential for novel medicines in the treatment of the behavioral dyscontrol of dementia. Because of the significant progress in the field, our task of picking and choosing publications was a difficult one. As space was limited, we decided to not include some of the older classics in the field when a more recent manuscript existed that was either immediately relevant for clinical practice or had important implications for future research. Some of the references were chosen because they were clear, comprehensive syntheses of complicated areas, whereas others were chosen because they were considered original, ground-breaking papers. Several books were included because we considered them essential resources that should be a part of any geriatrician's library. We categorized references based on diagnostic and therapeutic considerations but it should be noted that most areas have overlapping margins and therefore the reader may, for instance, find pertinent articles on diagnosis in a category on treatment. Finally, we wanted to emphasize that the references we have chosen are a representative sample of a large body of work. For those interested in geriatric psychiatry, this chapter should be the starting point, not the final destination, for pursuing an in-depth knowledge of the field.

General References

1. *Albert ML (ed): *Clinical Neurology of Aging*. New York, Oxford University Press, 1984

   Distinguishing the normal and pathologic neurologic processes of aging is a critical problem in geriatrics. This book surveys the field and includes clinical neurosciences, clinical examination and diagnostic studies, mental status, special senses, motor system, sensation, and common neurological disorders.

2. *Sadavoy J, Lazarus LW, Jarvik LF (eds): *Comprehensive Review of Geriatric Psychiatry*. Washington, DC, American Psychiatric Press, 1991

   This is one of the best current reviews of geriatric psychiatry. Each topic is comprehensively covered by an expert in the field.

Diagnosis and Diagnostic Procedures

3. **Abrams RC, Alexopoulos GS, Young RC:** Geriatric depression and DSM-III-R personality disorder criteria. *J Am Geriatr Soc* 35:383–386, 1987

   This article explores the relationship between late-life depression and personality traits.

4. **Addonizio G:** The patient with Parkinson's disease, in *Treatments of Psychiatric Disorders: A Task Force Report of the American Psychiatric Association*, Vol. 2. Edited by Karasu TB. Washington, DC, American Psychiatric Association, 1989, pp. 860–867

This is a thorough and comprehensive review of diagnostic and treatment issues in the psychiatrically impaired patient with Parkinson's disease.

5. **Alexopoulos GS, Mattis S:** Diagnosing cognitive dysfunction in the elderly: primary screening tests. *Geriatrics* 46:33–44, 1991

   This article provides a clear and comprehensive guide to the cognitive examination in geriatric patients.

6. *****Alexopoulos GS, Abrams RC, Young RC, Shamoian CA:** Cornell Scale for Depression in Dementia. *Biol Psychiatry* 23:271–284, 1988

   A scale is presented for rating depressive symptoms in patients with dementia. Both patient and caregiver are interviewed.

7. **Alexopoulos GS, Young RC, Shindledecker RD:** Brain computed tomography findings in geriatric depression and primary degenerative dementia. *Biol Psychiatry* 31:591–599, 1992

   The authors present evidence from computed tomography scans that late-onset depressive patients have structural brain changes that distinguish them from patients with early-onset depression.

8. *****Folstein MF, Folstein SE, McHugh PR:** Mini-Mental State: a practical method for grading the cognitive state of patients for the clinician. *J Psychiatr Res* 12:189–198, 1975

   This article provides a short, standardized form for performing a cognitive mental status examination. The Mini-Mental State has become a widely used gold standard for screening cognitive performance.

9. **Friedland RP, Jagust WJ:** Positron and single photon emission tomography in the differential diagnosis of dementia, in *Positron Emission Tomography in Dementia*. Edited by Duara R. New York, Wiley-Liss, 1990, pp. 161–177

   This is a review of positron-emission tomography and single photon emission computed tomography in the differential diagnosis of dementia.

10. **Johnson KA, Davis KR, Buonanno FS, Brady TJ, Rosen TJ, Growdon JH:** Comparison of magnetic resonance and Roentgen ray computed tomography in dementia. *Arch Neurol* 44:1075–1080, 1987

    The authors discusses findings on magnetic resonance imaging and computed tomography in dementia.

11. **Kalayam B:** The patient with sensory impairment, in *Treatment of Psychiatric Disorders,* Vol.2. Edited by Karasu TB. Washington, DC, American Psychiatric Association, 1989, pp. 948–960

Aging is often associated with a deterioration in sensory function. This chapter provides a comprehensive guide to sensory impairment and its psychiatric effects.

12. *****Lipowski ZJ:** Delirium in the elderly patient. *N Engl J Med* 320:578–582, 1989

This article is a concise fact-filled summary about delirium in the elderly.

13. **Margolin R, Daniel D:** Neuroimaging in geropsychiatry, in *Clinical and Scientific Psychogeriatrics,* Vol. 2. Edited by Bergener M, Finkel SI. New York, Springer, 1990, pp. 162–186

This chapter is a discussion of the role of neuroimaging in the diagnosis of psychiatric disorders in the elderly.

14. *****Mattis S:** Mental status examination for organic mental syndrome in the elderly patient, in *Geriatric Psychiatry.* Edited by Bellack R, Karasu B. New York, Grune & Stratton, 1976, pp. 77–121

In this comprehensive review, Mattis correlates neuroanatomy with the various cognitive functions of a mental status examination. This chapter also includes the Mattis Demention Rating Scale, widely used for in-depth neuropsychological evaluation.

15. **Reynolds CF, Hoch CC, Monk TH:** Sleep and chronobiologic disturbances in late life, in *Geriatric Psychiatry.* Edited by Busse EW, Blazer DG. Washington, DC, American Psychiatric Press, 1989, pp. 475–488

Sleep disturbances in late life are a common occurrence. Reynolds et al. have written an excellent overview of the field that includes physiology of sleep in elderly persons together with sleep disturbances and treatment interventions, both pharmacologic and nonpharmacologic.

16. *****Rovner BW, Kafoneck S, Filipp L, Lucas MJ, Folstein MF:** Prevalence of mental illness in a community nursing home. *Am J Psychiatry* 143:1446–1449, 1986

Psychiatric disorders in nursing homes have long been overlooked. This study identifies the high prevalence of mental and behavioral disorders found in nursing homes.

17. **Zimmerman RD, Fleming CA, Lee BCP, Saint-Louis LA, Deck MD:** Periventricular hyperintensity as seen by magnetic resonance: prevalence and significance. *AJR Am J Roentgenol* 7:13–20, 1986

This article helps to put in perspective the ubiquitous finding of periventricular hyperintensity on magnetic resonance imaging.

Psychopharmacologic Treatment and Electroconvulsive Therapy

18. *Abrams R: *Electroconvulsive Therapy.* New York, Oxford University Press, 1992

This is a book that beautifully synthesizes an enormous amount of diverse material.

19. *Alexopoulos GS, Shamoian CA, Lucas J, Weiser N, Berger H:** Medical problems of geriatric psychiatric patients and younger controls during electroconvulsive therapy. *J Am Geriatr Soc* 32:651–654, 1984

This study identifies medical complications of electroconvulsive therapy.

20. **Alexopoulos GS, Young R, Abrams RC:** ECT in the high-risk geriatric patient. *Convulsive Therapy* 5:75–87, 1989

This article is a useful guide to potential problems in high-risk electroconvulsive therapy patients and to strategies for reducing risk.

21. *Georgotas A, McCue RE, Hapworth W, Friedman E, Kim OM, Welkowitz J, Chang I, Cooper TB:** Comparative efficacy and safety of MAOIs versus TCAs in treating depression in the elderly. *Biol Psychiatry* 21:1155–1166, 1986

This article provides data that monoamine oxidase inhibitors are both effective and well tolerated in geriatric patients.

22. *Georgotas A, McCue RE, Cooper TB, Nagachandran N, Chang I:** How effective and safe is continuation therapy in elderly depressed patients? *Arch Gen Psychiatry* 45:929–932, 1988

This article presents factors affecting relapse rate in elderly patients treated with antidepressants.

23. **Jenike MA:** *Geriatric Psychiatry and Psychopharmacology: A Clinical Approach.* St. Louis, MO, Mosby-Year Book, 1989

This valuable book covers diagnostic tools, psychopathology, and treatment.

24. **Nelson JC, Jatlow P, Mazure C:** Desipramine plasma levels and response in elderly melancholic patients. *J Clin Psychopharmacol* 5:217–220, 1985

    Interpretations of tricyclic antidepressant levels are often misguided. This study determines the threshold concentration for response to desipramine.

25. **Ray WA, Griffin MR, Schaffner W, Baugh DK, Melton LJ 3rd:** Psychotropic drug use and the risk of hip fracture. *N Engl J Med* 316:363–369, 1987

    Falls and fractures in the elderly have become a major public health problem. This pivotal study examines the risk of hip fracture in elderly patients on psychotropic medication.

26. *Roose SP, Glassman AH, Giardina EGV, Walsh BT, Woodring S, Bigger JT:** Tricyclic antidepressants in depressed patients with cardiac conduction disease. *Arch Gen Psychiatry* 44:273–275, 1987

    This pivotal study documents that tricyclic antidepressants can slow conduction in patients with cardiac conduction disease.

27. *Salzman C (ed): *Clinical Geriatric Psychopharmacology,* 2nd Edition. Baltimore, MD, Williams & Wilkins, 1992

    This is an up-to-date and invaluable guide to those clinicians using psychotropic drugs in geriatric patients.

28. **Satel SL, Nelson JC:** Stimulants in the treatment of depression: a critical overview. *J Clin Psychiatry* 50:241–249, 1989

    This article provides a much-needed critical review of this controversial area.

29. **Shamoian CA** (ed): *Psychopharmacological Treatment Complications in the Elderly.* Washington, DC, American Psychiatric Press, 1992

    The cognitive and cardiac side effects of antidepressants and neurologic side effects of other psychotropic medications are examined in this book. An understanding of these potential side effects will allow the clinician to treat geriatric patients with the greatest measure of safety.

30. *Spiker DG, Weiss JC, Dealy RS, Griffin SJ, Hanin I, Neil JF, Perel JM, Rossi AJ, Soloff PH:** The pharmacological treatment of delusional depression. *Am J Psychiatry* 141:430–436, 1985

This article documents the efficacy of combined neuroleptic-tricyclic treatment in delusional depression.

31. **Sunderland T, Silver MA:** Neuroleptics in the treatment of dementia. *International Journal of Geriatric Psychiatry* 3:79–88, 1988

The history of neuroleptic treatment in dementia is reviewed.

32. *Young RC, Alexopoulos GS, Shamoian CA, Kent E, Dhar AK, Kutt H:** Plasma 10-hydroxynortriptyline and ECG changes in elderly depressed patients. *Am J Psychiatry* 142:866–868, 1985

Cardiac side effects are always a potential problem in elderly patients taking tricyclic antidepressants. This article helps to clarify the cause of conduction problems in elderly patients on nortriptyline.

Psychotherapy

33. **Birren JE, Schaie KW** (eds): *Handbook of the Psychology of Aging.* San Diego, CA, Academic Press, 1990

This is a uniquely important book that covers a wide range of topics: creativity and wisdom in aging; caregiving families; and cultural, racial, and ethnic minority influences on aging. This text is a critical resource for those who are interested in treating the whole individual.

34. *Lazarus LW** (ed): *Clinical Approaches to Psychotherapy With the Elderly.* Washington, DC, American Psychiatric Press, 1984

This book provides a discussion of the unique issues involved in doing psychotherapy with elderly patients.

35. **Myers WA:** Transference and countertransference issues in treatments involving older patients and younger therapists. *J Geriatr Psychiatry* 19:221–239, 1986

This is a helpful, insightful article for clinicians beginning to do psychotherapy with older patients.

36. **Sadavoy J, Leszcz M** (eds): *Treating the Elderly With Psychotherapy: The Scope for Change in Later Life.* Madison, CT, International Universities Press, 1987

In this book of great theoretical and practical importance in the psychotherapy of the aged, topics range from psychodynamic perspectives to specific treatment modalities.

Affective Disorders

37. *Alexopoulos GS:** Clinical and biological findings in late-onset depression, in *American Psychiatric Press Review of Psychiatry*, Vol. 9. Edited by Tasman A, Goldfinger SM, Kaufmann CA. Washington, DC, American Psychiatric Press, 1990, pp. 249–262

This chapter describes the hypothesis that late-onset depression is a syndrome distinct from early-onset geriatric depression and includes a large subgroup of patients with neurological brain disorders.

38. *Alexopoulos GS, Chester JG:** Outcomes of geriatric depression. *Clin Geriatr Med* 8:363–376, 1992

This review details factors affecting chronicity and relapse in geriatric depression.

39. **Baldwin RC, Jolley DJ:** The prognosis of depression in old age. *Br J Psychiatry* 149:574–583, 1986

This is an interesting study that follows the course of depressive symptoms in 100 elderly patients. Prognostic factors and treatment are also discussed.

40. *Blazer D:** Epidemiology of late-life depression and dementia: a comparative study, in *American Psychiatric Press Review of Psychiatry*, Vol. 9. Edited by Tasman A, Goldfinger SM, Kaufmann CA. Washington, DC, American Psychiatric Press, 1990, pp. 210–219

This chapter is a concise, up-to-date review of the epidemiology of late-life depression and dementia.

41. **Blazer DG, Bachar JR, Manton KG:** Suicide in late life. *J Am Geriatr Soc* 34:519–525, 1986

Elderly patients are at risk for suicide. This review provides epidemiologic data about suicide in the elderly.

42. **Emery VO, Oxman TE:** Update on the dementia spectrum of depression. *Am J Psychiatry* 149:305–317, 1992

This article reviews the area of depressive pseudodementia as well as depression occurring as part of neurologic brain disease.

43. *Murphy E:** The prognosis of depression in old age. *Br J Psychiatry* 142:111–119, 1983

In this 1-year prospective study of 124 elderly depressed patients, factors affecting outcome are identified.

44. **Nelson JC, Bowers MB Jr:** Delusional unipolar depression: description and drug response. *Arch Gen Psychiatry* 35:1321–1328, 1978

This study documents the need for combined antipsychotic and tricyclic antidepressant drug therapy in delusional depression.

45. **Roose SP, Glassman AH, Walsh BT, Woodring S, Vital-Herne J:** Depression, delusions and suicide. *Am J Psychiatry* 140:1159–1162, 1983

This article presents a study of the significant correlation between delusional depression and suicide.

46. **Roose SP, Dalack GW, Woodring S:** Death, depression, and heart disease. *J Clin Psychiatry* 52 (suppl):34–39, 1991

This article covers the effect of affective disorder on cardiac disease and use of antidepressants in patients with preexisting cardiac illness.

47. *Rovner BW, German PS, Brant LJ, Clark R, Burton L, Folstein MF:** Depression and mortality in nursing homes. *JAMA* 265:993–996, 1991

This article drew attention to the high prevalence of unrecognized depression in nursing homes and its association with increased mortality.

48. *Shulman K, Post F:** Bipolar affective disorder in old age. *Br J Psychiatry* 136:26–32, 1980

This is an important article documenting that first manic attacks may occur in patients over the age of 60.

49. **Young RC, Falk JR:** Age, manic psychopathology and treatment response. *International Journal of Geriatric Psychiatry* 4:73–78, 1989

This study discusses how aging may alter the psychopathology of mania and treatment response.

Paranoid States

50. **Harris MJ, Jeste DV:** Late-onset schizophrenia: an overview. *Schizophr Bull* 14:39–55, 1988

This review of the literature concludes that late-onset schizophrenia is a valid clinical entity.

51. **Harris MJ, Cullum CM, Jeste DV:** Clinical presentation of late-onset schizophrenia. *J Clin Psychiatry* 49:356–360, 1988

This report discusses late-onset schizophrenia and provides useful case vignettes.

52. **Jeste DV, Harris MJ, Pearlson GD, Rabins P, Lesser I, Miller B, Coles C, Yassa R:** Late-onset schizophrenia, studying clinical validity. *Psychiatr Clin North Am* 11:1–13, 1988

   Contrary to popular belief, this study concludes that late-onset schizophrenia may be no less valid an entity than early-onset schizophrenia.

53. *Miller NE, Cohen GD (eds): *Schizophrenia and Aging.* New York, Guilford, 1987

   This book represents a major contribution to the area of schizophrenia and aging. A compilation of chapters by experts in the field, it also includes an excellent chapter on aging and tardive dyskinesia.

54. **Raskind M, Alvarez C, Merlin S:** Fluphenazine enanthate in outpatient treatment of late paraphrenia. *J Am Geriatr Soc* 27:459–463, 1979

   Patients with "paraphrenia" may be a challenge to engage in outpatient treatment. This article offers helpful advice.

Substance Abuse

55. **Curtis JR, Geller G, Stokes EG, Levine DM, Moore RD:** Characteristics, diagnosis, and treatment of alcoholism in elderly patients. *J Am Geriatr Soc* 37:310–316, 1989

   Alcoholism is underrecognized in elderly patients.

56. **Schuckit MA:** A clinical review of alcohol, alcoholism, and the elderly patients. *J Clin Psychiatry* 43:396–399, 1982

   This article elucidates diagnostic and treatment considerations unique to older, alcoholic patients.

57. **Schweizer E, Case WG, Rickels K:** Benzodiazepine dependence and withdrawal in elderly patients. *Am J Psychiatry* 146:529–531, 1989

   This article reviews an often-neglected area in the evaluation of geriatric patients. The authors discuss benzodiazepine dependence and tapering of chronically administered benzodiazepines.

Dementia and Focal Brain Lesions

58. *Addonizio G, Shamoian CA: Depression and dementia, in *Neuropsychiatric Dementias*. Edited by Jeste DV. Washington, DC, American Psychiatric Press, 1986, pp. 73–109

This chapter extensively discusses the similarities and differences between depression and dementia from a historical, psychopathologic, and diagnostic perspective.

59. Chui HC: Dementia: a review emphasizing clinicopathologic correlation and brain-behavior relationships. *Arch Neurol* 46:806–814, 1989

Brain-behavior relationships are reviewed for Alzheimer's disease, Pick's disease, vascular dementia, and Parkinson's disease.

60. Cummings JL, Benson DF: *Dementia: A Clinical Approach*. Boston, MA, Butterworth, 1983

This book extensively covers all areas of the dementias in a highly organized way.

61. Cummings JL, Miller BL (eds): *Alzheimer's Disease: Treatment and Long-Term Management*. New York, Marcel Dekker, 1990

This is a valuable book that details disease-specific therapies, treatments of behavioral symptoms, and the long-term care of patients with Alzheimer's disease.

62. Mayeux R, Stern Y, Spanton S: Heterogeneity in dementia of the Alzheimer type: evidence of subgroups. *Neurology* 35:453–461, 1985

This article reports on an interesting study that subtypes Alzheimer's disease into four groups with different clinical courses.

63. *Reifler B, Larson E, Hanley R: Coexistence of cognitive impairment and depression in geriatric outpatients. *Am J Psychiatry* 139:623–626, 1982

Overlooking depression in a demented patient can be devastating. This report demonstrates that depression and dementia often coexist.

64. Robinson RG, Kubos KL, Starr LB, Rao K, Price TR: Mood disorders in stroke patients: importance of location of lesion. *Brain* 107:81–93, 1984

Interesting findings are presented that suggest that intrahemispheric lesion location is related to mood disorder in stroke patients.

65. *Robinson RG, Bolduc PL, Price TR: Two-year longitudinal study of post-stroke mood disorders: diagnosis and outcome at one and two years. *Stroke* 18:837–843, 1987

    This article explores the frequency and course of depression following a stroke.

66. *Wragg RE, Jeste DV: Overview of depression and psychosis in Alzheimer's disease. *Am J Psychiatry* 146:577–587, 1989

    The prevalence and phenomenology of affective and psychotic symptoms in patients with Alzheimer's disease are discussed. Thirty studies are reviewed.

Funding of Services

67. **Cutler J, Fine T:** Federal health care financing of mental illness: a failure of public policy, in *The New Economics of Psychiatric Care.* Edited by Sharfstein SS, Beigel A. Washington, DC, American Psychiatric Press, 1985, pp. 17–37

    This chapter is a walk through the historical development of federal funding of mental illness.

68. **Fogel BS, Gottlieb GL, Furino A:** Present and future solutions, in *Mental Health Policy for Older Americans: Protecting Minds at Risk.* Edited by Fogel BS, Furino A, Gottlieb GL. Washington, DC, American Psychiatric Press, 1990, pp. 257–277

    This chapter makes important recommendations for future policy development.

69. **Furino A, Fogel BS:** The economic perspective, in *Mental Health Policy for Older Americans: Protecting Minds at Risk.* Edited by Fogel BS, Furino A, Gottlieb GL. Washington, DC, American Psychiatric Press, 1990, pp. 23–36

    This chapter provides an enlightening view of the impact of the economy on the elderly.

70. **Gottlieb GL:** Financial issues affecting geriatric psychiatric care, in *Essentials in Geriatric Psychiatry.* Edited by Lazarus L. New York, Springer, 1988, pp. 230–248

    This remarkably lucid chapter explains the intricacies of Medicare and other funding sources.

Modalities in Child and Adolescent Psychiatry

Penelope Krener, M.D.
David A. Mrazek, M.D., F.R.C.Psych.

According to the Institute of Medicine (1989) report, between 12% and 17% of children and adolescents in the United States suffer from emotional or behavioral disorders. Because these conditions may adversely influence development and may evolve to more serious disorders, it is important to develop interventions.

Particular progress has been made in the psychopharmacological treatment of children during the last decade, and there has been increased recognition of treatable organic psychiatric conditions in childhood. Research for treatments of attention-deficit/hyperactivity disorder have produced the preponderance of articles on pharmacotherapeutics, and psychostimulants are the most frequently prescribed medications for psychiatric disorders in childhood. Increasing recognition and treatment of other externalizing syndromes, tic disorders, and affective disorders in childhood are further contributing to reports on the indications and use of other classes of medications. A new journal, the *Journal of Child and Adolescent Psychopharmacology,* is devoted to articles on pediatric pharmacotherapeutics of child and adolescent psychiatric disorders.

The psychotherapies encompass interpersonal interventions in specific treatment strategies that focus on the child, the adolescent, or the family—individually or in groups. Meta-analyses (Casey and Berman 1985; Weisz et al. 1987, both below) designed to compute effect size (the difference between the means of treated and nontreated groups) have been carried out to evaluate effectiveness of specific psychotherapeutic techniques such as behavioral, cognitive, or psychodynamic therapies.

A bibliographic resource is the series edited by Chess et al. (1993), now in its 25th year, which is a selection of the year's outstanding articles, with summary comments on each subject area and a brief synopsis of each article.

Because symptoms present in forms that are developmentally specific, the developmental progression during childhood presents specific challenges for establishing treatment objectives. Additionally, the presence of multiple symptoms that qualify a child for two or more DSM-IV disorders (comorbidity) is relatively common in childhood and has important implications for evaluating treatments. Given these caveats, the first part of this chapter offers general or overview references; the second part is organized by general treatment types; and the third part reviews treatment applications to specific disorders.

1. **Chess S, Thomas A, Hertzig ME:** *Annual Progress in Child Psychiatry and Child Development,* 25th Edition. New York, Brunner/Mazel, 1993

2. **Institute of Medicine:** Research on Children and Adolescents With Mental Behavioral and Developmental Disorders. Washington, DC, National Academy Press, 1989

General Overview and Outcome References

3. **Barrnett RJ, Docherty JP, Frommelt GM:** A review of child psychotherapy research since 1963. *J Am Acad Child Adolesc Psychiatry* 30:1–14, 1991

   The authors review 43 studies. They note that although there has been recent development of methodologies in adult psychiatry to study psychotherapy outcome, the comparable research in child psychiatry is flawed in research methodology, making generalizations difficult.

4. **Burns BJ:** Mental health service use by adolescents in the 1970s and 1980s. *J Am Acad Child Adolesc Psychiatry* 30:144–150, 1991

   Data from the Survey and Reports Branch, Division of Biometry and Applied Sciences, National Institute of Mental Health, between 1975 and 1986 indicate that although service use increased, less than 2% of adolescents in the United States received any sort of mental health service in 1986. Except for a higher level of affective disorders in hospitals, psychiatric diagnosis did not distinguish level of care received.

5. **Casey RJ, Berman JS:** The outcome of psychotherapy with children. *Psychol Bull* 98:388–400, 1985

A meta-analysis of 75 studies of psychotherapy outcome in children ages 3–15 is reported, which included psychodynamic, client-centered, cognitive, and behavioral treatments of children with a variety of clinical problems. The authors found that therapy improved symptoms for 76% of children (an effect size of 0.71 for all treatment versus nontreatment comparisons).

6. **Kazdin AE:** Effectiveness of psychotherapy with children and adolescents. *J Consult Clin Psychol* 59:785–796, 1991

This excellent review of outcome evidence for psychotherapy lays out the fundamental methodological issues. Factors that moderate treatment outcome, clarification of different features of psychotherapy as conducted in research versus in clinical practice, a clear explanation of effect size, and power analysis in assessing outcomes are reviewed. More than 100 citations are included.

7. [*]**Lewis M** (ed): *Child and Adolescent Psychiatry: A Comprehensive Textbook.* Baltimore, MD, Williams & Wilkins, 1991

In this comprehensive text with great depth of coverage, 139 contributors have brought together chapters in nine sections, of which one is devoted to treatment.

8. [*]**Rutter M, Hersov L** (eds): *Child and Adolescent Psychiatry: Modern Approaches.* Oxford, England, Blackwell Scientific Publications, 1993

This is a comprehensive and authoritative textbook with a commitment to explicate the scientific basis of the field.

9. **Strayhorn JM, Weidman CS:** Follow-up one year after parent-child interaction training: effects on behavior of preschool children. *J Am Acad Child Adolesc Psychiatry* 30:138–143, 1991

A preventive intervention with low-income parents who identified behavior problems in their preschoolers was carried out through group instruction and role playing as well as individual sessions. Children's improvements in classroom behavior were significantly correlated with improvements parents showed during the intervention in their behavior toward the children.

10. **Tharp RG:** Cultural diversity and treatment of children. *J Consult Clin Psychol* 59:799–812, 1991

    Tharp identifies basic questions germane to cultural differences between therapist and child patient that influence manifestation of symptoms. Approaches to culturally compatible treatment are presented, including modification of professional roles, recognition of status gaps within and between cultures, and choice of treatment levels and modalities.

11. **Weisz JR, Weis B, Alicke MD, Klitz ML:** Effectiveness of psychotherapy with children and adolescents: meta-analytic findings for clinicians. *J Consult Clin Psychol* 55:542–549, 1987

    In this meta-analysis of more than 100 controlled psychotherapy outcome studies, 26.9% of these studies overlapped with those reviewed by Casey and Berman (1985) above. A mean effect size (difference between means of treated and nontreated groups) was 0.79; that is, the outcome for the treated children was 79% of a standard deviation better than that of the untreated children. Behavioral treatments led to greater effect sizes.

12. *Wiener J (ed): *Textbook of Child and Adolescent Psychiatry*. Washington, DC, American Psychiatric Press, 1991

    In 56 chapters, the 75 contributors to this volume address every major issue in child and adolescent psychiatry clearly, in a straightforward tone and well-organized format. The 25-page chapter on pediatric psychopharmacology is comprehensive; there are chapters with detailed descriptions of behavioral, individual, family, and group therapies as well.

Treatment Modalities

Psychopharmacology

13. **Ambrosini PJ, Bianchi MD, Rabinovich H, Elia J:** Special article: antidepressant treatments in children and adolescents, I: affective disorders. *J Am Acad Child Adolesc Psychiatry* 32:1–6, 1993

    In this review of the efficacy of antidepressant treatment focusing on empirical findings, therapeutic group affects are modest or not present. Methodological shortcomings are carefully reviewed.

14. **August GJ, Raz N, Baird TD:** Brief report: effects of fenfluramine on behavioral, cognitive, and affective disturbances in autistic children. *J Autism Dev Disord* 15:95–106, 1985

Part of the multicenter coordinated study of fenfluramine in autistic patients, this study attempts to replicate the findings of Geller, Ritvo, Freeman, and Yuwiler in which significant improvements in sensory and motor behaviors were found in autistic children, associated with decreased platelet serotonin. A double-blind, placebo-controlled design was used. Hyperactivity and distractibility declined on medication; IQ measures remained stable; and serotonin levels declined. The authors conclude that fenfluramine is effective for symptomatic treatment of overactive distractible autistic children.

15. **Biederman J, Baldessarini RJ, Wright V, Knee D, Harmatz JS:** A double-blind placebo controlled study of desipramine in the treatment of ADD, I: efficacy. *J Am Acad Child Adolesc Psychiatry* 28:777–784, 1989

Clinically and statistically significant improvement in behavior resulted from desipramine over placebo for 68% of treated patients.

16. *Biederman J, Baldessarini RJ, Wright V, Knee D, Harmatz JS, Goldblatt A:** A double-blind placebo controlled study of desipramine in the treatment of ADD, II: serum drug levels and cardiovascular findings. *J Am Acad Child Adolesc Psychiatry* 28:903–911, 1989

In this study, 58 desipramine-treated children and adolescents were found to have wide variation of serum drug concentration at a given dose, with clinical improvement related to serum level. Small but statistically significant increases in diastolic blood pressure, heart rate, and electrocardiographic conduction parameters were found. The authors conclude that although treatment with doses above 3.5 mg/kg may be needed, caution and careful monitoring of serum levels and electrocardiogram are necessary.

17. **Campbell M, Spencer ED:** Psychopharmacology in child and adolescent psychiatry: a review of the past five years. *J Am Acad Child Adolesc Psychiatry* 27:269–279, 1988

The authors review 181 articles and identify developments in a 5-year period, organizing them by major diagnostic categories: schizophrenia, affective disorders, autism, mental retardation, tic disorders, attention-deficit/hyperactivity disorder, conduct disorders, parasomnias, and eating disorders.

18. **Campbell M, Perry R, Green WH:** Use of lithium in children and adolescents. *Psychosomatics* 25:95–106, 1984

This is a review of indications and usage of lithium in children and adolescents having parents who have responded to lithium. Treatment of mania, aggression, and externalizing behavior problems is considered.

19. **Coons HW, Klorman R, Borgstedt AD:** Effects of methylphenidate on adolescents with childhood history of attention deficit disorder, II: information processing. *J Am Acad Child Adolesc Psychiatry* 26:368–374, 1987

    This study characterizes the effects of methylphenidate and placebo on cognitive processing and event-related potentials in adolescents with childhood history of attention deficit disorder.

20. **Douglas VI, Barr KG, Aman K, O'Neill ME, Britton MG:** Dosage effects and individual responsivity to methylphenidate in attention deficit disorder. *J Child Psychol Psychiatry* 29:453–457, 1988

    Three dosages of methylphenidate (0.15, 0.30, and 0.60 mg/kg) were assessed in 19 children with attention-deficit/hyperactivity disorder on cognitive, academic, and behavioral measures in the laboratory and in the classroom. All children improved on multiple measures. The possibility that higher doses reduce stimulant effectiveness on some "high-level, high-load" tasks was raised by the observation that performances on one task—paired associate learning—decreased when dosage was increased from 0.30 to 0.60 mg/kg.

21. **Flament MF, Rapoport JL, Berg CZ, Sceery W, Kilts C, Mellstrom B, Linnoila M:** Clomipramine treatment of childhood obsessive compulsive disorder: a double-blind controlled study. *Arch Gen Psychiatry* 42:977–983, 1985

    Clomipramine led to 46% symptom reduction in 14 of 19 adolescent patients, with response related to platelet 5-hydroxytryptamine concentration and monoamine oxidase activity.

22. *Green WH: *Child and Adolescent Clinical Psychopharmacology.* Baltimore, MD, Williams & Wilkins, 1991

    This is a thorough treatment of the major pharmacological agents and their applications.

23. **Jacobitz D, Sroufe LA, Stewart M, Leffert N:** Treatment of attentional and hyperactivity problems in children with sympathomimetic drugs: a comprehensive review. *J Am Acad Child Adolesc Psychiatry* 29:677–688, 1990

    This article reviews studies of short-term medication effects. Discussion of dose-response curves and application to nonlaboratory settings is included. Atypical drug responses are discussed. The relation of attention-deficit/hyperactivity disorder to organic dysfunction is revisited; has been the theoretical justification for psychopharmacological treatment. Long-term effects of drug treatment on academic performance, peer relations, and antisocial behavior are reviewed. Drug effects are found not to generalize well or to produce lasting improvement on academic or behavioral outcome measures. Methodological limitations of cited studies may contribute to this conclusion.

24. **Klorman R, Coons HW, Brumaghim JT, Borgstedt AD, Fitzpatrick P:** Stimulant treatment for adolescents with attention deficit disorder. *Psychopharmacol Bull* 24:88–92, 1988

   The authors' double-blind treatment trial for placebo and methylphenidate demonstrated efficacy of methylphenidate for adolescents comparable with that for preadolescent patients with attention deficit disorder. Continuous performance task, home and school activities, and parent and teacher behavior scales were the variables followed.

25. **Leonard H, Swedo S, Rapoport JL, Coffey M, Cheslow D:** Treatment of childhood obsessive compulsive disorder with clomipramine and desmethylimipramine: a double-blind crossover comparison. *Psychopharmacol Bull* 24:93–95, 1988

   Following inpatient evaluation and a 2-week placebo-treatment period, two periods of 5-week treatment were administered with clomipramine and desmethylimipramine in a double-blind crossover design. Clomipramine showed striking superiority.

26. **Panksepp J, Lensing P:** Brief report: a synopsis of an open trial of naltrexone treatment of autism with four children. *J Autism Dev Disord* 21:243–249, 1991

   Naltrexone therapy is reported to have reduced hyperactivity, aggressiveness, self-injurious behavior, and stereotypies and to have promoted positive social behaviors and exploration. The role of social context in promoting the therapeutic effects of naltrexone is emphasized.

27. **Pelham WE, Walker JL, Sturges J, Hoa J:** Comparative effects of methylphenidate on ADD girls and ADD boys. *J Am Acad Child Adolesc Psychiatry* 28:773–776, 1989

   In an intensive summer camp setting, 12 boys and 12 girls matched for age and IQ received equal benefit from methylphenidate on a battery of behavioral measures. This is an important article because there are few studies of girls with attention deficit disorder, and it has been questioned whether the syndrome is similar in girls.

28. **Popper CW:** *Psychiatric Pharmacosciences of Children and Adolescents.* Washington, DC, American Psychiatric Press, 1987

In this book, of particular value is the chapter describing comprehensive guidelines for obtaining consent and following the progress of the child on medication.

29. **Popper CW, Razier SH** (eds): Special issue: the safe and effective use of psychotropic medications in adolescents and children. *Journal of Child and Adolescent Psychopharmacology* 1:1–102, 1990

The inaugural issue of this new journal presents definitive articles for the practitioner on practical use of each of the principal medication classes. This issue and the one immediately following it constitute a compact textbook of current clinical applications.

30. *Puig-Antich J, Perel JM, Luptakin W, Chambers WJ, Tabrizi MA, King J, Goetz R, Davies M, Stiller RL:** Imipramine in prepubertal major depressive disorders. *Arch Gen Psychiatry* 44:81–89, 1987

In this double-blind, placebo-controlled study of imipramine in 38 depressed children, the response rate was 56% in the 16 children treated with imipramine and 68% in the 22 receiving placebo.

31. **Realmuto GM, Jensen JB, Reeve E, Garfinkel BD:** Growth hormone response to L-dopa and clonidine in autistic children. *J Autism Dev Disord* 20:455–465, 1990

Clonidine and L-dopa were probes used to investigate neuroendocrine responses through changes in growth hormone. Premature and delayed growth hormone peaks were reported for clonidine and L-dopa, respectively, in seven autistic children ages 6.6–19.1. Possible abnormalities of both dopaminergic and noradrenergic neurotransmission are raised.

32. **Ryan ND, Puig-Antich J, Cooper T, Rabinovich H, Ambrosini P, Davies M, King J, Torres D, Fried J:** Imipramine in adolescent major depression: plasma level and clinical response. *Arch Psychiatr Scand* 73:275–288, 1986

A 6-week fixed-schedule treatment of imipramine titrated to 5.0 mg/kg/day in 34 adolescents resulted in modest response: 44% improved despite good compliance. Therapeutic response was found to be poorly correlated with plasma levels. Clinical factors, such as separation anxiety, were weakly associated with poor response as well.

33. *Satterfield JH, Cantwell DP, Satterfield BT:** Multimodality treatment: a two-year study of 61 hyperactive boys. *Arch Gen Psychiatry* 36:915–919, 1987

In this 3-year study, stimulants were assessed in combination with other forms of intervention. Significant improvements in academic performance over time were noted. Stimulants did not produce a positive effect on the academic performance of children with learning disabilities who did not have attention-deficit/hyperactivity disorder.

34. **Solanto MV, Wender EH:** Does methylphenidate constrict cognitive functioning? *J Am Acad Child Adolesc Psychiatry* 28:897–902, 1989

To evaluate the question of whether stimulants produce constriction or overfocusing of attention in children with attention deficit disorder, 19 children were tested on the Wallach-Kogan battery, which demands cognitive flexibility. Children increased their output on the medication and had decreased productivity on placebo days, indicating less, not more, cognitive constriction. A subgroup of 8 children appeared to be possibly overstimulated and perseverative on psychostimulant medication.

35. **Stewart JT, Myers WC, Burket RC, Lyles WB:** A review of the pharmacotherapy of aggression in children and adolescents. *J Am Acad Child Adolesc Psychiatry* 29:269–277, 1990

Based on the premise that aggressive behavior is heterogeneous and not explained by a single etiologic model, therapy may need to include psychotherapy, behavioral therapy, or pharmacological treatment. Adequate diagnostic characterization is critical. A combination of modalities is often indicated. Aggressive behavior arising in the contexts of conduct disorders, attention-deficit/hyperactivity disorder, depression, bipolar affective disorder, schizophrenia, organic mental disorders, epilepsy, mental retardation, and autism are discussed.

36. **Swanson JM, Cantwell D, Lerner M, McBurnett K, Hanna G:** Effects of stimulant medication on learning in children with ADHD. *Journal of Learning Disabilities* 24:219–255, 1991

A methodology for including and treating children with attention-deficit/hyperactivity disorder is presented. In the group with extreme symptoms, the percentage of favorable responders was 68.2%, whereas in the clinically referred group it was 46%. Dose-response curves indicate that an absolute-dose method may be superior to mg/kg dosing. Two reasons for inconsistency in the results of studies designed to demonstrate that stimulant medication improves learning or long-term academic achievement in children with attention-deficit/hyperactivity disorder may be 1) higher-than-optimal doses may be prescribed if behavioral control is used to titrate the endpoint, or 2) treatment may be overinclusive if diagnostic groups are targeted in which a significant proportion of cases do not have a favorable response to medication.

Psychotherapies and Other
Nonpharmacological Treatments

37. **Dulcan MK:** Brief psychotherapy with children and their families: the state of the art. *J Am Acad Child Adolesc Psychiatry* 23:544–551, 1984

    The literature on planned brief psychotherapy with children, adolescents, and families is reviewed. The prominent theoretical foundations and methods of intervention are characterized for psychodynamic therapies, crisis-oriented treatments, family systems therapies, and educational approaches. Clinical experience, published research, and changing constraints on practice are discussed.

38. **Greenspan SI, Wieder S, Nover RA, Lieberman AF, Louri RS, Robinson ME** (eds): *Infants in Multirisk Families: Case Studies in Preventive Intervention (Clinical Infant Reports Series of the National Center for Clinical Infant Programs)*. Madison, CT, International Universities Press, 1987

    This book includes careful case descriptions of Greenspan's theoretical model with applications of interventions illustrated by detailed clinical vignettes.

39. **Haworth MR:** *A Child's Therapy: Hour by Hour*. Madison, CT, International Universities Press, 1990

    This book is a detailed description of child psychotherapy.

40. **Kazdin AE:** *Child Psychotherapy: Developing and Identifying Effective Treatments*. New York, Pergamon, 1988

    The author brings together a thorough review of important work in the field and a scholarly discussion of theoretical issues.

41. **Kernberg PF, Chazan SE:** *Children With Conduct Disorders: A Psychotherapy Manual*. New York, Basic Books, 1991

    This is a systematic, staged description of the treatment of children with externalizing oppositional and antisocial behavior.

42. **Krall V:** *Play Therapy Primer: Therapeutic Approaches to Children With Emotional Problems*. New York, Human Sciences Press, 1989

    This book examines the literature on play therapy. Materials and techniques are described. Applications of the use of play therapy are included. Diagnostic categories discussed include autism, symbiotic psychosis, borderline personality organization, and neurosis.

43. **Marans S:** Psychoanalytic psychotherapy with children: current research trends and challenges. *J Am Acad Child Adolesc Psychiatry* 28:669–674, 1989

This article briefly reviews past and current efforts to collect and evaluate clinical data on psychoanalytic psychotherapy. A procedural scheme for organizing clinical data and planning therapy is presented.

44. **Sholevar GP, Burland JA, Frank JL, Etezady MH, Goldstein J:** Psychoanalytic treatment of children and adolescents. *J Am Acad Child Adolesc Psychiatry* 28:685–690, 1989

The usefulness of psychoanalytic psychotherapy in achieving optimal adaptation after neurotic and personality conflicts have been resolved is reviewed. Applications to preschool, latency-age, and adolescent children are illustrated.

Behavior Therapy and Cognitive-Behavioral Therapy

45. **Durand VM, Mindell JA:** Behavioral treatment of multiple childhood sleep disorders. *Behav Modif* 14:37–49, 1990

This article describes multiple baseline treatment for chronic night waking and nighttime disturbance in a 14-month-old child, using graduated extinction, a technique of gradually increasing the time before attending to the child's crying.

46. **Franko DP, Christoff KA, Crimmins DB, Kelly JA:** Social skills training for an extremely shy adolescent: an empirical case study. *Behavior Therapy* 14:568–575, 1983

This is one of the few reports on social skills training for young adolescents. This case demonstrates increasing social skills in a youth without social anxiety who had long-standing severe peer interaction difficulties.

47. **Kendall PC** (ed): *Child and Adolescent Therapy: Cognitive Behavioral Procedures.* New York, Guilford, 1990

The application of cognitive-behavioral therapy to a spectrum of psychiatric conditions in childhood is reviewed. It is not demonstrated to produce more than a marginal response in externalizing behavior disorders, but is more effective for internalizing disorders. The role of the family in participating in the child's cognitive-behavioral therapy is presented. A chapter on chronic illnesses and pain management is of interest to clinicians working with physically ill children.

48. *Werry JS, Wollersheim JP:** Behavior therapy with children and adolescents: a twenty year overview. *J Am Acad Child Adolesc Psychiatry* 28:1–18, 1989

Theories of neobehaviorist approaches and cognitive-behavioral approaches and social learning models are reviewed. Applications to specific DSM-III disorders—mental retardation; the autism continuum; speech and language disorders; disruptive disorders; anxiety, eating, elimination, and organic mood disorders; substance abuse; and somatoform and sleep disorders—are highlighted.

49. **Wilkes TC, Rush AJ:** Adaptations of cognitive therapy for depressed adolescents. *J Am Acad Child Adolesc Psychiatry* 27:381–386, 1988

Methods for adapting cognitive therapeutic techniques to the treatment of nonpsychotic depressed adolescents are described and illustrated.

Family Therapy

50. **Combrinck-Graham L** (ed): *Children in Family Contexts.* New York, Guilford, 1988

This is a valuable collection of chapters on aspects of family therapy, including less frequently addressed subjects like the very young child in family systems, the treatments of violent and incestuous families, the family and the school, and the family life cycle.

51. **Combrinck-Graham L:** Developments in family systems theory and research. *J Am Acad Child Adolesc Psychiatry* 29:501–512, 1990

This article summarizes advances in therapy with difficult clinical populations, chronic mental illness, conduct disorders, and depression. Theories of family therapy are considered in a review of several important developments in family therapy, such as increased awareness of the role of women, the inclusion of small children, and the application to families with a chronically ill family member.

52. **Sharff DE, Sharff JS:** *Object Relations Family Therapy.* Northvale, NJ, Jason Aronson, 1987

The authors present their theory and techniques of object relations family therapy. Active nondirective listening, personal communications, and interpretation are illustrated. This therapy makes use of the therapist's countertransference in direct involvement with family members during treatment.

53. **Textor M** (ed): *The Divorce and Divorce Therapy Handbook*. Northvale, NJ, Jason Aronson, 1989

This book deals with divorce both from the adults' and children's points of view. The second part contains chapters on psychotherapy for children after divorce, school intervention, and group intervention. The third part describes treating single-parent families, stepfamilies, and remarried families.

54. **Visher EB, Visher J:** *Old Loyalties, New Ties: Therapeutic Strategies With Step Families*. New York, Brunner/Mazel, 1988

Widely respected clinical techniques for dealing with the adjustment of the blended family are presented.

Milieu, Group, and Day Treatment and Other Modalities

55. **Gabel S, Finn M, Ahmad A:** Day treatment outcome with severely disturbed children. *J Am Acad Child Adolesc Psychiatry* 274:497–482, 1988

Preadmission variables of abuse, parental substance abuse, and suicidal and aggressive symptoms were dependent variables in analysis of outcome for 52 children referred to day treatment after discharge from a psychiatric hospital. Implications for admission criteria and program design of children's day-treatment programs are discussed.

56. **Harper G:** Focal inpatient treatment planning. *J Am Acad Child Adolesc Psychiatry* 28:31–37, 1989

The author describes focal inpatient treatment planning and provides guidelines for its use.

57. **Kaplan SL, Brent M, Gautier P, Busner J:** A comparison of three nocturnal enuresis treatment methods. *J Am Acad Child Adolesc Psychiatry* 28:282–286, 1989

The bell and pad used alone or with tangible rewards with fading or with the dry bed methods are described. There was a trend for the bell and pad with the dry bed method to lead to increased dryness, but the results did not achieve significance.

58. **Kiser LJ, Pruitt DB, McColgan EB, Ackerman BJ:** A survey of child and adolescent day treatment programs: establishing definitions and standards. *International Journal of Partial Hospitalization* 3:247–259, 1986

This article outlines the requirements for national standards and criteria for day-treatment facilities for children. Included are 1) development of treatment objectives; 2) necessary staffing; 3) daily treatment activities; and 4) provisions of individual, group, family, educational, and milieu therapies.

59. *Kliman G: Psychological Emergencies of Childhood.* New York, Grune & Stratton, 1991

This classic work is an excellent basis for practitioners unfamiliar with emerging child treatments, as well as a thoughtful summary for those who have years of experience.

60. **Nurcombe B:** Goal-directed treatment planning and the principles of brief hospitalization. *J Am Acad Child Adolesc Psychiatry* 28:26–30, 1989

This article presents steps in goal-directed planning and contrasts it with intuitive therapy in the context of a problem-oriented approach to inpatient treatment. On the basis of contemporary pressures to show efficacy of hospitalization, it justifies the use of goal-directed therapy.

61. **Scheidlinger S:** Short-term group psychotherapy for children: an overview. *Int J Group Psychother* 34:573–585, 1985

The sparse literature on short-term group psychotherapy of children is reviewed. A general framework to differentiate therapeutic group modalities is presented, and the structure of short-term children's psychotherapy groups is described.

62. **Stuber ML:** Psychiatric consultation issues in pediatric HIV and AIDS. *J Am Acad Child Adolesc Psychiatry* 29:463–467, 1990

This new, difficult area of pediatric consultation-liaison deals with 1) treatment decisions such as reentry into school setting, 2) family therapy when one member infects others, and 3) decisions about reproduction and primary prevention among adolescents. Case examples illustrate the points.

63. **Woolston JL:** Transactional risk model for short and intermediate term psychiatric inpatient treatment of children. *J Am Acad Child Adolesc Psychiatry* 28:38–41, 1989

A model for incorporating into treatment the transactional view of child psychopathology is presented. It presupposes interplay between the child and the environment. Family and school involvement in inpatient treatments is discussed.

Nonpharmacological Treatment Approaches to Specific Disorders

Attention-Deficit/Hyperactivity Disorder

64. **Abikoff H:** Cognitive training in ADHD children: less to it than meets the eye. *Journal of Learning Disabilities* 24:205–209, 1991

    This article is a careful review of studies of cognitive training.

65. ***Barkely RA:** *Attention Deficit Hyperactivity Disorder: A Handbook for Diagnosis and Treatment,* 2nd Edition. New York, Guilford, 1990

    This is a comprehensive handbook for clinical management of attention-deficit/hyperactivity disorders. Assessment with a developmental perspective is presented. A comprehensive review of the literature is included. Pharmacological and nonpharmacological treatments include training parents, family systems intervention, and social skills training approaches.

66. **Satterfield JH, Satterfield BT, Schell AM:** Therapeutic interventions to prevent delinquency in hyperactive boys. *J Am Acad Child Adolesc Psychiatry* 26:56–64, 1987

    Multimodality treatment approaches for a high-risk population of youngsters are reviewed.

67. **Silver LB:** *Attention Deficit Hyperactivity Disorder: A Clinical Guide to Diagnosis and Treatment.* Washington, DC, American Psychiatric Press, 1992

    This book contains six chapters on treatment, with a good explanation of multimodal treatment and a clear presentation of how to determine a child's specific treatment needs. The chapter on medication is well organized and categorizes the common pharmacological agents.

68. **Strayhorn JM, Weidman CS:** Reduction of attention deficit and internalizing symptoms in preschoolers through parent-interaction training. *J Am Acad Child Adolesc Psychiatry* 28:888–896, 1989

    A preventive mental health intervention with parents of disruptive preschoolers was carried out using standard treatment manuals. Parents' and children's behaviors together were videotaped and blindly rated to document improvement from the intervention.

69. **Whalen CK, Henker B:** Therapies for hyperactive children: comparisons, combinations, and compromises. *J Consult Clin Psychol* 59:126–137, 1991

Behavioral treatments and cognitive-behavioral self-regulation approaches are two alternative treatments to the use of stimulants. The relative advantages of different treatment modalities are evaluated. Methodological pitfalls include 1) subject sources, 2) clinical variability of symptom indicators, 3) constraints on full assessment of children's attention profiles, 4) multiple informants, and 5) heterogeneity in treatment responsiveness.

70. *Weiss G (ed): *Attention Deficit Disorder: Child and Adolescent Psychiatric Clinics of North America.* Philadelphia, PA, WB Saunders, 1992

This volume contains five excellent chapters on nonpharmacological treatment approaches for children with attention-deficit/hyperactivity disorder. Psychoeducational interventions are described and illustrated with case vignettes. Psychosocial interventions are described, as is behavior modification. The theoretical background supporting clinical applications of parent training groups and interventions to enhance social competence and social skills are included.

Conduct Disorder

71. **Bank L, Marlowe JH, Reid JB, Patterson GR, Weinrott MR:** A comparative evaluation of parent training interventions for families of chronic delinquents. *J Abnorm Child Psychol* 9:5–33, 1991

Boys in families who received parent training were found to have fewer offenses and to spend less time in institutional settings. Positive findings persisted at 1-year follow-up. Boys receiving services traditionally provided by juvenile court and community served as the comparison group. Average time of intervention was 44.8 professional hours. The emotional cost to the staff was described as high.

72. **Kazdin AE:** *Treatment of Antisocial Behavior in Children and Adolescents.* Homewood, IL, Dorsey Press, 1985

This is a review of the literature of treatments for antisocial children. Parent training techniques are considered most promising for treatment of preadolescent antisocial children.

73. **Lochman JE:** Cognitive-behavioral intervention with aggressive boys: three-year follow up and preventive effects. *J Consult Clin Psychol* 60:426–432, 1992

Three years after a preventive school-based intervention, boys receiving an anger-coping program had no difference from nonaggressive boys in drug and alcohol involvement, self-esteem, or social problem-solving skills. Overall intervention also did not have long-term effects on delinquency rates or classroom behaviors.

74. **Whitehead JD, Lab SP:** A meta-analysis of juvenile correctional treatment. *Journal of Research in Crime and Delinquency* 26:275–295, 1989

A meta-analysis of research reports from 1975 to 1984 indicates that interventions do not prevent recidivism and may exacerbate problems of incarcerated juveniles. System diversion (i.e., intervention in the community short of incarceration) appears to yield better results than does institutional/residential intervention.

Anxiety Disorders

75. **Barlow DH, Siedner AL:** Treatment of adolescent agoraphobics: effects on parent-adolescent relations. *Behav Res Ther* 21:519–526, 1983

Changes in the mother-child relationship for adolescents correspond with treatment changes in symptoms of phobia and avoidance.

76. **Blagg NR, Yule W:** The behavioral treatment of school refusal: a comparative study. *Behav Res Ther* 22:119–127, 1984

This article reports behavioral methods for treating fears and anxieties, including systematic desensitization and its variants, flooding-related procedures, modeling programs, and self-control procedures.

77. **Last CG, Straus CC:** School refusal in anxiety-disordered children and adolescents. *J Am Acad Child Adolesc Psychiatry* 29:31–35, 1990

School refusal is described clinically, and treatment approaches are laid out.

78. **Morris RJ, Kratochwill JR:** *Treating Children's Fears and Phobias: A Behavioral Approach.* New York, Pergamon, 1983

Behavioral approaches for fearful and anxious children are reviewed, including anxiety-inhibiting images through emotive imagery.

Obsessive-Compulsive Disorder

79. **Swedo SE, Rapoport JL, Leonard HL, Lenane M, Cheslow D:** Obsessive-compulsive disorder in children and adolescents. *Arch Gen Psychiatry* 46:335–345, 1989

This is a clinical study of 27 adolescents with obsessive-compulsive disorder treated with clomipramine and followed for 2–5 years. Symptoms of obsessive-compulsive disorder improved but the majority of adolescents remained symptomatic with depression or anxiety.

80. **Towbin KE, Leckman JF, Cohen DJ:** Drug treatment of obsessive compulsive disorder: a review of findings in the light of diagnostic and metric limitations. *Psychiatric Developments* 5:25–50, 1987

    This article reviews previous work on medication management of obsessive-compulsive disorder. Guidelines for use of pharmacological agents include careful assessment of presence of associated psychopathology.

Autism, Pervasive Developmental Disorder, and Childhood Schizophrenia

81. **Cantor S, Kestenbaum C:** Psychotherapy with schizophrenic children. *J Am Acad Child Adolesc Psychiatry* 25:623–630, 1986

    This article provides a description of the usefulness of supportive psychotherapy in schizophrenic children.

82. **Harris SL, Handleman JS, Gordon R, Kristoff B, Fuentes F:** Changes in cognitive and language functioning of preschool children with autism. *J Autism Dev Disord* 21:281–290, 1991

    Children with autism showed significant improvement on the Stanford-Binet and Preschool Language scale after 1 year of school, raising the controversial question that patients can make significant gains if offered intensive early education.

83. **Jenkins JR, Speltz ML, Odom SL:** Integrating normal and handicapped preschoolers: effects on child development and social interaction. *Except Child* 52:7–17, 1985

    The view is put forward that optimal outcomes for handicapped preschoolers require that typical children must be actively involved in their classroom experiences.

84. **Koegel RL, O'Dell M, Dunlap G:** Producing speech use in nonverbal autistic children by reinforcing attempts. *J Autism Dev Disord* 18:525–538, 1988

    A review of the literature on teaching speech to severely handicapped autistic children concludes that motivation as a central target behavior would be more effective than motor speech production. A new study using a repeated reversal design supported this conclusion; reinforcing attempts at speech was more effective than reinforcing motor speech sounds.

85. **Kydd RR, Werry JS:** Schizophrenia in children under 16 years. *J Autism Dev Disord* 12:343–357, 1982

    This is one of few studies of treatment of schizophrenia in young children. This article describes the role of major tranquilizers in diminishing positive symptoms such as hallucinations and delusions.

86. **Odom SL, McEvoy MA:** Integration of young children with handicaps and normally developing children, in *Early Intervention for Infants and Children With Handicaps.* Edited by Odom S, Karnes M. Baltimore, MD, Paul H Brooks Publishing, 1988

    Current developments in education for children with autism are described. Individualized group instruction combined with matching typical peers' social overtures to the repertories of autistic children in the classroom is illustrated.

87. **Rogers SJ, Lewis H:** An effective day-treatment model for young children with pervasive developmental disorder. *J Am Acad Child Adolesc Psychiatry* 28:207–214, 1989

    This article describes a structured milieu program using affective experiences to foster development of interpersonal relationships and increased use of play in children with pervasive developmental disorder.

Affective Disorders

88. **Cytryn L, McKnew DH:** Treatment issues in childhood depression. *Psychiatric Annals* 15:401–403, 1985

    This article provides a succinct summary of the principal issues in psychiatric treatment of a depressed child. Working with the family, individual therapy, and the provision of a corrective emotional experience in a climate allowing free expression of feelings are all described. The need of interacting with community agencies and the use of tricyclics and monoamine oxidase inhibitors and lithium are addressed.

89. **Fine S, Forth A, Gilbert M, Haley G:** Group therapy for adolescent depressive disorder: a comparison of social skills and therapeutic support. *J Am Acad Child Adolesc Psychiatry* 30:79–85, 1991

    Treatment in therapeutic support groups resulted in greater self-reported reduction in clinical depression and increase in self-concept than did treatment in social skills training groups. This difference was not seen after 9 months, although conclusions were limited by lack of a nontreatment control group, the addition of concurrent therapy for some patients, and the absence of solid duration and remission rates for base-rate comparison.

90. **Frank E, Prien RF, Kupfer DJ, Alberts L:** Implications of noncompliance on research in affective disorders. *Psychopharmacol Bull* 21:37–43, 1985

    The problem of medical noncompliance in the treatment of depression is reviewed. An approach to educate patients and families through a treatment seminar is described.

91. **Kestenbaum C, Kron L:** Psychoanalytic intervention with children and adolescents with affective disorders: a combined treatment approach. *J Am Acad Psychoanal* 15:153–174, 1987

    A comprehensive treatment approach is described in this article. The value of forming a therapeutic relationship with the depressed youngster within the context of which other treatments are incorporated is highlighted.

92. **Moreau D, Mufson L, Weissman MM, Klerman GL:** Interpersonal psychotherapy for adolescent depression: description of modification and preliminary application. *J Am Acad Child Adolesc Psychiatry* 30:642–651, 1991

    Interpersonal psychotherapy, developed for depressed adults, is a manualized, time-limited treatment that addresses specific tasks in the initial, middle, and termination phases. A modification of this therapy and its application to adolescents are described.

93. *Pfeffer CR:** *The Suicidal Child.* New York, Guilford, 1986

    This is a comprehensive volume, reporting clinical management and research findings for the clinician dealing with suicidally depressed children or adolescents.

94. **Robbins DR, Alessi NE, Colfer MV:** Treatment of adolescents with major depression: implications of the DST and the melancholic clinical subtype. *J Affect Disord* 17:99–104, 1989

    The authors describe a pilot treatment for hospitalized adolescents with major depression, using an open trial of psychotherapy similar to interpersonal psychotherapy; 47% responded with psychotherapy alone. Nonresponders were treated with tricyclic antidepressants and psychotherapy, and 92% responded. Dexamethasone suppression and melancholic subtype were associated with failure to respond to psychotherapy alone.

95. **Shaffer D, Garland A, Vieland V, Underwood M, Busner C:** The impact of curriculum-based suicide prevention programs for teenag-

ers: an 18-month follow-up. *J Am Acad Child Adolesc Psychiatry* 30:588–596, 1991

No convincing long-term effect was found for 174 students from two high schools who had been participants in a suicide prevention program. Nonetheless, the authors note that the adolescents were receptive to programs dealing with mental health issues, and, although expressing unwillingness to seek help for emotional problems from adult helpers, many would reveal that they had emotional problems or suicidal ideation, thus enabling referral.

Eating Disorders

96. **Anyan WR, Schowalter JE:** A comprehensive approach to anorexia nervosa. *J Am Acad Child Adolesc Psychiatry* 22:122–127, 1983

   The authors describe treatment of 137 female and 17 male patients meeting Feighner criteria for anorexia nervosa. A scheme for structured inpatient treatment is described in detail, and typical patients' responses to early, middle, and late phases of treatment are reported.

97. **Yates A:** Current perspectives on the eating disorders, II: treatment, outcome and research directions. *J Am Acad Child Adolesc Psychiatry* 29:1–9, 1990

   Yates describes general issues in the treatment of anorexia nervosa and bulimia nervosa, which are relatively distinct in their psychopathology and clinical manifestations. She notes that inpatient treatment is necessary for anorexia nervosa that has progressed to severe nutritional compromise. Treatment of underlying depression and obsessional thinking usually requires long-term psychotherapy and family involvement. Bulimia nervosa is effectively treated with cognitive-behavioral treatment and by establishing a therapeutic alliance in group settings. Pharmacological intervention studies are reviewed. Outcomes are discussed, and future directions of research are outlined.

Tourette's Syndrome

98. *Cohen DJ, Bruun RD, Leckman JF** (eds): *Tourette's Syndrome and Tic Disorders*. New York, Wiley, 1988

   This excellent volume contains chapters on both psychosocial management and treatment with medications.

99. **Leckman JF, Hardin MT, Riddle MA, Stevenson J, Ort SI, Cohen DJ:** Clonidine treatment of Gilles de la Tourette's syndrome. *Arch Gen Psychiatry* 48:324–328, 1991

Clonidine was shown to reduce tic symptoms in a double-blind, placebo-controlled trial. Clonidine improved tic severity, tic "noticeability," tic frequency, impulsivity, and hyperactivity.

100. **Price AR, Leckman JF, Pauls DL, Cohen DJ, Kidd KK:** Tics and central nervous system stimulants in twins and non-twins with Tourette syndrome. *Neurology* 36:232–237, 1986

A careful twin study addresses the controversial question of the potentiation of Tourette's syndrome by psychostimulants. Among monozygotic twins concordant for Tourette's syndrome and discordant for attention-deficit/hyperactivity disorder, where one twin was treated with stimulant medications, tics developed earlier. However, the fact that both twins went on to develop tics suggested that psychostimulants were not "causative."

101. **Shapiro AK, Shapiro ES, Young GG, Feinberg TE** (eds): *Gilles de la Tourette Syndrome*. New York, Raven, 1987

The medical history, epidemiology, clinical characteristics, and course of Tourette's syndrome are presented, together with detailed psychopathology, neuropsychology, genetics, clinical assessment and management techniques, and psychopharmacological treatments of this complex syndrome. Detailed reports of 1,610 patients using a data-oriented approach provide helpful clinical insights.

102. **Shapiro ES, Shapiro AK, Fulop G, Hubbard M, Mandeli J, Nordlie J, Phillips RA:** Controlled study of haloperidol, pimozide, and placebo for the treatment of Gilles de la Tourette's syndrome. *Arch Gen Psychiatry* 46:722–730, 1989

This is an important study that brings out the relative advantages of haloperidol and pimozide for youngsters with Tourette's syndrome.

Sequelae of Abuse

103. **Dell PF, Eisenhower JW:** Adolescent multiple personality disorder: a preliminary study of 11 cases. *J Am Acad Child Adolesc Psychiatry* 29:359–366, 1990

Eleven cases of previously traumatized adolescents with multiple personality disorder who were followed in therapy are described. The step-by-step approach was undertaken in sequence to 1) "detoxify" the patient's environment, 2) stabilize patient and family, 3) alter the family system, and 4) develop a therapeutic alliance. Four cases reached the stage of postintegration therapy.

104. **Hansen DJ, MacMillan VM:** Behavioral assessment of child-abusive and neglectful families. *Behav Modif* 14:255–278, 1990

This review article, in a special issue devoted to behavioral treatments of child abuse and neglect, discusses recent developments and current issues in the behavioral assessment of abusive and neglectful families. It also presents procedures and measures for assessment of progress.

105. **Kluft RP** (ed): *The Psychiatric Clinics of North America: Treatment of Victims of Sexual Abuse.* Philadelphia, PA, WB Saunders, 1989

This volume includes descriptions of a variety of treatment modalities successful in sexually abused children, such as individual psychotherapy, group psychotherapy for child victims, and minimization of the impact of legal procedures on child victims.

Normality and Development

52

Infant and Child Development

Linda C. Mayes, M.D.

T
he area of infant and child development readily lends itself to multiple perspectives ranging from a focus on specific symptoms, diagnoses, and interventions in the case of deviant or impaired development to an emphasis on what is expectable across developmental domains in different age groups. This biography was compiled with a specific reader in mind: trainees in psychiatry who wish to gain a basic functional understanding of the salient concepts that guide thinking about the normal and deviant development of infants and young children. To this end, the selected references are organized around broad areas (e.g., social development) and within those broad areas around selected key concepts (e.g., attachment) or clinical issues (e.g., assessment in infancy).

Several caveats are in order. First, the included key concepts or clinical issues are only a selection among many. What is key to one investigator or clinician may seem esoteric to another. But, by and large, the selected areas are those that cut across clinical and investigative pursuits and have a long tradition of consideration and debate within several disciplines considering child development.

Second, the bibliography represents work from several disciplines, including developmental psychology, psychoanalysis, and child psychiatry. Instead of categorizing areas by their primary field, I have chosen to provide the reader with representative articles about a concept regardless of the professional or theoretical orientation of the work. Where appropriate or necessary, I provide an annotated statement about how one discipline lends a somewhat different theoretical cast to the concept or issue.

Third, any bibliography of the field of infant and child development may tell several different although converging stories. One story that is fundamental for the developmental novice is gained through a thorough reading of the "classic" papers. However, I have chosen to make this listing more current than traditional and hope the reader will rely on the bibliographies of the works cited here to retrieve the related, older, sometimes classic works. Where appropriate, I point out the areas where a particularly salient classic and historical literature exists. As an area of study, infant and child development has burgeoned in the last decade, and the story highlighted in this bibliography reflects the more recent emphasis on mechanisms of genetic or biological-environmental interaction across all phases of development.

Finally, a practical word about the annotation. Some sections are annotated through an introduction that outlines the specific selection rules or themes highlighted by the cited references. Others, particularly when the references are classic ones, are specifically annotated. The annotation is meant to serve as a map to the themes of this bibliography but not consistently as a summary for each citation.

General References

Each of the references in this section offers the reader a different perspective and information base. Bornstein and Lamb (1992) provide a detailed and thoughtful summary and critique of the state of understanding about infancy and early childhood primarily from the view of developmental psychology, whereas Tyson and Tyson (1990) present the psychoanalytic view. Osofsky's (1987) handbook is a valuable resource for in-depth reviews of broad areas such as information processing and memory, again primarily from the standpoint of developmental psychology. Fraiberg's (1959) classic book is included as a general reference in part because of its wide circulation and familiarity to many child professionals and because it represents a translation of psychoanalytic concepts into an easily read basic "handbook" of development. Finally, two textbooks of child psychiatry, both recently published, are included. Noshpitz and King (1991; King and Noshpitz 1991) present an extensive review in two volumes that covers the child and adolescent psychiatric literature. Lewis's (1991) text is a similar compendium of relevant child and adolescent psychiatry but, because it is multi-authored, it contains chapters often reflecting the special expertise of the individual author.

1. *Bornstein MH, Lamb ME: *Development in Infancy: An Introduction.* New York, McGraw-Hill, 1992

2. *Fraiberg S: *The Magic Years: Understanding and Handling the Problems of Early Childhood.* New York, Scribner, 1959

3. **Kessen W, Haith MM, Salapatek PH:** Human infancy: a bibliography and guide, in *Carmichael's Manual of Child Psychology.* Edited by Mussen P. New York, Wiley, 1970, pp. 287–445

   Although the bibliography contained in this guide does not reflect the last two decades of work, the compilation is an excellent resource for many classic papers from early studies of infancy.

4. **King R, Noshpitz J:** *Pathways of Growth: Essentials of Child Psychiatry, Vol. 2: Psychopathology.* New York, Wiley, 1991

5. *Lewis M: *Child and Adolescent Psychiatry: A Comprehensive Textbook.* Baltimore, MD, Williams & Wilkins, 1991

6. **Noshpitz J, King R:** *Pathways of Growth: Essentials of Child Psychiatry, Vol. 1: Normal Development.* New York, Wiley, 1991

7. **Osofsky J:** *Handbook of Infant Development,* 2nd Edition. New York, Wiley, 1987

8. **Rutter M:** *Developmental Neuropsychiatry.* New York, Guilford, 1983

9. **Tyson P, Tyson RL:** *Psychoanalytic Theories of Development.* New Haven, CT, Yale Universities Press, 1990

Diagnostic Developmental Assessment of Infants and Young Children

General Theories of Development

The citations below complement the general references suggested in the previous section but are also intended to highlight several classic works. Notions of developmental stages or phases, of a linear approach to development, of the interdependency between different developmental domains, and of development through the life span are now implicit in much of developmental writing. The references cited below provide some sources for these critical developmental concepts.

10. *__Erikson EH:__ *Childhood and Society,* 2nd Edition. New York, WW Norton, 1963

    This book presents Erikson's psychosocial theory of sequential developmental stages, with each subsequent stage building on the achievements of the previous stage. Because the work is now a classic piece, all trainees working with children need some familiarity with Erikson's approach to a stage theory of development.

11. __Freud A:__ *Ego and Mechanisms of Defense.* New York, International Universities Press, 1937

    In this typology of the mechanisms of defense, Anna Freud extended the theory of developing ego functions.

12. *__Freud A:__ *Normality and Pathology in Childhood: Assessments of Development.* New York, International Universities Press, 1965

    Here Anna Freud outlines her notion of developmental lines. Instead of one integrated stage of development, she proposed that multiple developmental lines (e.g., body autonomy) contribute to the organization of mental functioning at any given age.

13. __Hinde RA:__ Ethology and child development, in *Handbook of Child Psychology, Vol. 2: Infancy and Developmental Psychobiology.* Edited by Haith MM, Campos JJ. New York, Wiley, 1983, pp. 27–94

    The ethological approach provides another perspective on children's development that focuses on the adaptive potential of behaviors across a number of species. The application to humans of bonding behavior at birth so critical among various species is one example of the ethological approach. Another is the study of attachment behaviors among infants and their parents. Although the ethological perspective is less often considered in any given clinical instance, it does provide a complementary view of development of which it is important to be cognizant.

Assessment Techniques

Much of assessment in infancy and early childhood is based on the implicit notions outlined above—a steady, stage-specific progression of emerging developmental capacities. To this end, beginning with the work of Buhler and Hetzer (1935) (which was expanded on by Arnold Gesell), a number of assessment techniques have been developed. Some, although by no means all, frequently used techniques are described in the references cited in this section. Also included are reviews and discussions about the notion of assessment and measurement of developmental functioning (e.g., Francis et al. 1987; Volkmar 1989).

14. **Brazelton TB:** *Neonatal Behavioral Assessment Scale (Clinics in Developmental Medicine, No. 50)*. Philadelphia, PA, JB Lippincott, 1984

This instrument is the most widely used neurobehavioral assessment scale for the neonate. Although it is rarely used by child psychiatrists, it is an important measure to understand conceptually because it contains notions of the regulation of states and the infants' early predisposition to social cues.

15. **Buhler C, Hetzer H:** *Testing Children's Development From Birth to School Age.* New York, Farrar & Rinehart, 1935

This book is a classic reference from two of the many infant observers (such as Arnold Gesell) who were contributing to the field in the 1920s and 1930s.

16. **Francis PL, Self PA, Horowitz FD:** The behavioral assessment of the neonate: an overview, in *Handbook of Infant Development*, 2nd Edition. Edited by Osofsky JD. New York, Wiley, 1987, pp. 723–779

17. **Sameroff AJ:** Organization and stability of newborn behavior: a commentary on the Brazelton Neonatal Behavior Assessment Scale. *Monogr Soc Res Child Dev* 43 (Serial No. 5–6):1–138, 1978

Although dated, this monograph provides the best summary at that time of the rationale behind using the Neonatal Behavior Assessment Scale and of the issues of reliability and predictive validity.

18. **Sparrow S, Balla DB, Cicchetti DV:** *The Vineland Adaptive Behavior Scales.* Circle Pines, MN, American Guidance Service, 1984

This scale is a widely used measure of adaptive behavior in several domains such as communication and daily living skills. In addition to showing robust psychometric properties, the Vineland provides an important, complementary addition to standard measures of development that assess what the child can do. Measures of adaptive behavior address what the child routinely does; for example, how does the child use the functional capacities he or she has adaptively?

19. **Volkmar FR:** Development assessment. *Semin Perinatol* 13:467–473, 1989

This article is a general review of the guiding concepts and historical context of a number of assessment techniques for infants and young children.

Neurobiological and Neurophysiological Contributions to Development

This section contains a number of classic papers that address issues of state regulation and autonomic nervous system maturation in early childhood (e.g., Fox and Fitzgerald 1990; Thoman 1991). Lester and Boukydis' (1985) work on cries is included because of the emphasis on the cry as a neurophysiologic measure of autonomic organization. Additionally, the last 10 years have brought to light a number of concepts about early brain development that are critical to understanding the early interface between experience and biologically determined maturation (e.g., Anderson and Cohen 1991; Leckman 1991). For example, as outlined by Black and Greenough (1986), Goldman-Rakic (1987), and Nowakowski (1987), sometime, probably in the first year of life, there is a marked remodeling of brain structure through synaptic pruning. The choice of synapses is in part use related; that is, those functions that are not supported by use are lost. Conversely, synaptic formation also continues long after birth, and there is an active remodeling process occurring through the first years of life that is apparently sensitive to environmental conditions and stimuli (e.g., Black and Greenough 1986). Finally, there has also been in the last decade a marked increase in the understanding of developmental neurochemistry and the effects of early neurotransmitters on brain development and on the timing of critical remodeling events in the central nervous system.

20. **Anderson GM, Cohen DJ:** The neurobiology of childhood neuropsychiatric disorders, in *Child and Adolescent Psychiatry*. Edited by Lewis M. Baltimore, MD, Williams & Wilkins, 1991, pp. 28–38

21. **Black JE, Greenough WT:** Induction of pattern in neural structure by experience: implication for cognitive development, in *Advances in Developmental Psychology*, Vol. 4. Edited by Lamb ME, Brown AL, Rogoff B. Hillsdale, NJ, Lawrence Erlbaum, 1986, pp. 1–50

22. **Fox NA, Fltzgerald HE:** Autonomic function in infancy. *Merrill-Palmer Quarterly* 36:27–52, 1990

23. ***Goldman-Rakic PS:** Development of cortical circuitry and cognitive function. *Child Dev* 58:601–622, 1987

24. ***Greenough WT, Black JE, Wallace CS:** Experience and brain development. *Child Dev* 58:539–559, 1987

25. *Leckman JF: Genes and developmental neurobiology, in *Child and Adolescent Psychiatry*. Edited by Lewis M. Baltimore, MD, Williams & Wilkins, 1991, pp. 3–10

26. **Lester BM, Boukydis CFZ** (eds): *Infant Crying: Theoretical Perspectives.* New York, Plenum, 1985

27. **Nowakowski RS:** Basic concepts of CNS development. *Child Dev* 58:568–595, 1987

28. **Thoman EB:** Sleeping and waking states in infants: a functional perspective. *Neurosci Biobehav Rev* 14:93–107, 1991

Social Development

In whatever setting the child professional works, issues of how the child relates to important others and how he or she adjusts to the social world will be, if not paramount, at least critical for understanding how the child's problems impact on his or her relationships with others as well as how he or she responds to interventions.

General Reviews

29. *Campos J, Barrett KC, Lamb ME, Goldsmith H, Stenberg C: Socioemotional development, in *Handbook of Child Psychology, Vol. 2: Infancy and Developmental Psychobiology*. Edited by Haith MM, Campos JJ. New York, Wiley, 1983, pp. 783–915

This is an extensive review of the field of social cognition as well as concepts of attachment and affective development. Although it is now dated, it remains an invaluable conceptual guide and review of the central issues in social development.

Attachment

The concept of attachment is an ascendant one in studies of social development. Beginning with Ainsworth et al.'s (1978) observations of the behaviors of children during myriad, everyday separations from their mothers, the concept was theoretically developed by Bowlby (1969, 1973, both later) and others to stand as a central force for development. Attachment to others and "internal working models" of others became basic to survival. There are differences in the types of attachments children form to their parents, and these differences affect the child's cognitive, social, and personality development. Additionally, the quality of the child's attachment to others is influenced by parental characteristics as well as child-related factors. The references contained in this section review the concept of attachment, cover some aspects of individual variability in attachments, and examine the predictive nature of the quality of the child's early attachments.

30. *Ainsworth MDS, Blehar MC, Walters E, Wall S:* Patterns of Attachment: A Psychological Study of the Strange Situation. *Hillsdale, NJ, Lawrence Erlbaum, 1978

   In this book, Ainsworth et al. outline their now widely used and discussed approaches to studying the child's attachments to important others.

31. *Bretherton I:* New perspectives on attachment relations: security, communication, and internal working models, in *Handbook of Infant Development.* Edited by Osofsky J. New York, Wiley, 1987, pp. 1061–1100

   This is an extensive review of the concept of attachment and its theoretical implications for later development. The bibliography is very useful for those wishing to review the attachment field in depth.

32. **Fox NA, Kimmerly NL, Schafer WD:** Attachment to mother/attachment to father: a meta-analysis. *Child Dev* 62:210–225, 1991

   This article investigates the concordance or lack of concordance between the child's attachment behaviors with mothers and fathers and raises important theoretical questions regarding the meaning of the attachment classification as obtained through the Ainsworth "strange situation" procedure (see also Lamb 1977 below).

33. **Lamb ME:** The development of mother-infant and father-infant attachments in the second year of life. *Developmental Psychology* 13:637–648, 1977

   This article presents a carefully done study of the differences in 2-year-old infants' attachment behaviors with mothers compared with fathers.

34. **Lamb ME, Hwang CP:** Maternal attachment and mother-neonate bonding: a critical review, in *Advances in Developmental Psychology,* Vol. 2. Edited by Lamb ME, Brown AL. Hillsdale, NJ, Lawrence Erlbaum, 1982, pp. 1–39

   This is a critical review of the literature on the importance of early mother-neonate contact for attachment between parents and infants. For a time, the notion of "bonding" between a parent and infant in the immediate perinatal period was considered critical for the formation of a successful relationship—a theoretical frame of reference that invoked concepts of critical periods and was taken from comparative ethological models. It is important for those working with young children to have a perspective on the weaknesses in the bonding notion.

35. **Vaughn B, Egeland B, Sroufe LA, Waters E:** Individual differences in infant-mother attachment at twelve and eighteen months: stability and chance in families under stress. *Child Dev* 50:971–975, 1979

This article addresses the critical methodological issue of whether so-called attachment classifications are stable for a given child across assessment periods. Additionally, this is an important article because the study sample is drawn from a different socioeconomic group than those children usually seen in attachment studies.

Parenting

Studying the parents' contribution to the child's development has been the focus of much research concerned with both individual differences in parental style and the modal behaviors between parents and children. The notions of synchrony and reciprocity in early dyadic relationships are important and presumed critical for the child's emerging social and affective development. References contained in this section cover detailed studies of early parent-child interactions as well as reviews of the presumed predictive and critical aspects of such interactions. From the standpoint of the parent, individual differences in parenting styles originate in parental beliefs, parental personality characteristics, the parents' psychological state, and the perceived characteristics of the child. The literature on parental depression is one such example of considering the effects of parental factors on the early interactions. Additionally, in much of the developmental literature, *parent* is synonymous with *mother*. However, a small but important literature exists about fathering (e.g., Lamb 1977; Yogman 1982, later). The references contained in this section are also relevant to considerations of early language development as well as to affective development. Finally, much has been written about the infant's predisposition to respond to social cues from parents. Included are references covering the infant's early capacities for imitation and for processing facial properties and cues (e.g., Caron et al. 1973; Haith et al. 1977; Meltzoff and Moore 1983).

36. **Adamson LB, Bakeman R:** Mothers' communicative acts: changes during infancy. *Infant Behavior and Development* 7:467–478, 1984

This is a descriptive study detailing how parents change their communications to their children as the child matures in the first year. The article also presents a useful theoretical overview of early communications between adults and children.

37. *Belsky J: The determinants of parenting: a process model. *Child Dev* 55:83–96, 1984

This is a classic article that outlines how individual differences in parental functioning are determined by interactions among three general domains: psychological resources of the parents, characteristics of the child, and sources of stress and support for the family.

38. **Caron AJ, Caron RF, Caldwell RA, Weiss SJ:** Infant perception of the structural properties of the face. *Developmental Psychology* 9:385–399, 1973

This article is a detailed study of infants' capacity to process facial information.

39. **Clarke-Stewart KA, Hevey CM:** Longitudinal relations in repeated observations of mother-child interaction from 1 to 2½ years. *Developmental Psychology* 17:127–145, 1981

This article addresses the issue of the continuity in interactive style for any given mother-infant dyad between 12 and 30 months.

40. **Dunn J, Kendrick C:** The arrival of a sibling: changes in patterns of interaction between mother and first-born child. *J Child Psychol Psychiatry* 21:119–132, 1980

This article is a detailed study of how interactions between mothers and their young children change with the arrival of a sibling. The study dramatically illustrates how, after the birth of a sibling, the now older child acquires more responsibility for initiating social interactions.

41. *Field T, Healy B, Goldstein S, Perry S, Bendell D, Schanberg S, Zimmerman EA, Kuhn CL:** Infants of depressed mothers show "depressed" behavior even with nondepressed adults. *Child Dev* 59:1569–1579, 1988

This is one of several studies addressing the pathogenic effects of early maternal depression on infants' interest in social interaction. The article is also important for its description of the still-face paradigm, another commonly used procedure in studies of the social development of infants and young children.

42. **Haith MM, Bergman T, Moore M:** Eye contact and face scanning in early infancy. *Science* 198:853–855, 1977

This is a classic study describing how infants scan faces and facial cues.

43. **Lamb ME:** Father-infant and mother-infant interaction in the first year of life. *Child Dev* 48:167–181, 1977 (see also Yogman 1982 below)

This is a descriptive study of the differences in interactive style and play between mothers and fathers with their young children.

44. ***Meltzoff AN, Moore MK:** The origins of imitation in infancy: paradigm, phenomena, and theories, in *Advances in Infancy Research,* Vol. 2. Edited by Lipsitt LP. Norwood, NJ, Ablex, 1983, pp. 266–301

This chapter provides a review of the literature on infants' capacities for imitation and cross-modal information processing.

45. **Yogman MW:** Development of the father-infant relationship, in *Theory and Research in Behavioral Pediatrics.* Edited by Fitzgerald HE, Lester BM, Yogman MW. New York, Plenum, 1982, pp. 221–280

Separation and Loss

Studies of separation and loss are clearly an extension of studies of attachment and the importance of early parenting. The topic is highlighted as a separate section in this bibliography for two reasons. First, mental health clinicians dealing with children will frequently find themselves considering how much weight to give to a prolonged or early separation from an important other in the child's symptomatic presentation. Issues of foster placement, parental divorce, multiple caretakers, and early parental depression are more and more frequently the central concerns for those caring for young children. Second, in a sense, the careful study of children's inner worlds and the recognition of the importance of early caretaking developed out of the classic studies of separation and loss (e.g., the studies of children in orphanages [Provence and Lipton 1962; Spitz 1945, 1946]).

46. ***Bowlby J:** *Attachment and Loss, Vol. 1: Attachment.* New York, Basic Books, 1969

47. ***Bowlby J:** *Attachment and Loss, Vol. 2: Separation.* New York, Basic Books, 1973

Bowlby's work is central to the concepts of attachment outlined earlier; these classic works address Bowlby's notion that attachment to a central figure was critical for the infant's survival.

48. ***Provence S, Lipton RC:** *Infants in Institutions.* New York, International Universities Press, 1962

49. **Rutter M:** Maternal deprivation, 1972–1978: new findings, new concepts, new approaches. *Child Dev* 50:283–305, 1979

    This article is an excellent review of what defines deprivation and how we think about the pathogenic effects of any given separation or loss.

50. *Spitz RA: Hospitalism: an inquiry into the genesis of psychiatric conditions in early childhood. *Psychoanal Study Child* 1:53–74, 1945

51. *Spitz RA, Wolf KM: Anaclitic depression: an inquiry into the genesis of psychiatric conditions in early childhood, II. *Psychoanal Study Child* 2:313–342, 1946

Affective Development

A critical aspect of social development is the interpretation of affective states in others. How young children gain the ability to distinguish differing affective states, to attribute individual as well as general meaning to such states, and to gauge their own responses based on the affects of others is an important conceptual area.

52. **Barrett K, Campos JJ:** Perspectives on emotional development, II: a functionalist approach to emotions, in *Handbook of Infant Development,* 2nd Edition. Edited by Osofsky JD. New York, Wiley, 1987, pp. 555–578

    This chapter provides an excellent review of early theories of affect recognition and expression as well as of what roles affects play in early development.

53. *Campos JJ, Stenberg C: Perception appraisal, and emotions: the onset of social referencing, in *Infant Social Cognition: Empirical and Theoretical Considerations.* Edited by Lamb ME, Sherrod LR. Hillsdale, NJ, Lawrence Erlbaum, 1981, pp. 273–314

    This chapter and the article by Hornik et al. (1987 below) address a by-now classic response of early childhood: social referencing. When faced with a novel, ambiguous, or frightening situation, young children look to their parents' affective responses for clues to their own responses. The notion of social referencing has been extended both conceptually and by analogy to a number of situations, including psychotherapy with young children as well as parents' role in facilitating children's exploration of novel material, situations, and persons.

54. **Campos JJ, Campos RG, Barrett KC:** Emergent themes in the study of emotional development and emotional regulation. *Developmental Psychology* 25:394–402, 1989

This review presents the reconceptualization of affects as not just indices of feeling states but also as processes for regulating the interaction between the child and the environment. The authors also address the issue of stability of emotional expressiveness.

55. **Caron AJ, Caron RF, MacLean DJ:** Infant discrimination of naturalistic emotional expressions: the role of face and voice. *Child Dev* 59:604–616, 1988

This article addresses the question of how early can infants reliably distinguish among different affective expressions and which cues (voices or facial expressions) are most salient.

56. *Harris P: *Children and Emotion.* Oxford, United Kingdom, Basil Blackwell, 1989

This book provides a comprehensive review of emotional development with a particular emphasis on how children come to understand the emotions of others.

57. **Hornik R, Risenhoover N, Gunnar M:** The effects of maternal positive, neutral, and negative affective communication on infant responses to new toys. *Child Dev* 58:937–944, 1987

58. **Izard CE, Malatesta CZ:** Perspectives on emotional development, I: differential emotions theory of emotional development, in *Handbook of Infant Development,* 2nd Edition. Edited by Osofsky JD. New York, Wiley, 1987, pp. 494–554

Izard and Malatesta have done considerable work on the detailed measurement of different affective expressions in early childhood.

59. **Malatesta CZ, Haviland JM:** Learning the display rules: the socialization of emotion expression in infancy. *Child Dev* 53:991–1003, 1982

This is a classic article addressing how children's use of affective expression adapts to fit the demands of their own family and are in part gender as well as culturally determined.

60. **Nelson CA:** The recognition of facial expressions in the first two years of life: mechanisms of development. *Child Dev* 58:889–909, 1987

This article returns to the question of how well do infants discriminate among different affective expressions. The article is an excellent example of a carefully done study in this area.

Self-Other Differentiation

How children develop the capacity to distinguish between themselves and others is an absolutely fundamental notion that cuts across several areas of child development research. Although a few studies have addressed the issue empirically (e.g., Lewis et al. 1989), most considerations of self-other development are psychoanalytically based. Readers are also referred to appropriate sections in the general references cited earlier.

61. **Lewis M, Sullivan MW, Stanger C, Weiss M:** Self development and self-conscious emotions. *Child Dev* 60:146–156, 1989

    This article provides an empirical approach to notions of self-recognition. It is also an excellent review of traditional methods for approaching the question of self-other differentiation.

62. ***Mahler MS, Pine F, Bergman A:** *The Psychological Birth of the Human Infant.* New York, Basic Books, 1975

    This is a major reference for understanding preverbal development of a concept of self. From Mahler's work comes the concepts of separation-individuation and rapprochement.

63. **Stern DN:** *The Interpersonal World of the Human Infant.* New York, Basic Books, 1985

    Stern presents a theoretical view of the stages of self-development. The book is particularly valuable for its review of the theories and empirical work behind the concept of self-other differentiation.

64. ***Winnicott DW:** Transitional objects and transitional phenomena: a study of the first not-me possession. *Int J Psychoanal* 34:89–97, 1953

    This is a classic, much-read article that addresses how internal objects are created in such a way as to facilitate the child's ability to be separate from others. The notion of transitional phenomena and objects pervades many clinical discussions of early development, and it is important that trainees gain a working understanding of what the concept does and does not apply to.

Language Development

The development of a capacity for verbal language is a significant milestone in the child's maturation. Verbal communication affords children broader opportunities for representing experiences and needs and simultaneously fosters further individuation and a different level of intimacy and togetherness with important others. Diagnostically, impairments or delays in language development are significant markers for a number of disorders and developmental disturbances (see section on psychopathology below).

General Reviews

Both Bruner (1983) and Nelson (1979) address the conceptual centrality of early language development for social development, the emerging capacity for symbolization, and the relationship between language and other developmental domains.

65. *Bruner JS: *Child's Talk: Learning to Use Language.* New York, WW Norton, 1983

66. Nelson K: The role of language in infant development, in *Psychological Development From Infancy: Image to Imitation.* Edited by Bornstein MH, Kessen W. Hillsdale, NJ, Lawrence Erlbaum, 1979, pp. 307–337

Preverbal Contributions to Language

How early social interactions contribute to language development and what constitutes the earliest forms of communication are outlined by the references in this section. Rheingold and Adams (1980) provide a detailed description of adults' speech to newborns. The differences in parental speech with young children is described by Papousek et al. (1985). Leung and Rheingold (1981) emphasize the importance of early pointing as a communicative act and a request for social interaction that necessarily precedes verbal interaction. Myers and Tronick (1985) underscore the importance of early turn-taking as the forerunner of verbal conversation.

67. **Leung E, Rheingold H:** Development of pointing as a social gesture. *Developmental Psychology* 17:215–220, 1981

68. **Myers NK, Tronick EZ:** Mothers' turn-giving signals and infant turn-taking in mother-infant interaction, in *Social Perception in Infants.* Edited by Field TM, Fox NA. Norwood, NJ, Ablex, 1985, pp. 199–216

69. **Papousek M, Papousek H, Bornstein MH:** The naturalistic vocal environment of young infants: on the significance of homogeneity and variability in parental speech, in *Social Perception in Infants.* Edited by Field TM, Fox NA. Norwood, NJ, Ablex, 1985, pp. 269–297

70. **Rheingold HL, Adams JL:** The significance of speech to newborns. *Developmental Psychology* 16:397–403, 1980

Emergence of Symbolic Play

Language development and the capacity for imaginative or symbolic play reflect the child's emerging capacity for mental representation. Language development and the capacity for symbolic play are closely related. With language, toddlers are beginning to say and to understand sound sequences that function as true naming as they shift from the contextually bound use of words to a more flexible use across contexts. The emergence of more flexible and generalizable language skills adds to the toddler's capacity for symbolic play. Whereas play in the first year of life is largely exploratory or nonsymbolic, play in the second year and afterward involves the capacity for substituting function (e.g., using a cup to stand for something other than a cup) and for pretend. The progression from nonsymbolic to symbolic play is not only a gradual one, but there are also marked individual differences in the amount of symbolic play shown by children. Besides serving as a marker of the child's capacity for symbolization, play is a reflection of a differentiated inner world of fantasy. Finally, included in this section are references to discussions of a child's emerging theory of mind, or the child's understanding that mental states such a beliefs, thoughts, or feelings, although not directly perceivable, nevertheless guide the actions of self and of others.

71. [*]**Astington JW, Harris PL, Olson DR:** *Developing Theories of Mind.* Cambridge, MA, Cambridge University Press, 1988

    Theory of mind is included under discussions of play because of the relationship with capacities for symbolization and representation.

72. **Belsky J, Most RK:** From exploration to play: a cross-sectional study of infant free play behavior. *Developmental Psychology* 17:630–639, 1981

    This article is a study of the developmental progression from simple exploration to symbolic play in a group of children followed longitudinally.

73. [*]**Fein G:** Pretend play: an integrative review. *Child Dev* 52:1095–1118, 1981

    This is a review of the social, cognitive, and linguistic competencies involved in the child's act of pretense.

74. **Tamis-LeMonda CS, Bornstein MH:** Habituation and maternal encouragement of attention in infancy as predictors of toddler, language, play and representational competence. *Child Dev* 60:738–751, 1989

This article discusses the relationship between early maternal activities such as naming objects and the child's later symbolic capacities.

75. **Ungerer JA, Zelazo P, Kearsley K, O'Leary K:** Developmental changes in the representation of objects of symbolic play from 18 to 34 months. *Child Dev* 52:186–195, 1981

   This article presents a study and a discussion of the child's emerging capacity to use objects in ways not related to the actual function and, vice versa, to represent in play functions not usually served in reality by the object. The article provides a format for discussing the child's developing capacity for metarepresentation.

Neuroperceptual and Cognitive Development

In the last three decades, the neuroperceptual capacities of infants and young children have been more clearly defined. The references in this section discuss the theories of information processing in early childhood, early neuroperceptual and neurocognitive development, and predicting later capacities from early performance.

General Reviews

76. **Aslin RN:** Visual and auditory development in infancy, in *Handbook of Infancy,* 2nd Edition. Edited by Osofsky JD. New York, Wiley, 1987, pp. 5–97

   This chapter provides a comprehensive review of both the methods for studying and the resulting evidence for staging visual and auditory capacities in early infancy.

77. **Harris PL:** Infant cognition, in *Handbook of Child Psychology, Vol. 2: Infancy and Developmental Psychobiology.* Edited by Haith MM, Campos JJ. New York, Wiley, 1983, pp. 689–782

   This chapter provides a detailed review of what the concept of "cognition" means for infants and what are the various theoretical approaches to studying cognitive processes in the preverbal years. This reference is also relevant to the subsequent section.

Information Processing and Memory in Infancy and Early Childhood

The references in this section address several key processes and issues in the study of early cognitive development. First is habituation, as represented in the works by Bornstein (1985) and Fantz (1964). Habituation is the process of declining attention on repeated presentation or exposure to novel information. The habituation response provides children (and adults) with a mechanism for sorting through familiar and novel information and as such has adaptive as well as cognitive significance. As noted in the next section on prediction, there is a relation between early habituation performance and later cognitive capacities (see Bornstein 1989 review). The second process addressed in this section is that of cross-modal information processing— that is, taking information from one sensory domain and associating it with information from a different domain, such as relating the sound of a person's voice to the correct facial image. Intermodal information processing is critical for early social development and is discussed by Bahrick (1988). Finally, the developmental stage when infants and young children evidence the capacity to remember persons and situations is a critical notion for studies of early development. Investigators such as Fagen and Ohr (1990) and Rovee-Collier (1987) address the evidence for emerging memory capacities in early childhood.

78. **Bahrick LE:** Intermodal learning in infancy: learning on the basis of two kinds of invariant relations in audible and visible events. *Child Dev* 59:197–209, 1988

79. **Bornstein MH:** Habituation of attention as a measure of visual information processing in human infants: summary, systematization, and synthesis, in *Measurement of Audition and Vision in the First Year of Postnatal Life: A Methodological Overview.* Edited by Gottlieb G, Krasnegor NA. Norwood, NJ, Ablex, 1985, pp. 147–170

80. ***Bornstein MH:** Stability in early mental development: from attention and information processing in infancy to language and cognition in childhood, in *Stability and Continuity in Mental Development: Behavioral and Biological Perspectives.* Edited by Bornstein MH, Krasnegor NA. Hillsdale, NJ, Lawrence Erlbaum, 1989, pp. 147–170

81. **Fagen JW, Ohr PS:** Individual differences in infant conditioning and memory, in *Advances in Infancy Research,* Vol. 2. Edited by Lipsitt LP. Norwood, NJ, Ablex, 1990, pp. 31–78

82. **Fantz RL:** Visual experience in infants: decreased attention to familiar patterns relative to novel ones. *Science* 146:668–670, 1964

83. *Olson GM, Sherman T:** Attention, learning, and memory in infants, in *Handbook of Child Psychology, Vol. 2: Infancy and Developmental Psychobiology.* Edited by Haith MM, Campos JJ. New York, Wiley, 1983, pp. 1001–1080

This is an excellent review of the guiding theories about the relationship between attentional processes and learning and memory in early childhood.

84. **Rose SA:** Measuring infant intelligence: new perspectives, in *Stability and Continuity in Mental Development: Behavioral and Biological Perspectives.* Edited by Bornstein MH, Krasnegor NA. Hillsdale, NJ, Lawrence Erlbaum, 1989, pp. 171–188

This chapter provides a discussion about what measuring cognitive capacities in early childhood implies.

85. **Rovee-Collier CK:** Learning and memory in infancy, in *Handbook of Infant Development,* 2nd Edition. Edited by Osofsky JD. New York, Wiley, 1987, pp. 98–148

Predicting Later Function From Infancy

In a sense, implicit in every section thus far is the notion of prediction. Attachment studies implicitly seek to predict later social adjustment. Early temperament characteristics are related to later personality. Early separations or losses are related to later psychopathology. This section includes primarily important studies of the prediction of later cognitive capacities (e.g., Bornstein and Sigman 1986; McCall 1989). Also included are discussions of the concepts of change in a developmental framework (e.g., Kagan 1971; Uzgiris 1989). Finally, embedded within any notion of prediction or continuities and discontinuities is the question of what moves development along. Motivation, defined in varying ways, has been a much-debated concept in child development; in one way or another, however, theorists and clinicians return to the concept (e.g., Yarrow and Messer 1983).

86. **Bornstein MH, Sigman MD:** Continuity in mental development from infancy. *Child Dev* 57:251–274, 1986

87. **Kagan J:** *Change and Continuity in Infancy.* New York, Wiley, 1971

88. **McCall RB:** Infancy research: individual differences. *Merrill-Palmer Quarterly* Special Issue, 1989

89. **Uzgiris IC:** Transformations and continuities: intellectual functioning in infancy and beyond, in *Stability and Continuity in Mental Development:*

Behavioral and Biological Perspectives. Edited by Bornstein MH, Krasnegor NA. Hillsdale, NJ, Lawrence Erlbaum, 1989, pp. 123–143

90. **Yarrow LJ, Messer DJ:** Motivation and cognition in infancy, in *Origins of Intelligence: Infancy and Early Childhood.* Edited by Lewis M. New York, Plenum, 1983, pp. 379–399

Environment and Maturation

The interaction between environmental factors and the expression of developmental functions has been an ongoing area of research and theory revision. Important current concepts include sensitive periods of development (i.e., times during which the child is more sensitive to the effects of a given environmental change). For example, very young children are more likely to suffer serious sequelae with primary object loss. Bornstein (1989) provides an in-depth discussion of the concept of sensitive periods. The second concept underscored in this section is genetic-environmental interaction or correlations (e.g., Goldsmith 1988; Plomin 1989; Scarr and McCartney 1983) in which it is posited that individuals guided by their endowments selectively experience and shape their own environments. In this view, it is the genotype both in its individual variability and its species specificity that shapes the effects of environment on development because the genotypic differences guide the individual's response to environmental opportunities. Such active or evocative genetic-environmental correlations occur because individuals seek out settings that fit their predilections and capacities best or because they evoke specific responses from the environments in which they find themselves. It is not just that environments and individuals come together in multideterminant ways, but that certain endowed factors in the individual affect how he or she experiences the world and how the world experiences the individual.

Sensitive Periods and Genetic-Environmental Interaction

91. *Bornstein MH** (ed): *Sensitive Periods in Development: Interdisciplinary Perspectives.* Hillsdale, NJ, Lawrence Erlbaum, 1987

92. **Goldsmith HH:** Human developmental behavioral genetics: mapping the effects of genes and environments. *Annals of Child Development* 5:187–227, 1988

93. **Plomin R:** Environment and genes: determinants of behavior. *Am Psychol* 44:105–111, 1989

94. *Scarr S, McCartney K: How people make their own environments: a theory of genotype-environment effects. *Child Dev* 54:424–435, 1983

Temperament and Individual Differences

The formation of personality has concerned child developmentalists for decades. Almost every area I have reviewed thus far also has something to say implicitly or explicitly about individual differences and the ultimate formation of what we call personality. Embedded in the concept of temperament is the notion that from the very beginning infants show differences in basic regulatory capacities such as sleep-wake cycles, quality of alertness, "engagibility," and capacity for self-soothing. How, or if, these early individual differences are reflected in later personality traits remains a subject of ongoing investigation from multiple perspectives, including psychoanalysis, developmental psychology, and developmental psychopathology.

95. **Bates JE:** The measurement of temperament, in *The Study of Temperament: Changes, Continuities, and Challenges*. Edited by Plomin R, Dunn J. Hillsdale, NJ, Lawrence Erlbaum, 1986, pp. 1–11

Bates, along with several others cited below, has created a useful instrument for assessing early temperament characteristics.

96. **Buss AH, Plomin R:** *Temperament: Early Developing Personality Traits.* Hillsdale, NJ, Lawrence Erlbaum, 1984

Buss and Plomin address the notion of temperament as a reflection of early neuroregulatory capacities (e.g., the regulation of states of arousal).

97. **Dibble ED, Cohen DJ:** Personality development in identical twins: the first decade of life. *Psychoanal Study Child* 36:45–70, 1981

This article is an excellent review of the issue of concordance in personality or temperament traits between monozygotic and dyzygotic twins.

98. *Horowitz FD: Developmental models of individual differences, in *Individual Differences in Infancy: Reliability, Stability, and Prediction*. Edited by Colombo J, Fagen J. Hillsdale, NJ, Lawrence Erlbaum, 1990, pp. 3–18

This chapter is an excellent review of the empirical and theoretical work about early individual differences.

99. **Hubert NC, Wachs TD, Peters-Martin P, Gandour MJ:** The study of early temperament: measurement and conceptual ideas. *Child Dev* 53:571–600, 1982

This article is an excellent review of the measurement issues involved in any study of temperament. The article details the comparative strengths and weaknesses among the various approaches to measuring temperament.

100. **Kagan J, Reznick JS, Gibbons J:** Inhibited and uninhibited types of children. *Child Dev* 60:838–845, 1989

The concept of inhibited and uninhibited children represents the results of much careful study from Kagan's group. The concept cuts across several others—temperament, the regulation of arousal, and modulation of anxiety. Because of its apparent predictive validity as well as the theoretical implications, it is an important concept for professionals working with children to follow.

101. **Rothbart MK, Posner MI:** Temperament and the development of self regulation, in *Neuropsychology of Individual Differences: A Developmental Perspective.* Edited by Hartlange H, Telzrow CG. New York, Plenum, 1986, pp. 93–123

Like Buss and Plomin (1984) above, Rothbart and Posner are concerned with tapping into early neuroregulatory capacities that underlie self-regulation and in turn affect how adults respond to the infant.

102. *Thomas A, Chess S: *Temperament and Development.* New York, Brunner/Mazel, 1977

Thomas and Chess represent the first to make a systematic study of the notion of temperament and the relation of early individual differences to later personality.

Effects of Culture and Context

Context and culture are two large topics that are less often considered when thinking about the individual child. In this section, I include two references that highlight the importance of keeping in mind other contextual variables that influence a child's individual presentation.

103. **Belsky J:** The "effects" of infant daycare reconsidered. *Early Childhood Research Quarterly* 3:235–272, 1988

Belsky addresses the debates surrounding the effect of early day-care experiences.

104. **Bornstein MH:** Approaches to parenting in culture, in *Cultural Approaches to Parenting.* Edited by Bornstein MH. Hillsdale, NJ, Lawrence Erlbaum, 1991, pp. 69–90

Bornstein addresses the broader issue of cultural differences in parenting.

Developmental Psychopathology

General Review

105. *Rutter M:* Developmental Psychiatry. Washington, DC, American Psychiatric Press, 1987

This book provides an extensive review of the presentations of childhood disorders across developmental phases (see also Rutter 1983 above).

Specific Disorders or Impairments

Although this bibliography in its entirety represents a highly selective distillation of possible topics and references, the following section is the most selective. In this section, I have chosen to highlight three disorders: autism and the pervasive developmental disorders, conduct disorders, and depression in childhood. For more in-depth coverage of the large number of specific disorders in childhood, readers are referred to the general child psychiatry references cited earlier. In particular, *Developmental Neuropsychiatry* (Rutter 1983) and *Pathways of Growth: Essentials of Child Psychiatry* (Noshpitz and King 1991; King and Noshpitz 1991) provide excellent, up-to-date reviews for these disorders as well as others (e.g., attention-deficit/hyperactivity disorder).

106. **Fleming JE, Offord DR:** Epidemiology of childhood depressive disorders: a critical review. *J Am Acad Child Adolesc Psychiatry* 29:571–580, 1990

107. **Offer D, Marohn RC, Ostrov E:** *The Psychological World of the Juvenile Delinquent.* New York, Basic Books, 1979

This is an extensive study of a large group of delinquent children. The investigators describe four distinctly different groups of conduct-disordered behavior.

108. **Rutter M, Schopler E:** Autism and pervasive developmental disorders: concepts and diagnostic issues. *J Autism Dev Dis* 17:159–186, 1987

109. **Volkmar FR, Cohen DJ:** Classification and diagnosis of childhood autism, in *Diagnosis and Assessment in Autism.* Edited by Schopler E, Mesibov G. New York, Plenum, 1988, pp. 71–89

Psychotherapeutic Interventions

The citations in this section address the issue of psychotherapeutic interventions as broadly defined with young children.

110. **Green WH:** *Child and Adolescent Clinical Psychopharmacology.* Baltimore, MD, Williams & Wilkins, 1991

Although the literature on psychopharmacology with children is a rapidly changing field, this recent text contains an extensive and useful bibliography.

111. **Lewis M:** Intensive individual psychodynamic psychotherapy: the therapeutic relationship and the technique of interpretation, in *Child and Adolescent Psychiatry.* Edited by Lewis M. Baltimore, MD, Williams & Wilkins, 1991, pp. 796–805

Lewis provides an excellent overview of the conceptual and clinical issues involved in a psychotherapeutic relationship with a school-age child.

112. **Meisels SJ, Shonkoff JP** (eds): *Handbook of Early Childhood Intervention.* New York, Cambridge University Press, 1990

Meisels and Shonkoff review the literature of the effectiveness of a number of early intervention techniques, some of which are educationally based.

113. **Minde KK, Minde R:** Psychiatric intervention in infancy: a review. *Journal of the American Academy of Child Psychiatry* 20:217–238, 1981

Minde and Minde review the technique of therapeutic interventions in early infancy, which necessarily involves working with parents and children together.

53

Adolescent and Young Adult Development

Aaron H. Esman, M.D.

The references in this chapter include both "classical" and more recent contributions to provide a broad survey of critical developmental issues as they have evolved over the century. The list is primarily psychoanalytic in its orientation, because the developmental point of view essential for the understanding of adolescence as a transitional stage in the life cycle has been most thoroughly studied and articulated by psychoanalysts and analytically oriented investigators. It is only recently that others, including psychiatric epidemiologists and biologically oriented psychiatrists, have come to focus on adolescent issues of psychopathology and its developmental implications. Accordingly, other approaches have been included where they seem helpful in illuminating areas of their special concern—especially cognitive and biological development.

Beginning, then, with Freud, the readings move from the work of his students and followers (Aichhorn 1948; Blos 1979; A. Freud 1958) to more "revisionist" views (Erikson 1966; Masterson 1968, 1978; Offer 1991) of normal development. Stress on sexual issues (Chilman 1979; Laufer 1976; Tanner 1971) is balanced by consideration of intergenerational conflicts (Anthony 1969; Blos 1979) and other phase-related and culturally determined concerns (Esman 1990). The papers on psychopathology tend to emphasize contemporary writings to benefit from newer ideas on diagnosis, ego psychology, and object relations theory. Since adolescents are on the front line of social and cultural change, such current issues as drug abuse (Meeks 1988; Wieder and Kaplan 1969), adolescent pregnancy (Group for the Advancement of Psychiatry 1986), cultism (Levine 1992), suicide (Kandel et al. 1991), and revisions of feminine psychology (Dalsimer 1986) are considered, as is the (by now essentially resolved) controversy about the "normality" of adolescent turmoil (Offer and Offer 1975). The works by Piaget (1969) and Overton et al. (1991) emphasize the importance of cognitive development as a central maturational factor in shaping adolescent behavior; they also address some current controversies surrounding this issue.

Finally, there is consideration of the recent efforts to conceptualize "youth" as a definable phase, distinct from adolescence on the one hand and adulthood on the other. Here again, social and technological changes are revealed as crucial determinants of our ways of seeing the evolution of personality.

General Considerations

1. **Feinstein SC, et al:** *Adolescent Psychiatry*, Vols. 1+. Chicago, IL, University of Chicago Press, 1971+

   This is an annual collection of papers on all aspects of adolescence.

2. **Caplan G, Lebovici S** (eds): *Adolescence: Psychosocial Perspectives.* New York, Basic Books, 1969

   This book is a collection of papers on various aspects of adolescent development, psychopathology, and therapy. Emphasis is placed on sociocultural issues and their influence on development.

3. **Esman A** (ed): *The Psychology of Adolescence: Essential Readings.* Madison, CT, International Universities Press, 1975

   This book contains a selection of classical and more recent papers on adolescent development and psychopathology, primarily from a psychoanalytic perspective. Historical and cross-cultural studies are also included.

4. **Esman A** (ed): *The Psychiatric Treatment of Adolescents.* Madison, CT, International Universities Press, 1983

   This is a selection of papers on various approaches to therapy for adolescent psychiatric disorders.

5. **Greenspan SI, Pollock GH** (eds): *The Course of Life, Vol. 4: Adolescence.* Madison, CT, International Universities Press, 1991

This book is a collection of original papers by major figures in child and adolescent psychiatry presenting current psychoanalytic views of normal and pathological personality formation.

6. **Kaplan L:** *Adolescence: Farewell to Childhood.* New York, Simon & Schuster, 1984

Kaplan provides a richly poetic but scientifically sound study of the history of adolescence and current views of its psychology and psychopathology.

Normal Development: Physical and Sexual

7. **Chilman C:** *Adolescent Sexuality in a Changing American Society: Social and Psychological Perspectives.* Washington, DC, Department of Health, Education, and Welfare, 1979

A thoroughgoing survey of current patterns of adolescent sexuality, based on a systematic review of basic and recent research, this book includes an annotated bibliography, suggestions for further research, and implications for social policy.

8. **Dalsimer K:** *Female Adolescence: Psychoanalytic Reflections on Works of Literature.* New Haven, CT, Yale University Press, 1986

Dalsimer provides a modern view of female adolescent development as it emerges from the critical study of a number of youthful protagonists.

9. *****Freud S:** The transformations of puberty (1905), in *The Standard Edition of the Complete Psychological Works of Sigmund Freud,* Vol. 7. Translated and edited by Strachey J. London, Hogarth Press, 1953, pp. 207–230

Freud discusses here his basic ideas about the primacy of genital sexuality, patterns of object choice, and the psychological differences between the sexes as they are consolidated during and after puberty.

10. **Laufer M:** The central masturbation fantasy, the final sexual organization, and adolescence. *Psychoanal Study Child* 31:297–316, 1976

Laufer regards the "central masturbation fantasy," conscious or unconscious, as the paradigm for personality organization, which is consolidated in adolescence.

11. *Tanner JM:** Sequence, tempo and individual variation in the growth and development of boys and girls aged 12 to 16. *Daedalus* 100:907–930, 1971; also in *New Directions in Childhood Psychopathology, Vol. 1: Developmental Considerations.* Edited by Harrison S, McDermott J. New York, International Universities Press, 1980, pp. 182–205

An illustrated review of the normal variations in pubertal development, with some reflections on the psychosocial consequences of deviations from the norm, this is an essential reference for the assessment of biological development and its emotional impact.

Normal Development: Cognitive and Psychosocial

12. **Anthony EJ:** The reactions of adults to adolescents and their behavior, in *Adolescence: Psychosocial Perspectives.* Edited by Kaplan G, Lebovici S. New York, Basic Books, 1969, pp. 54–78; also in *The Psychology of Adolescence.* Edited by Esman A. New York, International Universities Press, 1975, pp. 467–493

Anthony considers some of the factors that generate adult antagonism to adolescents. He demonstrates how adults stereotype adolescents to defend themselves against incompletely resolved impulses and conflicts.

13. **Anthony EJ:** Normal adolescent development from a cognitive viewpoint. *Journal of the American Academy of Child Psychiatry* 21:318–327, 1982

This article imaginatively integrates Piagetian with other approaches to cognitive development and demonstrates its central contribution to normal adolescent psychology.

14. *Blos P:** The second individuation process of adolescence. *Psychoanal Study Child* 22:162–186, 1967

Blos considers the phenomenon of disengagement from the parents during the adolescent process, analogizing it to Mahler's "separation-individuation" process in the young child. He emphasizes what he sees as the central role of regression in promoting normal adolescence.

15. **Blos P:** *The Adolescent Passage: Developmental Issues.* New York, International Universities Press, 1979

This book is a collection of Blos' major papers on adolescent psychological development. It includes some articles that propose revisions of classical psychoanalytic ideas on the basis of newer clinical and sociocultural findings.

16. **Brockman D** (ed): *Late Adolescence: Psychoanalytic Studies.* Madison, CT, International Universities Press, 1984

This is a collection of papers on various clinical and theoretical aspects of the 18- to 25-year period, including some excellent studies of learning problems in college students.

17. *Erikson E: The problem of ego identity. *J Am Psychoanal Assoc* 14:56–121, 1966

In this article, Erikson formulates his now-familiar concept of identity formation as the normative developmental crisis of adolescence, placing it in his epigenetic sequence. He further presents a number of pathological variants of the syndrome he calls identity diffusion.

18. *Freud A: Adolescence. *Psychoanal Study Child* 13:255–278, 1958; also in *The Psychology of Adolescence: Essential Readings.* Edited by Esman A. New York, International Universities Press, 1975, pp. 122–140

This is the classical statement of the psychoanalytic view of the ubiquity—even the necessity—of "adolescent turmoil" for normal development.

19. **Kaplan EH:** Adolescents, age fifteen to eighteen: a psychoanalytic developmental view, in *The Course of Life,* Vol. 4. Edited by Greenspan S, Pollock G. Madison, CT, International Universities Press, 1991, pp. 201–234

A comprehensive scholarly survey of midadolescent development within a modern psychoanalytic framework, this chapter incorporates cognitive, biological, and psychosocial perspectives. The "extensive intrapsychic reorganization" of this subphase is detailed.

20. *Lewis M: The phase of young adulthood, age eighteen-twenty-three years, in *The Course of Life,* Vol. 4. Edited by Greenspan S, Pollock G. Madison, CT, International Universities Press, 1991, pp. 493–498

This is a concise survey of the developmental issues in the transition between late adolescent and mature adult status.

21. *Offer D: Adolescent development: a normative perspective, in *The Course of Life,* Vol. 4. Edited by Greenspan S, Pollock G. Madison, CT, International Universities Press, 1991, pp. 181–200

This is a report of Offer's longitudinal study of adolescent development in "normal" populations, which effectively challenges the classical concept of normative "adolescent turmoil." It describes three modes of passage through this process, only one of which can be considered to show significant signs of turmoil.

22. *__Offer D, Offer J:__ *From Teenage to Young Manhood: A Psychological Study.* New York, Basic Books, 1975

   This work continues Offer and Offer's normative study of adolescent males into their young adult years, demonstrating the paths of personality consolidation and adaptive progress of the three groups defined in the earlier work.

23. __Overton W, Sterdl J, Rosenstein D, Horowitz H:__ Formal operations as regulatory context in adolescence. *Adolesc Psychiatry* 18:502–514, 1991

   This is a careful study of the effect of the acquisition of formal operational thought on adolescent mental function and self-regulation.

24. *__Piaget J:__ Intellectual development of the adolescent, in *Adolescence: Psychosocial Perspectives.* Edited by Kaplan G, Lebovici S. New York, Basic Books, 1969, pp. 22–26; also in *The Psychology of Adolescence.* Edited by Esman A. New York, International Universities Press, 1975, pp. 104–108

   This brief chapter presents a succinct statement of Piaget's views on cognitive development in adolescence—specifically the development of formal operational thought. It also raises important questions regarding the universality of this development and its possible effects under varying cultural conditions.

25. __Ritvo S:__ Late adolescence: developmental and clinical considerations. *Psychoanal Study Child* 26:241–263, 1971

   This article details the psychoanalytic view of the transformations of late-adolescent males in terms of object relations, ego ideal formation, psychopathology, and consequent treatment implications.

26. __Wallerstein J:__ The long-term effects of divorce on children: a review. *J Am Acad Child Adolesc Psychiatry* 30:349–360, 1991

   This article is a comprehensive critical review of research in the area of divorce and children, demonstrating the adverse effects of divorce on adolescent and young adult development.

27. __Weissman S, Barglow P:__ Recent contributions to the theory of female adolescent psychological development. *Adolesc Psychiatry* 8:214–230, 1980

   In this comprehensive review of classical and more recent ideas about the psychological development of female adolescents, emphasis is placed on contemporary research on aspects of the adolescent's cerebral and cortical functioning and its implications.

Psychopathology

28. *Aichhorn A: *Wayward Youth.* New York, Viking Press, 1948

This pioneering discussion of the psychopathology and psychoanalytic treatment of delinquency was originally published in 1917, and it continues to form the basis for much of the current work in this field. It provides impressive examples of virtuoso interview technique.

29. *Anthony EJ: Two contrasting types of adolescent depression and their treatment. *J Am Psychoanal Assoc* 18:841–859, 1970; also in *The Psychology of Adolescence.* Edited by Esman A. New York, International Universities Press, 1975, pp. 285–300

The distinction is made between a more phase-appropriate Oedipal "neurotic" type of depression and a more pervasive pre-Oedipally based depression, which may show a cyclical pattern.

30. **Bruch H:** *The Golden Cage: The Enigma of Anorexia Nervosa.* Cambridge, MA, Harvard University Press, 1978

In a concise presentation of her views on the syndrome of anorexia nervosa, derived from a lifetime of clinical study, Bruch emphasizes the ego-psychological and family relations aspects of the disorder.

31. **Cohen J:** Learning disabilities and adolescence: developmental considerations. *Adolesc Psychiatry* 12:177–196, 1985

Cohen delineates the ways in which learning disabilities adversely affect both cognitive and emotional development in adolescents, emphasizing their corrosive effects on self-esteem and the sense of identity.

32. **Esman A:** Borderline personality disorders in adolescence: current concepts. *Adolesc Psychiatry* 16:319–336, 1989

This article is a review of the literature on borderline personality disorders in adolescence, a controversial topic.

33. *Esman A: Mid-adolescence: foundations for later psychopathology, in *The Course of Life,* Vol. 4. Edited by Greenspan S, Pollock G. Madison, CT, International Universities Press, 1991, pp. 283–300

The author delineates a group of psychopathological reactions of older adolescents and young adults and demonstrates their roots in specific aspects of midadolescent development and/or failure to resolve earlier conflicts during this subphase.

34. *Feinstein SC, Miller D: Psychoses of adolescence, in *Basic Handbook of Child Psychiatry*, Vol. 2. Edited by Noshpitz J. New York, Basic Books, 1979, pp. 708–722

The authors review the phenomenology, dynamics, phase-specific characteristics, and treatment of psychotic disorders in adolescence.

35. **Group for the Advancement of Psychiatry:** *Crisis of Adolescence, Teenage Pregnancy and its Impact on Adolescent Development (Report No. 118).* New York, Brunner/Mazel, 1986

This book is a thorough review of teenage pregnancy, a major social problem.

36. **Holzman PS, Grinker RR Sr:** Schizophrenia in adolescence. *Adolesc Psychiatry* 5:276–292, 1977

Holzman provides a comprehensive view of schizophrenia and schizophrenia-like psychoses in adolescence, emphasizing the impact of maturational and social stresses on a biologically vulnerable organism.

37. **Kandel D, Raveis V, Davies M:** Suicidal ideation in adolescence: depression, substance use and other risk factors. *Journal of Youth and Adolescence* 20:289–309, 1991

This article is a thorough-going epidemiological study of suicidal thinking in adolescents and its correlation with some of the other major public health issues affecting adolescent development.

38. **Kernberg P:** Psychoanalytic profile of the borderline adolescent. *Adolesc Psychiatry* 7:234–256, 1979

This article is a systematic, developmentally based description of the borderline syndrome in adolescence and its differential diagnosis.

39. **Levine S:** Cults revisited: corporate and quasi-therapeutic cooptation. *Adolesc Psychiatry* 18:63–73, 1992

Levine provides a concise overview of the cult phenomenon and its more recent evolution.

40. *Masterson JF: The psychiatric significance of adolescent turmoil. *Am J Psychiatry* 124:1549–1554, 1968

This was one of the first articles to challenge the classical psychoanalytic view of the normality of "adolescent turmoil."

41. **Masterson JF:** The borderline adolescent: an object relations view. *Adolesc Psychiatry* 6:294–359, 1978

In this distilled statement of Masterson's ideas about the borderline syndrome in adolescence within the context of separation-individuation theory and the English school of object relations theory, special emphasis is placed on anorexia nervosa and its relationship to the borderline syndrome.

42. **Meeks J:** Adolescent chemical dependency. *Adolesc Psychiatry* 15:509–521, 1988

Meeks reviews the developmental, social, and clinical aspects of drug abuse in adolescence and describes a treatment approach that involves both short- and long-term psychodynamic components.

43. **Pfeffer CR:** Suicide, in *Recent Developments in Adolescent Psychiatry.* Edited by Hsu LKG, Hersen M. New York, Wiley, 1989, pp. 115–134

This chapter is a statement of current clinical and research views on suicide, a major public health problem.

44. **Strober M, Yager J:** Developmental perspectives on the treatment of anorexia nervosa in adolescents, in *Handbook of Psychotherapy for Anorexia Nervosa and Bulimia.* Edited by Garner D, Garfinkel P. New York, Guilford, 1985, pp. 363–390

This is a concise review of developmental issues that underlie eating disorders and a thorough depiction with case illustrations of a comprehensive treatment program based on these considerations.

45. **Strober M, McCracken S, Hanna G:** Affective disorders, in *Recent Developments in Adolescent Psychiatry.* Edited by Hsu LKG, Hersen M. New York, Wiley, 1989, pp. 201–232

The authors detail recent research on mood disturbances, including bipolar disorders in adolescence.

46. *Wieder H, Kaplan EH:** Drug use in adolescents: psychodynamic meaning and pharmacogenic effect. *Psychoanal Study Child* 24:399–431, 1969; also in *The Psychology of Adolescence.* Edited by Esman A. New York, International Universities Press, 1975, pp. 348–375

Adolescent drug use is not a random matter, but is determined by specific conflictual and developmental considerations. The adolescent's preference for a particular drug is a consequence of the correlation between the adolescent's specific psychological needs and the pharmacological property of the particular drug.

47. **Weiner IB:** *Psychological Disturbances in Adolescence,* 2nd Edition. New York, Wiley, 1992

This is an excellent textbook on adolescent psychopathology and its treatment, with detailed descriptions of clinical syndromes and extensive bibliographies.

Cultural Issues

48. **Arlow JA:** A psychoanalytic study of a religious initiation rite: Bar Mitzvah. *Psychoanal Study Child* 6:353–374, 1951

   This article illuminates the role of rites of passage in their relation to character and symptom formation in puberty and early adolescence. It emphasizes the changing relationship between father and son as the latter begins the process of detachment and individuation.

49. **Esman A:** *Adolescence and Culture.* New York, Columbia University Press, 1990

   This is a concise discussion of the reciprocal relationship of adolescence and society, based on a historical review and an analysis of cultural forces as they affect adolescent behavior and are affected by it.

50. **Muensterberger W:** The adolescent in society, in *Adolescents: Psychoanalytic Approaches to Problems and Therapy.* Edited by Lorand S, Schneer H. New York, Hoeber, 1961, pp. 346–368; also in *The Psychology of Adolescence.* Edited by Esman A. New York, International Universities Press, 1975, pp. 12–31

   Muensterberger, an anthropologist, provides a cross-cultural panorama of adolescent roles in non-Western societies and the rites of passage and other social institutions that promote them.

Adult Development

George E. Vaillant, M.D.

A lthough observations about stages of adult development have been made since ancient times, relatively few clinicians have utilized this perspective in modern psychology or psychiatry. In the early part of the 20th century, child psychiatrists and psychologists demonstrated the usefulness of a developmental framework. Such a framework not only allowed the intertwining strands of psychology, biology, and sociology to be combined, but it also was critical to understanding the psychopathology and the therapy of children. Only recently has this viewpoint been adopted by adult psychologists and psychiatrists to provide greater understanding of both health and illness in the adult years.

Focus on middle age has revealed these decades as a period of active biological and psychological change. As they reach their 40s and 50s, for example, as part of mastery of the tasks of generativity, women may get more in touch with assertiveness and men with capacity for tenderness. The necessity of adaptation to changing biology and to increasing awareness of one's vulnerability to a variety of major illnesses also enters into the complex developmental challenges of the fourth, fifth, and sixth decades. Since no consensus has yet emerged regarding the most important issues, the selected core readings in adult development fall in four rather different categories. First, there are readings rich in theory but without data (e.g., Erikson 1978; Jung 1933; Kegan 1982). Second, there are data-driven prospective studies of adult development that are atheoretical (e.g., Block

1971; Eichorn et al. 1981; Terman and Olden 1959). Third, there are method-driven studies that favor experimental rigor over biographical richness or theory (e.g., Baltes and Baltes 1990; Baltes and Smith 1990; Baltes et al. 1977; Schaie 1981, 1983). Finally, there are encyclopedic reviews that synthesize the theory and/or data of others (e.g., Neugarten 1977, 1980; Stevens-Long 1984; Young et al. 1991) but that lack a unifying point of view. In short, adult biopsychosocial development is a very young field that still needs a Darwin or a Piaget to provide an integrated overview.

Midlife Development: Normal and Abnormal

1. **Baltes PB, Smith J:** Toward a psychology of wisdom and its ontogenesis, in *Wisdom: Its Nature, Origins and Development.* Edited by Sternberg RJ. Cambridge, England, Cambridge University Press, 1990, pp. 87–120

   This is a thoughtful and empirical approach to the argument that increasing "wisdom" is one of the attributes of late midlife development.

2. **Baltes PB, Reese HW, Nesselroade JR:** *Life-Span Developmental Psychology: Introduction to Research Methods.* Monterey, CA, Brooks/Cole, 1977

   This text offers an unusually thorough discussion of life-span developmental psychology from the viewpoint of the "West Virginia" school of which Baltes, Reese, Schaie, and Nesselroade were among the founders. Although this viewpoint is based more on the view of academic psychology than clinical psychiatry, it brings a fresh and methodologically rigorous approach to the field.

3. **Block J (in collaboration with Haan N):** *Lives Through Time.* Berkeley, CA, Bancroft Books, 1971

   This book summarizes the personality changes over time of many of the subjects of the Institute of Human Development at Berkeley, California, from childhood to middle age. It provides the best single summary of the adult development of the children whose early study helped make the reputations of Harold Jones, Jean MacFarlane, and Erik Erikson. It is richer in data than in theory or clinical detail and introduces the reader to the Q-sort technique—a valuable methodology in longitudinal research.

4. **Brim OG, Kagan J** (eds): *Constancy and Change in Human Development.* Cambridge, MA, Harvard University Press, 1980

   Studies presented here reexamine the question of the permanence of early childhood psychological structures as they may affect later developmental events. It is interdisciplinary and contains scholarly considerations of biological, social, and, particularly, cognitive aspects of development. It is not easy reading, but contains interesting approaches to both cognitive and personality development in the midlife period.

5. **Clayton VP, Birren JE:** The development of wisdom across the life span: a re-examination of an ancient topic, in *Life-Span Development and Behavior*, Vol. 3. Edited by Baltes PB, Brimm OG. New York, Academic Press, 1980, pp. 104–135

This chapter is particularly interesting in that it presents its arguments in the form of assumptions that are presented and then challenged. There is an extensive bibliography.

6. **Colarusso CA, Nemiroff RA:** *Adult Development.* New York, Plenum, 1981

This is a well-written book, which opens with a review of the current psychodynamic theories of adult development and presents an integrated developmental diagnostic scheme. It is particularly useful in discussing transformations of narcissism. This work stands out from the majority of collections of essays in that it presents a unifying conceptualization of development.

7. **Colby A, Kohlberg L, Gibbs J, Lieberman MA:** A longitudinal study of moral judgement. *Monogr Soc Res Child Dev* 48:1–124, 1983

This article not only reviews the substance and the methodology underlying Lawrence Kohlberg's influential theory of moral development in adults, but it also, via a 20-year follow-up study, validates the theory prospectively.

8. **Eichorn DH, Clausen JA, Hahn N, Honzik MP, Munsen PH** (eds): *Present and Past in Middle Life.* New York, Academic Press, 1981

This is an anthology of the most important research papers from the Institute of Human Development at Berkeley, California—the longest and most thorough birth-to-maturity study in the world. The papers are data driven, come from many different disciplines, and reflect many different facets of life-span development.

9. *Erikson EH: *Childhood and Society,* 2nd Edition. New York, WW Norton, 1963

Erik Erikson was the first serious investigator to focus popular attention to adult development. Chapter 7, "Eight Ages of Man," remains a basic text of the ego-psychological approach to adult development. Here

Erikson reworks issues stressed by Freud, particularly in the *Three Essays on Sexuality,* and adds, importantly, the stages of young adulthood and middle adulthood, as well as those of the later years.

10. **Erikson EH** (ed): *Adulthood.* New York, WW Norton, 1978

    Chapters in this collection of essays contrast features of adulthood in a variety of cultures, including the United States, Russia, Japan, India, and China, in the search for those features that may be viewed as primarily cultural and those developmental features that appear universal.

11. **Farrell MP, Rosenberg SD:** *Men at Midlife.* Boston, MA, Auburn House, 1981

    This is a thoughtful book on men in midlife that is data driven and that seriously calls into question the idea of a midlife crisis being integral to adult development.

12. **Giele JZ:** *Women in the Middle Years.* New York, Wiley, 1982

    Authored by members of a study group at Brandeis University, Waltham, Massachusetts, this volume includes essays on normal developmental issues for women, including health, work, and marriage. This is a useful resource in the sparsely studied area of the life cycle of adult women.

13. **Goethals GW, Klos DS:** *Experiencing Youth.* Boston, MA, Little, Brown, 1976

    This book provides one of the best in-depth discussions of the development of intimacy in the literature. It is richly illustrated with clinical detail.

14. **Helson R, Moane G:** Personality change in women from college to midlife. *Journal of Personality and Social Behavior* 53:176–186, 1987

    This data-based article offers an introduction to a major prospective longitudinal study of the development of college women.

15. **Jung CG:** *Modern Man in Search of a Soul.* New York, Harcourt, Brace, 1933

    Carl Jung, another important early student of the life cycle, argues that the sense of self undergoes major changes in adulthood and that one can relate clinical phenomena, such as incidence of illnesses, to phases of adulthood. Although largely reflective personal speculation, his ideas remain both provocative and influential.

16. *Kegan R: *The Evolving Self.* Cambridge, MA, Harvard University Press, 1982

    Although lacking empirical data, this book is perhaps the best theoretical scheme of adult psychosocial development extant. Kegan builds on the ideas of Erik Erikson, Lawrence Kohlberg, Jean Piaget, and Jerome Bruner to provide an overarching vista of human development.

17. **Kotre JN:** *Outliving the Self: Generativity and the Interpretation of Lives.* Baltimore, MD, Johns Hopkins University Press, 1984

    This is a valuable addition to the literature on adult development. Kotre provides the most complete discussion of generativity available.

18. **Lamb ME, Sutton-Smith B:** *Sibling Relationships: Their Nature and Significance Across the Life Span.* Hillsdale, NJ, Lawrence Erlbaum, 1982

    This book specifically addresses the issue of sibling influence throughout the life span, and in Chapter 11 presents a review of social and developmental psychologists' studies of sibling relationships as they affect development in the adult years. Of particular interest is the focus on the fate of sibling relationships in adulthood.

19. **Levinson DJ, Darrow CN, Klein EB, Levinson MH, McKee B:** *Seasons of a Man's Life.* New York, Knopf, 1978

    Levinson's group made a cross-sectional study of men from three vocational groups and attempted to identify themes in common, related to adult development. Their views, centering on the importance of transitional periods and their relationship to fixed chronological points, are discussed in a rich theoretical context. Unfortunately, the data about these men's lives are retrospective.

20. *Loevinger J: *Ego Development.* San Francisco, CA, Jossey-Bass, 1976

    This is a well-written summary of the life's work of one of the most acute students of ego function and its development. Based on her Washington University Sentence Completion Test, Loevinger builds on the work of Piaget and Erikson to provide one the most comprehensive and clinically useful views of ego development in existence. The book is also valuable because the majority of her data come from women.

21. **Lowenthal MF, Fiske M, Chiriboga DA:** *Changes and Continuity in Adult Life.* San Francisco, CA, Jossey-Bass, 1990

    This book summarizes the data from a 12-year classic study of adult development. The book combines detailed case studies of men and women combined with quantitative data to trace stability and change as adults negotiate late adolescence, young adulthood, and early and late middle-age.

22. **McCrae RR, Costa PT Jr:** *Emerging Lives, Enduring Dispositions.* Boston, MA, Little, Brown, 1984

This book offers a concise, well-researched challenge to those who believe that adult personality evolves during adult development. The book embodies both the strengths and the weaknesses of "dust bowl" empiricism and of the prospective study of multiple-choice personality inventories.

23. **Nemiroff RA, Colarusso ED** (eds): *New Dimensions in Adult Development.* New York, Basic Books, 1990

This book of essays collected a wide variety of up-to-date viewpoints on adult development. Although there is no overarching theory, the collection offers recent viewpoints by some of the most thoughtful contributors to adult development, including Rangell, Stevens-Long, Gutmann, Cohler, Cath, Lifton, and Nadelson. Nemiroff and Colarusso have written brief integrating essays for each essay.

24. *Neugarten BL: Personality and aging, in *Handbook of the Psychology of Aging.* Edited by Birren JE, Schaie KW. New York, Van Nostrand, 1977, pp. 626–649

This wise literature review chapter remains as much a classic in the field as Erikson's (1963 above) Chapter 7 in *Childhood and Society.* Neugarten achieves a balance between theory and empirical data and between depth psychology and sociology that has not been surpassed in the last 15 years.

25. **Neugarten BL** (ed): *Personality in Middle and Late Life.* New York, Arno Press, 1980

Neugarten's important writings on personality development in the second half of life have contributed to a conceptualization integrating psychoanalytic, cognitive, and social perspectives. This book reports a series of studies carried out using a "normal" population drawn from the subjects of the Kansas City Study of Adult Life. The summary chapter by Neugarten is useful not only as a review of the results of the studies, but as a statement of the problems of social-psychological research related to adult development.

26. **Pollock GH, Greenspan SI** (eds): *The Course of Life, Vol. 5: Early Adulthood.* New York, International Universities Press, 1993; **Pollock GH, Greenspan SI** (eds): *The Course of Life, Vol. 6: Late Adulthood.* New York, International Universities Press, 1993

These two volumes represent an expanded and in some cases rewritten version of an earlier work (*Adulthood and the Aging Process*). The editors have gathered major psychoanalytic thinkers, who consider both normal and pathological conditions in adulthood. Pathological states are related to adult development. Although there is no continuity from one essay to another, the quality of these essays is high, and many reflect a contributor's most recent ideas on adult development.

27. **Schaie KW:** Psychological changes from midlife to early old age: implications for the maintenance of mental health. *Am J Orthopsychiatry* 51:199–218, 1981

    This is an inviting article that integrates biological, cognitive, and personality views in a careful manner. Of particular interest is the final section, which attempts to relate the findings of the adult life cycle theorists to mental health maintenance.

28. **Schaie KW:** *Longitudinal Studies of Adult Psychosocial Development.* New York, Guilford, 1983

    This book offers summaries of methodologically sophisticated studies of adult development by Schaie, Jarvik, Siegler, Thomas, Bray, Costa, and McCrae. These studies and authors provide an intellectual balance to studies by more clinically exciting but more speculative investigators.

29. *Stevens-Long J: *Adult Life.* Palo Alto, CA, Mayfield Publishing, 1984

    Stevens-Long comes as close as any writer other than Neugarten to having an encyclopedic and inclusive point of view toward adult development. Of any text listed in this section, this has the most complete and best indexed bibliography. Although this book has the limitations of a college textbook, it is a good place for any student of adult development to begin.

30. **Terman LM, Olden MH:** *The Gifted Group at Mid-Life.* Stanford, CA, Stanford University Press, 1959

    This book provides an entrée to the longest study of adult development in the world. Terman's study of more than 1,500 gifted children began in 1921 when the children were 10 and included both men and women. Terman's text, however, is richer in serial data than in case studies or in documentation of developmental change.

31. **Troyat H:** *Tolstoy.* Garden City, NY, Doubleday, 1967

    This is a literate psychobiography of Tolstoy. His social and occupational prominence, his own diaries, and the evolution of his creative productivity provide a rich prospective account of adult development. Using these sources creatively, Troyat has managed to describe the inner development of a man from childhood to old age in a way that is unusually valuable and provides a model for harvesting prospective studies of lives.

32. *Vaillant GE: *Adaptation to Life.* Boston, MA, Little, Brown, 1977

Vaillant presents data from a major longitudinal study of the male adult life cycle from an ego-psychological point of view. Drawing on the work of Erikson, Sigmund Freud, Anna Freud, and others, Vaillant reexamined, with a 40-year follow-up, the men of the Grant study (see Vaillant 1993 below). The book is well written and presents an important perspective on adult psychopathology, long-term adult adaptation, "health," and maturity.

33. **Vaillant GE:** *Wisdom of the Ego.* Cambridge, MA, Harvard University Press, 1993

This book focuses on the psychosocial and intrapsychic ego development of three psychosocially contrasting cohorts of adolescents prospectively followed for 50 or more years. These cohorts are the Harvard College students, or the Grant study, the Gluecks' inner-city control subjects for their study of delinquency, and the gifted women studied by Lewis Terman and his successors. The book links both the maturation of defense mechanisms and of creativity to an Eriksonian model of ego development.

34. **Young CH, Savola KL, Phelps E:** *Inventory of Longitudinal Studies in the Social Sciences.* Newbury Park, CA, Sage Publications, 1991

This is an inclusive compendium of almost 200 American longitudinal developmental studies. Carefully documented, it describes the instruments, the methodology, and the study of the demographics rather than the major research results of each of these studies.

Elderly Development: Normal and Abnormal

35. **Baltes PB, Baltes MM** (eds): *Successful Aging.* Cambridge, England, Cambridge University Press, 1990

This book is the summary of a conference sponsored by the European Science Foundation to look at healthy aging from a variety of points of view. Unlike many conference volumes, the final papers were the result of much cross-fertilization, and it provides a fresh view of aging from the point of health rather than from deterioration.

36. **Binstock RH, George LK** (eds): *Handbook of Aging and the Social Sciences,* 3rd Edition. San Diego, CA, Academic Press, 1990

37. *Birren JE, Schaie KW** (eds): *Handbook of the Psychology of Aging,* 3rd Edition. San Diego, CA, Academic Press, 1990

38. **Schneider EL, Rowe JW** (eds): *Handbook of the Biology of Aging,* 3rd Edition. San Diego, CA, Academic Press, 1990

These three volumes are the major resources for technical, comprehensive, up-to-date information about normal aging. Ranging from technical considerations of cellular aging to large social science studies regarding aging populations, they are authored by respected experts who provide detailed and thorough information. These three volumes constitute an encyclopedia.

39. **Busse E, Blazer D** (eds): *Handbook of Geriatric Psychiatry.* New York, Van Nostrand Reinhold, 1980

The title of this volume is deceiving; the first half of the book is largely about developmental processes in the older person. It is broad ranging and eclectic, with a good chapter on the epidemiology of mental illness in late life.

40. **Guttman D:** The cross-cultural perspective: notes toward a comparative psychology of aging, in *Handbook of the Psychology of Aging.* Edited by Birren JE, Schaie KW. New York, Van Nostrand, 1977, pp. 302–326

This is a well-documented, cross-culturally validated review article that supports Guttman's important, but unproved, hypothesis that after age 50, men became more stereotypically feminine, and women more stereotypically masculine.

41. **Jacques E:** Death and the midlife crisis. *Int J Psychoanal* 46:502–514, 1965

Jacques offers theoretical evidence that the *midlife crisis* (his term) is a period in which death and its meanings are critically important and become central in working through the crisis toward a renewed awareness of life and coming to terms with the presence of death.

42. **Karasu TB, Waltzman SA:** Death and dying in the aged, in *Geriatric Psychiatry: A Handbook for Psychiatrists and Primary Care Physicians.* Edited by Bellak L, Karasu TB. New York, Grune & Stratton, 1976, pp. 247–278

An overview of death from social, caretaker, patient, and institutional perspectives, this chapter discusses clinical management for the psychiatrist working with the dying patient and the patient's family. It is useful in its attention to issues for the caretaker in dealing with dying patients.

43. *Kubler-Ross E: *On Death and Dying.* New York, MacMillan, 1969

    Although it lacks a careful scientific base, Kubler-Ross's conceptualization of stages of dealing with death is useful in providing an approach to psychological work with the dying patient and the patient's family. This is a good resource for the psychiatrist working on a consultation-liaison service in general and on an oncology service in particular.

44. **Lieberman MA, Tobin SS:** *The Experience of Old Age.* New York, Basic Books, 1983

    This book provides rich clinical detail of the vicissitudes of stress, coping, and survival in old age. It studies the effects on 639 men and women during the year that they had to change their living arrangements. It provides a fresh view of postretirement aging as a life stage.

45. **Pollock GH:** Mourning and adaptation. *Int J Psychoanal* 42:341–361, 1961

    This article does not specifically address issues of adult development; it is, however, concerned with grieving and focuses on both normal and pathological grieving in relationship to adaptation. It relates psychoanalytic conceptualizations of mourning as a developmental process to those of ethology and social psychology.

46. **Streib GF, Schneider CJ:** *Retirement in American Society.* Ithaca, NY, Cornell University Press, 1971

    Although this book is now dated in terms of its demographic data, it still provides one of the broadest and most synthetic introductions to the process of retirement in our culture.

55

Gender Issues in Human Development Across the Life Cycle

Leah J. Dickstein, M.D.

This annotated bibliography includes references that span the general field of knowledge of the new psychology of gender issues as well as the major psychiatric treatment issues and techniques useful in recognizing and responding to female and male patients with these gender concerns. These materials have enabled psychiatric residents, medical students, and other health professionals to understand basic, broad diagnostic and treatment issues related to gender and the importance of the social, cultural, and political ramifications that must be considered as part of effective patient treatment viewed in the context of society with major unresolved gender issues.

The issues continue to be the basis of increased rigorous scientific research and may give rise to new information in the near and distant future. However, the obligation remains for all currently involved in treating patients and their gender issues to become as informed as possible so that patients, who are often unaware, may be guided in enlightened ways in their personal understanding of the impact gender may have on their personal and work lives and many relationships.

Reference selections extend from definitive scientific research as well as popular literature references; all are useful and applicable. Residents, students, and patients have benefited from them since 1976 here at the University of Louisville.

History and Current Psychology of Women's Developmental Issues

1. **Anderson SR, Hopkins P:** *The Feminine Face of God.* New York, Bantam, 1991

   From interviews with women in North America from varied spiritual choices, the authors reveal unique insights into women's religious understandings, choices, and beliefs. This book is useful for trainees and their patients.

2. **Baruch G, Barnett R, Rivers C:** *Life Prints: New Patterns of Love & Work for Today's Women.* New York, New American Library, 1984

   This is an excellent study of 300 women's lives that can assist trainees in guiding women (and men) patients in making choices that can guarantee nothing firm about happiness and worth except as individual decisions. This is good for a journal club.

3. **Belenky M, Clinchy B, Golderger N, Tarule J:** *Women's Ways of Knowing: The Development of Self, Voice, and Mind.* New York, Basic Books, 1986

   This is an excellent study of women and their use of and comfort with communication. It will enable trainees to understand and help female patients.

4. **Bem SL:** Masculinity and femininity exist only in the mind of the perceiver, in *Masculinity and Femininity: Basic Perspectives.* Edited by Reinisch JM, Rosenblum LA, Sanders SA. New York, Oxford University Press, 1987, pp. 304–311

   This is a succinct summary of how culture and environment impact differently on males and females in important ways and of the need for more discriminating projections of gender into only appropriate situations.

5. **Bernard J:** *Women, Wives, Mothers: Values and Options.* New York, Aldine Publishing, 1975

   This book provides an excellent explanation of poor sex-role socialization of women for the demanding roles of mother and wife—roles our culture has accepted. It includes an important section on adolescence.

6. **Coats PB, Overman SJ:** Childhood play experiences of women in traditional and nontraditional professions. *Sex Roles* 26:261–271, 1992

In this study, women in "nontraditional" professions had more male playmates, participated more in competitive sports, and had different forms of encouragement from their fathers than did women in "traditional" professions.

7. **Dickstein LJ, Symonds A, Braude M, Cohen CM, England MJ:** Women's issues: an integral part of social psychiatry. *The American Journal of Social Psychiatry* 6:99–106, 1986

This is a review article of the broad issues in our culture that affect female and male patients across the life cycle.

8. **Fausto-Sterling A:** *Myths of Gender: Biological Theories About Women and Men,* 2nd Edition. New York, Basic Books, 1985

These discussions of hormones, aggression, and brain differences are very useful in understanding basic gender differences.

9. **Gilligan C:** *In a Different Voice: Psychological Theory and Women's Development.* Cambridge, MA, Harvard University Press, 1982

This is a classic publication that must be read by all residents and can be suggested to many patients as a framework within which they can more readily and constructively understand women's socialization and value choices.

10. **Gilligan C, Ward IV, Taylor JM, Bardige B:** *Mapping the Moral Domain: A Contribution of Women's Thinking to Psychological Theory and Education.* Cambridge, MA, Harvard University Press, 1985

This book presents further research to assist therapists in understanding women's values and behaviors.

11. **Horney K:** *Feminine Psychology.* New York, WW Norton, 1967

This is the first work by the first therapist to accept Sigmund Freud's challenge that women figure out what they want and who they are.

12. **Jacklin CN, Baker LA:** Early gender development, in *Gender Issues in Contemporary Society.* Edited by Oskamp S, Costanzo M. Newbury Park, CA, Sage, 1993

This chapter is an overview of early gender development by the pioneer of describing gender development.

13. **Jardine A, Smith P:** *Men in Feminism.* New York, Methuen, 1987

An innovative collection of theoretical discourses by men about feminist issues, this is good journal club material.

14. **Kirkpatrick M:** *Women's Sexual Development: Explorations of Inner Space.* New York, Plenum, 1980

Kirkpatrick's work is a classic volume of information with which all residents must be familiar.

15. **Kopp C** (ed): *Becoming Female: Perspectives on Development.* New York, Plenum, 1979

Across the life cycle, women's unique developmental stages and experiences are thoughtfully detailed in this book. It includes excellent journal club topics vital to the knowledge base of all psychiatrists, such as female identity, father-daughter relationships, mother-daughter relationships, being a member of a minority group, and girls' play.

16. **Miller JB:** *Toward a New Psychology of Women,* 2nd Edition. Boston, MA, Beacon Press, 1987

One of the classic and most clear explanations of women's sex-role socialization, this volume is basic reading for all residents and most useful for many of their female and male patients.

17. **Sugar M** (ed): *Female Adolescent Development.* New York, Brunner/Mazel, 1979

This is an early collection of papers including research dilemmas regarding adolescent females, female pubertal development, changing body image, female delinquency, and the development of autonomy.

18. **Thorne B:** *Gender Play: Girls and Boys in School.* New Brunswick, NJ, Rutgers University Press, 1993

This book provides a current view of early childhood gender behavior; it is for both residents and patients.

History and Current Psychology of Men's Developmental Issues

19. **Boyd SB:** On listening and speaking: men, masculinity, and Christianity. *The Journal of Men's Studies: A Scholarly Journal About Men and Masculinities* 1:323–346, 1993 (from Harrimen, TN, Men's Studies Press)

This article is sensitive and useful. Religion for men is discussed.

20. **Chodorow NJ:** Being and doing: a cross-cultural examination of the socialization of males and females, in *Feminism and Psychoanalytic Theory.* Edited by Chodorow NJ. New Haven, CT, Yale University Press, 1989, pp. 23–44

The most important sex role socialization issues with lifelong repercussions are that girls are raised to BE and boys are raised to DO.

21. **Fasteau M:** *The Male Machine.* New York, Dell, 1975

An early classic describing stereotypic male behavior with insight, this book is excellent for trainees and their patients.

22. **Fogel GI, Lane FM, Liebert RS** (eds): *The Psychology of Men.* New York, Basic Books, 1986

Fogel et al. provide an excellent and in-depth review of the emerging field of the new psychology of men, from their earliest development to later fears, sexuality and new roles, and gender of their therapists.

23. **Garfinkel P:** *In a Man's World: Father, Son, Brother, Friend and Other Roles Men Play.* New York, New American Library, 1985

Clear explanations of important common issues in therapy with men (e.g., lack of ability to recognize and share vulnerable feelings) are discussed. This book is useful for journal clubs and trainees' patients.

24. **Gerzon M:** *A Choice of Heroes: The Changing Faces of American Manhood,* 2nd Edition. Boston, MA, Houghton Mifflin, 1992

Gerzon provides excellent descriptions of role models men face over a lifetime.

25. **Goldberg H:** The male condition, in *The Hazards of Being Male: Surviving the Myth of Masculine Privilege.* New York, New American Library, 1976, pp. 1–7

This chapter provides a clear foundation for understanding men's stressors consequent to our cultural values.

26. **Goldberg H:** *The New Male: From Macho to Sensitive But Still All Male.* New York, New American Library, 1979

This is a clear portrayal of changing men in the 1970s and beyond. It contains useful journal club material for trainees and their patients.

27. **Levinson D, with Darrow CN, Klein EB, Levinson MH, McKee B:** *The Seasons of a Man's Life.* New York, Ballantine Books, 1978

One of the earlier volumes in the first men's movement of the 1970s, this work is important for all trainees to understand men's development.

28. **Pleck J:** Sex role strain (SRS): an alternative paradigm, in *The Myth of Masculinity*. Cambridge, MA, MIT Press, 1981, pp. 133–135

    This excellent review of the male role since the 1930s enables us to understand men's traditional roles, which can be fraught with problems we continue to deal with in therapy.

29. **Pleck JH:** Husbands' psychological involvement in work and family, in *Working Wives/Working Husbands: New Perspectives on Family*. Edited by Pleck JH. Beverly Hills, CA, Sage, 1985

    This chapter provides important descriptions of men's and women's responsibilities and satisfactions from home and work, which are necessary for therapists to guide and understand many current marital conflicts.

30. **Pleck E, Pleck J** (eds): Men's power with women, other men and society: A Men's Movement Analysis, in *The American Man*. Englewood Cliffs, NJ, Prentice-Hall, 1980, pp. 417–433

    Pleck and Pleck provide an excellent cultural description of the problems of power and gender when inequality of power is the reality.

31. **Sanday PF:** The basis for male dominance, in *Female Power and Male Dominance: On the Origins of Sexual Inequality*. New York, Cambridge University Press, 1981, pp. 163–183

    This chapter is an excellent anthropological review of culture and sex roles.

Therapeutic Issues for Women Across the Life Cycle

32. **Baruch G, Brooks-Gunn J** (eds): *Women in Midlife*. New York, Plenum, 1984

    This is a good source on many topics faced in therapy (e.g., changing commitments, multiple roles, black women's issues). It is good journal club material.

33. **Chodorow NJ:** *Feminism and Psychoanalytic Theory*. New Haven, CT, Yale University Press, 1989

Chodorow, a leading theorist, continues her explanations of women's and men's development—in particular, how men can react to mothering with negative consequent attitudes to women, with an opposite positive reaction by women to women as a result of mothering. This work is very important for its clinical insights.

34. **Goodrich TJ** (ed): *Women and Power: Perspectives for Family Therapy.* New York, WW Norton, 1991

   Goodrich presents different arenas where the issue of women and power becomes a problem at work and at home, with 14 vignettes.

35. **Goulter B, Minninger J:** *The Father-Daughter Dance: Insight, Inspiration and Understanding for Every Woman and Her Father.* New York, Putnam, 1993

   This book provides useful examples of the variety of positive and negative relationships between fathers and daughters.

36. **Horney K:** The problem of feminine masochism, in *Psychoanalysis and Women.* Edited by Miller JB. New York, Penguin, 1973, pp. 21–38

   Masochism clearly continues to be a focus of concern for and about women. This chapter, along with the others in this collection, clarifies confusion about women's development.

37. **Laidlaw T, Malmo C (and associates):** *Healing Voices.* San Francisco, CA, Jossey-Bass, 1990

   This book will be enlightening to all trainees, who should be informed about the newer self-help and behavioral therapies, which can be very effective.

38. **Lerner H:** *Women in Therapy.* New York, Harper & Row, 1989

   This is a comprehensive volume about all the major issues and problems women need to and want to confront. It is good for trainees and their patients.

39. **Lerner H:** *The Dance of Deception.* New York, Harper Collins, 1993

   This is a clear and insightful text about women's communication with themselves. It is good for trainees and their patients.

40. **Morgan KS:** Caucasian lesbians' use of psychotherapy: a matter of attitude? *Psychology of Women Quarterly* 16:127–130, 1992

   A lesbian group had a significantly more positive attitude than the nonlesbian sample toward seeking counseling, regardless of whether they had experienced counseling. This is an important group for all residents to understand.

41. **Nadelson CC, Notman MT:** The impact on psychotherapy of the new psychology of men and women, in *American Psychiatric Press Review of Psychiatry,* Vol. 10. Edited by Tasman A, Goldfinger S. Washington, DC, American Psychiatric Press, 1991, pp. 608–622

    Psychotherapy issues for women and men are clearly delineated.

42. **Notman MT, Nadelson CC:** *The Woman Patient, Vol. 3: Aggression, Adaptations and Psychotherapy.* New York, Plenum, 1982

    This is one of several excellent volumes in which experts describe in detail the major health problems, including mental health, women and their therapists must understand.

43. **Prozan CK:** *Feminist Psychoanalytic Psychotherapy.* Northvale, NJ, Jason Aronson, 1992

    An excellent historical review of leading analysts' work, including feminists, in women's development, this book is useful for all areas of the psychiatric treatment of women. Reading this one volume can enable residents to understand early theory and recent modifications in the service of specific patients' problems.

44. **Symonds A:** Phobias after marriage: women's declaration of dependence. *Am J Psychoanal* 31:144–152, 1971

    A classic example of how adult women unconsciously resolve their ambivalence about their expected roles within marriage based on their mothers' lives and their current successful work roles.

Therapeutic Issues for Men Across the Life Cycle

45. **Biller H, Meredith D:** *Father Power.* Garden City, NY, Anchor Press/ Doubleday, 1975

    This is a useful "how-to" manual for male and female patients to understand the increasingly recognized parental role of fathers.

46. **Dickstein LJ:** Social change and dependency in university men: the white knight complex unresolved. *Journal of College Student Psychotherapy* 1:31–41, 1986

Young men are sex role socialized to deny vulnerable feelings, especially normal dependency and feelings of sadness when rejected. This denial can lead to suicidal behavior.

47. **Osherson S:** *Wrestling With Love: How Men Struggle With Intimacy.* New York, Fawcett Columbine, 1992

    Osherson provides excellent insight into the vulnerable feelings of men.

48. **Solomon K, Levy NB** (eds): *Men in Transition: Theory and Therapy.* New York, Plenum, 1982

    This is a classic volume of all the therapy issues facing men.

49. **Turkel AR:** Reflections on the development of male chauvinism. *Am J Psychoanal* 52:263–272, 1993

    This is a superb theoretical article on male chauvinism.

Violence and Trauma

50. **Adams D:** Stages of anti-sexist awareness and change for men who batter, in *Family Violence: Emerging Issues of a National Crisis.* Edited by Dickstein LJ, Nadelson CC. Washington, DC, American Psychiatric Press, 1989, pp. 61–97

    Adams presents a pioneering program in understanding the male abuser and an appropriate and effective treatment paradigm.

51. **Bart PB, Moran EG** (eds): *Violence Against Women: The Bloody Footprints.* Newbury Park, CA, Sage, 1993

    This is an up-to-date analysis of the continued violence toward women from many cultural areas that impact directly on treatment of women and men across the life cycle.

52. **Dickstein LJ:** Spouse abuse and other domestic violence. *Psychiatr Clin North Am* 11:611–628, 1988

    This article is an in-depth analysis of the broad although often hidden breadth of domestic violence in the United States today.

53. **Herman JL:** *Father-Daughter Incest.* Cambridge, MA, Harvard University Press, 1981

    The is a pioneering volume bringing incest "out of the closet" and describing its painful pervasiveness and repercussions. It is for residents and their patients.

54. **Herman JL:** *Trauma and Recovery: The Aftermath of Violence.* New York, Basic Books, 1992

   This is a new classic by an expert researcher-therapist who has led the field in working effectively with abused women.

55. **Kivel P:** *Men's Work: How to Stop the Violence That Tears Our Lives Apart.* New York, Ballantine Books, 1992

   Kivel presents a superb program that helps men identify their violent behavior and definite ways to end all violence in their lives. It is for residents and their patients.

Other Gender Therapy Issues

56. **Goodrich TJ** (ed): *Women and Power: Perspectives for Family Therapy.* New York, WW Norton, 1991

   This is an excellent discussion of a major gender issue: power.

57. **Thompson C:** Notes on the psychoanalytic significance of the choice of an analyst, in *Female Psychology: An Annotated Psychoanalytic Bibliography.* Edited by Schuker E, Levinson NA. Hillsdale, NJ, Analytic Press, 1991, p. 569

   This is a classic chapter about the selection of a therapist based on sex, a major issue for patients and therapists.

58. **Turkel AR:** Clinical issues for pregnant psychoanalysts. *J Am Acad Psychoanal* 21:117–131, 1993

   Specific issues for patients and pregnant therapists are clearly explained, as are several typical clinical vignettes.

Behavioral Aspects of Gender Issues

59. **Clark JM:** From gay men's lives: toward a more inclusive, ecological vision. *Journal of Men's Studies* 1:347–358, 1993

   This theoretical article articulates solid reasons for a gay-inclusive eco-theological paradigm that should foster clear directions about including issues of gays and lesbians in all psychiatric understanding and treatment.

60. **Greenberg S:** *Right From the Start: A Guide to Non-Sexist Child Rearing.* Boston, MA, Houghton Mifflin, 1978

Greenberg provides useful directions and insights for residents working both with parents who are aware and those who are unaware of the importance of early sex-role socialization.

61. **Pogrebin LC:** *Growing Up Free: Raising Your Child in the 80's.* New York, Bantam Books, 1980

Pogrebin's book is a clear guideline for all involved in helping young children develop healthy sex roles within and outside the home.

62. **Shaevitz M, Shaevitz M:** *Making It Together As a Two Career Couple.* Boston, MA, Houghton Mifflin, 1980

This is an early useful discussion recognizing important gender issues by two therapists involved in family therapy.

63. **Tannen D:** *You Just Don't Understand: Women and Men in Conversation.* New York, Ballantine Books, 1990

Tannen provides popular, carefully developed explanations of the most important gender issue: poor verbal communication. This is a good resource for residents and their patients.

64. **Tannen D:** *Talking From 9 to 5: How Women's and Men's Conversational Styles Affect Who Gets Heard, Who Gets Credit, and What Gets Done at Work.* New York, Morrow, 1994

Where Tannen's previous book, *You Just Don't Understand* (above), is extremely practical for personal conversation, *Talking From 9 to 5* offers superb understanding for residents and patients about major communication problems at work.

56

Socially Disadvantaged and Cross-Cultural Populations

Howard C. Blue, M.D.
Carlos Gonzalez, M.D.
Robin Johnson, M.D.
Ezra E. H. Griffith, M.D.

Psychiatric care of disadvantaged and cross-cultural populations continues to be a pressing area of importance. This is due at least partially to an increasing sociopolitical interest of our society in problems that concern "the underprivileged." Similarly, American psychiatrists have been forced to confront cross-cultural issues raised by the impact of heightened immigration to our shores of Cubans, Haitians, Puerto Ricans, Mexicans, Vietnamese, West Indians, and other groups. In addition, African Americans, Asian Americans, and Native Americans continue to emphasize their need for a type of psychiatric care that is appreciative of and founded on their unique sociocultural context. Similar arguments have been made about the special needs of women, hearing-impaired persons, and others in our society. Thus, the understanding of principles that must inform the psychiatric care of these groups of persons is now a serious and specialized enterprise.

It is not simple to structure core readings in these areas of psychiatry because of the multiplicity of problems and subgroups that exist. For example, there is ample literature that is specific to the needs of Mexican Americans and also to Puerto Ricans. Yet space does not allow the treatment of these groups separately. Neither will these readings address the psychiatric problems of Native Americans or Asian Americans.

Rather, emphasis has been placed on appreciating issues relevant to one or two groups in such a way that a model can be developed for thinking clinically about others. A similar style has been utilized in approaching the psychiatric care of the many unique groups in the "disadvantaged" category.

The readings are grouped into topics that reflect a developmental and longitudinal approach to working with these groups. Attention is drawn first to normal individual and family development of ethnically distinct groups and then to understanding the interaction of ethnicity, culture, and epidemiology. The focus is then turned to a discussion of the factors that inhibit certain groups' access to care before exploring how ethnicity, culture, and other factors complicate assessment and treatment.

Individual Development: Psychosocial Influences and Self-Concept

1. *Garcia Coll CT:** Developmental outcome of minority infants: a process-oriented look into our beginnings. *Child Dev* 61:270–289, 1990

   Garcia Coll reviews the literature on the development of minority infants (from birth to age 3 years) and suggests that development must be understood in the context of a synergism between five factors: cultural beliefs and caregiving practices, health status and health care practices, family structure and characteristics, socioeconomic factors, and biological factors. The author raises several important questions that challenge her readers to examine the extent to which differences in minority infant development are interpreted as deficits instead of as variations requiring understanding, respect, and accommodation.

2. **Spurlock J:** Development of self-concept in Afro-American children. *Hosp Community Psychiatry* 37:66–70, 1986

   Self-concepts of African American children are examined in the context of sociopolitical change. Spurlock challenges the early conclusions that suggested that African American children suffered significant diminutions of their self-esteem (self-concept) as a result of confrontations with societal attitudes that were devaluing and demeaning to African Americans. She counters these early conclusions by underscoring the role that family members and significant people from the child's immediate community play in ameliorating the impact of the broader community's negative attitudes and responses.

3. [*]**Taylor RL:** Psychosocial development among black children and youth: a reexamination. *Am J Orthopsychiatry* 46:4–19, 1976

Taylor highlights the weaknesses in empirical data of early studies about low self-esteem among blacks and squarely addresses factors that mediate the development of positive self-regard among blacks. He accentuates data suggesting that self-regard among blacks is influenced more by how one is treated by one's own family and community than how one is treated by those external to the community. He also refutes assumptions that blacks are passive recipients of self-destructive communications about themselves or that blacks, by virtue of prejudice and discrimination, are more psychologically vulnerable than whites.

Family Development: Ethnicity and Family Patterns

4. [*]**McGoldrick M:** Ethnicity and family therapy: an overview, in *Ethnicity and Family Therapy*. Edited by McGoldrick M, Pearce JK, Giordano J. New York, Guilford, 1982, pp. 3–30

This conceptual overview eloquently addresses how ethnicity influences the family life cycle and therapeutic processes. McGoldrick lays a template for working with ethnoculturally different families that highlights interethnic variations in family patterns and attitudes. A clear agenda is set that challenges clinicians to question their own ethnocentric assumptions and biases and to become open to the cultural variability in family structures and to the relativity of values and belief systems. This overview sets the tone for succeeding chapters, which focus on specific ethnic families. The range of ethnic families covered in the book is extensive (e.g., blacks, Cuban Americans, Puerto Ricans, German Americans, Jews, Irish Americans).

Epidemiology, Medical Research, Ethnicity, and Culture

5. [*]**Burnam MA, Hough RL, Karno M, Escobar JI, Telles CA:** Acculturation and lifetime prevalence of psychiatric disorders among Mexican Americans in Los Angeles. *J Health Soc Behav* 28:89–102, 1987

This is an important examination of the relationship between the level of acculturation and psychopathology. The authors seek to determine if acculturation and prevalence of psychiatric disorders is a function of place of birth (immigrant Mexican Americans versus native-born Mexican Americans) and if variation in acculturation helps predict the prevalence of psychiatric disorders.

6. *Guarnaccia PJ, Good BJ, Kleinman A:* A critical view of epidemiological studies of Puerto Rican mental health. *Am J Psychiatry* 147:1449–1456, 1990

The authors raise concerns about the validity of epidemiological studies on Puerto Rican mental health because they have lacked attention to cultural issues. The article reviews epidemiological studies of Puerto Rican mental health on the mainland United States and in Puerto Rico and argues that many of the findings of epidemiological studies indicating a high prevalence of psychiatric symptoms and disorders in Puerto Ricans can be understood in the context of two popular illness categories: nervios and ataque de nervios. This review challenges future researchers in this area to consider the cultural context of symptom expression and response styles.

7. *Osborne NG, Feit MD:* The use of race in medical research. *JAMA* 267:275–279, 1992

This important article reminds us all to be careful when we use racial classifications in medical research. The authors suggest that often racial classifications are unclear because the concept of race frequently varies with geography. Additionally, definitions of race regularly are a function of social class and nationality. The authors also point out that the reasons for race-linked research are not always openly stated, and bias may therefore dilute the objectivity and integrity of the work.

8. **Williams DH:** The epidemiology of mental illness in Afro-Americans. *Hosp Community Psychiatry* 37:42–49, 1986

Williams explores the literature on the rates of mental illness among African Americans and reports that community-wide studies have found no differences between racial groups that could not be accounted for by socioeconomic variables. He argues, quite convincingly, that epidemiological studies have not had a representative sample of a full spectrum of African American subjects to generate valid findings on the prevalence of specific disorders among African American people.

Factors Influencing Access to Health Care of Blacks and Hispanics

9. *Briones DF, Heller PL, Chalfant HP, Roberts AE, Aguirre-Hauchbaum SF, Farr WF: Socioeconomic status, ethnicity, psychological distress, and readiness to utilize a mental health facility. *Am J Psychiatry* 147:1333–1340, 1990

The authors consider the recurring assumption found in the literature that underutilization of services by the poor generally is taken to symbolize their alienation from mainstream society. Using the Mexican American population of El Paso, Texas, the authors advance a model that shows how a number of variables in combination influence an individual's readiness to seek professional help. They point out how sex, age, and ethnicity impact on one's readiness to utilize professional services, but through the intervening influence of socioeconomic status, stressful life events, and inclusion in a support network.

10. *Council on Ethical and Judicial Affairs: Black-white disparities in health care. *JAMA* 263:2344–2346, 1990

This article demonstrates that there is a differential use between black and white Americans of several medical treatments. Although these differences may be accounted for by the greater access of whites to health care, and by their superior educational status, the authors also suggest that another factor causing the difference may be the way the medical profession practices medicine.

11. **Ginzberg E:** Access to health care for Hispanics. *JAMA* 265:238–241, 1991

This article outlines several factors that are thought to influence the access of Hispanics to the health care system. Among these are the heterogeneity of the Hispanic population, their socioeconomic status, demographic and epidemiologic factors, other neighborhood problems, and the generally low number of Hispanic health professionals.

Diagnostic Assessment, Ethnicity, and Culture

12. **Greene RL:** Ethnicity and MMPI performance: a review. *J Consult Clin Psychol* 55:497–512, 1987

This is a thorough review of ethnicity and the Minnesota Multiphasic Personality Inventory, highlighting the need to consider such important moderator variables as degree of ethnic identity and socioeconomic status in cross-cultural comparisons. The author also stresses the need to find clinical correlates of interethnic differences in performance on this (and any other) inventory.

13. *Littlewood R, Lipsedge M:** The butterfly and the serpent: culture, psychopathology and biomedicine. *Cult Med Psychiatry* 11:289–335, 1987

The authors make an intriguing comparison between the cultural explanations of behavior in "small-scale, non-literate" societies versus the role of "biomedicine" as a cultural agency in larger-scale societies. They discuss the distinct possibility that male-oriented medicine (and psychiatry) has pathologized the reactions to oppression and inequality of women and other underprivileged groups.

14. *Neighbors HW, Jackson JS, Campbell L, Williams D:** The influence of racial factors on psychiatric diagnosis: a review and suggestions for research. *Community Ment Health J* 25:301–311, 1989

In reviewing recent research on the impact of race on psychiatric diagnosis, the authors caution against reliance on the interviewer's judgment alone, but rather suggest the development and use of racially tested diagnostic interviews as a way of reducing the variability of diagnosis.

15. *Westermeyer J:** Clinical considerations in cross-cultural diagnosis. *Hosp Community Psychiatry* 38:160–165, 1987

This article discusses a number of important concerns regarding the potentially confounding effect of ethnocultural difference on psychiatric assessment. The author presents interesting discussions on how elements such as language and the use of interpreters, interviewing style, and degree of self-knowledge of the interviewer impact on the establishment of a diagnosis.

Cross-Cultural Dimensions of Treatment

16. *Comas-Diaz L, Jacobsen FM:** Ethnocultural transference and countertransference in the therapeutic dyad. *Am J Orthopsychiatry* 6:392–402, 1991

This is a thorough review of transference and countertransference, through the use of clinical examples. The authors provide a division of each phenomenon into interethnic and intraethnic components that add to the article's clinical applicability. They suggest that ethnocultural difference may be a catalyst in therapy.

17. [*]**Gorkin M:** Countertransference in cross-cultural psychotherapy: the example of Jewish therapist and Arab patient. *Psychiatry* 49:69–79, 1986

The psychotherapeutic relationship is explored through clinical examples that focus on Jewish therapist–Arab patient dyads. The author stresses the special nature and meaning of countertransference in any cross-cultural treatment setting, as well as on the need to address countertransferential feelings in an active and culturally sensitive fashion.

18. **Javier RA:** The suitability of insight-oriented psychotherapy for the Hispanic poor. *Am J Psychoanal* 50:305–318, 1990

This article explores the role of prejudice in the perception of the poor, particularly the ethnoculturally different poor, as unable to benefit from insight-oriented psychotherapy. It makes special reference to the case of Hispanic Americans, providing one clinical illustration.

19. [*]**Wohl J:** Integration of cultural awareness into psychotherapy. *Am J Psychother* 43:343–355, 1989

The author describes all psychotherapeutic relationships as ultimately "cross-cultural." He advocates for the use of sound clinical judgment and honest curiosity as tools in exploring and using racial and ethnic differences in the therapy.

Psychopharmacologic Treatment, Ethnicity, and Gender

20. [*]**Lin K-M, Poland RE, Smith MW, Strickland TL, Mendoza R:** Pharmacokinetic and other related factors affecting psychotrophic responses in Asians. *Psychopharmacol Bull* 27:427–439, 1991

This article reviews the ethnic variability literature in enzyme polymorphism, such as the rate of acetylation, and the polymorphism of alcohol and aldehyde dehydrogenase. In addition, a review of the ethnic differences in pharmacokinetics of neuroleptics, tricyclic antidepressants, benzodiazepines, and lithium are presented.

21. [*]**Strickland TL, Ranganath V, Lin K-M, Poland RE, Mendoza R, Smith MW:** Psychopharmacologic considerations in the treatment of Black American populations. *Psychopharmacol Bull* 27:441–448, 1991

This is a thorough review of the sparse literature addressing psychotropic response differences in black Americans compared with white

Americans. There have been very few controlled studies; older studies suggest that black patients had 50% higher steady-state nortriptyline plasma levels compared with white patients. A few studies suggest that black patients are treated with substantially higher doses of neuroleptics than white patients.

22. *Wood AJ, Zhou H:** Ethnic differences in drug disposition and responsiveness. *Clin Pharmacokinet* 20:350–373, 1991

This article presents the ethnic differences in drug disposition and responsiveness, including acetylation polymorphism, polymorphism in hydrolysis of alcohol, and discussions of various classes of medications. However, the literature on tricyclic antidepressants and neuroleptic agents is limited. Most of the work in this area has been done with Asian Americans. The few studies with African Americans and Hispanics used a very small number of subjects. The authors suggest that drug licensing authorities should require dosage, efficacy, and toxicity data in different ethnic groups.

23. **Yonkers KA, Kando JC, Cole JO, Blumenthal S:** Gender differences in pharmacokinetics and pharmacodynamics. *Am J Psychiatry* 149:587–595, 1992

This article explores the theoretical potential differences in gender absorption, distribution, and metabolism of psychotropic medication. The literature is limited on this topic, but a review of the available literature is presented.

Issues in Family Therapy

24. *Boyd-Franklin N:** *Black Families in Therapy: A Multisystems Approach.* New York, Guilford, 1989

The author sets the stage first by explicating the cultural context that surrounds black families. Then she articulates major treatment theories and their applicability to black families. She focuses especially on the use of a multisystems approach to treating black families and illustrates the methodology impressively with appropriate case example material.

25. *Boyd-Franklin N, Shenonda NT:** A multisystems approach to the treatment of a Black, inner-city family with a schizophrenic mother. *Am J Orthopsychiatry* 60:186–195, 1990

This is a précis of some important principles encountered in Boyd-Franklin's (1989) book above. It does have the advantage of focusing sharply on how to approach multiproblem black families, particularly those who are underprivileged. However, the article lacks the comprehensive review of the culture that surrounds black families.

26. [*]Inclan J, Hernandez M: Cross-cultural perspectives and co-dependence: the case of poor Hispanics: *Am J Orthopsychiatry* 62:245–255, 1992

The authors argue cogently that economically disadvantaged, chemically dependent Hispanic patients and families are expected to recover from alcoholism in ways that conflict with Hispanic family values. The authors show how the concept of co-dependence is at odds with the Hispanic concept of familism. Consequently, the notion of co-dependence has to be culturally reframed if progress is to be made with Hispanic families.

Factors Complicating Treatment: Violence, Substance Abuse, and AIDS

27. [*]**Cheung YW:** Ethnicity and alcohol/drug use revisited: a framework for future research. *Int J Addict* 25:581–605, 1990–1991

This article provides a thoughtful and critical review of recent studies on chemical dependence and ethnicity. It discusses the difficulties encountered in attempting to define the concept of ethnicity, which is characterized as dynamic and multifaceted, rather than as a single, static variable.

28. [*]**Moore J:** Gangs, drugs, and violence. *NIDA Res Monogr* 103:160–176, 1990

Moore focuses on the contrast between beliefs about youth gangs propagated by the media and law-enforcement agencies and the small body of knowledge developed by research on the connections among said gangs, the sale and abuse of drugs, and the eruption of violence.

29. **Peterson JL, Marin G:** Issues in the prevention of AIDS among Black and Hispanic men. *Am Psychol* 43:871–877, 1988

The authors discuss the disproportionate number of acquired immunodeficiency syndrome (AIDS) cases among Hispanic Americans and African Americans, as well as the limited data available on AIDS risk behavior within each of these groups. They offer concrete suggestions on improving outreach and educational approaches for these underserved populations.

30. *Stark E:** Rethinking homicide: violence, race, and the politics of gender. *Int J Health Serv* 20:3–26, 1990

    This is a comprehensive review, highlighting the significant proportion of homicides that arise out of chronic domestic and other "friendly" violence. The author comments on institutional, racially based neglect of domestic violence and advocates for early and more effective intervention in incidents of "battering" as a means of homicide prevention.

Poverty, Homelessness, and Psychiatric Treatment

31. **Alisky JM, Iczkowski H:** Barriers to housing for deinstitutionalized psychiatric patients. *Hosp Community Psychiatry* 41:93–96, 1990

    A telephone survey was conducted of all managers of "Section 8 Housing" (low income) in St. Louis City and St. Louis County, Missouri: 1) 41.3% of managers surveyed refused to rent to a psychiatric patient, 2) 22% of the managers would refuse to rent to a psychiatric patient in a straightforward manner, and 3) 19% would either deny that a vacancy existed or change the price of the rental unit.

32. *Bachrach LL:** What we know about homelessness among mentally ill persons: an analytical review and commentary. *Hosp Community Psychiatry* 43:453–464, 1992

    The author considers all the basic questions one is likely to pose about the relationship between homelessness and mental illness, such as the question of prevalence, the problem of defining homelessness, and the difficulties that arise from the diversity of the homeless population. Finally, she considers the complexity of treatment planning for this obviously disadvantaged group.

33. **Koyanagi C:** The missed opportunities of Medicaid. *Hosp Community Psychiatry* 41:135–138, 1990

    This article reviews the essentials of the program of Medicaid and outlines the per capita cost, the amount spent annually, and who is covered. It additionally provides a detailed discussion of mental health coverage under Medicaid and activities not currently covered, such as halfway houses, group homes, and adult foster homes.

34. **Weissberg M:** Chained in the emergency department: the new asylum for the poor. *Hosp Community Psychiatry* 42:317–318, 1991

This is a brief review of the history of the treatment of mentally ill persons from 1789 to the present. The article focuses on the significantly decreased services to the mentally ill poor and the increased burden this places on the emergency room.

Gender and Psychiatric Care

35. *Carmen E, Russo NF, Miller JB: Inequality and women's mental health: an overview. *Am J Psychiatry* 138:1319–1330, 1981

This article argues that women's disadvantaged status, sex bias, and sex-role stereotyping contribute to the inferior quality of mental health services that women often receive. However, improvement of this state of affairs requires understanding of the complex processes that lead to the creation of barriers to women's access to appropriate and high-quality services.

36. *Dagg PK: The psychological sequelae of therapeutic abortion—denied and completed. *Am J Psychiatry* 148:578–585, 1991

The author did an extensive review of the abortion literature to ascertain whether women experience psychological distress as a consequence of abortion. The majority of women had positive psychological responses to therapeutic abortions. However, the study did identify three particular situations that seemed to account for an increased amount of distress following abortion: medically necessary abortions, previous psychiatric contact, or second-trimester abortions.

37. *Russo NF: Overview: forging research priorities for women's mental health. *Am Psychol* 45:368–373, 1990

This review of women's mental health research outlines the progress made in five priority areas: diagnosis and treatment of mental disorder, mental health issues for older women, violence against women, multiple roles, and poverty. The author draws special attention to the impact of violence and poverty on the mental health status of women. The author also provides an impressive bibliography on work done in these areas.

VI

Special Topics

57

Community Psychiatry

Kenneth S. Thompson, M.D.
Stephen D. Mullins, M.D., M.P.H.

For the past 50 years, since the term *community psychiatry* came into use, its meaning has been contested. Some, particularly its early advocates, have claimed it as the psychiatric analog of public health. They have seen it as a population-oriented (rather than individually directed) approach to psychiatric disorders that incorporates the principles of social psychiatry and systems theory. This definition has emphasized the psychiatric profession's obligation in a democratic society to be socially conscious in its particular role to focus on the psychiatric problems of disadvantaged and marginalized populations. Within this definition, some have identified a professional responsibility to engage, if necessary, in social activism to change oppressive and noxious social conditions viewed as detrimental to these populations.

Others have taken a less controversial and, perhaps, less ambitious approach. They have defined *community psychiatry* as simply being community-based (noninstitutional) clinical practice. Depending on the views of the particular writer, this definition can encompass varying degrees of emphasis on understanding the sociopolitical context of the patient and on the utilization of such "social" treatments as vocational rehabilitation and group and family therapies.

In recent times, the predominant trend in the profession has been to meld these two general approaches, albeit within a limited framework.

Adherents of this perspective view the primary task of community psychiatry as providing community-based care to a particularly vulnerable "target-population"—persons with chronic mental illness.

This chapter will not attempt to delineate the "true" domain of community psychiatry. Rather, we draw to some degree from all of the above conceptual traditions. We do this with the awareness that there are a number of other chapters in this volume containing writings of critical importance to community psychiatry theory and practice (e.g., Lidz, Chapter 8; Cutler, Chapter 20; Blue et al., Chapter 56). As a result, we have chosen to emphasize some issues not addressed elsewhere. In the process, we hope to demonstrate the diverse approaches and knowledge base of community psychiatry and its practical application in a variety of settings. Most importantly, we wish to highlight the spirit and values of community psychiatry. These are evidenced in its commitment to those with psychiatric disorders who are impoverished and dependent on public support and in its deliberate engagement in critical thought about the social forces that shape the construction of mental illness, society, psychiatric services, and the profession itself. They are further demonstrated by an active, integrated agenda of research-driven service system change and social reform.

Community psychiatry is a challenging field requiring tremendous creativity in its mission to make a difference in the lives of individuals, families, and communities. For psychiatrists, it promises a stimulating and varied practice. As a career, it guarantees the fulfillments and gratifications of shared work and struggle, sometimes on the hard edge of society, caring for those most in need.

Mission

1. **Eisenberg L:** Rudolf Ludwig Karl Virchow, where are you now that we need you? *Am J Med* 77:524–532, 1984

   Virchow, a German pathologist and social activist from the last century, is considered by many to be the father of social medicine. He is famous, among other things, for saying: "Medicine is a social science and politics nothing but medicine on grand scale" (p. 525). Eisenberg, himself an eminent social psychiatrist, holds Virchow up as an exemplar of the medical reformer and applies his spirit to the health problems of today.

2. **Roemer MI:** Medical ethics in education of social responsibility. *Yale J Biol Med* 53:251–266, 1980

   The social responsibilities of individual physicians and of the medical profession overall are examined in this article. Roemer, a noted authority on public health and on health care delivery systems, observes that the Hippocratic oath only spells out obligations to individual patients. He proposes, in its place, an oath that also highlights the responsibility of physicians to work to ensure the health of their communities.

History

3. **Caplan RB, Caplan G:** *Psychiatry and the Community in 19th Century America.* New York, Basic Books, 1969

   This book traces the rise and fall and rise and fall again in the 19th century of the notion of caring for patients in the community. Neither the idea nor the problems are entirely new. The epilogue, written by Gerald Caplan as a commentary on cycles of reform and on the prospects of community psychiatry, is worth the price of the book alone.

4. **Ewalt JR, Ewalt PL:** History of the community psychiatry movement. *Am J Psychiatry* 126:81–90, 1969

   This article, written during the heyday of community psychiatry in the late 1960s, traces the evolution of social psychiatric thought beginning in the early 1900s. Contributions of Adolf Meyer, Clifford Beer, and Harry Stack Sullivan, as well as those of others lesser known, are concisely outlined.

5. **Foley HA, Sharfstein SS:** *Madness and Government: Who Cares for the Mentally Ill?* Washington, DC, American Psychiatric Press, 1983

   This book is an excellent history of the changing roles, especially in the last 50 years, of local, state, and federal government in providing for the care of mentally ill persons. Foley and Sharfstein outline in detail the development of legislative policy and actions on mental health care up through President Reagan's decision to cut funding instead of implementing Jimmy (and Rosalyn) Carter's Mental Health Systems Act of 1980. John F. Kennedy's and Jimmy Carter's Messages to Congress are included in the appendix. They are essential reading.

6. **Goldman HH, Morrissey JP:** The alchemy of mental health policy: homelessness and the fourth cycle of reform. *Am J Public Health* 75:727–731, 1985

   Goldman and Morrissey, in a trenchant analysis of the historical evolution of public mental health policy, convey the underlying dreams and the eventual outcomes of the community mental health movement. In particular, they note what has been a major criticism of the movement in the 1960s and 1970s: its neglect of persons with chronic psychiatric illness. They suggest that the community mental health movement is now into a fourth cycle of reform, forced by the occurrence of homelessness to pay attention to this population and integrate fully clinical care with social services. It will be some time before we can know how we have done, what we have missed, and what we have gotten right.

7. **Grob GN:** *From Asylum to Community: Mental Health Policy in Modern America.* Princeton, NJ, Princeton University Press, 1991

This is undoubtedly the most extensive history written of psychiatry in the initial era of the community mental health movement and deinstitutionalization (1940–1970). It is crucial reading for anyone attempting to understand the array of social forces acting on and within psychiatry.

8. **Mollica RF** (ed): The unfinished revolution in Italian psychiatry: an international perspective. *The International Journal of Mental Health* 14:1–2, 1985

No doubt the most extensive psychiatric reform movement occurring anywhere in the last 50 years, "democratic psychiatry," the effort to close state hospitals in Italy, has been both a source of hope and of controversy. This special issue does an excellent job of presenting an overview of the movement and its successes and failures.

Concepts

9. **Astrachan BM, Levinson DJ, Adler DA:** The impact of national health insurance on the tasks and practice of psychiatry. *Arch Gen Psychiatry* 33:785–794, 1976

In the process of outlining the potential effects of a national health insurance plan then in the offing, the authors lay out a very useful categorization of the tasks of psychiatry in society. Anyone trying to think systematically and sort out the many agendas of psychiatry is well advised to consult this article for a framework.

10. **Banton R, Clifford P, Frosh S, Lousada J, Rosenthal J:** *The Politics of Mental Health.* London, Macmillan, 1985

Clinicians working in the community (versus those working in institutions) tend to have very ambivalent feelings about the power differential between them and their patients. At times they may try to pretend it is not there, whereas at other times they may purposefully exaggerate it. This book, by a group of radical therapists from England, examines this issue closely and suggests ways that this power may appropriately be used to the benefit of patients.

11. **Caplan G:** *Principles of Preventive Psychiatry.* New York, Basic Books, 1964

This is a classic work from the days when community psychiatry was in its golden years of promise. It is also a brilliant book, with Caplan picking up on the works of Lindemann and vastly expanding them. The potential of public health thinking in psychiatry has not been captured so fully since.

12. **Gartner A, Riessman F** (eds): *The Self-Help Revolution,* Vol. 10 (Community Psychology Series). New York, Human Sciences Press, 1984

One of the most significant changes since the early days of the community mental health movement has been the emergence of self-help groups of all kinds. Because of them, community psychiatry will be very different than it had been conceptualized. These authors have been at the forefront of this development and describe its multiple aspects and ramifications.

13. **Group for the Advancement of Psychiatry:** *Community Psychiatry: A Reappraisal.* New York, Mental Health Materials Center, 1983

Published by the Group for the Advancement of Psychiatry, the cohort of psychiatrists most responsible for developing and implementing community psychiatry, this monograph is an essential read. Well balanced and cogent, it examines the evolution of community psychiatry thoroughly at its midlife point. As have other critics, the authors of this report found that the attention paid to severely and persistently ill persons has been insufficient and that the expectations placed on community psychiatry have been excessive. They also note its successes, however, in expanding care and reorienting the mental health care system.

14. *Healthy People 2000: National Health Promotion and Disease Prevention Objectives.* Washington, DC, U.S. Department of Health and Human Services, 1990

Published by the Department of Health and Human Services, this document presents a public health strategy to improve the health of the nation. For mental health, it presents health status objectives, such as a reduction in the suicide rate; risk reduction objectives, such as making treatment more accessible to persons with depression; and service objectives, such as increasing the number of coordinated programs in the country aimed at preventing suicides in jails. Other topics of potential interest discussed include alcohol and other drugs, violence and abusive behavior, and human immunodeficiency virus infection.

15. **Henderson AS** (ed): *An Introduction to Social Psychiatry.* New York, Oxford University Press, 1988

   Simply put, this is the best book around on social factors in psychiatry and its implications for community psychiatric practice. In a step-by-step process, Henderson, who is Australian, elaborates on the methods, concepts, and interventions of psychiatrists practicing on the societal level, even when seeing an individual patient.

16. **Jones M:** The therapeutic community, social learning and social change, in *Therapeutic Communities: Reflections and Progress.* Edited by Hinshelwood RD, Manning N. London, Routledge & Kegan Paul, 1979, pp. 1–9

   Jones is credited as one of the originators of the concept of the therapeutic community during World War II in Britain. In this account, he traces his experiences with the concept and expresses his hopes for the spread of the democratic principles contained in therapeutic communities to other social organizations. Therapeutic communities are one advance of community psychiatry that we forget at our peril.

17. **Levine M, Perkins DV:** *Principles of Community Psychology: Perspectives and Applications.* New York, Oxford University Press, 1987

   As community psychiatry has "remedicalized" and focused more on biology and chronically mentally ill persons, it has paid less and less attention to issues like prevention, social action, and the impact of the environment. Now most of the research and writing in these arenas is produced by a prolific band of community psychologists. This is a very good example of their work.

18. **Macht LB, Scherl DJ, Sharfstein SS** (eds): *Neighborhood Psychiatry.* Lexington, MA, Lexington Books, 1977

   The concept of "neighborhood psychiatry," an offshoot of community psychiatry, never really stuck. Yet this book is compelling, calling as it does for service integration at the local level and for a broad view of psychiatric services. Perhaps its time will return.

19. **Mechanic D:** *Mental Health and Social Policy,* 3rd Edition. Englewood Cliffs, NJ, Prentice-Hall, 1989

   This book, by a sociologist and an esteemed thinker in the field, lays out a straightforward and pragmatic view of the intersection of functional sociology and mental health policy. His approach to the problems of severely mentally ill persons and those who would care for them or develop policy to address their needs is probably the most coherent and comprehensive of any writer on the subject.

20. **Mills CW:** *The Sociological Imagination.* New York, Oxford University Press, 1959

Mills was one of America's greatest and most innovative sociologists. Although this book does not directly address psychiatry, the thinking behind it is critical to concepts of community psychiatry. While making a critique of sociologic practices of the time, Mills conveys with passion the connection between personal troubles and shared social problems. It is a perspective that is antithetical to the notion of the rugged individual, who is entirely responsible for his or her own life, and therefore is a challenge to the American culture and to strains in American psychiatry. The last chapter on methods and ways to think creatively about social "facts" is a gem.

Epidemiology and Needs Assessment

21. **Bellah RN, Madsen R, Sullivan W, Swindler A, Tipton SM:** *Habits of the Heart: Individualism and Commitment in American Life.* Berkeley, CA, University of California Press, 1985

This is an exposé of American culture by a team of eminent sociologists. They examine the roots and manifestations of our cultural sense of the individual and contrast them with the absence of a sense of community. It raises a thought-provoking question for community psychiatrists: Where and how should individuals fit into the social system?

22. **Goldsmith HF, Line J, Bell RA, Jackson DJ** (eds): *Needs Assessment: Mental Health Service Systems Report.* Rockville, MD, U.S. Department of Health and Human Services

Epidemiology is very useful on the basic science level because it helps to highlight those characteristics in the population that may account for the distribution of disease. It can do more than that, however. It can also help systems planners determine how to allocate resources most efficiently and direct care to those in need. It can also determine who is "at risk" and focus preventive efforts. This report summarizes the promises and complexities of determining who needs what.

23. **Harrington M:** *The New American Poverty.* New York, Penguin, 1984

Poverty in America is not a static thing. This book, written by the author of *The Other America,* which helped launch the "war on poverty" in the 1960s, portrays the current face of this social scourge. Community psychiatrists focusing on the disadvantaged in the public sector can get a sense of the challenges their patients face.

24. **Mechanic D:** Medical sociology: some tensions among theory, method and substance. *J Health Soc Behav* 30:147–160, 1989

Epidemiology is a quantitative science, whereas the experience of persons with psychiatric illness and of their clinicians is qualitative. In this article, Mechanic makes the point that both qualitative and quantitative research on social phenomena can complement each other. This applies to the study of psychiatric disorders as well. Studies of cultural life and of subjective experience are critical aspects of the knowledge base of community psychiatry.

25. **Regester DC:** Community mental health: for whose community? *Am J Public Health* 64:886–893, 1974

One of the premises of the population-oriented approach to community psychiatry is that there is a community to serve. It did not take long for some to realize that there are many ways to define a community and that, in the real world, all these definitions apply simultaneously. The lesson extends to those now focused on providing care "in the community." What does that mean, exactly? Community psychiatric practice remains fuzzy around the edges, but this also allows for creative boundary breaking.

26. **Robins LN, Reiger DA** (eds): *Psychiatric Disorders in America: The Epidemiologic Catchment Area Study.* New York, Free Press, 1991

Epidemiology is one of the bedrock sciences of community psychiatry. This book is a compilation of findings of the Epidemiologic Catchment Area study, the most recent major undertaking in psychiatric epidemiology. A massive undertaking, it gives us our best estimate yet of the extent and distribution of psychiatric disorders in the United States. It also reveals some interesting findings, open to interpretation, such as the fact that rates of specific disorders seem to vary greatly from community to community. Are these real differences or study artifacts?

27. **Susko MA** (ed): *Cry of the Invisible.* Baltimore, MD, Conservatory Press, 1991

The dictum "listen to the patient. He/she is telling you what is wrong" is well known in medicine. Increasingly patients/consumers are finding their voices. This is an example, filled with heartfelt stories of life on the streets or in institutions.

28. **Strauss JS:** Subjective experiences of schizophrenia: toward a new dynamic psychiatry, II. *Schizophr Bull* 15:179–188, 1989

Persons with schizophrenia develop a relationship with the disease process. The illness is not them; it is something with which they live and with which they often learn to cope, sometimes in very creative ways. All it took Strauss to find this out was to ask and not dismiss their reports out of hand.

29. **Tischler GL, Aries E, Cytrynbaum S, Wellington SW:** The catchment area concept, in *Progress in Community Mental Health,* Vol. 3. Edited by Bellak L, Barten HH. New York, Brunner/Mazel, 1975, pp. 59–83

An often unappreciated component of the original versions of community psychiatry and the community mental health center was its willingness to accept responsibility for all patients in a geographic region, rather than to turn them away because they were unable to pay or had the "wrong" diagnosis. Minor irritants such as "turf" battles between agencies aside, this effort worked to maximize continuity of care, improve access for socially disadvantaged groups, and decentralize services.

Mental Health Care Services: Research and Systems Change

30. **Clarkin JF, Perry SW** (section eds): Differential therapeutics, in *Psychiatry Update: American Psychiatric Association Annual Review,* Vol. 6. Edited by Hales RE, Francis AJ. Washington, DC, American Psychiatric Press, 1987, pp. 327–441

Mental health services research has come into its own as the cost of health care has skyrocketed. Issues of efficiency and effectiveness are becoming paramount. This section of the annual review is a very good introduction to efforts to determine what kind of care in which setting should be offered to which patient.

31. **Goodrick D:** Mental health system strategic planning, in *Handbook on Mental Health Policy in the United States.* Edited by Rochefort DA. Westport, CT, Greenwood, 1988, pp. 449–473

Drawing on his experiences in Wisconsin in the public sector, Goodrich outlines an approach for directors of mental health service organizations to use to deal strategically with a changing environment. The deeper we get into mental health service reform, the clearer the necessity of this kind of thinking will be to community psychiatrists.

32. **Hollingshead AB, Redlich FC:** *Social Class and Mental Illness: A Community Study.* New York, Wiley, 1958

All mental health services research harkens back to this landmark study examining the differential utilization of mental health services by different social classes within the community. At the time it was published, it added greatly to the cause of those pushing to develop community mental health centers.

33. **Lewis DA, Shadish WR Jr, Lurigio AJ:** Policies of inclusion and the mentally ill: long-term care in a new environment. *Journal of Social Issues* 45:173–186, 1989

The authors attempt to place the care for mentally ill persons within the context of present social policy. "Policies of inclusion" refers to the present attempts to desegregate mentally ill persons and integrate them into mainstream society. The authors suggest that this has expanded what had been a mental health problem into a broader social welfare problem.

34. **Mechanic D, Aiken LH** (eds): *Paying for Services: Promises and Pitfalls of Capitation* (New Directions for Mental Health Services, No. 43). San Francisco, CA, Jossey-Bass, 1989

The public mental health system is typically underfinanced, fragmented, and inaccessible. The result is that many seriously mentally ill persons are neglected. This series of articles discusses capitation as a means of consolidating funding, developing necessary community services, and focusing responsibility and accountability. The authors offer a balanced view of this mechanism for financing services and a general introduction to the forces that appear to be defining the future of public mental health services.

35. **Mollica RF:** From asylum to community: the threatened disintegration of public psychiatry. *N Engl J Med* 308:367–373, 1983

Mollica offers a critical review of the status of publicly supported psychiatric services. He suggests that the threatened disintegration of public mental health services is due to the "over emphasis on social reform and political rather than clinical definition of treatment . . . and its inability to change psychiatry's historical assignment of low status to the public patient" (p. 367).

36. **Ridgway P, Zipple AM:** The paradigm shift in residential services: from the linear continuum to supported housing approaches. *Psychosocial Rehabilitation Journal* 13:11–31, 1990

With the decline in the availability of long-term hospital care, it has become increasingly imperative that appropriate housing be provided for mentally ill persons. The long-standing paradigm has been to move people from site to site as their condition changes. The authors turn this idea on its head, proposing that people move into long-term settings and that the level of support provided change as needed. It is a very good example of the flexibility of thinking needed in community psychiatry.

37. **Scott WR, Black BL** (eds): *The Organization of Mental Health Services: Societal and Community Systems.* Newbury Park, CA, Sage, 1986

This book begins with the hypothesis that organizations both create and attempt to alleviate mental illness. The focus is on understanding the "organizational arrangements by which society disperses mental health services" (p. 8) and how power relations determine the implementation of innovative programs.

38. **Stein LI:** Innovating against the current, in *Innovative Community Mental Health Programs* (New Directions for Mental Health Services, No. 56). Edited by Stein LI. San Francisco, CA, Jossey-Bass, 1992, pp. 5–22

This is a personal account of the development of the model of community care for chronically mentally ill persons that has now become the standard for all other programs. Stein discusses the difficulties in developing innovations and then disseminating them, noting the conflicts to be expected in this process.

39. **Surles RC, Blanch AK, Shern DL, Donahue S:** Case management as a strategy for systems change. *Health Aff (Millwood)* 9:151–163, 1990

Increasingly, community psychiatrists are faced with determining how to provide services more effectively in extremely complex social systems. This article describes an attempt to deliver mental health services to the most disenfranchised population. The authors offer one paradigm, termed a *non-synoptic* method of social change, as an approach to solving problems arising out of the complex interaction between mental illness and deprivation.

Underserved Populations

40. **Astrachan BM, Scherl DJ:** On the care of the poor and the uninsured. *Arch Gen Psychiatry* 48:481, 1991

The authors state clearly that "the poor tend to be sicker" (p. 481). They call for the development of research and new social models addressing the needs of the disadvantaged.

41. **Baumohl J, Hawks D, Hopper K:** Addiction and the American debate about homelessness (editorial and commentaries). *Br J Addict* 87:7–16, 1992

This editorial and accompanying commentaries provide a provocative yet lucid example of how social problems are defined by political and social forces. This determines whether these are treated as mental health problems needing psychiatric intervention or as system failures needing larger systemic solutions. The interplay between addiction and homelessness continues to be a neglected area of research.

42. **Brown DB, Parnell M:** Mental health services for the urban poor: a systems approach, in *Social and Political Contexts of Family Therapy.* Edited by Mirkin AP. New York, Gardner Press, 1990, pp. 176–215

    This chapter provides a firsthand look at the experience of providing care at an inner-city mental health center. It is described by elucidating the contextual forces that influenced the development and functioning of the clinical services program. A systems theory approach, as opposed to the individual clinical approach, is more effective in providing services in highly complex settings.

43. **Cheung FK, Snowden LR:** Community mental health and ethnic minority populations. *Community Ment Health J* 26:277–291, 1990

    These authors explore the current understanding of the impact of race on the utilization of mental health services along with recommendations for needed research. There continue to be barriers to adequate care, possibly due to organizational inadequacies and cultural incongruity.

44. **Cohen CI, Sokolovsky J:** *Old Men of the Bowery: Strategies for Survival Among the Homeless.* New York, Guilford, 1989

    The authors have provided an in-depth description and systemic study of older skid-row men. They examine pathways to homelessness, the available social supports, survival skills, and the physical and mental health problems in detail. The personal portraits of these men allow readers to experience the daily struggle of surviving on the streets.

45. **Dohrenwend BP:** Socioeconomic status (SES) and psychiatric disorders. *Soc Psychiatry Psychiatr Epidemiol* 25:41–47, 1990

    Despite the fact that socioeconomic status has become an increasingly ignored factor in research, Dohrenwend presents compelling and articulate evidence for continued research in this area. It seems particularly important to understand how socioeconomic status relates to normal personality characteristics such as locus of control, values and attitudes, and various stressful events.

46. **Federal Task Force on Homelessness and Severe Mental Illness:** *Outcasts on Main Street.* Rockville, MD, U.S. Department of Health and Human Services, 1992

    A distillation of all the recent efforts to address the problems of homeless mentally ill persons, this monograph is both enlightened and enlightening. Besides describing a comprehensive approach to the individual care of these persons, it suggests action steps at the federal level to begin to end this ongoing human tragedy.

47. **Imber-Black E:** *Families and Larger Systems: A Family Therapist's Guide Through the Labyrinth.* New York, Guilford, 1988

This is a vital text for any psychiatrist working in the public sector. It offers valuable insights into how to conceptualize the relationship between families and the complex social systems in which they must survive. Imber-Black specifically addresses the importance of gender issues in treating families.

48. **Jahiel RI** (ed): *Homelessness: A Prevention-Oriented Approach.* Baltimore, MD, Johns Hopkins University Press, 1992

This text is the most recent and comprehensive look at a social problem we have been struggling with for more than 15 years. Homelessness continues to have a devastating impact on large segments of the population. Particularly useful are the sections focusing on intervention directed at homeless people and those elucidating the social context of homelessness.

49. **Kaplan SR, Roman M:** *The Organization and Delivery of Mental Health Services in the Ghetto: The Lincoln Hospital Experience.* New York, Praeger, 1973

50. **Peck HB:** Psychiatric approaches to the impoverished and underprivileged, in *American Handbook of Psychiatry*, 2nd Edition, Vol. 2. Edited by Arieti S. New York, Basic Books, 1974, pp. 524–534

Community psychiatry has always been active in addressing the needs of impoverished populations. Peck describes innovative programs in the 1960s and gives practical approaches to effective individual and group therapy in inner-city populations. Kaplan and Roman describe in detail the project at Lincoln Hospital, which attempted to provide services to an impoverished area of the Bronx, New York, in an innovative manner. These two works dramatically illustrate both the successes and limitations of the activist approach.

51. **Mollica RF, Milic M, Bollini P:** Trends in mental health care: categorical treatment and the concept of "positionality." *International Journal of Mental Health* 18:31–47, 1990

This article focuses on the changes in mental health utilization in the population originally studied by Hollingshead and Redlich (1958) above. "Positionality" is the process by which an institution categorizes a patient, thus defining the patient's relationship to staff and setting. Obviously, this can have both a negative impact and a positive impact on the patient.

52. **Susser E, Valencia E, Goldfinger SM:** Clinical care of homeless mentally ill individuals: strategies and adaptation, in *Treating the Homeless Mentally Ill: A Report of the Task Force on the Homeless Mentally Ill.* Edited by Lamb HR, Bachrach LL, Kass FI. Washington, DC, American Psychiatric Press, 1992, pp. 127–140

This chapter describes the stages in developing a therapeutic relationship with those who are homeless and mentally ill. Understanding these stages will assist clinicians in promoting more stable housing situations. The authors point out that, to be more effective, it is always necessary to understand the context of homelessness.

53. **Tien L:** Determinants of equality and equity for special populations served by public mental health systems. *Hosp Community Psychiatry* 43:1104–1108, 1992

With decreased funding for public mental health services, allocation of resources becomes an increasingly difficult task. Tien proposes a conceptual framework in which two standards of fairness—equality and equity—are applied to three dimensions: utilization of services, funding for services, and access to services.

54. **Vega WA, Murphy JW:** *Culture and the Restructuring of Community Mental Health.* New York, Greenwood, 1990

This book focuses on mental health care for cultural minorities and the urban poor as illustrated by the community mental health movement. It begins with the Community Mental Health Center Act, with an emphasis on treatment in the "least restrictive environment" and "citizen participation" in planning, and traces the development and implementation of these ideas.

Community Care of Severely and Persistently Mentally Ill Persons

55. **Chamberlin J:** Speaking for ourselves: an overview of the ex-psychiatric inmates' movement. *Psychosocial Rehabilitation Journal* 8:56–61, 1984

Written by a former "mental patient," this article delineates the basic beliefs of the ex-inmate movement. This group has become an increasingly powerful voice in influencing mental health policy, and this article offers a unique perspective on the issues.

56. **Estroff SE:** *Making It Crazy: An Ethnographic of Psychiatric Clients in an American Community.* Berkeley, CA, University of California Press, 1981

This ethnography of persons with severe mental illness receiving psychiatric care in Dane County, Wisconsin, is the most compelling description of this group since Goffman's *Asylums.* It is crucial for anyone attempting to comprehend the daily existence of mentally ill persons since deinstitutionalization. Many disturbing questions are raised concerning the impact of mental health services on their clients.

57. **Hatfield AB:** *Family Education in Mental Illness.* New York, Guilford, 1990

The voice of the families of persons with mental illness has asserted itself with tremendous force in the last decade. This book was written as a curriculum on mental illness for families. It not only conveys the issues as families see them, but also suggests ways to help families learn how to deal with their ill relative and with the mental health care system.

58. **Mechanic D, Rochefort DA:** A policy of inclusion of the mentally ill. *Health Aff (Millwood)* 11:128–149, 1992

This is a concise yet lucid account of the current state of mental health services in this country. It particularly focuses on recent strategies of mental health funding and the impact of resource allocation on care for mentally ill persons. Is society willing to make available the resources to integrate these persons back into the community?

59. **Moxley D:** The practice of case management, in *Sage Human Services Guides Series,* Vol. 58. Edited by Lauffer A, Garvin CD. Newbury Park, CA, Sage, 1989

Case management has been suggested as the solution to persistent problems of fragmentation. There are key questions presented in this text that assist in developing more efficient use of this ever-expanding treatment strategy. This chapter provides an exhaustive list of service functions to be provided by case managers and is extremely useful for community mental health centers attempting to develop these services.

60. **Stroul BA:** Community support systems for persons with long-term mental illness: a conceptual framework. *Psychosocial Rehabilitation Journal* 12:10–26, 1989

The movement of persons with mental illness out of the institutions and into the community in recent years has been facilitated by the development of community support systems. Beyond providing psychiatric care, institutions fulfilled many other needs, such as housing, social and vocational opportunities, and a sense of community. The trick is to construct a system of resources and to develop a network of relationships to ensure the provision of these services. After disavowing its role in community organization in the 1970s, psychiatry is right back into it.

Primary Care

61. **Eisenberg L:** Treating depression and anxiety in the primary care setting. *Health Aff (Millwood)* 11:149–156, 1992

In a brief review, Eisenberg outlines the issues facing those who would try to take psychiatry to the patients in primary care. One fascinating aspect is that standard psychiatric nosology appears to be inadequate to capture the kinds of psychiatric disorders that present in primary care settings. It is an entirely different population from the one that shows up in psychiatric settings.

62. **Regier DA, Goldberg ID, Taube CA:** The de facto US mental health services system. *Arch Gen Psychiatry* 35:685–693, 1978

Psychiatrists sometimes assume that it is their job, and their job alone, to care for persons with psychiatric illness. This study is a strong refutation of that notion. It turns out that the vast majority of persons with psychiatric complaints are seen by a primary care physician. Since this article appeared, some efforts have been made to integrate psychiatry with primary care practitioners, but there is still much to be done if community psychiatrists want to be active and useful participants in primary care settings.

Disaster, Violence, and Prevention

63. **Barter J, Talbott SW** (eds): *Primary Prevention in Psychiatry: State of the Art.* Washington, DC, American Psychiatric Press, 1986

This primer is an excellent introduction to the current status of prevention in psychiatry. The promise is there. It is an area that suffers more than anything from neglect.

64. **Bell CC, Jenkins EF:** *Preventing Black Homicide: The State of Black American 1990.* New York, National Urban League, 1990

"Black-on-black" homicide has become a daily occurrence in most inner cities. This work explores the myths and realities of this epidemic and offers practical techniques for prevention and consciousness raising. It is a good example of the potential of a population-oriented psychiatric practice that focuses on a community problem outside the traditional definition of psychiatric disorders.

65. **Cooper B:** Epidemiology and prevention in the mental health field. *Soc Psychiatry Psychiatr Epidemiol* 25:9–15, 1990

This is a concise article that focuses on the promises and failures of epidemiological research to define the scope of prevention in the mental health field. The increasing predominance of concern for the impact of individual processes (diagnostic reliability and biological models) and a lack of interest in mental illness as the product of the ecosystem (poverty, disasters, political persecution) have limited our ability to make appropriate interventions.

66. **Lystad M, Sowder BJ** (eds): *Disasters and Mental Health: Contemporary Perspectives and Innovations in Services to Disaster Victims.* Washington, DC, American Psychiatric Press, 1986

This text presents the basics of "disaster" psychiatry: developing a taxonomy of disasters both natural and caused by humans, outlining their effects on people, and describing the efforts of mental health workers to address them. This is a clear example of the benefit of a population-oriented approach to community psychiatry, guided by social psychiatric principles.

Role of Psychiatrists

67. **American Psychiatric Association:** Guidelines for psychiatric practice in community mental health centers. *Am J Psychiatry* 148:965–966, 1991

These guidelines are the fruit of a movement begun by psychiatrists working in community mental health centers who did not want to leave and have fought to stay. They represent an effort to establish a domain for psychiatric practice in such settings and, in a sense, are a modern effort to reintegrate the medical and social approaches in psychiatry and mental health care.

68. **Cohen NL** (ed): *Psychiatry Takes to the Streets.* New York, Guilford, 1990

In this book, psychiatrists go everywhere, but especially to where those most in need of their help and services live. In addition to suggesting many fascinating programmatic and practice ideas, it challenges the image of the psychiatrists in their offices, isolated from the outside world.

69. **Knoedler W:** The continuous treatment team model: role of the psychiatrist. *Psychiatric Annals* 19:35–40, 1989

   Community treatment teams for persons with severe and persistent psychiatric disorders are clearly part of the future for community psychiatric practice. This article, written in a practical fashion by one of the original continuous treatment team's psychiatrists from Madison, Wisconsin, the heartland of assertive community treatment, conveys a sense of what the work is about and how to do it. It is a gem.

70. **Raphael B:** Psychiatry "at the coal-face." *Aust N Z J Psychiatry* 20:315–332, 1986

   Written "down under," this article concretely and effectively portrays the thought processes and practice of a community psychiatrist who cares for impoverished individual patients but also extrapolates the problems they face to the community level and plans community interventions.

71. **Sarason SB:** *The Creation of Settings and the Future Societies.* San Francisco, CA, Jossey-Bass, 1972

   This is a wonderful work by one of the founders of the community mental health movement. As community psychiatrists reassert themselves in the design, development, and management of community programming and services, they would be wise to consult this book. It contains a good deal of wisdom on being a leader, an architect, or just a participant in the construction of the social infrastructure of communities.

72. **Talbott JA:** Why psychiatrists leave the public sector, in *The Perspective of John Talbott* (New Directions for Mental Health Services, No. 37). Edited by Talbott JA. San Francisco, CA, Jossey-Bass, 1988, pp. 25–34

   Much has been written about the absence of psychiatrists in the public sector mental health care system. Talbott, who is noted for his advocacy for severely mentally ill persons, suggests some of the reasons a psychiatrist might want to work in some aspect of this system. He then describes the multiple work stressors in the system that seem to drive off even committed psychiatrists and offers a few proposals, including the privatization of public services, as a way to reverse this trend.

Training

73. **Brown DB, Goldman CR, Thompson KS, Cutler DL:** Training residents for community psychiatric practice: guidelines for curriculum development. *Community Ment Health J* (in press)

Developed by the training committee of the American Association of Community Psychiatrists, this article presents a model of the various aspects and levels of community psychiatric practice. From these it suggests a variety of didactic, clinical consultative, and administrative experiences to prepare tomorrow's community psychiatrists for the tasks ahead.

74. **Burt VK, Summit P, Yoger J:** Outpatient management team: integrating educational and administrative tasks. *Academic Psychiatry* 16:24–28, 1992

As community mental health services are reorganized, psychiatrists are increasingly finding themselves working on outpatient management teams or continuous treatment teams, providing supervision and medical backup. Working on such a team instead of on their own allows residents to get experience in providing care in the community and to do it in a less isolated, more structured way.

75. **Factor RM, Stein LI, Diamond RJ:** A model community psychiatry curriculum for psychiatric residents. *Community Ment Health J* 24:310–327, 1988

76. **Godard SL, Cutler DL, Pollack DA:** Education and training in public psychiatry, in *New Directions for Mental Health Services, State-University Collaboration: The Oregon Experience.* Edited by Bloom JD. San Francisco, CA, Jossey-Bass, 1989, pp. 5–16

These two works describe in detail two of the most advanced community psychiatry training programs in the country, representing the state of the art. Both focus almost entirely on persons with severe and persistent mental illness. Interestingly, they are both in cities known for being livable and progressive. Can such training be done in more socially stressed environments?

77. **Lurie N, Yergan J:** Teaching residents to care for vulnerable populations in the outpatient setting. *J Gen Intern Med* 5:S26–S34, 1990

Caring for disadvantaged, socially marginalized people is a challenge for all of medicine, not just psychiatry. This article describes the historically strong linkage between disadvantaged populations and the training of physicians. The authors discuss key aspects of learning to care for such populations, all of which are applicable to psychiatric training programs.

78. **Morrison AP, Shore MF, Grobman J:** On the stresses of community psychiatry and helping residents to survive them. *Am J Psychiatry* 130:1237–1241, 1973

Community psychiatry has been accused of breaking boundaries. There is no doubt that it diverges in many ways from "traditional" psychiatric practice. This article does a very good job outlining the stresses on residents involved in shattering the molds of tradition and learning how to do community psychiatry. It offers some useful suggestions for supervisors on helping them do this.

58

Administration in Psychiatry

Bradley M. Pechter, M.D.
Willie Earley, M.D.
Boris M. Astrachan, M.D.

I n a changing world of practice, the work of the psychiatrist increasingly takes place in organized settings. Administration organizes and structures the work of mental health professionals. The
work of administration is to identify and see to the execution of organizational tasks, to ensure the integration of tasks, to assign tasks appropriately
and to monitor them, to engage with groups with which the organization
must interact on behalf of the organization, and to plan for the future.
Whether we are aware of it or not, administrative concerns pervade our
professional lives.

In preparing this section, we have generally taken the sociologic perspective. We pay particular attention to the construction of organizations,
the relationship of organizations to their environment and to the individual, and, conversely, how individual roles influence the organization. We
hope to illustrate how these factors underpin administration and have
far-reaching implications for the accomplishments of any psychiatric organization. In all of our suggestions, we have tried to keep a progressive (and
appropriate) perspective. Alternative treatment settings, managed care,
ethics, and training issues are important concerns in psychiatric administration and are represented.

There have been many fundamental changes in this field in the past

20 years. In some sense, the values underpinning practice have changed; nevertheless, we remain confident in our abilities to adapt and retain a commitment to serving patients. The issues raised by this bibliography are important to residents and all mental health professionals. We may be more accustomed to or comfortable studying individuals or therapeutic dyads, but administration's focus on groups and organizations is essential. We no longer live in splendid isolation; we live and work in organizations.

Organization of Services

1. **Astrachan JH, Astrachan BM:** Medical practice in organized settings. *Arch Intern Med* 149:1509–1513, 1989

   The importance of the organized medical staff as an independent force in hospital management is described. Its significance as a voice for patient care issues is identified.

2. **Astrachan BM, Flynn HR, Geller JD, Harvey HH:** Systems approach to day hospitalization. *Arch Gen Psychiatry* 22:550–559, 1970

   This article relates the structure of day-hospital programs to their various goals. With constructs derived from systems theory, four possible primary tasks of day hospitals are identified: 1) an alternative to 24-hour inpatient hospitalization, 2) a transitional care setting whose task is to facilitate the reentry into the community of previously hospitalized patients, 3) a treatment and rehabilitative facility for chronically mentally disturbed persons, and 4) a structure that delivers those psychiatric services that a specified community defines as an overriding public need. These possible tasks are then examined in relation to openness of the system and boundary control.

3. **Bachrach LL:** The future of the state mental hospital. *Hosp Community Psychiatry* 37:467–474, 1986

   The author examines the state hospital from a systems approach and makes predictions regarding the state hospitals' future role in the psychiatric service system.

4. **Gudeman JE, Shore MF, Dickey B:** Day hospitalization and an inn instead of inpatient care for psychiatric patients. *N Engl J Med* 308:749–753, 1983

   This article describes one institution's attempt at providing alternatives to psychiatric hospitalization. By diverting patients to a day hospital (and for those with housing problems, to an inn), the Massachusetts

Mental Health Center demonstrated that aggressive outpatient management with appropriate follow-up is an excellent alternative to inpatient hospitalization.

5. **Hamilton EL:** The voluntary hospital in America: its role, economics and internal structure, in *Medical Care: Readings in the Sociology of Medical Institutions.* Edited by Scott WR, Volhart EH. New York, Wiley, 1966, pp. 393–405

This is an excellent overview from a historical standpoint on the ever-changing role and internal structure of hospitals in America. The author also describes how economics plays its role in shaping the delivery of modern health care.

6. **Moseley SK, Grimes RM:** The organization of effective hospitals. *Health Care Manage Rev* 1(3):13–23, 1976

This article is notable for its effort to glean the actual characteristics of organization that distinguish effective hospitals. Specialization of function and role, cooperation, integration, and standardization emerged as important features. Implications are drawn for hospital administration.

7. **Olfson M:** Assertive community treatment: an evaluation of the experimental evidence. *Hosp Community Psychiatry* 41:634–641, 1990

This article describes 10 versions of the assertive community treatment program originally described in Madison, Wisconsin, as the "Training in Community Living (TCL) Program." It illustrates how intensified outpatient management coupled with community and medical support can lessen the number of hospitalizations in a group of chronically mentally ill patients.

Leadership, Power, and Authority

8. **Kanter RM:** Power failure in management circuits. *Harvard Business Review* July/August 1979, pp. 65–75

This is an excellent and readable article in which the author argues that power resides in the position, not the person. Power in organizations can be productive or oppressive, and the use to which it is put is dependent on having open channels available to supplies, support, and information. Typically powerless positions (on all levels) are examined, as are issues of power failure for women.

9. **Kernberg OF:** Leadership in organizational functioning: organizational regression. *Int J Group Psychother* 28:3–25, 1978

    Problems attributed to failures in leadership may, in fact, reflect difficulties within the organization that lead to regressive group processes. Among the causes of such problems may be the failure to clarify priorities, poverty of resources, and even the impact of several severely regressed patients on staff group functioning.

10. *Levinson DJ, Klerman GL:** The clinician-executive: some problematic issues for the psychiatrist in mental health organizations. *Psychiatry* 30:3–15, 1967

    Identifying and formulating some of the problematic role issues for clinicians who function as administrators, the authors provide an excellent overview for the topic and a good starting point for any administrator in psychiatry.

11. *Munich RL:** The role of the unit chief: an integrated perspective. *Psychiatry* 49:325–336, 1986

    This article is an outstanding review of the multifaceted role of the psychiatric unit chief. Munich describes with vivid examples four interrelated tasks of the unit chief: boundary management, generation of resources, mobilization of consensus, and consultation and evaluation.

Role and Relationships in Organizations

12. *Benarroche CL, Astrachan BM:** Interprofessional role relationships, in *Psychiatric Administration: A Comprehensive Text for the Clinician-Executive.* Edited by Talbott JA, Kaplan R. New York, Grune & Stratton, 1983, pp. 223–236

    Administration in psychiatry must manage complex work relationships among professionals of various disciplines. This chapter examines the importance of role in these relationships by defining models and analyzing the tasks and perspectives that underpin such role relationships. It also includes discussion of particularly confounded role relationships in psychiatric work.

13. *Levinson DJ:** Role, personality, and social structure in the organizational setting. *Journal of Abnormal and Social Psychology* 58:170–180, 1959

    This is a somewhat theoretical but still useful article that draws distinctions between "role demands" of the organizations and "role definition" by the individuals in organizations. In this way, social structure and personality are bridged in personal role definition.

14. *Newton PM, Levinson DJ: The work group within the organization: a sociopsychological approach. *Psychiatry* 36:115–142, 1973

The authors argue that task, culture, social structure, and social process are the properties that primarily determine the nature and effectiveness of work in a work group. The example of a clinical team in a research ward is examined to illustrate the ways in which sociopsychological properties can help us understand dysfunctional behaviors in a work group.

15. Silver MA, Akerson DM, Marcos LR: Preferred management styles among psychiatrist-administrators. *Hosp Community Psychiatry* 41:321–323, 1990

This article identifies the importance that psychiatrist-administrators attribute to highly relationship–oriented management styles, suggesting that to some extent they view administration as a social process, rather than a process dependent on technology or policy. It addresses some of the problems of such a position.

Economics

16. Callaghan CT, Whalen WJ: Cost accounting for non-accountants. *Grantsmanship Center News* November-December 1981, pp. 27–32

This is a brief and informative article that "demystifies" accounting terminology and practices. It helps administrators to understand the workings of finance and budgetary restraints. A short, useful glossary for understanding cost accounting is included.

17. Feldman S: *Managed Mental Health Services,* 1st Edition. Springfield, IL, Charles C Thomas, 1992

This book is an early entry into the literature on the important, emerging field of managed mental health care. It recognizes its bias in favor of managed health care but discusses its drawbacks too. Chapters include applications, economics, the perspectives of buyers and insurer, quality, evaluation, clinical impact, and ethical and legal issues of managed mental health care.

18. Scherl DJ, English JT, Sharfstein SS: *Prospective Payment and Psychiatric Care,* 1st Edition. Washington, DC, American Psychiatric Press, 1988

This textbook provides useful and understandable information about the payment structure in modern health care. It also provides a historical perspective on federal government involvement in health care delivery.

Systems Theory

19. *Astrachan BM, Tischler GL:** A systems approach to the management of psychiatric facilities. *Administrative Mental Health* 8:225–236, 1981

   In this excellent introduction to understanding organization structure and processes, the authors argue that organization structure is related to organization tasks. They attempt to see if structure supports or inhibits tasks. Schematics are used to illustrate basic concepts and selected interesting examples.

20. **Miller EJ, Rice AK:** *Systems of Organization.* London, Tavistock, 1967

   This is a seminal work, delineating the approach to systems diagnosis developed at the Tavistock Institute. The examples primarily come from the world of industry and are worth reading and rereading.

21. **Schulberg HC, Baker F:** An open systems approach to mental health program development, in *The Mental Hospital and Human Services.* New York, Behavioral Publications, 1975, pp. 67–100

   This chapter is a useful overview of systems tasks and goals and their application to work within health organizations.

Quality Assurance

22. **Donabedian A:** The quality of care: how can it be assessed? *JAMA* 260:1743–1748, 1988

   In this thoughtful discussion of the problems associated with accurate monitoring of care, Donabedian specifies what quality is and speaks to the importance of assessment of outcome.

23. **Enthoven AC:** What can Europeans learn from Americans. *Health Care Financing Review: Annual Supplement* 11 (suppl):49–63, 1989

   Enthoven provides an overview of some of the exciting quality-focused and organizational initiatives in American medical practice. These include uniform data reporting, uniform hospital cost accounting, studies of practice variation, risk-adjusted measures of outcomes, outcomes management, and new ways of organizing and paying for service. This is an article worth rereading.

24. **Kritchovsky SB, Simmons BP:** Continuous quality improvement. *JAMA* 266:1817–1823, 1991

Continuous quality improvement is a systems approach to improving quality, and quality is measured against the ability to meet the needs and wants of the customers. This article, despite being somewhat technical, gives some very useful ideas for implementing continuous quality improvement in the health care industry.

Ethics

25. **Bayer R, Callahan D, Caplan AL, Jennings B:** Toward justice in health care. *Am J Public Health* 78:583–588, 1988

This article grapples with the tough ethical issue of health care distribution in American society. By pointing out some of the efficient and inefficient uses of our health care resources, the authors believe that changes can be made to ensure adequate health care for all Americans.

26. *Eisenberg L:** Health care: for patients or for profits? *Am J Psychiatry* 143:1015–1019, 1986

In this consciousness-raising review of the physician's responsibility in the ever-increasing monetarization of health care, Eisenberg concludes that physicians have an ethical imperative to join together in protecting the equity and quality of health care.

27. **Engelhardt HT Jr, Rie MA:** Morality for the medical-industrial complex. *N Engl J Med* 319:1086–1089, 1988

A brief discussion of various problems with mass marketing of health care in our contemporary economic milieu is presented.

28. **Ginzberg E:** The monetarization of health care. *N Engl J Med* 310:1162–1165, 1984

Ginzberg describes the increasing emphasis of profit in the current health care system and highlights the continual necessity of physician involvement in advocating health care over profit.

29. *Relman AS:** The new medical-industrial complex. *N Engl J Med* 303:963–970, 1980

This article reviews some ethical issues facing the proprietary medical industry. In an era when profit is all too often placed before the patient's benefit, Relman concludes that the physician should have no conflicting financial interests and should always put the interests of the public before those of the stockholders.

30. *Towery OB, Sharfstein SS:* Fraud and abuse in psychiatric practice. *Am J Psychiatry* 135:92–94, 1978

    In this concise yet informative review of the sometimes confusing issues of fraud and abuse within psychiatry, the authors attempt to clarify the differences between fraud and abuse by using various case vignettes.

31. **Webb WL:** Ethical aspects of the continuum of care concept. *The Psychiatric Hospital* 18:147–151, 1987

    This article describes some of the ethical issues that inevitably seem to surface in providing continual health care for the chronically mentally ill population. The author believes that by providing alternative structured treatment programs, health care is ultimately improved for this population.

Training Issues

32. **Arce AA:** Psychiatric training issues: the Puerto Rican perspective. *Am J Psychiatry* 139:461–465, 1982

    This article critically reviews mental health care delivery to the Hispanic population. The author states that two factors are crucial in understanding the inadequacies of mental health delivery to Hispanics: underrepresentation of Hispanic mental health care professionals and curriculum deficits in training programs.

33. **Borus JF:** Teaching residents the administrative aspects of psychiatric practice. *Am J Psychiatry* 140:444–448, 1983

    With the ever-increasing bureaucratic demands placed on psychiatric practice, the author maintains that administrative psychiatry is an often-overlooked and undervalued part of psychiatric training. The author believes that administrative issues should be integrated into psychiatric training. He also provides a blueprint of how he believes this integration could take place.

34. *Griffith EE, Delgado A:* On the professional socialization of black residents in psychiatry. *Journal of Medical Education* 54:471–476, 1979

    Although written about the unique demands placed on the socialization of black residents in psychiatric training, this article provides useful and thoughtful information for any minority group going through psychiatric training.

35. **Jellinek MS:** Recognition and management of discord within house staff teams. *JAMA* 256:754–755, 1986

The management of discord within a house staff team is an essential part of leadership during residency. Jellinek states that the leader must first possess the ability to recognize the conflict early and then make timely and well thought out interventions.

36. **Jones BE, Lightfoot OB, Palmer D, Wilkerson RG, Williams DH:** Problems of black psychiatric residents in white training institutes. *Am J Psychiatry* 127:798–803, 1970

In this somewhat dated, yet still poignant discussion of racial issues in psychiatric training, the authors contend that psychiatric training programs fail to produce psychiatrists, black or white, who are willing or prepared to address the mental health needs of the black community. A number of useful recommendations are suggested to help alleviate this problem.

37. *Lowy FH, Thornton JF:** To be or not to be a psychiatric chief resident. *Can J Psychiatry* 25:121–127, 1980

This article offers some practical ideas about the sometimes confusing and poorly defined role of the psychiatric chief resident and describes some factors in selecting the chief resident and helping the resident define realistic goals.

38. **Sharaf MR, Levinson DJ:** The quest for omnipotence in professional training: the case of the psychiatric resident. *Psychiatry* 27:135–149, 1964

The article provides an excellent description of the maturational process of residents. Although written about psychiatric residents, the article would be useful for other medical specialties as well. Early in training, residents essentially believe that their teachers and supervisors are all-knowing and all-powerful. They aspire to a degree of knowledge that cannot be mastered. As they mature as clinicians, they develop more reasonable expectations about their capabilities.

39. **Yager J:** Psychiatric residency training and the changing economic scene. *Hosp Community Psychiatry* 38:1076–1081, 1987

The current medical trend toward cost containment has created a profound effect on psychiatry and psychiatric training alike. This article describes that change, and several suggestions are made on what programs can do to meet the challenges of training psychiatrists in an era of increased bureaucracy.

General Texts

40. **Feldman S:** *The Administration of Mental Health Services,* 2nd Edition. Springfield, IL, Charles C Thomas, 1980

    This is a text that covers a wide range of administrative issues as they relate specifically to mental health services.

41. **Talbott JA, Hales RE, Keill SL** (eds): *Textbook of Administrative Psychiatry.* *Washington, DC, American Psychiatric Press, 1992*

    This is a comprehensive text for explaining the many facets of psychiatric administration.

59

Ethics

Roger C. Sider, M.D.

Ethics—the inquiry into the nature of morality, of human conduct where values are concerned, and of vice and virtue—is a subject of central concern to psychiatrists. Although it overlaps with questions of law and of professional codes of conduct, ethics should be distinguished from each of these. For beyond the legality or consistency with professional codes of any professional act, one looks for deeper evidence that it is ethically justified.

Before 1960, there was remarkably little interest in the formal study of ethical issues in psychiatry and medicine. Biomedical ethics has since become a growth industry, however, and psychiatric ethics is taking its place within that domain. Ethical issues that have received special attention in psychiatry include the physician-patient relationship, informed consent, involuntary treatment, therapeutic modality choice, values in psychotherapy, confidentiality, suicide, behavior control, therapist-patient sex, double agency, and research with human subjects.

At the risk of oversimplification, it is possible to discern three periods in the development of this literature: pre-1960, 1960–1980, and post-1980. The first period we might label traditional. Characterized by an ethic of beneficence, psychiatrists, like other physicians, justified their treatment in terms of patient best interest. The second period, 1960–1980, witnessed the ascendancy of autonomy ethics, with patient choice, informed consent, and respect for autonomy the cardinal benchmarks of ethical practice.

Since 1980, the field has moved rapidly in several directions. Reflective of the dynamic changes in this field is the fact that the large majority of citations in this chapter are new, many of them not yet published when the first edition of this book appeared in 1984. Of particular note is the renewed interest in the place of virtue and character in professional ethical practice, the growing influence of economics in determining access to and quality of care, and the question of physician-assisted suicide. Renewed attention is also being given to the clarification of standards of and the procedures for dealing with violations of professional ethical conduct. This is a direct result of the unfortunate tarnishing of psychiatry's public image that has occurred in recent years. Most damaging has been widespread media scrutiny of alleged sexual indiscretions between psychiatrists and their patients. Survey data document that these violations of professional ethical standards are not uncommon. An additional problem area has been the involvement of psychiatrists in abuses of inpatient hospitalization, particularly in the for-profit hospital sector. Charges of unnecessary hospitalization, hospitalization without prior psychiatric assessment, and the tailoring of treatment primarily to maximize insurance benefits have all given the appearance that in these cases psychiatrists and administrators of the hospitals involved were more interested in enhancing their incomes than in the best interests of their patients.

Obviously, there is much yet to be done. The readings identified in this chapter are best considered as representative of work now in progress in our field. Since ethics is inherently a contentious subject, allowing for deep differences of opinion, these references should be approached as stimuli to further reflection, not as a compendium of moral certainties.

Textbooks and Monographs

1. *Beauchamp TL, Childress JF:** *Principles of Biomedical Ethics,* 3rd Edition. New York, Oxford University Press, 1989

   One of the most widely used textbooks in medical ethics, this book covers the major topics: ethical theories, the major principles of biomedical ethics, and the place of virtue. Included are 38 case studies.

2. *Bloch S, Chodoff P** (eds): *Psychiatric Ethics,* 2nd Edition. Oxford, England, Oxford University Press, 1991

   This highly recommended book is the most comprehensive reference in psychiatric ethics. Most of the chapters are written by leading psychiatrists rather than philosophers.

3. **Brody H:** *The Healer's Power.* New Haven, CT, Yale University Press, 1992

In this new treatment of medical ethics from the perspective of the power disparity in the physician-patient relationship, Brody helpfully extends the medical ethics dialogue beyond rights and autonomy.

4. **Browning DS, Evison IS** (eds): *Does Psychiatry Need A Public Philosophy?* Chicago, IL, Nelson-Hall, 1991

This book, although not technically an ethical text, examines psychiatry's interface with religion, ethics, law, and philosophy.

5. **Dyer AR:** *Ethics and Psychiatry: Toward Professional Definition.* Washington, DC, American Psychiatric Press, 1988

This book is particularly helpful in examining what it means to practice as a psychiatric professional from an ethical point of view. Dyer is concerned to show that virtue, idealism, and altruism are integral to fulfilling our professional responsibilities to our patients.

6. **Gabbard G** (ed): *Sexual Exploitation in Professional Relationships.* Washington, DC, American Psychiatric Press, 1989

This book—multiauthored by mental health professionals, clergy, and attorneys—provides a broad overview of the empirical, clinical, ethical, and medicolegal aspects of the vexing problem of professional sexual exploitation.

7. **Group for the Advancement of Psychiatry:** *A Casebook in Psychiatric Ethics.* New York, Brunner/Mazel, 1990

This brief volume, designed as a discussion guide, contains 17 case vignettes clustered around major ethical issues in psychiatry.

8. **Engelhardt HT Jr:** *Bioethics and Secular Humanism: The Search for a Common Morality.* Philadelphia, PA, Trinity Press International, 1991

Engelhardt, perhaps the foremost proponent of a secular, libertarian medical ethics, provides the most recent formulation of his views.

9. **Lakin M:** *Ethical Issues in the Psychotherapies.* New York, Oxford University Press, 1988

This is a comprehensive examination of ethical issues in individual, group, marital, and family psychotherapies.

10. **Lidz CW, Meisel A, Zerubael E, Carter M, Sestak RM, Roth LH:** *Informed Consent: A Study of Decision Making in Psychiatry.* New York, Guilford, 1984

This is an excellent report of informed consent in psychiatric clinical settings with the best empirical data to date on the complexity and difficulty in applying this ethical principle in clinical practice.

11. **London P:** *The Modes and Morals of Psychotherapy*, 2nd Edition. Washington, DC, Hemisphere Publishing, 1986

    In this well-written overview of psychotherapy as an ineluctably moral enterprise, both insight- and action-oriented therapies are examined.

12. *May WF: *The Patient's Ordeal*. Bloomington, IL, Indiana University Press, 1991

    This book views medical ethics from a relational and ultimately a religious perspective. Psychiatrists will benefit from the author's understanding of the patient's experience and his insights into how this perspective supplements an ethics based on duties, rights, and principles.

13. **Reiser SJ, Burszajn HJ, Appelbaum PS, Gutheil TG:** *Divided Staffs, Divided Selves: A Case Approach to Mental Health Ethics.* Cambridge, MA, Cambridge University Press, 1987

    Organized into clusters of cases illustrative of major ethical issues in psychiatric practice, this book provides excellent questions to stimulate group discussion.

Official Statements

14. AIDS policy: guidelines for outpatient psychiatric services. *Am J Psychiatry* 149:721, 1992; AIDS policy: guidelines for inpatient psychiatric units. *Am J Psychiatry* 149:722, 1992

    These two statements provide specific advice regarding patient care, protection of patients and staff, and confidentiality.

15. **American Psychiatric Association:** *Guidelines on Confidentiality.* Washington, DC, American Psychiatric Association, 1988

    These official guidelines offer assistance in balancing the duty to preserve confidentiality against competing goods, such as duties toward the public welfare or the patient's good.

16. *The Principles of Medical Ethics With Annotations Especially Applicable to Psychiatry.* Washington, DC, American Psychiatric Association, 1993; Addendum to the 1993 edition of *The Principles of Medical Ethics With Annotations Especially Applicable to Psychiatry.* Washington, DC, American Psychiatric Association, 1993; *Opinions of the Ethics Committee on the Principles of Medical Ethics With Annotations Especially Applicable to Psychiatry.* Washington, DC, American Psychiatric Association, 1992

These official publications are small booklets summarizing current interpretations of the ethical code of the profession, procedures for handling complaints of unethical conduct, and specific answers to a wide range of ethical questions that have come before the American Psychiatric Association Ethics Committee.

Confidentiality and Duty to Protect

17. **Appelbaum PS:** Tarasoff and the clinician: problems in fulfilling the duty to protect. *Am J Psychiatry* 142:425–429, 1987

Using case examples, this article outlines legal requirements in violating confidentiality to protect others.

18. **Siegler M:** Confidentiality in medicine: a decrepit concept. *N Engl J Med* 307:1518–1521, 1982

Confidentiality has been severely compromised because of the large number of persons now having authorized access to hospitalized patients' medical records. Siegler suggests ways of coping ethically with this situation.

Economics

19. **Dougherty CJ:** Mind, money and morality: ethical dimensions of economic change in American psychiatry. *Hastings Center Report* 18:15–20, 1988

Psychiatrists are especially vulnerable to ethical conflicts resulting from cost-containment pressures. They will face complex double-agent roles that may compromise their commitment to the patient's good.

20. **Reagan MD:** Physicians as gatekeepers: a complex challenge. *N Engl J Med* 317:1731–1734, 1987

This article provides a thorough review of the ethical implications of the gatekeeper role.

21. ***Relman AS:** Dealing with conflicts of interest. *N Engl J Med* 313:749–751, 1985

Relman asserts the fundamental distinction between business and professional practice.

Informed Consent, Competence, and Refusal of Treatment

22. Appelbaum PS: The right to refuse treatment with antipsychotic medications: retrospect and prospect. *Am J Psychiatry* 145:413–419, 1988

The evolution of the right to refuse treatment over the past 15 years is reviewed, and its future prospects are predicted.

23. Appelbaum PS, Grisso T: Assessing patients' capacities to consent to treatment. *N Engl J Med* 319:1635–1638, 1988

This article is a practical guide for assessing competency.

24. *Dyer AR, Bloch S: Informed consent and the psychiatric patient. *J Med Ethics* 13:12–16, 1987

In this article, consent is viewed as a process, modeled after the partnership of the therapeutic alliance.

25. Winslade WJ: Informed consent in psychiatric practice: the primacy of ethics over law. *Behavioral Sciences and the Law* 1:47–56, 1983

In this article, we are advised to think in terms of respect for persons rather than minimal legal requirements in obtaining ethically valid informed consent.

Involuntary Treatment

26. Chodoff P: Involuntary hospitalization of the mentally ill as a moral issue. *Am J Psychiatry* 141:384–389, 1984

This article provides an analysis of the philosophic basis of disagreements about the moral justification for involuntary hospitalization.

27. Szasz T: The religion called psychiatry. *Second Opinion* 6:50–61, 1987

This is a brief and polemical statement of the author's now-familiar view that psychiatry, masquerading as science, unethically deprives patients of basic human rights.

Professional Responsibility and Unethical Conduct

28. Appelbaum PS, Jorgenson L: Psychotherapist-patient sexual contact after termination of treatment: an analysis and a proposal. *Am J Psychiatry* 148:1466–1473, 1991

This controversial article proposes that therapist-patient sexual contact be considered unethical if it occurs within 1 year of the termination of treatment.

29. **Fink PJ:** Presidential address: on being ethical in an unethical world. *Am J Psychiatry* 146:1097–1104, 1989

The author calls on psychiatrists to reassert their primary ethical obligation to the patient.

30. **Gartrell N, Herman JL, Olarte S, Feldstein M, Localio R:** Psychiatrist-patient sexual contact: results of a national survey, I: prevalence. *Am J Psychiatry* 143:1126–1131, 1986

31. **Herman J, Gartrell N, Olarte S, Feldstein M, Localio R:** Psychiatrist-patient sexual contact: results of a national survey, II: psychiatrists' attitudes. *Am J Psychiatry* 144:164–169, 1987

These are two empirical reports of the continuing problem of psychiatrists' unethical sexual involvement with patients.

32. **Gutheil TG, Gabbard GO:** The concept of boundaries in professional practice: theoretical and risk-management dimensions. *Am J Psychiatry* 150:188–196, 1993

This article will rapidly become a classic. By clearly defining the necessity of boundaries in the therapeutic relationship, it establishes a clear framework for ethical and legally defensible practice. A major tenet of the article is that sexual exploitation in the therapeutic relationship is almost always preceded by a series of progressively more serious boundary violations.

Suicide and Euthanasia

33. **Gaylin W, Kass L, Pellegrino E, Siegler M:** Doctors must not kill. *JAMA* 259:2139–2140, 1988

The authors articulate their opposition to euthanasia.

34. *Hendin H, Klerman G:** Physician-assisted suicide: the dangers of legalization. *Am J Psychiatry* 150:143–145, 1993

This excellent article views the euthanasia debate from a specifically psychiatric perspective.

35. **Wanzer SH, Federman DD, Adelstein SJ, Cassel CK, Cassem EH, Cranford RE, Hook EW, Lo B, Moertel CG, Safar P, Stone A, van Eys J:**

The physician's responsibility toward hopelessly ill patients: a second look. *N Engl J Med* 320:844–849, 1989

The authors, who formulated this statement under the sponsorship of the Society for the Right to Die, discuss the care of terminally ill patients, including the view of all but two of the authors that physician-assisted suicide or euthanasia may not always be unethical.

The Impaired Psychiatrist

36. **Swearingen C:** The impaired psychiatrist. *Psychiatr Clin North Am* 13:1–11, 1990

    The author surveys the complex issues of psychiatrist impairment and advocates a balance between sanction and rehabilitation.

Forensic Psychiatry

Seymour L. Halleck, M.D.

Forensic psychiatry has two major dimensions. First, it deals with the manner in which psychiatric practice is regulated by statutes, administrative agencies, and the courts. In working with patients who may be incompetent or nonconsenting, psychiatrists assume certain legal obligations and must practice within certain constraints. Psychiatrists must also be aware of the regulatory aspect of malpractice litigation and learn to provide the most beneficial treatment to their patients while at the same time avoiding the painful consequences of a lawsuit. The second aspect of forensic psychiatry deals with the matter in which psychiatry can assist society in resolving complex legal problems. The law is often concerned with the state of mind of various participants in the litigation process. Psychiatrists assist the criminal courts by testifying and consulting on issues such as competency to stand trial, insanity, sentencing, and release. They assist the civil courts in assessing psychological damages, in determining various competencies, and in resolving child custody disputes.

There is a rich forensic psychiatry literature, much of which deals with complicated theoretical inquiries into the relation of law and psychology. The emphasis in this bibliography is on material the practicing psychiatrist needs to know. Sources are listed on the basis of their accuracy and readability. Although most of the listings are recent publications, a few classic texts and articles have been included to provide some sense of the scope of the field and to allow the reader the option of delving into some of the more complex and fascinating issues.

Children

1. **Brinson P, Hess KD:** Mediating domestic law issues, in *Handbook of Forensic Psychology.* Edited by Weiner IR, Hess AK. New York, Wiley, 1987, pp. 86–154

   This is an excellent although lengthy chapter on basic issues in family law and child custody. It helps the psychiatrist understand the legal issues involved in marital disputes and in what has been referred to as the "ugliest litigation," child custody.

2. **Burton K, Myers WC:** Child sexual abuse and forensic psychiatry: evolving in controversial issues. *Bull Am Acad Psychiatry Law* 20:439–455, 1992

   This article summarizes problems in this difficult area very well, focusing on such issues as psychic damages, false allegations, improper investigatory techniques, use of anatomical dolls, admissibility of expert testimony, hearsay testimony, and the competency of minors to testify.

3. **Walker CE, Bonner BL, Kaufman KL:** *The Physically and Sexually Abused Child: Evaluation and Treatment.* Elmsford, NY, Pergamon, 1988

   This book provides a comprehensive and practical approach to assessments, intervention, and prevention of child abuse. Much of the material is relevant to dispositional issues that have forensic consequences.

Competency

4. *Appelbaum PS, Grisso T:** Assessing patients' capacities to consent to treatment. *N Engl J Med* 319:1635–1638, 1988

   This is a brief but extremely useful article on practical means of assessing competency to choose to be treated. It is especially useful in defining the assessments the psychiatrist must note in determining the nonpsychiatric patient's capacity to accept or refuse treatment.

Commitment

5. **Johnson AB:** *Out of Bedlam: The Truth About Deinstitutionalization.* New York, Basic Books, 1990

   Johnson traces the history of hospitalization of mentally ill persons throughout the past 40 years with an effort to determine the causes and consequences of deinstitutionalization. She provides fascinating insights into a most important facet of contemporary psychiatric history.

6. *Miller RD: *Involuntary Commitment of the Mentally Ill in the Post Reform Era.* Springfield, IL, Charles C Thomas, 1987

This is a thorough, scholarly review of how the process of civil commitment has changed during the 1970s and 1980s. The impact of these changes on patients, on psychiatrists, and on psychiatrists working in the public sector is carefully and methodically described.

7. Szasz TS: *Law, Liberty and Psychiatry: An Inquiry Into the Social Uses of Mental Health Practices.* New York, Macmillan, 1963

This book was one of the first to expose psychiatric practices that allegedly compromised the rights of mentally ill persons. It became the rallying point for a generation of civil liberties attorneys who radically changed commitment practices and treatment of mentally ill patients.

Confidentiality

8. **Beck JC** (ed): *Confidentiality Versus the Duty to Protect.* Washington, DC, American Psychiatric Press, 1990

Beck presents a series of excellent articles that describe basic principles of confidentiality in psychiatric practice and consider situations in which confidentiality must be compromised to protect patients. A special advantage of the format is that it discusses the duty to protect in various settings, including hospitals, outpatient clinics, and emergency rooms. It also deals with current issues of confidentiality with the patient positive for the human immunodeficiency virus antibody.

Ethics

9. **Strasburger LH, Jorgenson L, Randles R:** Mandatory reporting of sexually exploitive psychotherapists. *Bull Am Acad Psychiatry Law* 18:379–384, 1990

This article synopsizes some of the effects of sexual exploitation of patients, but focuses primarily on the difficult issue of requiring subsequent treating psychotherapists to report the abuse of a former therapist to a licensing agency. The authors conclude that there are some advantages to mandatory reporting.

10. **Weinstock R** (ed): *Bull Am Acad Psychiatry Law* Vol. 20, No. 2, 1992

This is a memorial issue dedicated to Bernard L. Diamond. Much of the material deals with one of Diamond's major interests: ethics in forensic psychiatry. Some of the most esteemed practitioners of forensic psychiatry, including four Isaac Ray Award winners, discuss a variety of issues that were of interest to Diamond.

Expert Testimony

11. **American Psychiatric Association:** Peer review of psychiatric expert testimony: American Psychiatric Association's Council on Psychiatry and Law. *Bull Am Acad Psychiatry Law* 20:343–352, 1992 (also available from the office of the American Psychiatric Association)

This report represents a pioneer effort by a group of eminent forensic psychiatrists to try to determine if standards of competence can be developed in regard to forensic testimony. The authors suggest that the process of peer review holds promise for developing ethical standards in this area.

12. **American Psychiatric Association:** The use of psychiatric diagnoses in the legal process: Task Force of the American Psychiatric Association's Council on Psychiatry and Law. *Bull Am Acad Psychiatry Law* 20:481–499, 1992 (also available from the office of the American Psychiatric Association)

This work attempts to describe both the value and the potential misuse of psychiatric diagnosis in the legal process. It is particularly useful in clarifying the relevance and usefulness of the official diagnostic and statistical manuals in resolving legal disputes.

13. **Binder RL:** Sexual harassment: issues for forensic psychiatrists. *Bull Am Acad Psychiatry Law* 20:409–418, 1992

This is an excellent overview of the problem of sexual harassment and the role of the forensic psychiatrist in litigation involving harassment.

14. **Faust D, Ziskin J:** The expert witness in psychology and psychiatry. *Science* 241:31–35, 1988

This article questions the credibility of psychiatric and psychological testimony in the courtroom. It is frequently cited by attorneys in an effort to discredit psychiatric testimony. It should heighten the psychiatrist's awareness of how proposed testimony might be attacked.

15. **Hoge SK, Grisso T:** Assessing the accuracy of expert testimony. *Bull Am Acad Psychiatry Law* 20:67–76, 1992

This article is a critique of the Faust and Ziskin (1988) article above, pointing out some of its fallacies. The article supports the reliability and validity of psychiatric expert testimony in various contexts.

16. **Usdin J:** Psychiatric participation in court. *Psychiatric Annals* 7:42–51, 1977

This is a brief article that offers practical advice on being an expert witness.

General Texts

17. **Davidson HA:** *Forensic Psychiatry*, 2nd Edition. New York, Roland Press, 1965

This is a classic textbook in forensic psychiatry, noteworthy for its comprehensive discussion of civil as well as criminal issues. It is still a useful text for any psychiatrist planning to be a witness.

18. *Hodgins S (ed): *Mental Disorder and Crime.* Newbury Park, CA, Sage, 1993

This is the most modern collection of articles on this subject. It includes the research of many of the most prominent investigators working in forensic psychiatry. The research perspective provides a sharp contrast to earlier theoretical treatises on this subject.

19. **McDonald JM:** *The Murderer and His Victim.* Springfield, IL, Charles C Thomas, 1961

This is easy reading covering issues related to homicide. The case illustrations are excellent, and the style is lively. This is a comfortable way to learn about the criminal justice system.

20. **Simon RI** (ed): *Review of Clinical Psychiatry and the Law,* Vol. 2. Washington, DC, American Psychiatric Press, 1991

This volume includes several in-depth articles on malpractice, civil commitment, violence, and relationships with nonmedical professionals and an update of recent developments in psychiatry. It is scholarly and readable.

21. **Stone AA:** *Law, Psychiatry and Morality.* Washington, DC, American Psychiatric Association, 1984

This is a series of essays by Stone, an author who has presented stimulating ideas in the area of forensic psychiatry for the last 20 years. His insights, although often controversial, provide a broad social perspective to the field of forensic psychiatry.

Insanity and Competency to Stand Trial

22. **Callahan LA, Steadman HJ, McGreevy MA, Robbins PC:** The volume and characteristics of insanity defense pleas: an eight state study. *Bull Am Acad Psychiatry Law* 19:331–338, 1991

    This is a classic article illustrating some of the difficulties of doing research in forensic psychiatry and collecting such elementary data as the actual incidence of insanity defenses. It reminds us of the complexity of the research process in forensic psychiatry and the need for carefully defined studies, such as this one they have produced.

23. *Goldstein AS:** *The Insanity Defense.* New Haven, CT, Yale University Press, 1967 (also available from Westport, CT, Greenwood, 1980)

    Primarily a legal treatise on the difficult issue of criminal responsibility, it is, however, a must for psychiatrists who need to understand the historical, moral, and legal meaning of the insanity defense.

24. **Halleck SL:** *The Mentally Disordered Offender.* Rockville, MD, National Institute of Mental Health, 1986

    This monograph focuses attention on a number of legal and clinical issues at the interface of the criminal justice and mental health systems. It includes a detailed discussion of issues involved in the management and treatment of offenders found incompetent to stand trial, offenders not guilty by reason of insanity, offenders who become ill during the course of imprisonment, and offenders who are subject to specialized treatment.

25. **Morris N:** *Madness in the Criminal Law.* Chicago, IL, University of Chicago Press, 1982

    In a delightful book, Morris has written a series of short stories that illustrate some of the thorny principles involved in dealing with issues such as criminal competency and insanity. The stories are followed by illuminating discussion of the theoretical issues involved.

26. **Warren JI, Fitch LW, Deitz P, Elliott E, Rosenfeld BD:** Criminal offense, psychiatric diagnoses and psycho legal opinion: an analysis of 894 pre-trial referrals. *Bull Am Acad Psychiatry Law* 19:63–69, 1991

This article relies on experience with evaluating a large group of former patients to delineate issues in determining criminal responsibility and competency to stand trial. Diagnostic considerations played a major role in the evaluator's finding of both incompetency and legal insanity.

Malpractice

27. **Klerman GL:** A debate: the psychiatric patient's right to effective treatment: implications of Osheroff vs. Chestnut Lodge; **Stone AA:** Law, science, and psychiatric malpractice: a response to Klerman's indictment of psychoanalytic psychiatry. *Am J Psychiatry* 147:409–427, 1990

    This debate between two prominent psychiatrists illustrates how changing paradigms of treatment can influence malpractice litigation. In the course of their lively argument, both authors clarify a number of critical issues related to malpractice in psychiatry.

28. **Modlin HC:** Forensic psychiatry and malpractice. *Bull Am Acad Psychiatry Law* 18:153–163, 1990

    Modlin describes the process of evaluation of malpractice cases by a psychiatric team at the Menninger Clinic. The focus is on how the forensic expert deals with the issues of standards of care and the clinical problems of evaluating patients for harm or disability related to presumed negligence by medical personnel.

29. *Simon RI: *Clinical Psychiatry and the Law.* Washington, DC, American Psychiatric Press, 1987

    This is a highly practical and detailed text covering all areas of forensic psychiatry in a comprehensive and clear manner. The material, for the most part, is up to date. The sections on malpractice are particularly useful.

Treatment of Offenders

30. **Adson PR** (ed): Paraphilias, and related disorders. *Psychiatric Annals* 22:22–26, 1992

    This is a group of articles on the diagnosis and treatment of paraphiliac disorders. The lead article on treatment of paraphilias is especially useful for anyone working in the correctional setting.

31. **Berlin FS:** The paraphilias and Depo-provera: some medical, ethical and legal considerations. *Bull Am Acad Psychiatry Law* 17:233–239, 1989

This article discusses the use of antiandrogens in the treatment of paraphiliac behavior. Berlin concludes that the use of antiandrogen medication to suppress sexual appetite constitutes an ethical and useful adjunct in treatment.

32. **Forer LG:** *Criminals and Victims.* New York, WW Norton, 1980

Forer draws on her experiences as a criminal court judge to present a very intimate and humanistic perspective of those who commit crimes and of those who are victimized by crime. Although she does not use the language of psychiatry, her perspectives of human suffering should provide the psychiatric reader with many new insights into the problems of crime in American society.

33. **Menninger KA:** *The Crime of Punishment.* New York, Viking, 1968

This is a classic argument for a rehabilitative rather than a punitive approach to criminal behavior. It is a powerful reminder of the moral responsibilities of the psychiatrist.

34. **Rennie YF:** *The Search for Criminal Man.* Lexington, MA, DC Heath, 1978

This is a comprehensive study of theoretical criminology. The historical role of psychiatry in the study and treatment of the criminal is presented in useful perspective and with remarkable clarity.

35. **Roth LH:** Correctional psychiatry, in *Modern Legal Medicine, Psychiatry and Forensic Science.* Edited by Curran W, McGarry L, Petty C. Philadelphia, PA, FA Davis, 1980, pp. 677–719

This is a comprehensive description of mental health service in jails and prisons. It describes limits of treatment in the custodial setting, but also emphasizes the possibility of useful intervention.

Violence

36. **Monahan J:** Mental disorder and violent behavior: perceptions and evidence. *Am Psychol* 47:511–521, 1992

In this article, Monahan, who is perhaps the most prominent researcher on the relationship between violence and mental illness, concludes that some of his earlier comments on this relationship may well have been wrong. He notes that there could be a modest relationship between mental disorder and violence and delineates those rare situations in which the correlation is evident.

37. **Tardiff K:** *Concise Guide to Assessment and Management of Violent Patients.* Washington, DC, American Psychiatric Press, 1989

   This is an excellent guide that begins with a discussion of seclusion and restraint. It considers the major issues in the diagnosis of violence and contains an excellent and up-to-date section on the use of medication in the management of violent patients.

61

Economic Issues in Psychiatry

Joseph T. English, M.D.
Richard G. McCarrick, M.D., M.H.A.

D espite the fundamental importance of economics in shaping virtually all aspects of health care, ranging from what drugs are developed by pharmaceutical companies to what specialties are chosen by graduating medical students, the field of medical economics is a relatively neglected one in the curricula of medical schools and residency training programs. Although joint degree programs in the basic sciences aimed at producing physicians-scientists are now a well-established feature of medical education, the need to offer conjoint graduate training to future physician-economists has yet to be recognized. The support of the Robert Wood Johnson Foundation's Clinical Scholars Program, notably at the University of Pennsylvania, is a rare exception that attempts partially to remedy this deficiency, albeit at the postresidency level. Unfortunately, most physicians will approach economics with a limited or rapidly receding background and, quite possibly, a feeling of intimidation from the often elaborately quantitative nature of the field.

With these considerations in mind, the references listed in this chapter have been selected on the assumption that the reader possesses no prior knowledge of the subject beyond that of the average citizen of high intelligence and keen curiosity. All of the selections should be comprehensible without any familiarity with specialized technical information beyond that which is explained within the text. A particular premium has been placed on selections that provide a conceptual framework that enables the clinician to arrange the specific details into a readily understood context. Selections have been included on the basis of being current and topical. It is hoped that they are relevant not only to what is occurring on the national level at the present time, but to what may happen in the near future during a period of anticipated rapid transition in the organization and delivery of health care. A number of classic articles have been included because they continue to shed light on contemporary issues despite the lapse of time since their publication.

Another selection criterion is that articles should provide a balanced presentation of the material, giving the reader an understanding of the complexities of the arguments and data involved, even when refuting an opposing position. Despite a mass of empirical research, the field of economics is fragmented among a variety of competing theoretical "schools" with strongly held viewpoints, so that even leading authorities may come to widely divergent conclusions about the same issue (a situation not unfamiliar to psychiatrists). Ideally, selections will encourage the reader to learn more about the subject and stimulate ideas for future investigation, rather than offer doctrinaire prescriptions.

Finally, selections have been made on the basis of accessibility of sources to medical students, residents, and practicing psychiatrists. Most selections should be available in medical libraries or through commonly existing interlibrary loan programs. Each of the selections contains informative bibliographies and references that will greatly assist the reader who wishes to pursue a subject in greater depth or breadth.

It is our conviction that psychiatric economics can be understood only in the context of developments in general medical economics. In this respect, of primary importance is the decision of society as reflected in the policies of the major federal agencies to regard health care as an ordinary business and to allow market mechanisms freely to operate with the expectation that financial competition will reduce medical costs. Diagnosis-related groups for payment of hospitals and the resource-based relative value scale for payment of individual physicians are a direct reflection of this governmental philosophy. A negative consequence of this approach is a de-emphasis on professional responsibility for standards of care, service to the community, and self-regulation.

It is likely that the second half of the 1990s will be an era of landmark legislation with regard to health care, similar to the mid-1960s but with greater potential for effecting a fundamental alteration in the nature of the medical profession. Furthermore, the impetus for this change, along with the urgent demands for health care reform and decisive government intervention, is largely the result of economic considerations. To safeguard the interests of their patients and the ideals of their profession, it has become all the more imperative that physicians stay fully informed about economic issues and take a proactive stance through their professional organizations in determining the health care agenda for the 21st century. To achieve this objective, the serious student of psychiatric economics who wishes to keep abreast of current developments should regularly peruse the table of contents of a number of key publications for articles of interest. By far the best source of timely and accurate information on medical economics among general interest publications is the *Wall Street Journal*. The most important in-depth articles on relevant economic subjects in a general medical journal are those found in the *New England Journal of Medicine*. The principal specialized journals with an emphasis on analysis of economic issues in medicine are *Health Policy* and *Health Affairs*. Of most direct relevance to the practicing psychiatrist are the scholarly and practical articles on mental health economics contained in two publications of the American Psychiatric Association: the occasional feature item in the *American Journal of Psychiatry* and the regularly appearing economic grand rounds in *Hospital and Community Psychiatry*. Finally, it should be noted that the American Psychiatric Association Office of Economic Affairs has compiled comprehensive bibliographies on selected economic topics in mental health and also publishes a bimonthly newsletter, *Eco-Facts*, that provides concise summaries, helpful perspectives, and clear information on the latest economic research, changes in regulations, and proposed legislation.

History and General Background

1. **Angell M:** The presidential candidates and health care reform. *N Engl J Med* 327:800–811, 1992

   This combination editorial and "sounding board" features the positions of the two major political parties in the United States on health care reform. Louis Sullivan, Secretary of Health and Human Services, presents the plans of the Bush administration, and Governor Clinton submits his own proposal. Noted health economists Alain Enthoven and Uwe Reinhardt offer their analysis of the specific proposals, and Angell gives six general criteria for evaluating any possible reforms of health care.

2. *English JT, Kritzler ZA, Scherl DJ:** Historical trends in the financing of psychiatric services. *Psychiatric Annals* 14:321–331, 1984

   This article demonstrates that the economics and financing of psychiatric facilities and services have been important and constant concerns of the physicians and administrators who have directed mental hospitals in the United States since colonial times.

3. **Gibson R:** The use of financing to control the delivery of services. *Psychiatric Annals* 4:22–41, 1974

   Gibson surveyed the existing state of mental health care financing and foresaw many of the developments and problems of the next two decades, including the rapid growth of managed care and the consequent infringements on professional autonomy and quality of care.

4. **Ginzberg E:** The monetarization of medical care. *N Engl J Med* 310:1162–1165, 1984

   Ginzburg laments the transformation of American medicine from a profession into a business. Faulty public policy with regard to reimbursement of hospitals and physicians has set the stage for the explosive growth of for-profit health care.

5. **Grob GN:** Mental health policy in America: myths and realities. *Health Aff (Millwood)* 11:7–22, 1992 (Fall)

   Before World War II, the focus of government-sponsored efforts to treat mentally ill persons was individuals who suffered from severe and chronic problems. More recently, the target population has become diffuse and the service provision has become decentralized. This article explores the forces behind this shift, including changes in patient populations, funding patterns, character of hospitals, and the role of psychiatry.

6. **Relman AS:** The new medical-industrial complex. *N Engl J Med* 303:963–970, 1980

   Relman notes that health care has become a huge and changed industry that supplies services for profit. This has created problems of overuse, fragmentation of services, overemphasis on technology, and undue influence on national health policy. The interests of stockholders should not be put before those of the public.

7. **Rosenheck R, Astrachan B:** Regional variation in patterns of inpatient psychiatric care. *Am J Psychiatry* 140:1180–1183, 1990

   District regional variation in length of stay and ratio of psychiatric beds to population exists in the United States, even in centrally organized health care systems, such as the Veterans Administration. The authors examine this phenomenon and offer possible explanations for the existing pattern.

8. **Sharfstein SS, Beigel A** (eds): *The New Economics and Psychiatric Care.* Washington, DC, American Psychiatric Press, 1985

Although now in need of updating, this book still provides the best general introduction to current issues in mental health economics.

9. ***Starr P:** *The Social Transformation of American Medicine.* New York, Basic Books, 1982

In this insightful and highly readable account of the development of medicine in the United States from a semiskilled trade to a prestigious profession, Starr makes clear the importance of economic considerations in all phases of the history of American medicine.

10. **Staton D:** Mental health care economics and the future of psychiatric practice. *Psychiatric Annals* 19:421–427, 1989

Staton provides a concise and informative overview of many of the current important issues in mental health economics, summarizes trends of the last 20 years, and projects likely scenarios for the future.

Hospital Payment Systems

11. **English JT, McCarrick RG:** DRG's: an overview of the issues. *Gen Hosp Psychiatry* 8:359–364, 1986

This article provides a summary of many of the problematic areas that need to be addressed in the design of any modified system of financing for psychiatric care. These issues include the potential for premature discharge, code manipulation, cost shifting, and lack of equitable patient access to psychiatric services.

12. ***English JT, Sharfstein SS, Scherl DJ, Astrachan B, Muszuynski IL:** Diagnosis-related groups and general hospital psychiatry: the APA study. *Am J Psychiatry* 143:131–139, 1986

The American Psychiatric Association study of the potential impact of diagnosis-related groups (DRGs) used a database of 1.7 million hospital discharges. It showed that diagnosis alone explains only about 5% of the variance in length of stay for psychiatric admissions. It conclusively demonstrated that the DRG payment mechanism, as it then existed, was a poor predictor of resource consumption when applied to psychiatric services, would result in a disproportionate number of outlier cases, and would place hospitals at undue financial risk.

13. **Essock-Vitale S:** Patient characteristics predictive of treatment costs on inpatient psychiatric wards. *Hosp Community Psychiatry* 38:263–269, 1987

Utilizing a database of more than 1,100 discharges, this study examined length of stay and nursing care time as measures of resource consumption. It found that age; medical comorbidities; and presence of procedures such as computed tomography scans, electroencephalograms, and electroconvulsive therapy were valuable predictors of increased costs.

14. **Fetter RB, Shin Y, Freeman JL, Averill RF, Thompson JD:** Case mix definition by diagnosis-related groups. *Med Care* 18 (suppl):1–53, 1980

This article explains the original methodology used to categorize all medical illnesses into 468 diagnosis-related groups. According to the authors, this classification system was designed to be medically meaningful, manageable, applicable to existing hospital discharge abstracts, comparable across different coding schemes, and fair in determining amount of reimbursement for resources utilized as approximated by the length of stay.

15. **Freiman MP, Mitchell JB, Rosenbach ML:** An analysis of DRG-based reimbursement for psychiatric admissions to general hospitals. *Am J Psychiatry* 144:603–609, 1987

Actual payments under Medicare for nonexempt psychiatric services are based on a diagnosis-related group (DRG) category, which is adjusted for outliers, hospital location, area wage levels, and teaching status. This article reports a simulation of how hospitals in four states would fare in a fully phased-in DRG-based payment system. On average, general hospitals with psychiatric units not currently included in the DRG payment methodology would fail to recover the actual costs for psychiatric care and become net financial losers under a DRG system.

16. **Leibenluft E, Leibenluft RF:** Reimbursement for partial hospitalization: a survey and policy implications. *Am J Psychiatry* 145:1514–1520, 1988

The authors contacted major third-party payers to determine reimbursement policies for partial hospitalization. Private insurers are interested mainly in acute care partial hospitalization. An extracontractual agreement is suggested as the method to overcome reimbursement barriers for chronic care.

17. **McGuire TG, Dickey B, Shively GE, Sturmvasser I:** Differences in resource use and cost among facilities treating alcohol, drug abuse and mental disorders: implications for design of a prospective payment system. *Am J Psychiatry* 144:616–620, 1987

The authors examined 30,000 inpatient admissions. Three diagnosis-related groups (DRGs) accounted for the majority of admissions, but there was significant variation in resource use both across and within

DRGs. General hospitals with "scatter bed" psychiatric services were systematically overpaid, whereas specialized psychiatric units were systematically underpaid. More costly patients are likely to be treated on distinct-part psychiatric units.

18. **Mitchell JB, Dickey B, Liptzin B, Sederer LI:** Bringing psychiatric patients into the Medicare prospective payment system: alternatives to DRG's. *Am J Psychiatry* 144:610–615, 1987

   The authors used Medicare data from four states to examine two patient classification systems as alternatives to diagnosis-related groups (DRGs) in determining prospective payments. Both disease staging and clinically related groups were superior to DRGs in explaining variation in hospital costs and length of stay, but both had severe limitations for reimbursement purposes.

19. **O'Connell RA:** Time-limited treatment: the DRG challenge, in *Common Treatment Problems in Depression*. Edited by Schatzberg AF. Washington, DC, American Psychiatric Press, 1985, pp. 101–117

   O'Connell discusses the impact of diagnosis-related groups (DRGs) on the actual clinical work of the individual practicing psychiatrist from initial decision of whom to admit to the increased importance of discharge planning, along with the issues of "skimming" and "DRG creep."

20. **Scherl DJ, English JT, Sharfstein SS** (eds): *Prospective Payment in Psychiatric Care*. Washington, DC, American Psychiatric Association, 1988

   This collection of articles and reviews summarizes the implications for policy directions of the major research studies on prospective payments, including those done by the American Psychiatric Association, the National Alliance for the Mentally Ill, and the National Association of Private Psychiatric Hospitals and the results of the New Jersey experience. Other topics include the impact of pricing, the role of caps, and the function of peer review and quality assurance in changing reimbursement schemes.

Physician Payment Systems

21. *Dorwart RA, Chartock LR:** Psychiatry and the resource-based relative value scale. *Am J Psychiatry* 145:1237–1242, 1988

   The authors describe the derivation of a resource-based relative value scale physician payment system and the difficulties of operationalizing such a system for psychiatry. There is a dearth of procedures. Cross-specialty comparisons are difficult. It promotes subspecialization, and it leads to rigidly standardized treatment approaches.

22. **Hsiao W, Braun P, Becker ER, Thomas SR:** The resource based relative value scale: toward the development of an alternative physician payment system. *JAMA* 258:799–802, 1987

    The authors propose a system for determining physicians fees based on time spent performing a service, the practice costs, the lost opportunity costs during years of training, the intensity and complexity of the physical and mental effort involved, and the level of stress including potential liability. These components are combined into a relative value determination by a mathematical formula.

23. **Mechanic D, Aiken LH** (eds): Paying for services: promises and pitfalls of capitation. *New Dir Ment Health Serv* 43:1–122, 1989

    This entire book-length issue is devoted to a discussion of the capitation approach to financing mental health services. It presents capitation from the perspective of both theoreticians and implementers, and many examples of both positive and negative results using a capitation model are given. Of particular note is an article by Stein on the Wisconsin system of mental health financing and an article by Babigian and Marshall on the Rochester Comprehensive Mental Health Capitation experiment.

Managed Care and Utilization Management

24. **American Psychiatric Association Committee on Managed Care:** *Utilization Management: A Handbook for Psychiatrists.* Washington, DC, American Psychiatric Association, 1992

    This book is the most complete and easily understood guide to utilization management. It provides a step-by-step explanation of the process of utilization management. It has chapters on frequently encountered problems and their solutions; confidentiality and the handling of medical records; and a review of the legal, financial, organizational, and operational considerations that need to be taken into account when contracting. Appendices give a listing of chief executive officers and medical directors of major insurance and managed care companies.

25. **Bennett MJ:** The Greening of the HMO: implications for prepaid psychiatry. *Am J Psychiatry* 145:1544–1549, 1988

    Bennett contrasts the sound practices of long-established health maintenance organizations with the volatility and profit orientation of newer ones. An earlier idealistic emphasis on making equitable and affordable health care more available has been replaced by preoccupation with technical dimensions of practice and exclusion of high-risk patients. Mental health benefits are a particular target for limitation.

26. **England MJ, Vaccaro VA:** New systems to manage mental health care. *Health Aff (Millwood)* 10:129–137, 1991

The authors provide a description of the models and unique features of managed mental health care that have been developed by a number of the largest corporate purchasers of care, such as McDonnell Douglas, First Chicago, Pacific Bell, IBM, Chevron, and Digital. The concerns about quality, which commonly arise in managed care systems, are discussed.

27. **Fink PJ, Health WR:** No free lunch: limitations on psychiatric care in HMO's. *Hosp Community Psychiatry* 42:363–365, 1991

The authors examine the means by which some health maintenance organizations (HMOs) seek to provide less mental health care. The type and extent of services are limited by narrowing the diagnostic groups treated, contracting with nonpsychiatrist therapists, serving institutions that agree to cut benefits, paying bonuses to providers for delivering less care, and using HMO-generated utilization review criteria.

28. **Hodgkin D:** The impact of private utilization management on psychiatric care: a review of the literature. *Journal of Mental Health Administration* 19:143–157, 1992

Despite the impressive growth of third-party management of mental health care during the last decade, this comprehensive review article makes clear how little is known about its impact on quality of care, outcome, or economics. In the privately insured sector, limited evidence exists of decreased costs to the payer. There have been few rigorous studies of the effect of utilization management on patients, providers, and society.

29. **National Association of Private Psychiatric Hospitals:** *1991 Survey on Utilization Management Firm's Conducting Psychiatric Review.* Washington, DC, National Association of Private Psychiatric Hospitals, 1991

This is a report of the results of a yearly survey conducted by the National Association of Private Psychiatric Hospitals of member facilities concerning their experiences with outside utilization review. More than 70% of admitted patients now require outside preadmission approval and continued-stay review for reimbursement. Frequently cited problems included reviewers lacking expertise or experience, inconsistent application of review criteria, failure to explain criteria, and increased demands on staff time.

30. **Norquist GS, Wells KB:** How do HMO's reduce outpatient mental health care costs? *Am J Psychiatry* 148:96–101, 1991

The authors compared a group of health maintenance organization (HMO) enrollees with a group covered by a fee-for-service plan. Both groups were drawn from a similar demographic group and had similar prevalence of psychiatric disorder and access to specialty mental health care. The HMO group had fewer visits per user, suggesting the provision of a less intensive style of care.

31. **Sederer LI, St. Clair RL:** Managed health care and the Massachusetts experience. *Am J Psychiatry* 146:1142–1148, 1989

The authors review precedents for organized psychiatry's role in managed care in Philadelphia (Pennsylvania) and New Haven (Connecticut) and nationally before reporting on the activities of the Massachusetts Psychiatric Society. These include certification of managed mental health plans, monitoring of utilization review organizations, and development of a second opinion service.

32. *Tischler GL:** Utilization management of mental health services by private third parties. *Am J Psychiatry* 147:967–973, 1990

Tischler describes the current process of utilization management and examines some of the sources of friction that frequently arise when applied to psychiatric services. The differing models of mental illness and the varying theoretical orientations of clinicians leave much room for professional uncertainty and discretionary behavior in psychiatric care. Significant geographic variations in service capacity and coordination leave gaps in availability of alternatives to inpatient care. Concern for privacy of patients leads to incomplete or vague reporting of symptoms and diagnoses. Liability risks outweigh cost-containment concerns in physician decision making.

33. **Wilenseky GR, Rossiter LF:** Coordinated care and public programs. *Health Aff (Millwood)* 10:62–77, 1991

The authors report on the current status of the Health Care Financing Administration's efforts to promote managed care as an alternative to traditional fee-for-service medicine. The full continuum of choices are outlined from health maintenance organizations to primary care case management, and recipient incentives to choose these options are described.

The Offset Effect and Cost Effectiveness

34. **Borus JF, Olendzki MC, Kessler LG, Burns BJ, Brandt UC, Broverman CA, Henderson PR:** The "offset effect" of mental health treatment on ambulatory medical care utilization and charges. *Arch Gen Psychiatry* 42:573–580, 1985

    The authors conducted a 5-year ambulatory medical care study of 400 patients with mental disorders. Psychiatric treatment was associated with significant offset savings for medical care. However, the costs of the psychiatric care boosted the overall care charges above those of patients treated solely by their primary physicians.

35. **Krupnick JL, Pincus HA:** The cost-effectiveness of psychotherapy: a plan for research. *Am J Psychiatry* 149:1295–1305, 1992

    The authors point out the paucity of research in this area and the conceptual issues that would need to be addressed in methodologically sound cost-effectiveness studies. These include the target population, type of psychotherapy, length of treatment, type of clinician, treatment context, outcome measures, health care costs and utilization, and social costs and social service utilization.

36. **Levitan SJ, Kornfeld DS:** Clinical and cost benefits of liaison psychiatry. *Am J Psychiatry* 138:790–793, 1981

    This study found that the availability of liaison psychiatric services considerably shortened the postoperative course of elderly patients who had undergone surgical repair of hip fractures compared with a control group. Psychiatric intervention resulted in a saving of 12 days of hospitalization on average and contributed to better outcome as measured by patients able to return home. This is the classic study establishing that psychiatric services can contribute to efficiency and cost savings in institutional settings.

37. **Roper WL, Winkenwerder W, Hackbarth GM, Krakauer H:** Effectiveness in health care: an initiative to evaluate and improve medical practice. *N Engl J Med* 319:1197–1202, 1988

    The authors give their views on deficiencies in research on effectiveness of medical interventions resulting in wide variations in practice patterns and unnecessary costs. They propose a new science of health care evaluation based on rigorous outcome studies, epidemiologic statistics, and mathematical modeling leading to greater standardization of practice. They report on such efforts being undertaken by the Health Care Financing Administration and the Public Health Service.

38. **Schlesinger HJ, Mumford E, Glass GV:** Mental health treatment and medical care utilization in a fee-for-service system. *Am J Public Health* 73:422, 1983

    The authors studied federal employees' insurance claims for care in fee-for-service private medical practices. Savings were achieved for patients suffering from chronic medical illnesses who received mental health treatment within 1 year of their medical diagnosis.

Insurance Coverage for Mental Health Services

39. **Fein R:** *Medical Care, Medical Costs: The Search for a Health Insurance Policy.* Cambridge, MA, Harvard University Press, 1986

    This book provides both history and analysis of the evolution of private health insurance and government third-party payment through Medicare and Medicaid. It deals extensively with the particular problems in coverage specific to middle class, elderly, and poor patients. The author outlines his proposal for a universal insurance program with cost-containment mechanisms.

40. **Keeler EB, Wells KB, Manning WG:** *The Demand for Episodes of Mental Health Services* (R-3432-HHS/NIMH). Santa Monica, CA, Rand Corporation, 1986

    The health insurance experiment conducted by the Rand Corporation starting in 1974 involved more than 6,000 subjects in a randomized controlled study of the effect of insurance on demand for health services. It demonstrated that increases in the price of services, such as co-payments and deductibles, result in a decrease in utilization. Although the authors initially concluded that mental health services are no more price sensitive than general health services, this reexamination of the data indicates greater price-responsiveness for outpatient mental health services.

41. **Sharfstein SS, Taube CA:** Reductions in insurance for mental disorders: adverse selection, moral hazard, and consumer demand. *Am J Psychiatry* 139:1425–1430, 1982

    The authors examine the cause for severe cutbacks in the federal employees health benefit program for psychiatric care. These include the accumulation of high-risk consumers, the carelessness of enrollees in running up large charges, and the lack of overt consumer demand due to reluctance of psychiatric patients to speak up and let their needs be known.

Private Practice

42. **Astrachan B, Sharfstein SS:** The income of psychiatrists: adaptation during difficult economic times. *Am J Psychiatry* 143:885–887, 1986

   Psychiatrists have lower earnings than physicians in procedurally oriented specialties. However, the authors demonstrate that relative to other cognitive medical specialists, such as pediatrics and internal medicine, psychiatrists do better on an hourly basis. Psychiatrists have had to become more efficient, productive, and diverse in their treatments to remain competitive. Subspecialization and multiple work settings have become trends.

43. **Sharfstein SS, Beigel A:** How to survive in the private practice of psychiatry. *Am J Psychiatry* 145:723–727, 1988

   The authors note that patients are paying more out-of-pocket for psychiatric care through demand-side cost sharing, and health care providers are being forced to assume more of the financial risk of treatment through supply-side cost sharing. Specific suggestions for adaptation include joining health maintenance organizations and preferred payment organizations, increased medical staff activity, broadening of patient case mix, and participation in research studies.

Planning for Mental Health Services

44. **Allen JG, Coyne L, Lyle J, Spohn HE:** Assessing need for extended psychiatric hospitalization. *Compr Psychiatry* 33:346–352, 1992

   The authors assessed a wide range of variables that possibly influence length of hospital stay. Longer stays were correlated with a more chronic course, worse premorbid functioning, organic impairment, and poorer outside support. Severity of impairment in the current episode was not related to length of stay.

45. **de Figueiredo J, Boerstler H:** The relationship of presenting complaints to the use of psychiatric services in a low-income group. *Am J Psychiatry* 145:1145–1148, 1988

   The authors examined the relationship between type of presenting complaint, race, ethnicity, gender, age, marital status, diagnosis, source of referral, and previous use of psychiatric services. Individuals presenting with social complaints tended to be low users of services, whereas those presenting with medical complaints were likely to be high users.

46. **Hillard JR, Slomowitz M, Deddens J:** Determinants of emergency psychiatric admission for adolescents and adults. *Am J Psychiatry* 145:1416–1419, 1988

    The authors identified a combination of variables that predicted odds of hospitalization. For adolescents, these were suicidal tendencies, physical abuse, schizophrenia, and age. For adults, these were delusions, aggressive behavior, suicidal tendencies, and either schizophrenia or affective disorder.

47. **Klerman GL, Olfson M, Leon AC, Weissman MM:** Measuring the need for mental health care. *Health Aff (Millwood)* 11:23–33, 1992

    The authors address the complexity of determining the need for mental health services as a prerequisite for planning. Account must be taken of epidemiology and the prevalence of mental illness, clinical research on the effectiveness of treatment, and mental health policy research on financial and organizational issues.

48. **Regier DA, Boyd JH, Burke JD Jr, Rae DS, Myers JK, Kramer M, Robins LN, George LK, Karno M, Locke BZ:** One month prevalence of mental disorders in the United States. *Arch Gen Psychiatry* 45:977–986, 1988

    The authors report the prevalence results of the five-site National Institute of Mental Health Epidemiologic Catchment Area (ECA) study. More than 15% of the population 18 years and older met criteria for a substance abuse or mental disorder during the preceding month. Epidemiologic studies such as the ECA form the basis for public health policy planning. The identified sociodemographic correlates of mental disorders are essential to construction of sound financing schemes for mental health care.

49. **Rice DP, Kelman S, Miller LS, Dunmeyer S:** *The Economic Costs of Alcohol and Drug Abuse and Mental Illness: 1985.* San Francisco, CA, Institute for Health and Aging, University of California, 1990

    The staggering cost attributable either directly or indirectly to mental illness and substance abuse are well outlined in this book-length report submitted to the Office of Financing and Coverage Policy of the Alcohol, Drug Abuse and Mental Health Administration (ADAMHA). Separate chapters deal with the conceptual issues related to cost-of-illness studies, morbidity and mortality costs, and special groups (e.g., those with acquired immunodeficiency syndrome or fetal alcohol syndrome and the homeless population).

50. **Taube CA, Goldman HH, Burns BJ, Kessler LG:** High users of outpatient mental health services, I: definition and characteristics. *Am J Psychiatry* 145:19–24, 1988

The authors present data from the National Medical Care Utilization and Expenditure Survey for the year 1980. Of individuals who utilized mental health outpatient visits during the year, less than 10% accounted for more than 50% of mental health expenditures through multiple visits. One-third of the high-users group were significantly disabled and had multiple medical disorders, rather than the stereotype of the healthy, high-functioning individual in long-term psychoanalytic therapy.

51. **Taube CA, Goldman HH, Burns BJ, Kessler LG:** High users of outpatient mental health services, II: implications for practice and policy. *Am J Psychiatry* 145:24–28, 1988

The authors present data to refute widely held beliefs in the insurance industry that psychiatric outpatient treatment is discretionary, ill-defined, and interminable. They suggest that different types of treatment episodes vary in their responsiveness to price. The most efficient mechanism to control costs is intensive case management and clinical review of the high-user group.

Privatization

52. *Dorwart RA, Schlesinger M:** Privatization of psychiatric services. *Am J Psychiatry* 145:543–553, 1988

The authors provide an overview of the privatization trend in mental health policy. They examine the reasons for the rapid growth of the private hospital sector and the balance between the for-profit and nonprofit hospitals.

53. **Eisenberg L:** The case against for-profit hospitals. *Hosp Community Psychiatry* 35:1009–1012, 1984

Eisenberg sees for-profit hospitals as a departure from the historic goal of medical care: the maximization of the health status of the general population. He raises concerns about access to care; quality of care; costs of care; and the impact on public sector programs, research, and training.

54. **Fisher WH, Dorwart RA, Schlesinger M:** The role of general hospitals in the privatization of inpatient treatment for serious mental illness. *Hosp Community Psychiatry* 43:1114–1119, 1992

The authors examined general hospitals' practices in accepting referrals from community mental health centers and emergency rooms.

Half of all general hospitals now treat patients with serious mental illness. However, significant, although decreasing, differences exist between public and private general hospitals with regard to payer mix. Many patients formerly treated at state hospitals now go to public general hospitals.

55. **Levenson AI:** The growth of investor owned psychiatric hospitals. *Am J Psychiatry* 139:902–907, 1982

Levenson expresses concern about proprietary psychiatric hospital chains with regard to their admitting practices, quality of care, treatment approaches, and philosophy.

56. **Rafferty FT:** The case for investor-owned hospitals. *Hosp Community Psychiatry* 10:1013–1016, 1984

Rafferty views investor-owned hospitals as a natural development within a capitalist democracy. Good and bad hospitals exist in all ownership categories. Quality depends more on good management, personnel, and fiscal and physical resources, rather than type of ownership.

62

Military Psychiatry

David R. Jones, M.D.

M ilitary psychiatric practice is qualitatively different from its civilian counterpart in some important respects; these writings focus on the differences. Medical care in the service occurs in an authoritarian and judgmental societal subsegment that maintains an active third-party role in the patient-therapist relationship. The military psychiatrist is concerned with maintaining a person's ability to function in worldwide settings, often with very little medical support. Some military people must work in chronically severely stressful situations involving extremes of personal and group danger. Frequently the military psychiatrist must predict the degree of incapacity for productive work resulting from personality disorders of varying severity. Overt psychotic and severe anxiety-based mental diseases disqualify a person for military duty. The military psychiatrist must also deal with two unique manifestations of stress—combat reactions and aviators' fear of flying—which are almost never seen in the civilian world. Military life also imposes unusual demands on families, and some references address family moves, recurrent separations, and the continuing subtheme of possible violent death of the military member. The focus is thus on occupational decisions, stress tolerance, healthy psychological defenses, the ability to handle fear, and the affirmation of mental health.

On the more proactive side, the needs of military psychiatrists have produced some concepts of community mental health programs, group support systems, rapid and goal-directed therapeutic techniques, and preventive mental health programs that have been integrated into the mainstream of American psychiatry. These writings provide a reasonably broad introduction to military psychiatry, and their references will carry the interested reader into the mainstream of this literature.

General Military Psychiatry

1. **Belenky G** (ed): *Contemporary Studies in Combat Psychiatry.* New York, Greenwood Press, 1987

   Drawing especially on work done at the Walter Reed Army Institute of Research, this volume, edited by one of the United States Army's experts in this field, is an excellent introduction to their findings and doctrine.

2. *__Bey DR, Chapman RE:__ Psychiatry: the right way, the wrong way, and the military way. *Bull Menninger Clin* 38:343–354, 1974

   The authors present an even-handed comparison of the differences in focus, goals, and methods of military and civilian psychiatric practice. Some of the military approaches may be useful in civilian organizational or industrial applications, such as balancing the needs of the worker against those of the organization, or working with employees who face danger as a part of their jobs (e.g., oil rig, pararescue, mining).

3. *__Blaustein M, Proctor WC:__ The active duty conscientious objector: a psychiatric-psychological evaluation. *Milit Med* 142:619–621, 1977

   This article reviews the life stories, clinical presentations, and psychological assessments of a group of conscientious objectors, as well as the administrative procedures necessary to establish conscientious objector status.

4. **Garfield RM, Neugut AI:** Epidemiologic analysis of warfare: a historical review. *JAMA* 266:688–692, 1991

   This article is an overview of the direct health effects of various wars on military and civilian populations during the last 200 years. Risk factors for injury and death are analyzed. Indirect effects, including crowding, deprivation, lack of sanitation, and shortage of medical care, are considered. Specific examples include the influenza outbreak following World War I, discarded ordnance, the 3-to-2 ratio of civilian to military casualties in low-intensity warfare, and the relatively recent recognition of posttraumatic stress disorder.

5. **Goldman NL, Segal DR:** *The Social Psychology of Military Service* (Sage Research Progress Series on War, Revolution and Peacekeeping, Vol. 6). Beverly Hills, CA, Sage, 1976

This series of excellent presentations covers areas of military stress: basic training, combat, the organizational environment, family pressures, reentry into the civilian community, and civil-military relations. The extensive bibliography will allow the interested reader to follow up any of these topics in depth.

6. *In the service of the state: the psychiatrist as double agent (spec suppl). *Hastings Cent Rep* 8:1–24, 1978

This article reports on a conference sponsored by the American Psychiatric Association and by the Institute of Society, Ethics, and the Life Sciences in 1977. It is a responsible and articulate look at the dilemma of the psychiatrist who must serve not only the interests of the patient, but also the interests of an institution or organization. Addressing issues of loyalty, confidentiality, societal interests, and individual rights, it offers no specific answers, but certainly clarifies the questions.

7. *Jones DR:** Aeromedical transportation of psychiatric patients: historical review and present management. *Aviat Space Environ Med* 51:709–716, 1980

Jones traces the history of aeromedical evacuation of psychiatric patients in war and in peace. Present indications and cautions are considered from the aeromedical and from the psychiatric points of view.

8. **Lande RG:** Military psychiatry and criminal law. *Milit Med* 157:392–397, 1992

This article provides guidance for performing clinical psychiatric evaluations of criminally accused persons within the United States military court martial system. As in the civilian world, the boundary between law and psychiatry is difficult to traverse. Lande reviews military regulations and case law and provides suggestions to enhance the control, quality, and value of the consultation. The clinician needs honest and comprehensive disclosure from the accused to ensure a complete forensic assessment, and this may conflict with legal concerns. Confidentiality and compliance are specifically discussed, along with their practical ramifications.

9. **Shanfield SB:** The military psychiatrist: themes of separation and dislocation. *Psychiatric Annals* 8:255–260, 1978

Shanfield discusses his experiences (and those of some of his peers) in his 2 years as a "Berry Plan" drafted military psychiatrist. This is a thoughtful article about the dynamics of adjustment to military psychiatry for psychiatrists trained in civilian institutions.

10. *United States Medicine* Vol. 27, No. 15–16. August 1991

This entire issue is dedicated to medicine in the Gulf War. Psychiatric problems were not a major factor, but morale was not always high during the 6-month build-up. Morale has a reciprocal relationship to combat fatigue.

11. *Watson P: *War on the Mind: The Military Uses and Abuses of Psychology.* New York, Basic Books, 1978

This is a very readable and complete review of psychological factors in military endeavors, covering combat factors, stress research, loyalty (and its dark side, treason), and counterinsurgency. Specific attention is paid to psychological warfare, combat psychiatry (preventive and therapeutic measures), and issues of leadership. Watson is far from being a military apologist, and sees his viewpoint as a moderate attitude. If you can read only one book on the interface between emotional factors and military life, this is the book to read.

12. **Wise MG:** The past, present and future of psychiatric training in the U.S. Armed Services. *Milit Med* 152:550–553, 1987

This article traces the history of military psychiatry and its training programs, from the first reports of "nostalgia" during the Civil War down through Vietnam. The "90-day wonders," general medical officers given a brief crash course in psychiatry, served their country well in World War II, and many of them took residencies in the specialty after the war. The lessons of the past, particularly those regarding the lag time required in each war to learn about the unique aspects of military and combat psychiatry, point toward the necessity of maintaining a sufficient core of career military psychiatrists in peacetime. Recent experiences in mobilizing an expeditionary force for the Gulf War underscore the author's concerns.

Combat Psychiatry

13. **Fox RP:** Narcissistic rage and the problem of combat aggression. *Arch Gen Psychiatry* 31:807–811, 1974

Fox distinguishes between individual aggression as a response to combat dangers and as a quest for personal revenge for a significant loss. This dynamic distinction may be of use in working with issues of guilt and grief in combat veterans.

14. **Fullerton CS, Ursano RJ:** Behavioral and psychological responses to chemical and biological warfare. *Milit Med* 155:54–59, 1990

Chemical warfare is sometimes regarded as causing all-or-none casualties: you either survive or you die. In fact, acute exposure to nerve agents and to other organo-phosphates, especially at repeated low-dose levels (as with crop dusters), may lead to a symptomatic picture of acute psychiatric complaints and performance disruptions. This article reviews the literature on long-term consequences of acute and chronic exposures to such agents. In addition, stress-related responses to chemical warfare training are considered: casualties may run as high as 15%, especially if the psychological stress is accompanied by significant heat stress. (As an added note, six Israeli civilians were asphyxiated during the Iraqi Scud attacks because their gas masks' inlet ports were jammed, and they were so frightened of the threat of gas that they died rather than pull off the masks.)

15. **Grinker RR Sr, Spiegel JP:** *Men Under Stress.* New York, McGraw-Hill, 1945

This book is mainly concerned with the reactions of United States troops to the campaign in North Africa in World War II and is one of the classics of combat psychiatry. Its discussion of the dynamics of the individual case histories is particularly valuable.

16. *Hausman W, Rioch D:** Military psychiatry: a prototype of social and preventive psychiatry in the United States. *Arch Gen Psychiatry* 16:727–739, 1967

This superb historical review summarizes the evaluation of Army doctrine on the care of men with combat neurosis. Some of these principles were applied to community psychiatry after World War I and are still used in primary, secondary, and tertiary preventive settings and in evaluating some aspects of the relationship between the individual and the environment.

17. **Hendin H, Haas AP:** Combat adaptations of Vietnam veterans without posttraumatic stress disorders. *Am J Psychiatry* 141:956–960, 1984

Perhaps the question should be not "Why do some veterans have posttraumatic stress disorder?," but "Why don't they all?" The authors studied 10 veterans of intense combat who did not and found a consistent adaptation pattern. During combat, these men had been calm, maintained intellectual control, accepted their fear, and did not engage in excessively violent or guilt-arousing behavior. The authors conclude that the telling factor is not the combat experience alone, but "how those events and situations were perceived, integrated and acted upon that bears the primary relationship to the postcombat response" (p. 959).

18. **Holsenbeck LS:** "PSYCH-FORCE 90": the OM (combat stress) team in the Gulf. *Journal of the U.S. Army Medical Department* PB-8-92-3/4:32–36, 1992

    The activation of the 528th Medical Department during Operation Desert Shield/Storm marked the first time that the United States Army has sent a combat stress team into a combat operation. During its 171 days in the theater, this multidisciplinary mental health team of 25 officers and 33 enlisted troops evaluated 514 soldiers, holding 124 for treatment and evacuating 18 from the theater. They also performed 811 command consultations with company-sized units, briefing them on the importance of early recognition and treatment of combat stress symptoms. As is always true with medical innovation, a number of lessons were learned the hard way, but it seems clear that this tactical approach to the prevention and treatment of combat stress disorders will be refined and reapplied in future conflicts.

19. **Ingraham LH, Manning FJ:** Psychiatric battle casualties. *Military Review* 60:19–29, 1980

    This summary reviews the roles of the commander and of the mental health professional in preventing or at least minimizing losses from combat exhaustion in a fluid battle situation such as anticipated in a major conventional war.

20. **Kalinowsky LB:** Problems of war neuroses in the light of experiences in other countries. *Am J Psychiatry* 107:340–346, 1950

    This unique article compares and contrasts some of the English, American, German, and Japanese experiences with the psychological effects of combat on civilian and military populations in World War I and World War II. Such an epidemiologic approach allows for an assessment of the role of secondary gain and compensation factors in judging the long-term effects of "war neuroses," with concomitant implications for treatment.

21. *Milgram NA** (ed): *Stress and Coping in Time of War: Generalizations From the Israeli Experience.* New York, Brunner/Mazel, 1986

    Seventh in the "Psychological Stress Book Series," this collection of 22 chapters deals with the role of attribution in stressful situations, risk factors, treatment of acute and posttraumatic stress disorders, performance under stress, and the effects of war on civilian populations. Because much of the combat stress literature since the Vietnam War has come from the careful work of Israeli investigators, this book provides, in one source, a general survey of their results.

22. **Noy S:** Battle intensity and the length of stay on the battlefield as determinants of the type of evacuation. *Milit Med* 152:601–607, 1987

This scholarly view of the usually chaotic scene of battle concerns the factors involved in a soldier's leaving and returning to the battlefield for many different reasons, including psychiatric symptoms. Factors studied include length of stay in combat, number of casualties, days away, and the risk of chronic or "permanent" symptoms. Noy equates successful return to the unit with avoidance of later posttraumatic stress disorder.

23. **Richardson FM:** *Fighting Spirit: A Study of Psychological Factors in War.* New York, Crane, Russak, 1978

Written by a British Army physician with extensive combat experience and a thorough grounding in medical and military history, this is an articulate and convincing presentation of the author's views on the causes, treatment, and (most important) prevention of combat fatigue. This book is a basic text for any military physician who may face combat.

24. *Salmon TW:** War neuroses ("shell shock"). *Military Surgery* 41:674–693, 1917

This is truly a classical reference. Salmon had visited the psychiatric hospitals of several allied nations and distilled their experiences with "war neurosis" and its treatment into a formulation that has consistently been successful in rapidly returning to duty about 75% of soldiers thus affected. His epidemiologic point of view was remarkably advanced and accurate.

25. **Scurfield RM, Tice SN:** Interventions with medical and psychiatric evacuees and their families: from Vietnam through the Gulf War. *Milit Med* 157:88–97, 1992

The authors present a personalized and dramatic picture of combat psychiatry, much of it in patients' words. Integrating family concerns and patient management issues, they review the way psychiatric problems in combat were experienced in Vietnam, Panama, and the Persian Gulf. Specific stressors faced by women, ethnic minorities, and National Guard and reserve returnees are highlighted. The presentation ends with clinical considerations and some of the stressors that can affect therapists. Well written and well referenced, this article is an excellent summary of nonpharmaceutical issues involved in combat stress reactions today.

26. **Sokol RJ:** Early mental health intervention in combat situations: the USS *Stark*. *Milit Med* 154:407–409, 1989

   On May 17, 1987, the USS *Stark* was struck by two Iraqi Exocet missiles, which killed 37 of its crew of 212 and wounded dozens more. This sudden and unexpected attack combined elements of combat stress and disaster stress, and part of the United States Navy's response was to dispatch a stress management team to the ship. This brief article outlines the team's observations of the clinical effects and the group process.

27. **Steiner M, Neumann M:** Traumatic neurosis and social support in the Yom Kippur War returnees. *Milit Med* 143:866–868, 1978

   The authors conclude that lack of social support, poor unit identification, lack of trust in leadership, displacement, and rotation all contribute to the condition of late-onset posttraumatic combat reactions. In contrast, positive social support helps prevent "traumatic neurosis of war," even in conditions of severe stress.

28. **True PK, Benway MW:** Treatment of stress reaction prior to combat using the "BICEPS" model. *Milit Med* 157:380–381, 1992

   BICEPS, an acronym for brevity, immediacy, centrality, expectancy, proximity, and simplicity, was coined by D. R. Jones for the United States Air Force's Medical Red Flag Exercises in the early 1980s. It brings together the principles identified by Salmon during World War I, disseminated by Army psychiatrists in World War II, and augmented by F. D. Jones during and after the Vietnam War. This case report describes a classic acute stress reaction in a young marine who was quickly and appropriately treated by medical authorities, aided by the cooperation of his unit. Following 3 days of brief therapy, he was returned to his unit, where he was restored to full duties without stigma or any feeling of failure. One hopes that such early and vigorous treatment will forestall later development of posttraumatic symptoms.

Aerospace Psychiatry

29. **Bond DD:** *The Love and Fear of Flying*. New York, International Universities Press, 1952

   An often-cited classic, this book summarizes the World War II experience with combat stress disorders and fear of flying in the fliers of that day. Of particular note is the psychoanalytical perspective on the emotional components of flying, the development of fear of flying, and aspects of treatment. This volume is the starting point for any knowledgeable discussion of aviation psychiatry.

30. **Deakins DE, Baggett JC, Bohnker BK:** Brief reactive psychosis in naval aviation. *Aviat Space Environ Med* 62:1166–1170, 1991

Although psychotic disorders are almost always permanently disqualifying for fliers, a few persons with brief reactive psychoses have been considered for a return to flying privileges. This article presents five case studies and considers the aeromedical factors involved in reaching such decisions. These include the need for clear distinction between functional and organic psychoses and determining whether an organic psychosis is completely reversed without residue and with no increased chance for recurrence. The final decision must be jointly made by physicians skilled in aerospace medicine and in psychiatry.

31. **Fine PM, Hartman BO:** *Psychiatric Strength and Weaknesses of Typical Air Force Pilots* (Report No. SAM-TR-68-121). San Antonio, TX, Brooks Air Force Base, 1968

This is an extensive report of psychodynamic and psychometric studies of Air Force pilots, comparing them with the "super pilots" chosen as astronaut candidates in the early 1960s. These characterizations are of particular value to anyone who routinely deals with professional fliers.

32. **Jones DR:** Psychiatric assessment of female fliers at the U.S. Air Force School of Aerospace Medicine (USAFSAM) *Aviat Space Environ Med* 54:929–931, 1983

During 1976–1982, 3,669 male and 34 female fliers were referred for medical evaluation. Of the men, 570 (15%) were referred for psychiatric evaluations, compared with 17 (50%) of the women. Of the 570 men, 367 (64%) were returned to flying, compared with 9 (53%) of the 17 women. The circumstances of referral and the small numbers of females make the interpretation of these numbers difficult to evaluate for trends, but women sent to the U.S. Air Force School of Aerospace Medicine during that era had a significantly higher ($P = .025$) chance of being grounded than men. Jones presents a few clinical vignettes to illustrate the particular pressures that affected these women fliers.

33. *Jones DR:** Flying and danger, joy and fear. *Aviat Space Environ Med* 57:131–136, 1986

What motivates people to undertake a profession as dangerous as flying high-performance military jet aircraft? This formulation proposes a continuum stretching between a purely emotional (and largely subconscious) attraction to flying as a means of assuming power over death and a purely rational decision that it is a pretty good way to earn a living. Those who decide to fly may later decide to cease flying without paying any particular emotional price, but those who are deeply attracted may experience marked symptoms of anxiety or depression when their motivation weakens or when their defenses against fear are over-whelmed. Too, some motivation is counterphobic or displaced and may give way quickly when the stresses of actual flight supersede the fanta-sies of power found in some pilot trainees. Illustrated with six case histories, this article considers the nature of motivation to fly, its various modes of failure, and some clinical aspects of fear of flying in aviators.

34. *Jones DR, Perrien JL:** Neuropsychiatry in aerospace medicine, in *Fundamentals of Aerospace Medicine.* Edited by DeHart RL. Philadelphia, PA, Lea & Febiger, 1985, pp. 538–570

This textbook chapter serves as a basic introduction to the interface between the aerospace milieu and the disciplines of psychiatry, psychol-ogy, and neurology.

35. **Leiman Patt HO:** The right and wrong stuff in civil aviation. *Aviat Space Environ Med* 59:955–959, 1988

Most of the "fear of flying" literature concerns either military aviators or airline passengers; this article discusses the civil aviation pilot. The author discusses the interplay of motivation to fly, defenses against anxiety, and aviation stress to explain the manifestations of flight adap-tation and maladaptation seen in some aviators.

36. **Little LF, Gaffney IC, Rosen KH, Bender MM:** Corporate instability is related to airline pilots' stress symptoms. *Aviat Space Environ Med* 61:977–982, 1990

A "symptoms of stress" questionnaire was administered to three samples of commercial airline pilots: one group represented an airline with a history of corporate instability, and two groups represented more stable airlines. The first group reported significantly more symptoms of stress and depression. Considering the present turmoil in the airline industry, the authors conclude that the relationship between corporate instabil-ity and pilots' distress should be further investigated from a health and safety standpoint.

37. *Perry CJ** (ed): *Psychiatry in Aerospace Medicine* (International Psychiatry Clinics, Vol. 4). Boston, MA, Little Brown, 1967

The editor brought together a highly qualified panel of authors who covered this complex field in depth. Among the subjects covered are the emotional considerations in selecting a flying career, the psychophysiology of aerospace medicine, normative psychological data, fear of flying, emotional factors in aircraft accidents, psychiatric aspects of being in space, and clinical aspects of psychiatric illness in flying. This is a solid background text for those who must deal with the emotional aspects of flying.

38. **Picano JJ:** Personality types among experienced military pilots. *Aviat Space Environ Med* 62:517–520, 1991

Using a sample of 170 experienced United States Army pilots, Picano identifies three clusters of personality subtypes. The variety of personalities found among these experienced and successful pilots reminds those who treat them to be careful about stereotypical expectations.

39. *Reinhardt RF: The outstanding jet pilot. *Am J Psychiatry* 127:732–736, 1970

This study of 105 Navy pilots, selected by their peers as the best, showed most to be firstborn, with unusually good father-son relationships. They were self-confident, were not introspective, and tended toward interpersonal distance. It is a fine study of a mentally healthy and successful population.

40. **Retzlaff PD, Gilbertini M:** Air Force pilot personality: hard data on the "Right Stuff." *Multivariate Behavioral Research* 22:383–399, 1987

Using a sample of 350 United States Air Force student pilots, the authors identified three distinct personality types; these correspond well with the types later defined by Picano (1991) above. These two articles help to translate the dime-novel "right stuff" folklore into a more conventional and professional description of fliers' personality traits, thus increasing our understanding of the people who undertake such exciting, dangerous, and responsible careers.

41. **Roberts RJ:** Passenger fear of flying: behavioural treatment with extensive in-vivo exposure and group support. *Aviat Space Environ Med* 60:342–348, 1989

Fear of flying in passengers has proven amenable to classic behavioral modification techniques: relaxation, systematic desensitization, cognitive restructuring, education, in vivo exposure, and group support. This article, based on the use of these techniques on 158 passengers, reports 90% were flying with greater ease afterward among the 42% who responded to a questionnaire.

42. **Sledge WH:** Aerospace psychiatry, in *Comprehensive Textbook of Psychiatry/III,* Vol. 3. Edited by Kaplan HI, Freedman AM, Sadock BJ. Baltimore, MD, Williams & Wilkins, 1980, pp. 2902–2914

This chapter furnishes an introduction to aerospace psychiatry, providing sufficient information for anyone seeking a brief, broad overview. The references, which cover the field through 1977, furnish greater length on specific subjects.

43. **Sledge WH, Boydstun JA:** Vasovagal syncope in aircrew: psychosocial aspects. *J Nerv Ment Dis* 167:114–124, 1979

Comparing 24 aviators who had vasovagal syncope with 26 control subjects, the "fainters" were found to be younger and slightly less adaptable and to have significantly more negative feelings about their work. This article demonstrates the utility of considering the psychosocial perspective, as well as the physiological and pathological, when evaluating such episodes.

44. **Sledge WH, Boydstun JA:** The psychiatrist's role in aerospace operations. *Am J Psychiatry* 137:956–959, 1980

The authors emphasize the special stressors and occupational requirements of aviation and "the ambiguous role of the aerospace psychiatrist" (p. 956). Two case reports of fliers with vasovagal syncope illustrate the influence of occupational factors on the world of the aviator.

45. **Strongin TS:** A historical review of the fear of flying among aircrewmen. *Aviat Space Environ Med* 58:263–267, 1987

Strongin reviews the use of the term *fear of flying* to describe 65 years of data concerning anxiety disorders, traumatic stress, exhaustion, psychosis, and changes in motivation to fly in peace and in war. He suggests three basic questions to ask in such instances: Do the symptoms arise from a preexisting disorder? Was the ego overwhelmed from situational stress, or exhausted from overwork? Have changes in the life situation temporarily altered the flier's motivational and defensive structure? These factors may occur alone or in combination. (The reader must remember that fear of flying that occurs in a flier who previously enjoyed aviation is considerably different in etiology, course, treatment, and prognosis from that prevalent in some 15% of the general population.)

Space Psychiatry

46. **Kanas N:** Psychological and interpersonal issues in space. *Am J Psychiatry* 144:703–709, 1987

Reviewing more than 60 United States and Soviet space simulator studies performed on earth, along with space mission reports, Kanas identified nine psychological and seven interpersonal issues. The psychological issues were sleep problems; time sense disturbances; demographic effects; career motivation; stages of reaction to isolation; transcendent experiences; postflight personality changes; psychosomatic reactions; and anxious, depressive, and psychotic reactions. Interpersonal issues were tensions, problems resulting from crew heterogenicity, anger displaced to outside persons, need for dominance, decreased cohesiveness over time, task-neutral interactions, and types of leadership. Several research areas are suggested: rapid screening methods for motivation, for covert psychopathology, and for predicting crew cohesion factors. Education of crew members about psychological and interpersonal factors should be emphasized. Crew interactions should be studied at different stages of the mission, especially types of interactions, signs of developing interpersonal tensions, and formal versus informal leadership. Finally, we need to develop and test strategies for dealing with psychiatric emergencies in space (e.g., psychoses, suicidality). Methods that could be considered include speech stress analysis, training a lay crew member, or working through ground communications to validate their use.

47. *Santy P: The journey out and in: psychiatry and space exploration. *Am J Psychiatry* 140:519–527, 1983

Santy reviews much of the literature concerning clinical psychiatry and psychology available at the time and summarizes it well. This literature is considered as it pertains to astronaut and crew selection, isolation and confinement, hyperarousal and sensory overload, group interactions, human-machine interactions, psychophysiological studies, stress-related responses, and biological rhythms. She closes with speculations on future information necessary for successful long-duration space flight and how to get it.

48. **Santy PA, Holland AW, Faulk DM:** Psychiatric diagnoses in a group of astronaut applicants. *Aviat Space Environ Med* 62:969–973, 1991

In an attempt to systematize the "select-out" portion of the psychiatric examination of astronaut applicants, a standardized, semistructured clinical interview was developed to evaluate the presence or absence of psychiatric disorders. Some 117 applicants underwent this clinical interview as a part of their 1-week comprehensive medical evaluation. Of the 117, 9 (7.7%) met DSM-III-R criteria for marital problem (2); adjustment disorder (2); and (1 each) parent-child problem, phase of life problem, uncomplicated bereavement, and anxiety disorder (Axis I). Under Axis II, one each had compulsive personality disorder, narcissistic personality disorder, and schizotypal personality disorder. (Two individuals had one diagnosis on each axis.) Of the 9 with diagnoses, only 1, who had a nondisqualifying resolving adjustment disorder, was chosen to become an astronaut. Once selected into the astronaut corps, applicants who passed this evaluation will be "selected-in" to a specific crew or mission. These select-in criteria are considerably different from the select-out process and are presently under investigation to validate their use.

Prisoners of War

49. **Beebe GW:** Follow up studies of World War II and Korean war prisoners. *Am J Epidemiol* 101:400–422, 1975

    This is a large and rather carefully controlled follow-up study of the morbidity, disability, and maladjustments of three groups of United States prisoners of war: those captured by the Germans in World War II, by the Japanese in World War II, and by the Koreans in the Korean War. Data are given on both somatic and psychiatric conditions. The role of malnutrition is especially emphasized.

50. **Segal J, Hunter EJ, Segal F:** Universal consequences of captivity: stress reactions among divergent populations of prisoners of war and their families. *International Social Science Journal* 28:593–609, 1976

    This study compares data on individual and family reactions to wartime captivity, drawing on data from World War II, the Korean War, and the Vietnam War. Children suffer too, not only as prisoners, but within the families where the father has been absent because of captivity. This is an excellent review article.

51. **Ursano RJ:** The Viet Nam era prisoner of war: precaptivity personality and the development of psychiatric illness. *Am J Psychiatry* 138:315–318, 1981

    This unique study of six fliers with extensive pre- and postcaptivity psychiatric and psychological evaluations indicates that the presence of precaptivity psychiatric symptoms is neither necessary nor sufficient for the development of psychiatric illness after repatriation.

52. **Ursano RJ, Rundell JR:** The prisoner of war. *Milit Med* 155:176–180, 1990

    Ursano was one of the Air Force psychiatrists who followed the Air Force fliers who were repatriated from the Hanoi prisoner of war

(POW) camp in 1973. This review concerns the role of environmental and cultural factors in the POW experience. Communication, maintenance of the military social structure, and personal flexibility are crucial coping mechanisms, and their presence or absence, along with the severity of the captivity experience, play major roles in postrepatriation mental health or illness. The most common disorders seen include the sequelae of illness, injury, or malnutrition; posttraumatic stress disorder; adjustment disorders; depression; anxiety disorders; substance abuse; and family problems. The excellent reference list will be of particular value to anyone interested in these issues.

53. **Ursano RJ, Wheatley R, Sledge W, Rahe A, Carlson E:** Coping and recovery styles in the Vietnam era prisoner of war. *J Nerv Ment Dis* 174:707–714, 1986

United States Air Force prisoners used four general coping styles in captivity, with varying degrees of success. No style is clearly associated with an increased risk of psychiatric morbidity after repatriation. This article summarizes much of the work of these investigators to date, and its references offer a wide range of citations to their previous publications.

Military Families

54. **Beckman K, Marsella AJ, Finney R:** Depression in the wives of nuclear submarine personnel. *Am J Psychiatry* 136:524–526, 1979

Nuclear submarine crews live in a continuing cycle of 3 months at sea and 3 months at home. Their wives, studied in a crossover research design, showed evidence of increased depressive symptoms during the cruise months. Anecdotal data (including use of medical facilities) support this report.

55. **Bey DR, Lange J:** Waiting wives: women under stress. *Am J Psychiatry* 131:283–286, 1974

This is an excellent report of a seldom-mentioned subject: the stresses and conflicts of wives whose husbands are away in combat or on other prolonged absences (such as remote overseas tours). The authors suggest some specific support structures that might lessen the personal and marital stresses.

56. **Lagrone DM:** The military family syndrome. *Am J Psychiatry* 135:1040–1043, 1978

This study compares 792 juvenile military family members with a comparable civilian group and concludes that the former group has a predominance of behavioral disorders. Lagrone cites several possible causes, although these are admittedly theoretical, and suggests several possible alleviating programs.

57. **Lagrone DM:** More on the military family syndrome (letter). *Am J Psychiatry* 139:133–134, 1982

This letter, and Morrison's reply (same page), continue the dialogue begun in their articles in 1978 (above) and 1981 (below), respectively. The questions raised are applicable to much that has been published about military families and highlight the epidemiologic problems inherent in comparing spouses or children of military members with their civilian counterparts.

58. **Morrison J:** Rethinking the military family syndrome. *Am J Psychiatry* 138:354–357, 1981

Written in reply to Lagrone's (1978) article above, this report cites data on children of military and nonmilitary families seen in the author's practice. No denominator data are given for the population base from which these patients are drawn. Morrison is skeptical about any "military family syndrome" and raises some significant questions.

63

Occupational Psychiatry

Jay B. Rohrlich, M.D.

A t least one-third of our lives is spent at work. Our jobs can trigger physical and mental disorders. They can also be instrumental in recovering from illness. We can feel loved through the admiration our work earns, as well as rejected and emotionally disabled from job loss. Occupational goals and accomplishments are central to our identities. Work organizations structure our lives. We discharge aggression when we "attack" tasks and feel masterful when we "conquer" them. We earn our places in civilization through our work. We reduce guilt through hard labor. We defy time with productivity. The people we love, hate, fear, and need come as importantly from our offices, factories, and shops as from our families and communities. Occupational psychiatrists focus clinically on the human psyche in the workplace. They may enter the work setting directly or indirectly to examine or treat individual, group, or large-scale organizational problems that arise there. They may be called on to consult with executives on the psychological implications of corporate structure and policy. Occupational psychiatrists are concerned not only with the psychological impact of the workplace on the emotional health of individuals or groups, but also with the impact of people's behavior on the quality of life in the workplace and its optimal functioning.

I am indebted to Barrie Greiff, M.D., for his generous assistance in the preparation of this chapter.

Although psychiatrists who work with employees of government agencies, hospitals, prisons, colleges, and the armed forces can rightly be called "occupational psychiatrists," these specialists have organized separately. Because the historical origins of occupational psychiatry are in profit-oriented industrial organizations, those people who call themselves "occupational psychiatrists" for the most part continue to function in private sector settings.

The greatest contribution of occupational psychiatry to the overall field of psychiatry is the idea that the internal and external dynamics of people's work lives are of equal importance to understanding and treating them as are the dynamics of their personal lives.

I have emphasized references in this chapter that introduce occupational psychiatry to readers who are relatively unfamiliar with the field. Moreover, there is an abundance of citations that deal with the intrapsychic dimensions of work—work as a state of mind and not simply as a state of employment. The works by Fenichel (1938), Hendrick (1943), Kramer (1977), Lantos (1943, 1952), Menninger (1942), and Oberndorf (1951) have been generally overlooked in most surveys of the occupational psychiatry literature.

I have also inserted a section on "Stress and Psychopathology in the Workplace." Two of these citations discuss the specifics of particular occupations—pilots and air traffic controllers—in terms of 1) the unique stresses involved in them, 2) the personality profiles that optimize adjustment, and 3) the types of psychopathology that are most commonly found. I included these works primarily because they serve as prototypes for psychiatric thinking and involvement in the problems of specific occupations.

History and Overview

1. *Brodsky C: Occupational psychiatry, in *Review of General Psychiatry.* Edited by Goldman HH. Los Altos, CA, Lange Medical Publications, 1984, pp. 667–676

   This is a concise overview of the role of the psychiatrist functioning in the work setting. This is a nontheoretical presentation of the variety of psychiatric activities in the workplace. Particularly interesting is the discussion of the management of "special problems," such as evaluation for disability, absenteeism and malingering, mass psychogenic illness, and industrial accidents. There is also a section on forensic consultations.

2. *Greiff B: The history of occupational psychiatry. *Psychiatric Opinion* 12:10–18, 1978

This article is an excellent review of historical developments in the practice of psychiatry in the industrial workplace. Greiff addresses the impact of the industrial revolution, which changed the nature of work in the United States from 90% farming in 1790 to less than 4% in 1980. He discusses the psychological and sociological impact of Frederick Taylor's (born 1856, the same year as Freud) "scientific management," which broke industrial work down into the smallest mechanical components and rearranged them to maximize efficiency. He also makes reference to the dehumanizing effect of Frank Gilbreth's (1868–1924) very influential "motion economy," whose sole objective was to maximize productivity. The survey moves through the early 20th century and World War II to the present, making references to the enormous variety of corporate and academic programs that dealt with the mental health of men and women in the workplace.

3. *Group for the Advancement of Psychiatry: *An Introduction to Occupational Psychiatry*. Washington, DC, American Psychiatric Press, 1994

This is a comprehensive overview of the current state of occupational psychiatry, including specific recommendations about entry into the field and techniques of practice. Five models of occupational consultation (from the dyadic relationship with an individual to involvement in corporate policy making) are discussed. Some of the conflicts inherent in the work (e.g., issues of confidentiality) are described. Profiles of several practitioners, outlines for work and organizational history taking, and a comprehensive bibliography are included.

4. **Herzberg F:** *Work and the Nature of Man*. New York, World Publishing, 1966

A professor of management argues that industry must satisfy its workers' inner as well as external needs, or else take a painfully high human toll, and demonstrates how work organizations must make work meaningful and enriching. Herzberg has been a very influential thinker about the optimal work environment.

5. *Mayo E: *The Human Problems of an Industrial Civilization*. New York, Macmillan, 1934

This is an early classic from the Harvard Business School defining the social systems and clinical approaches appropriate to a work setting. Landmark research was conducted at the Hawthorne plant of Western Electric from 1929 to 1933. Mayo decries the dehumanizing effect of then-popular "time in motion" and "human engineering" approaches to people in the workplace and argues that sensitivity to the psychological dimension of workers is humane and also good business.

6. **McLean AA:** Report of the Task Force on Psychiatry and Industry. *Am J Psychiatry* 141:1139–1144, 1984

   This article is a position paper promoting the need for psychiatry to be proactive in forming relationships with industry. McLean was regional medical director of IBM for many years, and his extensive writing and innovative programs have been of critical importance to the growth of occupational psychiatry.

7. *****Neff W:** Psychoanalytic conceptions of the meaning of work. *Psychiatry* 28:324–333, 1965

   This article is a detailed survey of the evolution of psychoanalytic thinking on work. Starting with Freud, whose references are scattered and sparse because of a belief that work represented a renunciation of the instincts and was ruled by the reality principle, Neff goes on to discuss the contributions of Erik Erikson, whose developmental approach addressed work's influence on such issues as mastery and identity. Neff surveys the works of Hendrick, Lantos, Menninger, and Oberndorf and concludes that "work behavior appears to be too complex to be satisfactorily accounted for within the framework of psychosexual development" (p. 333) and that its unique qualities await a comprehensive psychology of its own.

8. **Sherman M:** A review of industrial psychiatry. *Am J Psychiatry* 6:701–710, 1927

   The first overview of the field of psychiatric consultation in the workplace, this article is written by the former chairman of the Department of Psychiatry at Northwestern University. Sherman discusses a number of intrapsychic theories dealing with work situations, but places strong emphasis on a developmental approach.

9. **Southard EE:** The modern specialist in unrest: a place for the psychiatrist in industry. *Mental Hygiene* 4:550–563, 1920

   This is a plea from the early years of our profession that psychiatric insights be actively applied to people in their work setting. "Industrial medicine exists, industrial psychiatry ought to exist. It is important for the psychiatrist not to hide his light under a bushel, but to step forth to new community duties" (p. 563).

10. **Sperry L:** *Psychiatric Consultation in the Workplace.* Washington, DC, American Psychiatric Press, 1993

    Sperry heads an occupational psychiatry program at the Medical College of Wisconsin. His comprehensive book focuses on clinical challenges with rank-and-file employees to senior executives. It is divided into three sections. The first section, "Occupational Psychiatry," deals with the needs and conflicts of occupational psychiatrists as they encounter the organizational arena. His treatment of the translation of traditional clinical psychiatric expertise to the workplace is particularly illuminating. The second section, "The Practice of Workplace Psychiatry," deals with four main issues: executive consultations, employee consultations, organizational consultation, and transitional consultation. The third section, "Special Issues in Workplace Psychiatry," focuses on executive stress; neurotic behavior in executives and organizations; job loss; balancing personal, family, and work life; women executives; family-owned businesses; cultural diversity in the workplace; and confidentiality and ethical issues. This is an extremely well-written and comprehensive overview of the field.

11. *Terkel S: *Working*. New York, Pantheon Books, 1972

This book contains moving personal accounts of people describing their jobs. Interviews include those with farmers, waitresses, factory workers, salespersons, poets, executives, stockbrokers, grave diggers, and others.

12. *Work in America: Report of a Special Task Force to the Secretary of Health, Education, and Welfare*. Cambridge, MA, MIT Press, 1973

This landmark document had a great impact on public policy with regard to the fundamental role of work in adult life and the ways in which jobs that do not address people's needs for individual responsibility and autonomy can lead to "declining physical and mental health, greater family and community instability . . . and an increase in drug abuse, alcohol addiction, aggression, and delinquency" (p. xvi). This was very influential in the implementation of programs for mental health in corporate settings.

Intrapsychic Dynamics

13. *Fenichel O: The drive to amass wealth. *Psychoanal Q* 7:69–95, 1938

The drive to accumulate money is integral to understanding a central motivation for work. Fenichel took Freud's theoretical perspective and applied it to an analysis of the unconscious meanings of money. His thinking goes beyond traditional anal dynamics and begins to look at ego-psychological perspectives. He discusses rational motives, power needs, the desire for possessions, and sociological sources. This is an important article on understanding the dynamics of ambition.

14. *Freud S:* Those wrecked by success (1915), in *Some Character Types Met With in Psychoanalytic Work: Collected Papers,* Vol. 4. Edited by Jones E. New York, Basic Books, 1959, pp. 323–342

This work by Freud discusses several clinical cases—and Lady Macbeth—in which the achievement of something consciously wished for leads to emotional catastrophe. Freud's formulation centered on superego conflicts and Oedipal guilt arising from the gratification of forbidden impulses. His ideas have since been extended by numerous other authors on success neuroses to include not only guilt but conflicts over dependency, identity diffusion, responsibility, and other factors.

15. **Furman E:** Thoughts on pleasure in working. *Bulletin of the Philadelphia Psychoanalytic Association* 19:197–212, 1969

This article presents a child analyst's summary of the developmental evolution of work gratifications from the toddler stage, ages 3–5, latency, and adolescence.

16. *Hendrick I:* Work and the pleasure principle. *Psychoanal Q* 12:311–329, 1943

This is the first of Hendrick's landmark papers proposing a "work principle . . . the need of human beings for the pleasure afforded by effective integration of the neuromuscular and intellectual functions" (p. 327). Hendrick believed that a fundamental drive, separate from the pleasure and reality principles, needed to be postulated to understand the intrapsychic motivation to work. I do not believe that this is necessary, but Hendrick's thinking is provocative.

17. *Jaques E:* *Creativity and Work.* Madison, CT, International Universities Press, 1990

This is a brilliant series of papers on a variety of work-related topics by a psychoanalyst and professor of management. Jaques coined the term *mid-life crisis* in an article contained herein. Jaques is an extremely literate writer who treats the subject of work with great originality and philosophical breadth. There are 17 articles in this book whose titles range from "The Conscious, Preconscious, and Unconscious Experience Called Time" to the "Work-Payment-Capacity Nexus."

18. *Kramer Y:* Work compulsion: a psychoanalytic study. *Psychoanal Q* 46:361–385, 1977

Kramer explores a cases of compulsive work with unconscious castration and homosexual dynamics and extends the discussion into a general treatment of the unconscious meanings of work.

19. **Lantos B:** Work and the instincts. *Int J Psychoanal* 24:114–119, 1943

Lantos distinguishes between "three principles of activity: the principle of playing; the principle of learning; and the principle of working" (p. 118) and sees play as activity for its own sake, work as serving ends of self-preservation, and learning as preparatory to work.

20. **Lantos B:** Metapsychological considerations on the concept of work. *Int J Psychoanal* 33:439–443, 1952

This is a later article by Lantos that sees work as "the voluntary submission to hardship and boredom for the sake of self-preservation. . . . It is not the object or the skill of the activity which makes the difference between work and play, but the participation of the super-ego, which changes play activities into work activities" (p. 442).

21. *__**Menninger K:**__ Work as a sublimation. *Bull Menninger Clin* 6:170–182, 1942

This is a very important and lucid article that relates work to the aggressive instinct and contradicts the need for Hendrick's mastery instinct. It explores the vicissitudes of aggression. "All work represents a fight against something, an attack upon the environment. . . . All this is done in order to create something, for which reason we can call it work and not rage. . . . Destructiveness is . . selectively directed, and a net 'product' is obtained" (p. 171).

22. **Oberndorf CP:** Psychopathology of work. *Bull Menninger Clin* 15:77–85, 1951

In this analysis of work inhibition, Oberndorf sees libidinal cathexis of work as a cornerstone of adult maturation.

Organizational Dynamics

23. *__**Brown W, Jaques E:**__ *The Glacier Project Papers*. London, Heinemann, 1965

Anything by Jaques is must reading. This book resulted from a 17-year study of the operations of the Glacier Metal Company, of which Brown was chairman of the board. The authors bring psychoanalytic insight to bear on such issues as the meanings of work, organizational policy, job performance, and union negotiations.

24. *__**Hirschhorn L:**__ *The Workplace Within*. Cambridge, MA, MIT Press, 1990

Hirschhorn examines the rituals that organizations develop to cope with change and uses the work of Bion and his concepts of "social defenses" as the theoretical underpinning of this very illuminating book, which bridges the intrapsychic and the organizational.

25. *Levinson H: *Organizational Diagnosis*. Cambridge, MA, Harvard University Press, 1972

This book provides a template for analyzing and diagnosing an organization's history, current actions, and direction. It uses psychoanalytic approaches integrated into systems theory. Levinson believes that by using this system, one can determine the strengths and weaknesses of an organization. This is must reading for a psychiatrist working in an organizational structure.

26. **Speller J:** *Executives in Crisis*. San Francisco, CA, Jossey-Bass, 1989

Extensive case histories illustrate psychopathology in people at the top of corporations. Written for a popular audience as a guide to recognizing mental illness, alcoholism, and drug addiction, this book nevertheless provides helpful insights for psychiatrists about the process of dealing with troubled people within organizations.

Work-Family Dynamics

27. *Greiff G, Munter P:* Tradeoffs: Executive, Family, and Organizational Life.* New York, New American Library, 1980

Grieff and Munter, psychiatrists to the Harvard Business School and Harvard Law School, respectively, explore the compromises between personal harmony and occupational success essential to healthy adaptation. This book was the culmination of a landmark business school course that Greiff taught for many years on "the executive family."

28. **Kates M, Greiff B, Hagen D:** *The Psychosocial Impact of Job Loss*. Washington, DC, American Psychiatric Press, 1989

In this integrative study of the impact of unemployment on the individual and the family, the authors discuss strategies of psychiatric intervention after job loss and present psychologically informed approaches to public policy on unemployment.

29. *Rohrlich JB:* Work and Love: The Crucial Balance.* New York, Summit Books, 1980

Rohrlich defines the opposing psychological dynamics of working and loving. Work is goal directed, structured, ego oriented, and fed by the aggressive drive. Love is sensory, present oriented, ego transcending, and fed by the erotic drive. This book explores the psychopathology of those "addicted" to work at the expense of family relationships, love, and leisure.

Stress and Psychopathology in the Workplace

30. *Davidson MJ, Cooper CL: A model of occupational stress. *J Occup Med* 23:564–574, 1981

   In this multidisciplinary approach to work stress involving the interaction of demands from psychological, sociological, and physiological areas, Davidson and Cooper use coronary-prone individuals as the clinical focus to demonstrate the pathological influence of organizational and extraorganizational factors.

31. **Rose RM:** Predictors of psychopathology in air traffic controllers. *Psychiatric Annals* 12:925–933, 1982

   In this 6-year multidisciplinary study of 416 air traffic controllers, 15% of the subjects had significant psychopathology, and another 20% experienced milder symptomatology but significant subjective distress. Rose discusses the host of psychosocial predictors that identified those susceptible to psychopathology, such as impulse control, sense of responsibility, low marital support, and alcohol consumption. The author mentions the issue of preventive intervention at the individual and workplace level. Increased support from co-workers and supervisors was central to prevention.

32. *Sledge WH: Aerospace psychiatry (Chapter 46.2), in *Comprehensive Textbook of Psychiatry/III*, 3rd Edition, Vol. 3.   Edited by Kaplan HI, Freedman AM, Sadock BJ. Baltimore, MD, Williams & Wilkins, 1980, pp. 2092–2914

   In great detail, this chapter documents the range of physical stressors (e.g., acceleration forces that cause motion sickness and spatial disorientation) and psychological stressors that distinguish the work of fliers and astronauts. Personality characteristics of those best equipped to function as aviators are detailed: ability to balance compliance to rules and routines with responsibility and initiative, freedom from impulsiveness with adaptive quickness in the face of danger, tolerance for long hours of work at a stretch alternating with long periods of rest, and ability to withstand long periods of separation from home and family. Psychiatric problems most frequently encountered are psychophysiological disorders, anxiety and depressive disorders, alcoholism, and paranoid personality disorders (grandiose and persecutory). Special problems such as prisoners of war and hijacking are discussed.

Psychiatric Research

Charles A. Kaufmann, M.D.
Vajramala Bhatia, M.D., M.A., M.Ed.

This chapter is intended as a general introduction to the art and science of psychiatric research. In it, we introduce the reader to basic principles of scientific reasoning, of statistical inference, and of study design and analysis. Both theoretical and pragmatic considerations in the conduct of psychiatric research are entertained, and the promises and pitfalls of various designs and analytic approaches are outlined. Subsequently, we provide an overview of the variety of investigational strategies currently available to the psychiatric researcher. This overview focuses on books, chapters, and papers that our consultation with acknowledged experts in each of the represented fields has suggested best highlight the strategy, its capabilities, and its limitations. It presents a panoply of approaches to understanding the brain and the mind in health and disease, approaches that explore the range of phenomena from the molecular to the societal level. It is intended to be broad, but shallow, in its scope, and to serve as an entree to the relevant literature. The chapter concludes with a discussion of three topics of practical concern to beginning and established psychiatric researchers alike: research ethics, research training, and research funding. We hope that this chapter will enable the reader to become a more critical practitioner and/or consumer of psychiatric research.

Basic Principles

1. **Kuhn TS:** *The Structure of Scientific Revolutions*, 2nd Edition. Chicago, IL, University of Chicago Press, 1970

   This monograph is a landmark introduction to the history and sociology of "normal" science, in which underlying "paradigms," which direct scientific theorizing and experimentation, are not themselves subject to scientific inquiry (and falsification), but may be overturned by new paradigms they spawn to explain otherwise inexplicable "anomalous" phenomena. It serves as a sobering commentary on how the scientific method can simultaneously facilitate and inhibit discovery.

2. ***Platt JR:** Strong inference. *Science* 146:347–353, 1964

   This is another classic contribution attempting to explain those circumstances under which the scientific method is most productive: when alternative hypotheses are clearly articulated and when critical and readily interpretable experiments refuting some of these hypotheses are performed. It purports to provide a blueprint for scientific success, based on formulating falsifiable hypotheses, with examples drawn from disciplines ranging from high-energy physics to molecular biology.

3. **Popper KR:** *The Logic of Scientific Discovery*. New York, Harper & Row, 1968

   This epistemological manifesto similarly stresses the centrality of falsifiable hypotheses and provides a lucid discussion of the inductive generation of theories, the deductive testing of theories, and the role of probability in "corroborating" theories.

Study Design and Analysis

Basic Statistics, Study Design, and Bias

4. **Bailar III JC, Mosteller F:** *Medical Uses of Statistics*, 2nd Edition. Waltham, MA, NEJM Books, 1991

   This volume is an excellent, user-friendly introduction to biostatistics, with special emphasis on medical research applications. In addition to presenting elementary topics in research design and analysis, it guides the reader through more advanced topics, like meta-analysis and survival analysis, which have of late increasingly appeared in the medical literature.

5. **Begg CB, Berlin JA:** Publication bias: a problem in interpreting medical data. *Journal of the Royal Statistical Society A* 151:419–463, 1988

This is a commentary on the practice of investigators being more likely to submit, and editors being more likely to publish, studies with significantly positive results. It identifies those features of studies (e.g., small sample size) that render them especially sensitive to publication bias, the impact of this practice on meta-analysis, and the changes in editorial policy that might diminish its effect.

6. **Halbreich U, Bakhai Y, Bacon KB, Goldstein S, Asnis GM, Endicott J, Lesser J:** The normalcy of self-proclaimed "normal volunteers." *Am J Psychiatry* 146:1052–1055, 1989

This study emphasizes the high rates of current, past, and familial psychopathology among volunteer research subjects and the influence of this self-selection bias on the generalizability of research results.

7. **Spohn HE, Fitzpatrick T:** Informed consent and bias in samples of schizophrenic subjects at risk for drug withdrawal. *J Abnorm Psychol* 89:79–92, 1980

Spohn and Fitzpatrick highlight the biases inherent in studying neuroleptic-withdrawn patients with schizophrenia—biases that are introduced during recruitment, informed consent screening, and attrition due to early relapse—and bring into question the generalizability of data derived from drug-withdrawal "surviving" subjects.

ANOVA and MANOVA

8. **Ekstrom D, Quade D, Golden RN:** Statistical analysis of repeated measures in psychiatric research. *Arch Gen Psychiatry* 47:770–772, 1990

This survey of 343 articles published in major psychiatry research journals reveals the rarity with which appropriate multivariate statistics (11%)—or univariate statistics with appropriate adjustments (6%)—are applied to the analysis of repeated measures data from parallel groups designs.

9. **Lavori P:** ANOVA, MANOVA, my black hen. *Arch Gen Psychiatry* 47:775–778, 1990

This accompanying commentary provides a balanced response to Ekstrom et al. (1990) above, defining the variety of repeated measures and exploring both the possibilities and the problems inherent in their analysis with multivariate analysis of variance; among the latter are the sensitivity of this approach to missing data and its inability, even when it can detect that groups differ in some way, to specify the ways in which those groups differ.

Comparisons Among Means

10. **Keppel G:** Analytical comparisons among treatment means, in *Design and Analysis: A Researcher's Handbook*, 2nd Edition. Englewood Cliffs, NJ, Prentice-Hall, 1982, pp. 103–125

   This chapter provides a comprehensive, albeit technically sophisticated, overview of the variety of statistical approaches for comparing subsets of variables, and hence specific hypotheses, within complex parallel groups designs.

Decision Analysis and Receiver Operating Characteristic Analysis

11. **Murphy JM, Berwick DM, Weinstein MC, Borus JF, Budman SH, Klerman GL:** Performance of screening and diagnostic tests: application of receiver operating characteristic analysis. *Arch Gen Psychiatry* 44:550–555, 1987

   This article represents the introduction of receiver operating characteristic analysis—a statistical approach deriving its name from its initial application to radar studies during World War II—to the psychiatric literature. This approach, which has come to play an important role in the field of clinical decision analysis, permits the diagnostic utility of various instruments or tests to be compared and allows threshold scores on these instruments or tests that optimize diagnostic sensitivity and specificity to be determined.

12. **Pauker SG, Kassirer JP:** Decision analysis. *N Engl J Med* 316:250–258, 1987

   This review discusses decision analysis, a statistical approach based on characterizing the decision-making process as a probabilistic decision tree, specifying several potential outcomes, assigning these outcomes valences and likelihoods, and optimizing the result. It considers the potential of this approach to provide a quantitative guide to clinical decision making for both practitioners and patients.

13. **Sandercock P:** The odds ratio: a useful tool in neurosciences. *J Neurol Neurosurg Psychiatry* 52:817–820, 1989

   This article describes the odds ratio as a measure of association between an exposure or a treatment and a particular outcome and discusses its relative utility, compared with more traditional measures like the chi-square statistic, in aiding the interpretation of case-control studies, descriptive studies, and comparisons among studies.

Measurement and Reliability

14. *Bartko JJ, Carpenter WT Jr: On the methods and theory of reliability. *J Nerv Ment Dis* 163:307–317, 1976

This classic article provides a very readable introduction to the most frequently used (and misused) interrater reliability measures and an important guide to choosing the most suitable measure given the nature of the data being analyzed (be they categorical or quantitative) and the number of raters being compared.

15. Snaith RP: Measurement in psychiatry. *Br J Psychiatry* 159:78–82, 1991

This report offers a helpful overview of the variety of measures used in psychiatry, ranging from self-report and direct observation to physiological indices and psychological test results, and presents a rational basis for evaluating such measures according to the scope of the phenomena they assess, as well as their sensitivity, specificity, reliability, and validity.

Meta-Analysis

16. Dickersin K, Berlin JA: Meta-analysis: state-of-the-science. *Epidemiol Rev* 14:154–176, 1992

This review examines meta-analysis, an emerging statistical approach that allows the outcomes of a large collection of individual studies to be compared, contrasted, and integrated. While emphasizing the potential of this approach, even to the point of suggesting that "prior to embarking on any research study, a meta-analysis should be attempted in order to establish reliably what is already known" (p. 156), the article also attends to possible problems in its application, namely, the lack of combinability of studies, publication bias, underascertainment (via electronic means) of those studies that make it to publication, and the uncertain reliability of meta-analysis itself.

Multiple Regression

17. Cohen J, Cohen P: Applied multiple regression, in *Correlation Analysis for the Behavioral Sciences*. Hillsdale, NJ, Lawrence Erlbaum, 1975, pp. 73–122

This chapter discusses the extension of bivariate linear regression and correlation techniques to the case where two or more independent variables are linearly related to a dependent variable. It offers a lucid exposition of the variety of approaches to multiple regression that exist, considers issues of statistical power, and provides worked examples.

Multivariate Statistics

18. **Nunnally JC:** Fundamentals of factor analysis, in *Psychometric Theory*, 2nd Edition. New York, McGraw-Hill, 1978, pp. 327–404; **Nunnally JC:** Special issues in factor analysis, in *Psychometric Theory*, 2nd Edition. New York, McGraw-Hill, 1978, pp. 405–436

These two chapters present an extraordinarily readable introduction to the fundamentals of factor analysis, the broad category of mathematical procedures for determining groupings or clusterings of variables. They cover hypothesis-independent methods for "condensing" variables (exploratory factor analysis) and hypothesis-dependent methods for testing groupings (confirmatory factor analysis), related approaches such as cluster and image analysis, and an extensive list of caveats that should be borne in mind in the interpretation of factors derived from these procedures.

19. *Stevens J:** Discriminant analysis, in *Applied Multivariate Statistics for the Social Sciences*, 2nd Edition. Hillsdale, NJ, Lawrence Erlbaum, 1992, pp. 273–302

This chapter focuses on discriminant analysis, a statistical approach that may be used to describe major differences among groups analyzed in a multivariate analysis of variance, as well as to classify subjects into groups on the basis of a battery of measurements. As with other chapters in Steven's text, a clear theoretical discussion is paired with a practical implementation of the approach using popular statistical packages such as SAS and BMDP.

Power Analysis

20. *Cohen J:** The concepts of power analysis, in *Statistical Power Analysis for the Behavioral Sciences*, 2nd Edition. Edited by Cohen J, Cohen P. Hillsdale, NJ, Lawrence Erlbaum, 1988, pp. 1–17

Type II errors (false acceptance of the null hypothesis, based on the mistaken conclusion that an absence of proof constitutes a proof of absence) have received relatively little attention when compared with type I errors (false rejection of the null hypothesis, based on the mistaken conclusion that the presence of proof constitutes a proof of presence). Nonetheless, their assessment is critical to the evaluation of research results and may be achieved through a statistical method known as power analysis. This introductory chapter in the acknowledged bible of power analysis, written by its acknowledged prophet, provides a cogent overview of the method.

21. **Pulver AE, Bartko JJ, McGrath JA:** The power of analysis: statistical perspectives, part 1. *Psychiatry Res* 23:295–299, 1988

The power of a statistical test refers to the probability of its detecting a difference or effect, should one truly exist. It represents the converse of the type II error (when type II error is high, statistical power is low). Despite the importance of statistical power considerations in the interpretation of studies, this survey of 154 published articles reporting nonsignificant Student's *t* test results suggests that less than half had sufficient power to reject the null hypothesis, owing to small numbers of subjects, small differences between means, or both.

Single Case Designs

22. **Guyatt GH, Heyting A, Jaeschke R, Keller J, Adachi JD, Roberts RS:** N of 1 randomized trials for investigating new drugs. *Controlled Clin Trials* 11:88–100, 1990

Although this article considers single subject study designs in pharmacological research, it has clear implications for the evaluation of other treatments (such as psychotherapy and psychoanalysis).

Research Approaches

Animal Models and Neuroethology

23. **Willner P:** Methods for assessing the validity of animal models of human psychopathology, in *Animal Models in Psychiatry, I*. Edited by Boulton AA, Baker GB, Martin-Iverson MT. Clifton, NJ, Humana Press, 1991, pp. 1–23

This introductory chapter to a text on animal models in psychiatry suggests a variety of criteria against which such models may be validated, including face validity (i.e., phenomenological similarity between the animal model and the human condition being modeled), construct validity (i.e., basing the model on a sound theoretical foundation), and predictive validity (i.e., observing comparable responses to manipulation in both the model and the condition). Having suggested these criteria, the chapter goes onto to evaluate how a number of animal models of, for example, anorexia, depression, and medication responsiveness, fare.

Cognitive and Computational Neuroscience

24. **Churchland PS, Sejnowski TJ:** Perspectives on cognitive neuroscience. *Science* 242:741–745, 1988

This theoretical overview of approaches to how the "mind-brain" works draws rough parallels between levels of analysis in computer science (the level of problem solving, the level of algorithms used in problem solving, and the level of physical implementation of those algorithms) and the levels of organization in the nervous system (the level of systems and maps, the level of networks and layers, and the level of neurons, synapses, and molecules). Using color vision as an example, it displays the transition from (and convergence of) physiology and psychology and discusses various experimental windows (ranging from anatomic lesions and positron-emission tomography to patch clamp techniques and single unit recordings) on the functioning of the brain at its various levels.

Epidemiology

25. **Eaton WE:** Epidemiology of schizophrenia. *Epidemiol Rev* 7:105–126, 1985

This review of the epidemiology of schizophrenia clearly demonstrates the wide range of questions asked by epidemiologists (such as disease prevalence and incidence and the role of genetic and mutable/immutable sociodemographic risk factors), as well as the wide range of research approaches aimed at answering them (including the survey, the record-based, the case-control, the high-risk, and the genetic approaches), each with its own strengths and weaknesses.

Genetics

26. **Martin JB:** Molecular genetics: applications to the clinical neurosciences. *Science* 238:765–772, 1987

Although somewhat outdated by recent findings in, for example, amyotrophic lateral sclerosis, Huntington's disease, and neurofibromatosis, this review outlines the rationale behind molecular genetic approaches to neuropsychiatric disorders, summarizes chromosomal localization and gene abnormality findings for a number of diseases, and suggests future directions for the field (including transgenic animal models of disease and gene therapy).

Imaging

27. **Andreasen NC:** Brain imaging: applications in psychiatry. *Science* 239:1381–1388, 1988

Beginning with a discussion of potential brain mechanisms underlying psychiatric disorders, this article surveys brain imaging techniques for elucidating such mechanisms. These include both structural brain imaging (such as computed tomography and magnetic resonance imaging) and functional brain imaging (such as regional cerebral blood flow, single photon emission computed tomography, and positron-emission tomography), each with its own temporal and spatial limitations.

Molecular Biology and Neurobiology

28. **Black IB:** *Information in the Brain: A Molecular Perspective.* Cambridge, MA, MIT Press, 1991

Starting with a systems theory framework, this monograph identifies the molecular components of the brain (e.g., neurotransmitters in synapses and neurotrophic factors in brain systems), the ways in which combinatorial and modular strategies use these building blocks to construct the nervous system, and ultimately, mentation.

29. **Hyman SE, Nestler EJ:** *The Molecular Foundations of Psychiatry.* Washington, DC, American Psychiatric Press, 1992

This textbook provides a readable introduction to the central role of molecular biology in the modern neuroscience of psychiatry, considering applications ranging from molecular genetics to molecular pharmacology.

30. **Yool AJ, Schwarz TL:** Alteration of the ionic selectivity of a K^+ channel by mutation of the H5 region. *Nature* 349:700–704, 1991

This modest "letter to *Nature*," combining molecular manipulation of single amino acids with electrophysiology of channel proteins, typifies an enormously enlightening approach to uncovering structure/function relationships in the nervous system.

Neurochemistry

31. **Moore KE:** Biochemical correlates of the behavioral effects of drugs: difficulties in studying functional biochemistry of the central nervous

system, in *An Introduction of Psychopharmacology*. Edited by Rech RR, Moore KE. New York, Raven, 1971, pp. 82–85

This introductory chapter from a classic textbook details the special difficulties—including inaccessibility, critical dependence on in vivo connectivity diminishing the utility of in vitro preparations, and marked functional and anatomical heterogeneity—inherent in studying the functional biochemistry of the brain.

Neuroendocrinology

32. **Nemeroff CB, Krishnan KRR:** Neuroendocrine alterations in psychiatric disorders, in *Neuroendocrinology*. Edited by Nemeroff CB. Boca Raton, FL, CRC Press, 1992, pp. 413–441

In describing alterations in three major hormonal axes (the hypothalamic-pituitary-adrenal, hypothalamic-pituitary-thyroid, and growth hormone systems) in psychiatric illness, this chapter demonstrates the variety of neurochemical and neuropharmacological approaches available to study endocrine function in the nervous system.

Neuroimmunology and Neurovirology

33. **Waksman BH:** Autoimmunity in demyelinating diseases. *Ann N Y Acad Sci* 540:13–24, 1988

Using multiple sclerosis and other demyelinating disorders as examples, this review discusses the different immune mechanisms (e.g., autoimmunization to cross-reacting viruses versus immune response to persistent viral infection) causing neuropsychiatric disease. It also discusses the different kinds of evidence (ranging from circumstantial epidemiological findings to more direct measurement of immune parameters) that may be adduced in support of these immune mechanisms of disease.

Neuropathology

34. **Casanova MF, Kleinman JE:** The neuropathology of schizophrenia: a critical assessment of research methodologies. *Biol Psychiatry* 27:353–362, 1990

This article highlights a number of techniques (ranging from gross pathology, to morphometry, to shape analysis, to automated cell counting) that are available to the modern neuropathologist for the study of neuropsychiatric disorders, as well as a number of methodological considerations that must be entertained to ensure maximally reliable and valid results.

Neuropsychology

35. **Posner MI, Petersen SE, Fox PT, Raichle ME:** Localization of cognitive operations in the human brain. *Science* 240:1627–1631, 1988

This article, integrating anatomical neurology with cognitive psychology, provides a schema for localizing mental operations in the brain through specification of elemental components, selective activation, and functional brain imaging.

Nosology

36. **Balla JI, Iansek R, Elstein A:** Bayesian diagnosis in presence of pre-existing disease. *Lancet* 1:326–329, 1985

This article offers a statistical approach to improving the ability of diagnostic tests to discriminate disease complications from new disease in the setting of preexisting disease through the application of Bayes' theorem.

37. **Dawes RM, Faust D, Meehl PE:** Clinical versus actuarial judgment. *Science* 243:1668–1674, 1989

This report contrasts two approaches to clinical decision making: actuarial judgment (based on the systematic, empirical, and statistical establishment of relationships between predictors and outcomes of interest) and clinical judgment (based on less systematic processing of such relationships). Moreover, it suggests that the former approach may be superior to the latter in providing psychiatric diagnoses and predicting outcomes and indicates factors that may underlie this superiority.

38. *Kendell RE: Clinical validity. *Psychol Med* 19:45–55, 1989

This article proposes a variety of research approaches to improving and validating our definitions of psychiatric disorders, short of discovering their distinct etiologies. These include identifying syndromes through cluster analysis; identifying boundaries between syndromes through discriminant analysis; and validating these syndromes through prospective outcome studies, treatment response studies, or family recurrence studies applied to populations chosen to represent a broad range of psychopathology.

39. **Schwartz WB, Patil RS, Szolovits P:** Artificial intelligence in medicine: where do we stand? *N Engl J Med* 316:685–688, 1987

This "sounding board" article documents the evolution of computer-aided diagnosis, from rule-based systems linking specific symptoms to specific diseases, to more sophisticated systems linking symptoms and diseases through intervening pathophysiological models or hypotheses. It goes on to suggests ways in which the predictive accuracy of such systems can be improved through the introduction of data on prior probabilities and the use of statistical analyses.

Psychoanalysis

40. **Bachrach HM, Galatzer-Levy R, Skolnikoff A, Waldron S Jr:** On the efficacy of psychoanalysis. *J Am Psychoanal Assoc* 39:871–916, 1991

    This study critically reviews the psychoanalytic literature attempting to identify clinical factors predicting successful treatment outcome. It suggests that "suitability" for analysis and "analyzability" are not good predictors of therapeutic benefit, although this negative result must be weighed against the methodological limitations of the studies reviewed, limitations that have plagued research into other psychotherapies and that include specification and operationalization of predictor and outcome variables and assurance that the treatment being studied is actually being administered.

41. **Jones EE, Windholz N:** The psychoanalytic case-study: toward a method for systematic inquiry. *J Am Psychoanal Assoc* 38:985–1015, 1990

    This article represents an attempt to put psychoanalytic research on a firmer footing by developing a standardized, psychometrically sound scale for rating a wide range of phenomena during the analytic hour, including transference manifestations, resistance, the analyst's activity, and the analysand's affective state. Indirect support for the validity of the scale includes its gradual evolution over the course of a 6-year analysis to which it has been applied.

Psychophysiology

42. **Venables PH:** Overview of psychophysiology in relation to psychopathology with special reference to schizophrenia, in *Handbook of Schizophrenia, Vol. 5: Neuropsychology, Psychophysiology and Information Processing.* Edited by Steinhauer SR, Gruzelier JH, Zubin J. Amsterdam, Elsevier, 1991, pp. 3–37

    This chapter provides an overview of the variety of roles that psychophysiological measures may serve (as episode markers, vulnerability markers, or genetic markers); discusses the current status of such measures in schizophrenia research; and considers areas that have been relatively neglected in psychophysiological research, such as the effects of gender and age, the diagnostic specificity of the measures, and their underlying neuroanatomic substrates.

Social Psychiatry

43. **Dohrenwend BP, Levav I, Shrout PE, Schwartz S, Naveh G, Link BG, Skodol AE, Stueve A:** Socioeconomic status and psychiatric disorders: the causation-selection issue. *Science* 255:946–952, 1992

   This study, examining the relative contributions of social causation (exposure to increased adversity and stress) and social selection (downward mobility of at-risk individuals) to the observed inverse relationship between social class and mental illness, highlights the research designs and analyses available to social psychiatrists.

Therapeutics

Psychotherapy and Other Nonsomatic Treatments

44. **Fiske DW, Hunt HF, Luborsky L, Orne M, Parloff MB, Reiser MF, Tuma AH:** Planning of research on effectiveness of psychotherapy. *Arch Gen Psychiatry* 22:22–32, 1970

   This classic article outlines some general considerations in the design and implementation of studies directed at examining the effectiveness of psychotherapy. These considerations include the choice of research subjects (broadly or narrowly defined) and of appropriate controls (between or within subject), the specification of the treatment parameters and of the therapist's attributes and qualifications, the choice of adequate outcome measures (both within and outside of the therapy context), and the choice of a meaningful research design and statistical treatment.

45. **Kazdin AE:** Comparative outcome studies of psychotherapy: methodological issues and strategies. *J Consult Clin Psychol* 54:95–105, 1986

   Additional considerations arise in comparing two psychotherapeutic approaches, including identification of treatment-specific ingredients; elimination of therapist-specific factors, which may be confounded with treatment (i.e., different sorts of therapists may be attracted to different treatments); and attention to clinically, as opposed to statistically, significant differences.

46. **Wilson GT, Rachman SJ:** Meta-analysis and the evaluation of psychotherapy outcome: limitations and liabilities. *J Consult Clin Psychol* 51:54–64, 1983

This critique of meta-analysis as applied to the evaluation of psychotherapy outcome questions the practices of assigning methodologically weak and strong studies equal weight and of arbitrarily lumping together theoretically and procedurally diverse treatments.

Psychopharmacology

47. **Greenblatt M, Grosser GH, Wechsler H:** Differential response of hospitalized depressed patients to somatic therapy. *Am J Psychiatry* 120:935–943, 1964

This milestone publication, comparing the response of 281 severely depressed patients with varying diagnoses to electroconvulsive therapy, tricyclic antidepressants, or monamine oxidase inhibitors, demonstrated, for the first time, an important diagnosis-by-treatment interaction.

48. **Klerman GL:** Treatment of recurrent unipolar major depressive disorder: commentary on the Pittsburgh study. *Arch Gen Psychiatry* 47:1158–1162, 1990

The Pittsburgh studies on long-term treatment of recurrent unipolar major depression compare the individual and combined use of medication and psychotherapy. This commentary on these studies highlights a number of methodological refinements contained therein (such as advances in the classification of depression, in the effective use of antidepressants, in the assessment of outcome, and in the statistical treatment of outcome studies) and suggests that prevention of relapse (a frequent occurrence at 1-year follow-up for the untreated control group) may be achieved with either imipramine (especially in high dosages) or interpersonal psychotherapy, with possibly some additional benefit with combined treatment.

49. **Quitkin FM, Rabkin JG, Ross D, McGrath PJ:** Duration of antidepressant drug treatment: what is an adequate trial? *Arch Gen Psychiatry* 41:238–245, 1984

This meta-analysis examines another important methodological question in psychopharmacology research: How long must a medication trial last to consider it adequate? A significant portion of subjects showing no clear response to antidepressants at 4 weeks do show a noticeable response at 6 weeks.

50. **Robinson DS, Nies A, Ravaris CL, Ives JO, Bartlett D:** Clinical pharmacology of phenelzine. *Arch Gen Psychiatry* 35:629–635, 1978

This important contribution to the drug treatment literature showed, for the first time, a significant effect of antidepressant dose on treatment outcome.

Research Ethics

51. **Gallant DM, Eichelman B:** Ethical dilemmas in neuropsychopharmacologic research, in *Psychopharmacology: The Third Generation of Progress.* Edited by Meltzer HY. New York, Raven, 1987, pp. 1–15

This chapter begins by considering a variety of ethical concerns in psychiatric research, codified in "A Statement of Principles of Ethical Conduct for Neuropsychopharmacologic Research in Human Subjects" developed by the American College of Neuropsychopharmacology, including issues related to choosing research subjects, obtaining informed consent, and minimizing risk. Adopting a case study approach, it goes on to explore a number of ethical dilemmas that face psychiatric researchers when studying special populations, such as children, prisoners, nonpatient volunteers, and patients who lack capacity.

52. **Howard-Jones N:** Human experimentation in historical and ethical perspectives. *Soc Sci Med* 16:1429–1448, 1982

As a prologue to the development of an international consensus for the ethical conduct of biomedical research involving human subjects, this article details the historical evolution of human experimentation and the circumstances under which formal ethical codes arose.

53. ***Levine RJ:** *Ethics and the Regulation of Clinical Research,* 2nd Edition. New Haven, CT, Yale University Press, 1988

This encyclopedic tome offers a survey of the ethical and legal duties of clinical researchers. Although intended for the novice member of an institutional review board (be they physician or layperson), it serves as an excellent guide for even the experienced researcher to a wide variety of ethical issues, including those involving randomized clinical trials, "deception" in research (such as occurs with placebo treatment, with misrepresentation of the researcher's true identity, or with covert observation), and research with human embryos and fetuses.

Research Training

54. **Ledley FD:** The physician-scientist's role in medical research and the mythology of intellectual tradition. *Perspect Biol Med* 34:410–420, 1991

    This thought-provoking article portrays the critical cultural challenges confronting the identity of the physician-scientist, who must not be distracted from his or her interest in health and disease because of the "radiant potential" of basic science. It identifies physicians as essential members of the community of scientists and medicine not as the antithesis but as the wellspring of biotechnological advance.

55. **Nevin J, Pincus HA** (eds): *Directory of Research Fellowship Opportunities in Psychiatry, 1992.* Washington, DC, Office of Research, American Psychiatric Association, 1992

    The introductory chapter to this directory provides prospective psychiatric researchers with wonderfully practical advice regarding clarifying their research interests, choosing research training programs, and identifying potential research mentors.

56. **Pincus HA:** Research and clinical training in psychiatry: inputs and outputs. *Psychiatr Q* 62:121–133, 1991

    This article details the potential for psychiatric research created by the succession of scientific advances and the advent consumer advocacy, reviews public policies and funding that have shaped psychiatric research over the past several decades, and proposes a number of strategies aimed at recruiting medical students with the greatest scientific interest, talent, and ambition into careers in psychiatric research.

Research Funding

57. **Pincus HA:** "Anatomy" of research funding of mental illness and addictive disorders. *Arch Gen Psychiatry* 49:573–579, 1992

    This systematic survey of the public and private sources of research support extant in fiscal 1988 concludes that the study of mental illnesses and addictive disorders is disproportionately underfunded given their profound impact on society, that nearly two-thirds of all support is derived from the three institutes that formerly made up the Alcohol, Drug Abuse and Mental Health Administration (ADAMHA), and that greater coalition building and advocacy will be necessary to diversify and protect the funding portfolio for psychiatric research.

65

Psychiatric Education
and Supervision

James W. Lomax, M.D.

P sychiatric education is a marvelous business. Educators get paid
for telling other people what they know or believe and best of
all for the tremendously gratifying experience of being a men-
tor to a group of mostly bright, dedicated men and women of great integrity, energy, and enthusiasm for learning. Medical students and residents
are in an environment orchestrated to enhance their knowledge, skills,
attitudes, and some of the most precious of human qualities: empathy and
compassion.

There *are* also endless hours of preparation to teach and lecture; the
agony of deciding whether a resident or student is troubled and incompetent or troubling and creative; and the need to respond to the scrutiny of
hospital administrators, residency review committees, due process, and a
public more interested in funding the repair of potholes in the present than
education for the future. For residents, there is the coming to grips with the
personal and individual tragedy of severe mental illness, seeing too much of
oneself in patients with character disorder and neurotic conflict, too many
nights on call after long regular working days, and coming to one's own
place in a field enriched by pluralism but that looks like "sustained muddle-
headedness" to most students and to much of the general public (including
the student's family and friends).

There are many ways to slice the pie of psychiatric education. The following readings begin with a focus on the content and attitudes about psychiatric education, mostly written from the perspective of faculty members. Some selections are overviews of medical education and leadership. Others offer very specific advice for the common problems that emerge in academic centers.

The next section relates to the resident's perspective in the educational process. Our present decade has brought new challenges (e.g., acquired immunodeficiency syndrome and managed care) to a developmental process that is rarely trouble free and never simple. Psychiatric residency is different from the rest of graduate medical education. The 4 years of residency on the one hand involve a steady stream of personal and professional development. On the other hand, most residents experience a predictable sequence of developmental concerns and themes that are compelling and pervasive enough so that each postgraduate year tends to take on a "life of its own." These themes are different enough from each other that there is a sense of starting a new residency each year. The first-year resident is generally preoccupied by the enormity of responsibility for decisions that greatly influence either life itself or the quality of life for our patients. This is not different per se for residents in other specialties, but medical student education in psychiatry is rarely as comprehensive as that for other specialties. Psychiatric residents accurately feel unprepared in terms of exposure to the basic sciences of our field. In the second postgraduate year, residents struggle to understand character pathology in their patients and develop the basic knowledge and skills required for doing psychotherapy. The combination of the limits of our field and the slowness of response of the central nervous system to psychotherapeutic efforts often leads to a period of significant disillusionment, self-doubt, and doubt about career choice. In the third postgraduate year, most residents have their first experience with children and families on the one hand and the longitudinal outpatient care of significant numbers of people with severe and persistent mental illness on the other. The hard-won sense of personal efficacy obtained in the first 2 years is a necessary but not sufficient repertoire for dealing with these new and challenging problems. Although educational abilities of the residents should begin with their very first rotations, PGY-IV brings a focused opportunity for generativity in the form of senior or chief residency experiences on teaching wards for medical students and more junior residents. Simultaneously, residents become aware that a difficult but supportive environment will no longer be available in a matter of months. Articles in this section touch various aspects of the above in a way that offers empathic understanding, a sense of universality or inevitability, and occasional welcome bits of humor.

The third section emphasizes medical student experiences in psychiatric education. Questions about recruitment are particularly pressing matters for psychiatry faculty at present. Articles in this section, however, are selected with the bias that excellence in our teaching activities with a particular emphasis on the junior year clerkship is our best bet to recruit the (hopefully) 5% of medical students interested in psychiatry while ensuring that the other 95% remember us favorably after they graduate from medical school.

The final section is dedicated to the psychotherapy curriculum and supervision in psychiatry. Several major educational conferences and a variety of references in the literature have recently reaffirmed competence in psychotherapy as a core clinical skill of the psychiatrist. There is less consensus about how to accomplish this ability in a curriculum overfilled with new information and undersupported for outpatient treatments in general and psychotherapy in particular. These citations range from comprehensive overviews to specific strategies to address very particular problems and opportunities.

Psychiatric Education: Readings for Every Faculty Member

1. **Arif A, Westermeyer J:** Guidelines for teaching and training, in *Manual of Drug and Alcohol Abuse.* New York, Plenum Medical, 1988, pp. 9–33

   Teaching about substance abuse requires special skills because of the common attitudes of medical practitioners about substance abuse and the way those attitudes interact with patient denial and other resistances. Knowledge, attitudes, and skills are systematically considered in a comprehensive curriculum in drug dependence.

2. **Bowden CL, Sledge WH, Humphrey FJ, Kromer M:** Educational objectives in psychiatric residency training: a survey of training directors and residents. *Am J Psychiatry* 140:1352–1355, 1983

   This article builds on a previous survey that defined 120 educational objectives determined to be of essential importance for psychiatric residency training. This article reports a substantial discrepancy between residents and residency directors as to the importance and to the accomplishment of those essential objectives. Residents have a more narrow view of what is essential in psychiatric residency training and are less sanguine than training directors about what residency accomplishes. The authors report that a similar disparity exists in family medicine, which may be some small solace. However, this disagreement introduces a predictable tension during residency and suggests an obligation for psychiatric educators not only to educate but also to explain and engage their trainees in an educational alliance.

3. **Brown GR:** The inpatient database as a technique to prevent junior faculty burnout. *Academic Psychiatry* 14:224–229, 1990

   Assignment of new faculty members to a busy inpatient rotation for first- or second-year residents is often the first step down a dead end street. Prevention of burnout or seduction into a more lucrative private practice can result from the rapid simultaneous involvement of new faculty in the more rewarding aspects of academic life. Developing an excited anticipation about research, teaching, mentoring, professional public speaking, representing the department to the community, and so on, is a "must" for the successful development of faculty. This article should be a part of an orientation meeting with the chairperson, educational director, and research guru of the department for the new faculty members shortly after their appointment.

4. **Glick ID, Janowsky DS, Salzman C, Shader RI:** *A Model Psychopharmacology Curriculum for Psychiatric Residents.* Washington, DC, American College of Neuropsychopharmacology and National Institute of Mental Health, 1984

   This is a most extensive model curriculum. It reflects not only an ad hoc committee of the American College of Neuropsychopharmacology but also substantial input from individual psychiatric educators as well as the American Association of Directors of Psychiatric Residency Training and the Association for Academic Psychiatry. Even though the specific reading list and psychopharmacology books are now dated, the organizational plan and curriculum elements sequenced over the years of residency are useful to departments and programs reviewing their educational endeavors in this core element of psychiatric residency.

5. **Katzelnick DJ, Gonzales JJ, Conley MC, Shuster JL, Borus JF:** Teaching psychiatric residents to teach. *Academic Psychiatry* 15:153–159, 1991

   Recruitment is a major issue for all of psychiatry. Most medical students make their decision to enter or not to enter psychiatry during their required clinical rotation on psychiatry, and medical students spend about as much time learning from residents as from faculty during their core clerkship. For all these reasons, it is important that we prepare our residents to teach. This article describes a carefully thought out approach to this important activity. The references provide entrees to a variety of other concepts and formats for teaching about teaching.

6. **Kay J:** *Handbook of Psychiatry Residency Training.* Washington, DC, American Psychiatric Press, 1991

   This volume emerged after 20 years of incubation within the American Association of Directors of Psychiatric Residency Training. It reflects the systematic consideration of 23 senior residency training directors regarding the major topic areas in psychiatric education. Each topic (from curriculum planing to evaluation to special events and special problems) is considered in great detail. The volume is of particular interest to faculty and senior residents in administrative positions.

7. **Nemiah JC:** The idea of a psychiatric education. *Journal of Psychiatric Education* 5:183–194, 1981

   This article is a literate and personal account of the shifting perspectives required of the psychiatrist and the resulting pluralism of conceptual frameworks required in good psychiatric education. Nemiah's personal encounter with this fundamental requirement of the competent psychiatrist is particularly useful for the resident beginning to learn psychotherapy skills at the expense of intermittently and temporarily relinquishing hard-won "objective" perspectives valued or demanded during most of medical education.

8. **Reiser MF:** Are psychiatric educators "losing the mind"? *Am J Psychiatry* 145:148–153, 1988

   This written version of the 1986 Vestermark Lecture argues for a middle ground of clinical synthesis of neurobiology and psychoanalysis. It is an important complement to a more limited "diagnostic" perspective, which might turn the psychiatric encounter into a detached and mechanistic enterprise. This article is useful for first-year residents wondering why we have seminars on interviewing and for those faculty who provide clinical or didactic instruction about the same topic.

9. **Rittelmeyer LF:** Leadership in an academic department of psychiatry. *Academic Psychiatry* 14:57–64, 1990

   Leadership remains elusive to define. This article makes an attempt at definition, delineates various categories and qualities of leadership, and puts enough detail in the definitions to stimulate useful discussion. Although focused on the chairperson and residency director, the article would be useful for anyone assuming leadership of the section, division, or team within the department of psychiatry.

10. **Scheiber SC:** Graduate psychiatric education (Chapter 48), in *Comprehensive Textbook of Psychiatry/II,* 5th Edition, Vol. 2. Edited by Kaplan HI, Sadock BJ. Baltimore, MD, Williams & Wilkins, 1989, pp. 2099–2106

    The title of this chapter should be "Regulation and Evaluation of Graduate Psychiatric Education." As might be expected from the vice president of the board, it is an excellent review of the American Board of Psychiatry and Neurology in terms of its history, its relationship with other national organizations, and its function as the national certifying entity. A section on the Residency Review Committee/Accreditation Council for Graduate Medical Education would have been a useful addition.

11. **Schwenk T, Whitman N:** *The Physician as Teacher.* Baltimore, MD, Williams & Wilkins, 1987

Although not specifically oriented to psychiatry, this book systematically reviews the elements of teaching ranging from defining roles and relationships to specific suggestions regarding lectures, small group teaching, and teaching rounds. Pros and cons of various styles of teaching are considered in various contexts. The book is particularly useful for senior residents and junior faculty starting their careers. However, many senior academicians who have never had the benefit of an opportunity to consider educational issues systematically may find it just as valuable.

12. **Shemo JP, Ballenger JC, Yazel JJ, Spradlin WW:** A conjoint psychiatry–internal medicine program: development of a teaching and clinical model. *Am J Psychiatry* 139:1437–1442, 1982

Ten years before a combined internal medicine and psychiatry program was approved by the American Board of Psychiatry and Neurology, this article described one version of such a program at West Virginia University and Virginia University. The program described is one model for such combined programs. The authors advocate an intentional blurring of the boundaries between internal medicine and psychiatry to produce what they espouse as a "hybrid" as opposed to "grafted" practitioner. The article is worth reviewing for those programs and departments considering a combined program in internal medicine and psychiatry.

13. **Sparr LF, Bloom JD, Marcel LJ, Shore JH:** The organization and regulation of voluntary faculty. *Academic Psychiatry* 15:61–68, 1991

This article is a carefully considered approach to the utilization and role of voluntary faculty members. The criteria for achieving, maintaining, and advancing voluntary faculty are particularly useful. Comments about the legal responsibilities of clinical faculty are controversial and provocative but worthy of serious consideration. The article ends with raising the question of clinical faculty development but does little to help address this latter important problem.

14. **Yager J, Borus JF:** A survival guide for psychiatric residency training directors. *Academic Psychiatry* 14:180–187, 1990

Although geared toward the training director and associate, this article is also useful for the chairperson and key faculty members of any child or general residency program. Simply having a label for common phenomena and destroying the illusion that one is uniquely beleaguered are among the possible benefits from a careful reading of this article.

15. **Yager J, Linn LS, Winstead DK, Leake B:** Characteristics of journal clubs in psychiatric training. *Academic Psychiatry* 15:18–32, 1991

   This article is a comprehensive and databased approach to the roles and formats of journal clubs in psychiatric residency. It delineates the characteristics of successful journal clubs and offers helpful guidelines for those who organize or participate in them.

Resident and Student Perspectives in the Education Process: How to Survive and How to Thrive

16. **Auchincloss EL:** Conflict among psychiatric residents in response to pregnancy. *Am J Psychiatry* 139:818–821, 1982

   Nearly one-half of psychiatric residents are women. This article is timely reading for both residents and program administrators. It details what happens when neither the administration nor the residents directly discuss the implications of pregnancy for a task-oriented group. Auchincloss seems to disagree with viewing pregnancy as an illness from the administrative perspective but does not offer a better alternative.

17. **Barbee JG, Kasten AM, Rosenson MK:** Toward a new alliance: psychiatric residents and family support groups. *Academic Psychiatry* 15:40–49, 1991

   In the past decade, psychiatry and psychiatrists have made an important rapprochement with the families of our patients. Faculty and supervisors of residents grew up in an educational environment in which there was often an unfortunate tendency to blame families for the illnesses of our patients. This tendency colluded with family guilt over the emergence of psychiatric illness in offspring or family members to form a most unfortunate misalliance. This article provides not only a curriculum for helping residents collaborate with families, but also specifies problems and goals in establishing a working collaborative relationship.

18. **Borenstein DB:** Should physician training centers offer formal psychiatric assistance to house officers? a report on the major findings of a prototype program. *Am J Psychiatry* 142:1053–1057, 1985

This article recounts the experience of a program offering psychiatric evaluation and brief treatment for University of California at Los Angles house staff during the first 3 years of its existence. Some of the article's conclusions are erroneous. (It was neither the first such comprehensive program nor the only one in existence at the time of the report.) Its main value is in documenting the utilization rate and potential value of such programs. For a variety of reasons, it is important that psychiatry departments and psychiatrists take leadership roles in initiatives aimed at addressing psychiatrically ill physicians.

19. **Campbell HD:** The prevalence and ramifications of psychopathology in psychiatric residents: an overview. *Am J Psychiatry* 139:1405–1411, 1982

    This is a well-conceived review article of the topic described in its title. It includes helpful distinctions between program interventions to facilitate negotiation of predictably stressful residency experiences from treatment interventions for psychopathological states that may be present independent from the particular context of training.

20. **Clark DC, Salazar-Grueso E, Grabler P, Fawcett J:** Predictors of depression during the first 6 months of internship. *Am J Psychiatry* 141:1095–1098, 1984

    This article expands the Valko and Clayton study of a decade earlier by a prospective study of the predictors of mood disturbance during the first 6 months of internship. A family history of depression and high scores of "trait neuroticism" identify interns at unusual risk for developing depression. More than one-fourth of the medicine, pediatrics, surgery, and ob-gyn house staff who participated in this study developed a major depression during the first 6 months of PGY-I. This article is useful in our efforts to build a case for accessible and affordable psychiatric services for all house staff.

21. **Fink D, Shoyer B, Dubin WR:** A study of assaults against psychiatric residents. *Academic Psychiatry* 15:94–99, 1991

    This article reports on a survey of psychiatric residents in Pennsylvania, delineating their collective experience with assaults and threats on residents. It is a useful addition to resident training in aggression management to put this serious educational, clinical, and personal problem in perspective.

22. **Kris K:** Distress precipitated by psychiatric training among medical students. *Am J Psychiatry* 143:1432–1435, 1986

    This article focuses on an unanticipated result of psychiatric training: Identifying with patients or overstimulating encounters with patients or teachers may lead to the development of psychiatric symptomatology in medical students. The description of interactions with instructors is particularly informative, if somewhat of an embarrassment to our field. The article serves a useful purpose by raising the consciousness of faculty about the implications of their instruction and the instructional situation for medical students.

23. **Roback HB, Crowder MK:** Psychiatric resident dismissal: a national survey of training programs. *Am J Psychiatry* 146:96–98, 1989

   This is a short but databased report on the negative outcome of the troubled or troubling resident. Most dismissed residents had been identified as potentially problematic in their interviews, which is far and away the most powerful screening instrument. Dismissal of residents is a rare but disturbing event for residents and programs alike. A substantial percentage of dismissed residents are able to enter another program.

24. **Sacks MH:** When patients kill themselves, in *American Psychiatric Press Review of Psychiatry*, Vol. 8. Edited by Tasman A, Hales RE, Francis AJ. Washington, DC, American Psychiatric Press, 1989, pp. 563–579

   This chapter is an expanded version of one originally published in the *Journal of Psychiatric Education* in 1987. It documents the high frequency of patient suicide during the education and subsequent professional life of psychiatrists. It also documents that patient suicide is an extremely stressful event, particularly if it occurs early in the psychiatrist's education. The article describes characteristic responses to patient suicide and valuable specific recommendations to educational and clinical programs when such important events occur.

25. **Shapiro MF, Hayward RA, Guillemot D, Jayle D:** Residents' experiences in, and attitudes toward, the care of persons with AIDS in Canada, France, and the United States. *JAMA* 268:510–515, 1992

   The acquired immunodeficiency syndrome (AIDS) epidemic has changed the character of medicine and medical education in dramatic ways. One element of that change is reflected by this survey of the attitudes of physicians toward their patients that suffer from AIDS. The striking national differences in attitudes toward patients with AIDS and the incidence of AIDS patients who have been refused care by medical specialists reveal information important in both health care planning and medical education.

26. **Werner A, Riessinger CA, Gibson G, Hughes L:** Part-time residency training in psychiatry. *Academic Psychiatry* 15:180–187, 1991

A positively biased but reasonably balanced piece on a topic of interest to faculty and residents alike, this article poses the value of part-time residency to the residents and the advantages to programs while at least indicating some of the difficulties encountered when part-time residency is allowed or pursued.

27. **Yager J:** A survival guide for psychiatric residents. *Arch Gen Psychiatry* 30:494–499, 1974

There have been many articles written about the downside of the rich pluralism of psychiatry. This article helps residents to appreciate that their dilemmas are universal. It also helps faculty members who have lost empathic connection with the position of psychiatry residents attempting to find their way in a field complicated by "overchoice." The concluding section of the article offers advice to faculty and residents that remains timely about two decades later.

A Snapshot of Medical Student Education: How to Educate 95% and Recruit 5%

28. **Kay J:** Child psychiatry recruitment and medical student education. *Academic Psychiatry* 13:208–212, 1989

This article is from the 1989 Child and Adolescent Psychiatry Recruitment Conference. It focuses on medical student education and offers very specific suggestions for the involvement of child psychiatrists in that curriculum. Additionally, there is a skeleton outline of topics to be included in that curriculum for medical students.

29. **Kay J, Bienenfeld D:** The role of the residency training director in psychiatric recruitment. *Academic Psychiatry* 16:127–133, 1992

This article begins with a basic review of our recruitment difficulties. It follows with a brief summary of critical recommendations from the 1980 Recruitment Conference and highly specific advice for residency training directors in regard to recruitment of medical students. Most "survivors" in the residency director job will have found these excellent recommendations on their own. However, this article should be required reading for new training directors trying to develop a comprehensive approach to this critical component of their job. The article updates a 1985 piece in the *Journal of Psychiatric Education* by Kay and Langsley and foreshadows the recommendations of the 1992 American Association of Directors of Psychiatric Residency Training and National Institute of Mental Health Recruitment Conference report, which appeared in *Academic Psychiatry* in 1993.

30. **Reiser LW, Sledge WH, Edelson M:** Four-year evaluation of a psychiatric clerkship 1982–1986. *Am J Psychiatry* 145:1122–1126, 1988

    This article describes the transition from a loose affiliation of clerkships to a medical school clerkship with a clearly defined core experience carried out in a variety of different sites. Over the 4 years of the evaluation, the clerkship was rated as outstanding or excellent by nearly three-fourths of the students, and 10% of the medical school graduates during this period elected to go into psychiatry.

31. **Scully JH, Dubovsky SL, Simons RC:** Undergraduate education and recruitment into psychiatry. *Am J Psychiatry* 140:573–576, 1983

    These authors conclude their article with a caution that merits our attention given our present preoccupation with recruitment: Self-conscious efforts at recruitment may backfire. This article describes changes in an undergraduate medical school curriculum in psychiatry that correlated with increased recruitment into psychiatry over a several-year period. Increased involvement of senior faculty in small group teaching activities of the basic science years and an orientation to providing rigorous teaching aimed at the nonpsychiatric practitioner during the clerkship are recommended.

32. **Yager J, Lamotte K, Nielsen A, Eaton JS:** Medical students' evaluation of psychiatry: a cross-country comparison. *Am J Psychiatry* 139:1003–1009, 1982

    This article compares evaluations of psychiatric teaching by medical students in Los Angeles, California, and Washington, DC. Relevance, rigor, and role models who are active and available over time are the enduring principles identified here and repeated in many subsequent studies.

Supervision and the Psychotherapy Curriculum: Swimming Upstream With Grace

33. **Altshuler KZ:** Common mistakes made by beginning therapists. *Academic Psychiatry* 13:73–80, 1989

    This article offers help in recognizing mistakes and avoiding them. It is useful for both beginning residents and their supervisors. There is an increasing need for the help offered by this article with the increasing discrepancy between the residency experience of clinical faculty supervisors and that of current residents.

34. Arlow JA: The supervisory situation. *J Am Psychoanal Assoc* 11:576–594, 1963

Supervision of psychiatry residents is very different from psychoanalytic supervision of psychoanalytic candidates. However, the latter can inform part of our work with the former. This classic analytic article is a clear statement of a central function of psychoanalytic supervision. The principles elucidated by Arlow are useful if appropriately modified for the situation of psychotherapy supervision of graduate trainees.

35. Betcher RW, Zinberg NE: Supervision and privacy in psychotherapy training. *Am J Psychiatry* 145:796–803, 1988

This article deals not only with the differences between "didactic" and "countertransference"-based theories of supervision, but also with the implications of making supervision more "objective" through the use of recording instruments and direct examination of the patient by the supervisor. Several questions raised by the article are worth discussion in a meeting of the program's supervisors.

36. Borus JF, Groves JE: Training supervision as a separate faculty role. *Am J Psychiatry* 139:1339–1342, 1982

Some programs appoint a faculty member to have an overall relationship with a resident to enhance the trainee's general professional development. Borus and Groves define this as "training supervision." They elaborate this faculty role and describe a meeting of individuals fulfilling this program function.

37. Buckley P, Conte HR, Plutchik R, Karasu TB, Wild KV: Learning dynamic psychotherapy: a longitudinal study. *Am J Psychiatry* 139:1607–1610, 1982

This article uses an instrument previously developed by the authors to study what changes can be detected by psychotherapy supervisors and their supervisees during the first year of a psychotherapy curriculum. The article delineates what changes can be reasonably expected with 1 year of supervised psychotherapy experience. It also raises the interesting question of whether empathy and awareness of countertransference reflect innate qualities that require something other than an educational experience to effect change in therapeutic abilities.

38. Goldberg DA: Resistance to the use of video in individual psychotherapy training. *Am J Psychiatry* 140:1172–1176, 1983

This article delineates factors that interfere with using videotape in the psychotherapy curriculum. The explicit elaboration of each reluctance, acknowledging the grains of truth therein, and examining the experiences of using videotape in education help trainee and supervisor to proceed in an informed manner. Guidelines about the differential use of videotape, audiotape, process notes, and direct observation in the educational curriculum would be useful.

39. **Kline F, Goin MK, Zimmerman W:** You can be a better supervisor! *Journal of Psychiatric Education* 1:174–179, 1977

This is one of the first articles to study the supervisory process in a reliable and databased manner. Certain findings have been repeated and confirmed by Shanfield et al. (1992) below. Outstanding supervisors rarely talk about themselves. Outstanding supervisors stick to the case in mind, are specific and active, and direct the supervisory process in an authoritative but not authoritarian way.

40. **Lewis JM:** *To Be a Therapist: The Teaching and Learning.* New York, Brunner/Mazel, 1978; **Lewis JM:** *Swimming Upstream.* New York, Brunner/ Mazel, 1991

In the first book, Lewis outlines his "structured approach" to the teaching and learning of psychodynamic psychotherapy. The experiential conference described in this book has been modified for use in many programs. It is also useful for the beginning psychotherapist to appreciate the central role of empathic connectedness to patients in psychotherapy. Lewis' second book is an interesting counterpart and reflection on suggestions made by the author more than a decade later.

41. **Mohl PC, Lomax J, Tasman A, Chan C, Sledge WH, Summergrad P, Notman MT:** Psychotherapy training for the psychiatrist of the future. *Am J Psychiatry* 147:7–13, 1990

This article describes a comprehensive curriculum for training in psychodynamic psychotherapy for psychiatry residents. The rationale for including psychotherapy, learning goals and objectives for each PGY level, learning experiences to achieve those goals, and a means to evaluate whether learning has taken place are elucidated. The format for curricula in psychiatric education used by this article is also helpful in the development of curricula in other content areas.

42. **Nestler EJ:** The case of double supervision: a resident's perspective on common problems in psychotherapy supervision. *Academic Psychiatry* 14:129–136, 1990

This article describes a resident's experience presenting the same patient and case notes to two individual supervisors and a case conference. The widely differing responses and recommendations of the supervisors reported by this resident provide useful information for resident and supervisor alike. Supervision is implicitly defined as an educational consultation and distinguished sharply from clinical supervision provided by an attending responsible for patient care.

43. **Pate LA, Wolff TK:** Supervision: the residents' perspective. *Academic Psychiatry* 14:122–128, 1990

This is a databased article of the determinants of residents' satisfaction with their supervisory experiences comparing residents from one United States program with those of a previous Canadian resident survey. The supervisor's teaching ability, rapport between the supervisor and the trainee, and the supervisor's fund of knowledge are identified as the three most important factors. This article is a good companion to Shanfield et al.'s (1992) work below evaluating supervision from the perspective of external observers.

44. **Shanfield SB, Mohl PC, Matthews KL, Hetherly V:** Quantitative assessment of the behavior of psychotherapy supervisors. *Am J Psychiatry* 149:352–357, 1992

This is the most recent product of Shanfield's ongoing databased study of the process of psychotherapy supervision. Rater-perceived quality of supervision is related to the supervisor's empathy, the capacity to focus on the resident's immediate experiences, and making synthesizing comments in depth about those experiences. The Psychotherapy Supervision Inventory Rating Scale developed by Shanfield et al. can be used by programs to orient supervisors and provide feedback about their behavior.

45. **Verhulst J:** The psychotherapy curriculum in the age of biological psychiatry: mixing oil with water? *Academic Psychiatry* 15:120–131, 1991

This article describes one attempt to accommodate to the pluralism of contemporary psychiatry by developing a series of complementary strategies within the psychotherapy curriculum. The article is useful for its delineation of competing educational paradigms, the clarity of goals it espouses for various elements of the psychotherapy curriculum, and strategies to accomplish these goals over the 4 postgraduate years.

66

Books for Families About Serious Mental Illness

Harriet Baldwin, M.A.

This chapter is a resource for professionals in their work with families. The role of families in the treatment of mental illness has changed since the mid-1980s. Once viewed by professionals as the source of pathology, families are increasingly seen as essential partners in the treatment program of mentally ill family members. To fill this new role, families need to be supported and encouraged by professionals, educated about mental illness, and trained in coping skills. Suggesting that families read appropriate books will help professionals achieve these goals.

The books listed in this chapter are drawn from the reading lists of the National Alliance for the Mentally Ill (NAMI). NAMI is a national organization mainly of families with mentally ill members, but its membership also includes professionals and consumers of mental health services who serve them. NAMI was organized in 1979. It has about 150,000 members, 1,000 local affiliates, and umbrella organizations in all 50 states. Its mission is to eradicate serious mental illnesses and improve the quality of life for those who suffer from those diseases. NAMI members believe that serious mental illnesses are no-fault brain diseases. NAMI members engage in family support, educate their members and the community at large about serious mental illnesses, and advocate for more research and better services.

Since it began, NAMI has operated a literature review and sales service. NAMI's literature committee evaluates nontechnical books about serious mental illnesses, measuring books by such criteria as readability, reliability, and helpfulness to families. Books judged to meet the committee's criteria by at least three readers are sold by NAMI at a 5% discount. Books sold by NAMI are reviewed in NAMI's newsletter, *The Advocate,* and are listed in NAMI's reading lists, which are included in this chapter.

NAMI's literature committee perceives two trends over the years in book publishing about serious mental illnesses. The number of books published each year has increased dramatically, and their quality, generally, has improved. Books help to reduce the burden of families ravaged by mental illnesses, and they also help to reduce the stigma the public associates with them. It is NAMI's hope that these trends will strengthen public acceptance of mental illnesses as a national public health problem and that this acceptance, in turn, will speed the day when these illnesses will be fully understood and—finally—cured.

For this chapter, the asterisk (*) in an annotation identifies core readings, those in NAMI's Basic Library About Serious Mental Illness for 1992.

General

1. **American Psychiatric Association:** Diagnostic and Statistical Manual of Mental Disorders, 4th Edition. Washington, DC, American Psychiatric Association, 1994

   This is a classification system of serious mental illnesses that is widely used by American psychiatrists as a diagnostic tool. Known as DSM-IV, it describes precisely and objectively the observable symptoms that underlie accurate and reliable diagnosis and is a valuable addition to any library.

2. *__Andreasen NC:__ *The Broken Brain: The Biological Revolution in Psychiatry.* New York, Harper & Row, 1984

   An excellent explanation of advances in brain research and their impact on understanding and treating mental illness, this book is clearly organized and written; even the technical explanations are understandable. This is the single best book available about state-of-the art psychiatry.

3. *__Andreasen NC, Black DW:__ *Introductory Textbook of Psychiatry.* Washington, DC, American Psychiatric Press, 1991

   This is an excellent introductory textbook on psychiatry by the author of *The Broken Brain.* Although it is intended for medical students and residents, its clarity makes it useful to family members who want a research-based, up-to-date yet readable reference work on the diagnosis and treatment of mental illnesses.

4. **Shiffrin J:** *Pathways to Partnership: An Awareness and Resource Guide on Mental Illness.* St. Louis, MO, Interfaith Ministries and Prolonged Mental Illness, 1990; **Shiffrin J:** *Pathways to Partnership: An Awareness and Resource Guide on Mental Illness for the Jewish Community.* St. Louis, MO, Interfaith Ministries and Prolonged Mental Illness, 1992

These are two guidebooks for religious congregations that want to reach out to persons with serious mental illnesses and integrate them into congregational life. The first is for Protestants; a book for Catholics is in preparation. The books contain practical and realistic suggestions about congregational activities.

Specific Conditions

Children and Adolescents

5. *McElroy E:** *Children and Adolescents With Mental Illness: A Parents' Guide.* Kensington, MD, Woodbine House, 1988

A realistic and practical guidebook for dealing with the problems parents face when mental illness strikes a child, this book provides guidance in deciding about therapists and hospitals, working with professionals, coping with crises, asserting the educational and legal rights of children, and planning ahead.

6. *Peschel E, Peschel R, Howe JW, Howe C** (eds): *Neurobiological Disorders in Children and Adolescents.* San Francisco, CA, Jossey-Bass, 1992

Chapters by some of the country's leading clinicians and neuroscientists summarize the evidence for the neurological basis of 13 mental disorders in children. The book also discusses the implications of research findings for treatment, services, and the management of educational and legal systems.

7. **Wender PH:** *The Hyperactive Child, Adolescent, and Adult: Attention Disorder Through the Lifespan,* 3rd Edition. New York, Oxford University Press, 1987

This is a book about attention deficit disorder by a distinguished psychiatrist, who discusses the symptoms and asserts that the disorder is a disorder of brain chemistry. Treatment requires medication and psychological and educational management. Practical suggestions for parents and teachers are included.

Depressive Illnesses (Affective Disorders)

8. **Goodwin FK, Jamison KR:** *Manic-Depressive Illness.* New York, Oxford University Press, 1990

   A landmark book for physicians and scientists by a leading psychiatrist and clinical psychologist, this is comprehensive, authoritative, and readable; it will be the leading book on the subject for many years. Goodwin and Jamison show great sensitivity to the suffering that accompanies manic-depression.

9. **Mondimore FM:** *Depression: The Mood Disease,* Revised Edition. New York, Harper & Row, 1992

   In this authoritative and comprehensive presentation of evidence that serious depression is a biochemical disorder in the brain, Mondimore explains the complexity of medications, their side effects, and the need for close monitoring. He is optimistic about the future for those with depressive illnesses.

10. *Papolos D, Papolos J:** *Overcoming Depression,* Revised Edition. New York, Harper & Row, 1992

    A comprehensive, up-to-date treatment of depression, this book describes symptoms, discusses diagnosis and research, and considers various forms of treatment. A closing section on "living with the illness" is practical and realistic. Appendices list resources in the various states.

11. **Schou M:** *Lithium Treatment of Manic Depressive Illness: A Practical Guide,* 3rd Edition. New York, Karger, 1986

    Written by a Danish scientist who was a pioneer in using lithium to treat manic-depressive illness, this book deals with practical, day-to-day questions about lithium treatment—laboratory tests, dosage, side effects, risks. It is concise and clearly presented.

Dual Diagnosis

12. *Minkoff K, Drake RE** (eds): *Dual Diagnosis of Major Mental Illness and Substance Disorder.* San Francisco, CA, Jossey-Bass, 1991

    In chapters written mainly for professionals that assert that coexisting mental illness and substance abuse must be treated simultaneously, the authors are authorities on the condition and pioneers in its treatment. They discuss various aspects of treatment and describe four innovative treatment programs.

Homelessness

13. **Interagency Council on the Homeless:** *Outcasts on Main Street.* Washington, DC, Interagency Council on the Homeless, 1992

This report of the Federal Task Force on Homelessness and Severe Mental Illness reviews the roles of federal, state, and local governments; service providers; mental health consumers; family members; and voluntary agencies in ending homelessness among seriously mentally ill persons and asserts principles and goals for program development.

14. *Torrey EF: *Nowhere to Go: The Tragic Odyssey of the Homeless Mentally Ill.* New York, Harper & Row, 1988

This is a forceful history of the failure of deinstitutionalization of mentally ill persons and its relationship to homelessness. The ideas that underlay community mental health centers were abandoned in practice. Discharged hospital patients rarely find aftercare, housing, or rehabilitation programs.

Obsessive-Compulsive Disorder

15. *Greist JH: *Obsessive Compulsive Disorder: A Guide,* Revised Edition. Madison, WI, Lithium Information Center, University of Wisconsin, 1991

In this compact guide in question-and-answer format that asserts the biological cause of obsessions and compulsions, Griest explains medications and suggests coping strategies. Because the disorder is treatable, the book is hopeful and encouraging.

16. **Rapoport JL:** *The Boy Who Couldn't Stop Washing: The Experience of Obsessive-Compulsive Disorder.* New York, EP Dutton, 1988

This is a discussion of obsessive-compulsive disorder by the chief of child psychiatry at the National Institute of Mental Health. Rapoport believes that obsessive-compulsive disorder is a hereditary brain disorder and that effective treatment combines medication and behavioral therapy.

Schizophrenia

17. **Gottesman II:** *Schizophrenia Genesis: The Origins of Madness.* New York, WH Freeman, 1990

    A geneticist of world standing presents state-of-the-art views of the genetic elements in the origin of schizophrenia. Gottesman sees the origin of schizophrenia in a complex genetic predisposition, together with environmental stressors that are still unknown. The book is fascinating, meticulous, and highly technical.

18. *****Torrey EF:** *Surviving Schizophrenia: A Family Manual,* 3rd Edition. New York, Harper & Row, 1995

    This is the revised edition of NAMI's all-time bestseller that deals with schizophrenia in understandable terms and covers the subject comprehensively. It contains practical and realistic suggestions for families for managing an ill family member. Each chapter has a helpful annotated list of further reading.

19. **Wash M:** *Schizophrenia: Straight Talk for Families and Friends.* New York, Warner Books, 1985

    This book is written by a NAMI member who is the mother of a schizophrenic son. After discussing the disease and its effect on patients and families, Wash deals with treatment and services in realistic and practical terms. She urges families to become agents of change.

Family and Coping Strategies

20. *****Hatfield A:** *Coping With Mental Illness in the Family: A Family Guide,* 2nd Edition, Revised (NAMI Book No. 6). Arlington, VA, National Alliance for the Mentally Ill, 1991

    In this new edition of a NAMI classic that helps families understand and cope with mental illness, Hatfield discusses diagnoses, causes, treatment, and rehabilitation and suggests coping strategies—creating a supportive environment, managing disturbing behavior, and using community resources. This is useful for family education.

21. **Woolis R:** *When Someone You Love Has a Mental Illness.* New York, Putnam, 1992

    Realistic and practical suggestions are presented by the director of a family support program at the University of California at Los Angeles. Both a textbook for a family education program and a handbook for families, the book describes the main mental illnesses, suggests coping strategies, helps family members deal with their own feelings, and directs them to community resources.

See also books listed under "Specific Conditions."

Legal and Financial Considerations

22. *Turnbull JR: *Disability and the Family: A Guide to Decisions for Adulthood.* Baltimore, MD, Paul H. Brookes Publishing, 1989

An up-to-date and comprehensive guidebook for families of disabled persons about planning for the future, this book covers legal issues, government disability programs, wills and trusts, housing and employment, and advocacy. Designed mainly for mentally retarded persons, it is immediately applicable to persons with mental illness.

Medications

23. *Bouricius JK: *Psychiatric Drugs and Their Effects on Mentally Ill Persons* (NAMI Book No. 3). Arlington, VA, National Alliance for the Mentally Ill, 1989

In this handbook about medication for patients and families, Bouricius discusses a wide range of psychoactive drugs and includes information about dosages, side effects, and interactions with other drugs and food. The book is a meticulous treatment of the subject with extensive references and a helpful index.

24. *Gorman J: *The Essential Guide to Psychiatric Drugs.* New York, St. Martin's Press, 1990

An authoritative and readable book for consumers, family members, and professionals by a national authority on psychopharmacology, this book covers specific drugs used in the treatment of anxiety, depression and manic-depression, schizophrenia, sleep disorders, and drug abuse. It discusses side effects and costs.

25. Snyder S: *Drugs and the Brain.* New York, WH Freeman, 1986

An outstanding contribution to the literature about psychopharmacology and the brain written by a leading neuroscientist, this book is technical but readable and is illustrated with photographs and diagrams. Snyder relates scientific discovery to the treatment of mental illness.

Services and Facilities

26. Farkas M, Anthony WA (eds): *Psychiatric Rehabilitation Programs: Putting Theory Into Practice.* Baltimore, MD, Johns Hopkins University Press, 1989

Chapters by authorities in rehabilitation discuss a philosophy of rehabilitation and outline successful programs. Written mainly for professionals, this book contains technical language and concepts that will be difficult for families to grasp, but the effort is rewarding.

27. Liberman RP (ed): *Psychiatric Rehabilitation of Chronic Mental Patients.* Washington, DC, American Psychiatric Press, 1991

In chapters written at a cluster of California institutions that form an important center for research and practice in rehabilitation, the authors stress careful assessment, closely monitored medication, social skills training, vocational rehabilitation, and family participation in treatment.

28. Liberman RP (ed): *Effective Psychiatric Rehabilitation.* San Francisco, CA, Jossey-Bass, 1992

This book contains accounts of 10 innovative rehabilitation projects in 9 research-oriented community-based treatment centers and 1 hospital. By combining medication, skills training, social support, cognitive and behavioral therapies, case management, and transitional and supported employment, the projects greatly improve the quality of life of mentally ill persons.

29. Torrey EF, Erdman K, Wolfe S, Flynn L: *Care of the Seriously Mentally Ill: A Rating of State Programs,* 3rd Edition. Washington, DC, Public Citizen Health Research Group and National Alliance for the Mentally Ill, 1990

The third—and last—annual survey of state programs for seriously mentally ill persons, this book identifies the components of good programs and describes problems in care that are of crisis proportions. It proposes improvements in services, cites meritorious persons and programs, and rates state programs.

For Professionals and Families

Although the books below are written mainly for professionals, they have been found to be helpful also to families.

30. Duke P, Hochman G: *A Brilliant Madness: Living With Manic Depressive Illness.* New York, Bantam Books, 1992

This book, written by actress Patty Duke, is the account of her suffering until her mid-30s with manic-depression and of the stabilization brought about by lithium treatment. Hochman, a medical writer, contributes well-rounded and accurate material on manic-depression. The two writers have produced an informative, perceptive, and readable presentation.

31. Gerhart U: *Care for the Chronic Mentally Ill.* Itasca, IL, FE Peacock Publishers, 1991

In this first textbook for social workers about caring for chronic mentally ill persons, Gerhart presents sound social work principles and sees increasing independence and improvement in the quality of life as goals of treatment. The chapter on medication contains errors and inaccuracies.

32. *Hatfield AB: *Family Education in Mental Illness.* New York, Guilford, 1990

This is a book that provides the content and methodology for educating families about serious mental illness. The content is based on family needs as identified by the author's research (knowledge of mental illness, coping skills, and support) and suggests helpful strategies for teaching adults.

33. Hatfield AB, Lefley H (eds): *Families of the Mentally Ill: Coping and Adaptation.* New York, Guilford, 1987

This is a scholarly work that suggests coping and adaptation as a theoretical framework for understanding and interpreting the behavior of families with mentally ill members. The authors cite research on families' perceptions of their needs and explore the implications of their model for future research.

34. March D: *Families and Mental Illness: New Directions in Professional Practice.* New York, Praeger, 1992

In this overview of new developments in working with families of mentally ill persons, March discusses the impact of mental illnesses on families and its implications for professional practice. She believes that families are central in community-based care.

35. Moorman M: *My Sister's Keeper.* New York, WW Norton, 1992

In this account of serious mental illness in a sister, Moorman experiences the dreads, doubts, and worries of all siblings and slowly assumes the responsibility of managing her sister's care. She knows pain and sadness, courage, resilience, and love as she and her sister learn to accept each other.

36. **National Alliance for the Mentally Ill:* *Experiences of Patients and Families* (NAMI Book No. 2). Arlington, VA, National Alliance for the Mentally Ill, 1990

    This is a collection of short accounts by patients and family members of their experiences with schizophrenia, most of them reprinted from *Schizophrenia Bulletin.* The accounts illustrate the range and complexity of the disease and enhance the understanding of patients, families, and professionals.

37. **North CS:** *Welcome, Silence: My Triumph Over Schizophrenia.* Dresden, TN, Avon Books, 1989

    This is the autobiography of a woman who became schizophrenic as a child. She describes crises, hospitalizations, medications, and her intensifying struggle with auditory hallucinations and distorted thinking. The book is a brilliant description of the experience of schizophrenia.

38. **Sheehan S:** *Is There No Place on Earth For Me?* New York, Random House, 1983

    This is a journalist's detailed account of a woman with schizophrenia. Sheehan portrays in realistic and unrelenting terms the failure of hospital treatment and of the community to provide appropriate care. The book is both an indictment of the system of care and a humane portrait of a deeply troubled woman.

39. **Styron W:** *Darkness Visible: A Memoir of Madness.* New York, Random House, 1990

    This is a brilliant and penetrating account by a bestselling author of his experience of unipolar depression. His literary skill gives the reader extraordinary access to the experience of worthlessness and gloom that characterize the disorder. He believes the illness has genetic and environmental roots.

40. **Wechsler J:** *In A Darkness,* 2nd Edition. Miami, FL, Pickering Press, 1988

    This is an account by a distinguished journalist of his son's schizophrenia in the 1960s. Wechsler writes of frustrating experiences with psychiatrists and mental hospitals, recurring crises, and gathering hopelessness. He pays tribute to his son's valiant struggle. This heartbreaking book was first published in 1972.

Research

The publications below present the research plans of the National Institute of Mental Health in four areas: the brain, schizophrenia, children and adolescents, and services. The National Institute of Mental Health supports and directs 80% of the nation's research on serious mental illness. The four plans thus define the direction in which most publicly and privately funded research about serious mental illness will move in the 1990s. All publications are reports to the U.S. Congress from the National Advisory Mental Health Council.

41. **National Institute of Mental Health:** *A National Plan for Schizophrenia Research* (DHHS Publ. No. ADM-88-1571). Rockville, MD, National Institute of Mental Health, 1988

    This is the plan that makes schizophrenia a research priority for the National Institute of Mental Health. It reviews research accomplishments and new technologies and promises rapid advances in understanding the disease in the near future. The book is a helpful framework for those who follow research developments closely.

42. **National Institute of Mental Health:** *Approaching the 21st Century: Opportunities for NIMH Neuroscience Research* (DHHS Publ. No. ADM-81-580). Rockville, MD, National Institute of Mental Health, 1989

    This technical report is generally understandable to the attentive lay reader. It delineates prospects in basic and clinical neuroscience and points to major breakthroughs that increased research will make possible. It notes the need for more grants to individual investigators and new and improved research facilities.

43. **National Institute of Mental Health:** *National Plan for Research on Child and Adolescent Mental Disorders* (DHHS Publ. No. ADM-90-1683). Rockville, MD, National Institute of Mental Health, 1990

    This is a review of current knowledge about the cause of the mental disorders that affect 12% of the nation's children and adolescents. The plan discusses existing treatments and services and cites the need for more research and research training.

44. **National Institute of Mental Health:** *Caring for People With Severe Mental Disorders: A National Plan of Research to Improve Services* (DHHS Publ. No. ADM-91-7262). Washington, DC, National Institute of Mental Health, 1991

    This plan for an integrated program of research on the delivery of care to severely and persistently mentally ill persons summarizes the state of knowledge and points to future research in clinical services, community services and systems, and research resources.

Reading Lists

45. **National Alliance for the Mentally Ill:** *Annotated Reading List 1990* (NAMI Book No. 4). Arlington, VA, National Alliance for the Mentally Ill, 1990; **National Alliance for the Mentally Ill:** *Supplement for 1991* (NAMI Book No. 5). Arlington, VA, National Alliance for the Mentally Ill, 1991

    These works provide annotations of books about serious mental illness that NAMI sold between 1984 and 1991, other books of merit, journals and periodicals, and free or low-cost United States government publications. The list is frequently updated.

46. *National Alliance for the Mentally Ill: *NAMI's Basic Library About Serious Mental Illness.* Arlington, VA, National Alliance for the Mentally Ill, annually since 1991

    This is a list of books NAMI sells that it considers "must" reading for NAMI families and "must" acquisitions for affiliate and public libraries. The list is updated annually and contains 12 to 15 titles.

47. *National Alliance for the Mentally Ill: *NAMI's Resource Catalog.* Arlington, VA, National Alliance for the Mentally Ill, quarterly since 1992

    This is a catalog for ordering books, pamphlets, brochures, and specialty items useful to NAMI members and others.

Author Index

Citations are referred to by the chapter number plus a decimal and then the reference number within that chapter (e.g., "15.59" refers to Chapter 15, reference 59).

Subject Index

AA (Alcoholics Anonymous), 24.34,
43.34
Abortion, 56.36
Absenteeism, 63.1
Abuse. *See* Child abuse; Physical abuse;
Sexual abuse; Trauma
Access to health care. *See also*
Community psychiatry
blacks and Hispanics, 56.9–56.11,
57.43
capitation and, 57.34
emergency room use, 56.34
ethics of, 58.25–58.26
Medicaid, 56.33
positionality and, 57.51
socioeconomic class and,
57.49–57.50
underserved populations,
57.40–57.54
women, 56.35
Accidental death
bereavement and, 25.39
ACoA syndrome, 33.35
Acquired immunodeficiency syndrome
(AIDS). *See also* Human
immunodeficiency virus
AZT therapy, 18.11
children and adolescents,
30.115–30.117
consultation-liaison psychiatry,
18.27, 46.11, 46.12, 51.62
counseling, 18.32–18.35,
24.56–24.57
cross-cultural issues, 56.29
epidemiology and risk behavior,
18.12–18.15
guidelines for outpatient psychiatric
services, 59.14
health care workers' risk,
18.16–18.17

hope and, 18.30
impact on gay community, 18.15
intravenous drug use and, 18.14,
24I, 24.52, 24.56–24.57
legal and ethical issues, 18.27, 18.41
mother-infant transmission of, 18.13
neuropsychiatric complications,
18.18–18.24
overview, 18I, 18.1–18.8
pediatric, 51.62
prevention, 18.14, 18.32, 18.35,
24.56–24.57, 56.29
psychiatric disorders associated
with, 18.25–18.31
residents' experiences with AIDS
patients, 65.25
severe mental illness and,
19.36–19.40
suicide and, 18.28
survival, 18.10
transmission of, 18.9, 18.13, 18.14,
24.52
Adaptation. *See* Stress, coping, and
adaptation
Addiction. *See also* Alcoholism;
Substance use and abuse
homelessness and, 57.41
models of, 24.24–24.31
pharmacology of, 24.15
Adjustment disorders
children and adolescents, 30.61,
30.97–30.98, 30.107
Administration
economics, 58.16–58.18
ethical issues, 58.25–58.31
leadership, power, and authority,
58.8–58.11
organization of services, 58.1–58.7
overview of, 58I, 58.40–58.41
quality assurance, 58.22–58.24

Citations are referred to by the chapter number plus a decimal and then the
reference number within that chapter (e.g., "15.59" refers to Chapter 15, reference
59). Citations that consist of a chapter number plus "I" (e.g., "24I") refer to the
introduction to that chapter.